T0135331

# Springer Proceedings in Mathematics & Statistics

Volume 259

This book series features volumes composed of selected contributions from workshops and conferences in all areas of current research in mathematics and statistics, including operation research and optimization. In addition to an overall evaluation of the interest, scientific quality, and timeliness of each proposal at the hands of the publisher, individual contributions are all refereed to the high quality standards of leading journals in the field. Thus, this series provides the research community with well-edited, authoritative reports on developments in the most exciting areas of mathematical and statistical research today.

More information about this series at http://www.springer.com/series/10533

D. Marc Kilgour · Herb Kunze
Roman Makarov · Roderick Melnik
Xu Wang
Editors

# Recent Advances in Mathematical and Statistical Methods

IV AMMCS International Conference,
Waterloo, Canada, August 20–25, 2017

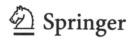 Springer

*Editors*
D. Marc Kilgour
Department of Mathematics &
  MS2Discovery Interdisciplinary
  Research Institute
Wilfrid Laurier University
Waterloo, ON, Canada

Roderick Melnik
Department of Mathematics &
  MS2Discovery Interdisciplinary
  Research Institute
Wilfrid Laurier University
Waterloo, ON, Canada

Herb Kunze
Department of Mathematics & Statistics
University of Guelph
Guelph, ON, Canada

Xu Wang
Department of Mathematics &
  MS2Discovery Interdisciplinary
  Research Institute
Wilfrid Laurier University
Waterloo, ON, Canada

Roman Makarov
Department of Mathematics &
  MS2Discovery Interdisciplinary
  Research Institute
Wilfrid Laurier University
Waterloo, ON, Canada

ISSN 2194-1009          ISSN 2194-1017   (electronic)
Springer Proceedings in Mathematics & Statistics
ISBN 978-3-030-07626-9          ISBN 978-3-319-99719-3   (eBook)
https://doi.org/10.1007/978-3-319-99719-3

Mathematics Subject Classification (2010): 15-XX, 34-XX, 35-XX, 37-XX, 60-XX, 45-XX, 49-XX, 62-XX, 65-XX, 68-XX, 74-XX, 76-XX, 91-XX, 92-XX

This Springer imprint is published by the registered company Springer Nature Switzerland AG
The registered company address is: Gewerbestrasse 11, 6330 Cham, Switzerland

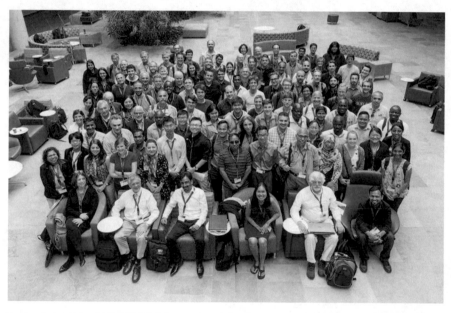

Group photo of the AMMCS-2017 International Conference: Applied Mathematics, Modeling and Computational Science Conference

# Preface

AMMCS-2017 was an international conference on Applied Mathematics, Modeling and Computational Science held at Wilfrid Laurier University from August 20 to 25, 2017. The conference was intentionally interdisciplinary, aiming to promote research and collaboration involving mathematical and computational sciences across many fields, and to showcase recent advances within an international community of researchers, practitioners, and students.

Mathematical methods have been fundamental components of human knowledge for millennia. Now sophisticated mathematical and statistical methods make essential contributions to progress in an amazing range of application areas—in the natural and social sciences, engineering, and even the arts. Mathematics, statistics, and the associated computational techniques play a fundamental role in the modern world, addressing human problems and contributing to human well-being.

Today's most challenging human problems have arisen not only in the traditional areas of mathematical application, physical sciences, and engineering, but also in life, the social sciences, and finance. They are being addressed with mathematical reasoning of great subtlety and power, augmented by data collection on a scale so massive that only recently has statistical analysis been possible, and by computation utilized not only to support analysis but also to explore new combinations and structures. These developments have forged new connections among disciplines that were once widely separated, and are expanding ever further the horizons of mathematical and computational modeling.

AMMCS-2017 was a major international forum for the exchange of ideas in an interdisciplinary setting with a focus on the mathematical and computational sciences and their applications in natural and social sciences, engineering and technology, industry and finance. It followed the traditions of previous events in the AMMCS series, particularly in its emphasis on the interdisciplinary aspects of mathematical and statistical methodologies and the role of computational modeling.

This book exhibits a broad selection of examples of current research, all of which was presented at AMMCS-2017. It illustrates how mathematics, statistics, and modeling are contributing to a range of disciplines. The 57 selected contributions are organized into eight parts, as follows:

I. Advances in Mathematical and Statistical Modelling
II. Analytical and Computational Methods in Inverse Problems
III. Computational Methods and Modelling in Engineering and Mechanics
IV. Mathematical Modelling and Computation in Physical and Chemical Sciences
V. Mathematical Modelling in Biological and Environmental Sciences
VI. Mathematical Modelling in Medical and Health Sciences
VII. Mathematics and Computation in Finance, Economics, and Social Sciences
VIII. Theory and Applications of Dynamical Systems

The titles of the parts make the breadth of the topics clear. This wide-ranging selection is appropriate to the emerging role of mathematical, statistical, and computational sciences.

The editors of this volume extend their thanks to all of the contributors to AMMCS-2017, to all of the attendees, to the Organizing, Scientific, and Technical Committees, and to all of the volunteers, without whom the conference would never have been held. We are also grateful to our sponsors and to Wilfrid Laurier University. We give special thanks to the contributors who chose to submit their papers to this volume, and the referees whose guidance was essential to us as we evaluated the proposed contributions. We also thank Ruth Allewelt of Springer, who assisted us with the editorial work and production. We are proud of this volume, and pleased to acknowledge all of those who helped to bring it to fruition. As always, however, views presented in each article are those of the authors and do not necessarily reflect those of the editors of this volume or the referees. Any remaining errors are the sole responsibilities of the authors.

Waterloo, ON, Canada                                            D. Marc Kilgour
Guelph, ON, Canada                                                   Herb Kunze
Waterloo, ON, Canada                                           Roman Makarov
Waterloo, ON, Canada                                           Roderick Melnik
Waterloo, ON, Canada                                                   Xu Wang
July 2018

# Contents

**Part I   Advances in Mathematical and Statistical Modelling**

**Reuse Method for Quantum Circuit Synthesis** . . . . . . . . . . . . . . . . . . . .   3
C. Allouche, M. Baboulin, T. Goubault de Brugière and B. Valiron

**Robust Reliable $H_\infty$ Control and Input-to-State Stabilization
for Uncertain Hybrid Systems** . . . . . . . . . . . . . . . . . . . . . . . . . . . . .   13
Mohamad S. Alwan, Xinzhi Liu and Taghreed G. Sugati

**Exact Coloring of Sparse Matrices** . . . . . . . . . . . . . . . . . . . . . . . . . . .   23
Shahadat Hossain and Ahamad I. Khan

**A General Method for Selection Function Optimization
in Genetic Algorithms** . . . . . . . . . . . . . . . . . . . . . . . . . . . . . . . . . .   37
Nawar Ismail and Matthew Demers

**Exploring the Method of Colour Stealing for Contractive
Iterated Function Systems** . . . . . . . . . . . . . . . . . . . . . . . . . . . . . . . .   47
Eva Kasanda and Matthew Demers

**Infinite Products Involving Binary Digit Sums** . . . . . . . . . . . . . . . . . . .   59
Samin Riasat

**Part II   Analytical and Computational Methods in Inverse Problems**

**Image-Driven Two-Point Boundary Value Inverse Problems:
A Case Study** . . . . . . . . . . . . . . . . . . . . . . . . . . . . . . . . . . . . . . .   71
Victoria Brott and Herb Kunze

**Circle Inversion IFS** . . . . . . . . . . . . . . . . . . . . . . . . . . . . . . . . . . .   81
Maxwell Fitzsimmons and Herb Kunze

**Inverse Problems and Total Variation Minimization**
**for Iterated Function Systems on Maps** . . . . . . . . . . . . . . . . . . . . . . .   93
Herb Kunze and Davide La Torre

**Using the Collage Method to Solve Inverse Problems**
**for Vector-Valued Variational Problems on a Perforated**
**Domain in Reflexive Banach Spaces** . . . . . . . . . . . . . . . . . . . . . . . . . . .  105
Herb Kunze, Davide La Torre and Manuel Ruiz Galán

**Inverse Problems Using Iterated Function Systems**
**with Place-Dependent Probabilities** . . . . . . . . . . . . . . . . . . . . . . . . . . .  115
Davide La Torre, Erik A. Maki, Franklin Mendivil and Edward R. Vrscay

**Solving Inverse Problems for Fractional ODEs via the Collage**
**Theorem** . . . . . . . . . . . . . . . . . . . . . . . . . . . . . . . . . . . . . . . . . . . . . . . . . . .  127
Kimberly M. Levere and Brent Van De Walker

**Part III   Computational Methods and Modelling in Engineering**
**and Mechanics**

**Characterization of Fluid Dynamics in Capillary Vessels:**
**Applications for Drug Delivery** . . . . . . . . . . . . . . . . . . . . . . . . . . . . . . . .  139
Seraphin C. Abou

**Large Eddy Simulation of Turbulent Flow Over a Hill**
**Using a Canopy Stress Model** . . . . . . . . . . . . . . . . . . . . . . . . . . . . . . . . . .  151
Md. Abdus Samad Bhuiyan and Jahrul M. Alam

**A Computational Model for Adjusting Surface Tension Coefficient**
**in Pseudo-potential Lattice Boltzmann Method** . . . . . . . . . . . . . . . . . . .  161
Mahmud Ashrafizaadeh and Seyyed Meysam Khatoonabadi

**Magnetohydrodynamic Flow in a Rectangular Duct** . . . . . . . . . . . . . . .  171
Canan Bozkaya

**The Effects of Thermal Radiation on a Reactive Hydromagnetic**
**Internal Heat Generating Fluid Flow Through Parallel**
**Porous Plates** . . . . . . . . . . . . . . . . . . . . . . . . . . . . . . . . . . . . . . . . . . . . . . . .  183
Anthony R. Hassan, Jacob A. Gbadeyan and Sulyman O. Salawu

**Exponential Stability of Discrete Impulsive Switched Singular**
**Systems with Time Delay** . . . . . . . . . . . . . . . . . . . . . . . . . . . . . . . . . . . . . .  195
Humeyra Kiyak, Mohamad S. Alwan and Xinzhi Liu

**Experimental Investigation of ABB Effect on Unbalanced**
**Rotor Vibration** . . . . . . . . . . . . . . . . . . . . . . . . . . . . . . . . . . . . . . . . . . . . . .  207
Michael Makram, Mohamed K. Khalil, Ahmed F. Nemnem
and Guirguis Samer

**Optimization of a Flanged DAWT Using a CFD Actuator
Disc Method** . . . . . . . . . . . . . . . . . . . . . . . . . . . . . . . . . . . . . . . . . . . . . . 219
Mohammad Hassan Ranjbar, Seyyed Abolfazl Nasrazadani
and Kobra Gharali

**Axisymmetric Simulations of Nonlinear Sound Propagation
in a Trumpet** . . . . . . . . . . . . . . . . . . . . . . . . . . . . . . . . . . . . . . . . . 229
Janelle Resch, Andrew Giuliani, Lilia Krivodonova and John Vanderkooy

**Turbulent Diffusion of Inertial Particle Pairs Such as in Pollen
and Sandstorms** . . . . . . . . . . . . . . . . . . . . . . . . . . . . . . . . . . . . . . . . 239
Syed M. Usama and Nadeem A. Malik

**Coupled Axial, In Plane and Out of Plane Bending Vibrations
of Cable Harnessed Space Structures** . . . . . . . . . . . . . . . . . . . . . . . . 249
Karthik Yerrapragada and Armaghan Salehian

**Part IV   Mathematical Modelling and Computation in Physical
and Chemical Sciences**

**A Comparison of the Magnus Expansion and Other Solvers
for the Chemical Master Equation with Variable Rates** . . . . . . . . . . . . 261
Khanh Dinh and Roger Sidje

**Temperature Effect on Sound Scattering by Fine Bubbles
in Viscoelastic Liquid** . . . . . . . . . . . . . . . . . . . . . . . . . . . . . . . . . . 271
S. Levitsky

**A Fourth-Order Compact Numerical Scheme for Three-Dimensional
Acoustic Wave Equation with Variable Velocity** . . . . . . . . . . . . . . . . . 279
Wenyuan Liao and Ou Wei

**On Global Properties of Gowdy Spacetimes in Scalar-Tensor
Theory** . . . . . . . . . . . . . . . . . . . . . . . . . . . . . . . . . . . . . . . . . . . . . . 291
Makoto Narita

**A Computational Resolution of the Inverse Problem of Kinetic
Capillary Electrophoresis (KCE)** . . . . . . . . . . . . . . . . . . . . . . . . . . . 303
József Vass and Sergey N. Krylov

**Part V   Mathematical Modelling in Biological and Environmental
Sciences**

**A Simulation Study of the Effect of Meso-Scopic Sinusoidal
Surface Roughness on Biofilm Growth** . . . . . . . . . . . . . . . . . . . . . . . 315
Md. Afsar Ali, Hermann J. Eberl and Rangarajan Sudarsan

**Dynamics of a Stage Structured Intraguild Predation Model** . . . . . . . . . 327
Juancho A. Collera and Felicia Maria G. Magpantay

**A Conceptual Model for the Pliocene Paradox** . . . . . . . . . . . . . . . . . . .  339
Brady Dortmans, William F. Langford and Allan R. Willms

**First Order Versus Monod Kinetics in Numerical Simulation
of Biofilms in Porous Media** . . . . . . . . . . . . . . . . . . . . . . . . . . . . . . . .  351
Harry J. Gaebler and Hermann J. Eberl

**Predictability of Marine Population Trajectories Affected
by Birth and Harvest Pulses** . . . . . . . . . . . . . . . . . . . . . . . . . . . . . . . .  363
Anna S. J. Frank and Sam Subbey

**Phage Therapy and Antibiotics for Biofilm Eradication:
A Predictive Model** . . . . . . . . . . . . . . . . . . . . . . . . . . . . . . . . . . . . . .  375
Amjad Khan, Lindi M. Wahl and Pei Yu

**A Simple Model of Between-Hive Transmission of Nosemosis** . . . . . . . .  385
Nasim Muhammad and Hermann J. Eberl

**Spreading of Nearshore Effluent Discharges on Eroded Sloping
Sandy Beaches** . . . . . . . . . . . . . . . . . . . . . . . . . . . . . . . . . . . . . . . . .  397
Anton Purnama, Huda A. Al-Maamari and E. Balakrishnan

**Part VI   Mathematical Modelling in Medical and Health Sciences**

**Using Social Media to Improve Knowledge Sharing among
Healthcare Practitioners** . . . . . . . . . . . . . . . . . . . . . . . . . . . . . . . . . .  411
Haitham Alali

**Model Based Economic Assessment of Avian Influenza Vaccination
in an All-in/All-out Housing System** . . . . . . . . . . . . . . . . . . . . . . . . . .  419
Meagan Coffey, Hermann J. Eberl and Amy L. Greer

**Estimating the Crossover Point of a Fuzzy Willingness-to-Pay/
Accept for Health to Support Decision Making** . . . . . . . . . . . . . . . . . .  431
Michał Jakubczyk

**Fuzzy Approach to Elicitation of Preferences for Health States** . . . . . . .  441
Bogumił Kamiński and Michał Jakubczyk

**Optimal Control of Breast Cancer: Investigating Estrogen
as a Risk Factor** . . . . . . . . . . . . . . . . . . . . . . . . . . . . . . . . . . . . . . . .  451
S. I. Oke, M. B. Matadi and S. S. Xulu

**Part VII  Mathematics and Computation in Finance, Economics, and Social Sciences**

**Dynamical Analysis of a Modified Prey-Predator Model for Venture Capital Investment** . . . . . . . . . . . . . . . . . . . . . . . . . . . . . 467
Letetia Mary Addison, Balswaroop Bhatt and David Owen

**Modelling Asynchronous Assets with Jump-Diffusion Processes** . . . . . . . 477
Yuxin Chen and Roman N. Makarov

**Efficient Hedging in Bates Model Using High-Order Compact Finite Differences** . . . . . . . . . . . . . . . . . . . . . . . . . . . . . . . . . . . . 489
Bertram Düring and Alexander Pitkin

**An Explicit Optimal Strategy for Flow Trades at NASDAQ Around Its Close** . . . . . . . . . . . . . . . . . . . . . . . . . . . . . . . . . . . 499
Christoph Frei and Chad Yan

**Optimal Selection of Assets and Portfolios** . . . . . . . . . . . . . . . . . . . . . 509
Bowen Hu and Roman N. Makarov

**Kinetic Models of Need-Based Transfers** . . . . . . . . . . . . . . . . . . . . . . 521
K. Kayser, D. Armbruster and C. Ringhofer

**Optimal Static Hedging of Non-tradable Risks with Discrete Distributions** . . . . . . . . . . . . . . . . . . . . . . . . . . . . . . . . . . . . . . 531
Adam W. Kolkiewicz

**Population and Pollution Interactions in a Spatial Economic Model** . . . . . . . . . . . . . . . . . . . . . . . . . . . . . . . . . . . . . . . . . . . 543
Davide La Torre, Danilo Liuzzi and Simone Marsiglio

**Price Bounds in Jump-Diffusion Markets Revisited via Market Completions** . . . . . . . . . . . . . . . . . . . . . . . . . . . . . . . . . . . . . . 553
Anne MacKay and Alexander Melnikov

**Part VIII  Theory and Applications of Dynamical Systems**

**Error Expansion for a Symplectic Scheme for Stochastic Hamiltonian Systems** . . . . . . . . . . . . . . . . . . . . . . . . . . . . . . . . 567
Cristina Anton

**Rogue Waves in the Generalized Davey-Stewartson System** . . . . . . . . . . 579
Mervenur Belin and Irma Hacinliyan

**Linearization and Local Topological Conjugacies for Impulsive Systems** . . . . . . . . . . . . . . . . . . . . . . . . . . . . . . . . . . . . . . . . . 591
Kevin E. M. Church and Xinzhi Liu

**Oscillations in Low-Dimensional Cyclic Differential Delay Systems** . . . . . . . . . . . . . . . . . . . . . . . . . . . . . . . . . . . . . . . . . . . . . 603
Anatoli F. Ivanov and Zari A. Dzalilov

**Asynchronous Control of Switched Nonlinear Systems** . . . . . . . . . . . . . 615
Jiaojiao Ren, Xinzhi Liu, Hong Zhu and Shouming Zhong

**FMPS of Master-Slave Dynamical Networks with Hybrid Feedback Control** . . . . . . . . . . . . . . . . . . . . . . . . . . . . . . . . . . . . . . . . . 625
Xin Wang, Xinzhi Liu, Kun She and Shouming Zhong

**Implicit State Dependent Delay in Range-Based Position Estimation and Navigation** . . . . . . . . . . . . . . . . . . . . . . . . . . . . . . . . . . . . . . . . . . 637
Erik I. Verriest

# Part I
# Advances in Mathematical and Statistical Modelling

# Reuse Method for Quantum Circuit Synthesis

## C. Allouche, M. Baboulin, T. Goubault de Brugière and B. Valiron

**Abstract** The algebraic decomposition of a unitary operator is a key operation in the synthesis of quantum circuits. If most methods factorize the matrix into products, there exists a method that allows to reuse already existing optimized circuits to implement linear combinations of them. This paper presents an attempt to extend this method to a general framework of circuit synthesis. The method needs to find suitable groups for the implementation of new quantum circuits. We identify key points necessary for the construction of a comprehensive method and we test potential group candidates.

**Keywords** Circuit synthesis · Quantum computation · Reuse method

## 1 Introduction

The notion of *quantum circuit* has emerged from the beginning of the field of quantum computing [3] and so far remains the most widespread description of a quantum algorithm. Contrary to conventional algorithms that manipulate bits (0 or 1) using boolean gates, a *quantum algorithm* operates on quantum bits, or *qubits*, using a series of quantum gates which are generally desired as simple as possible. A quantum

C. Allouche
Atos-Bull, Les Clayes-sous-Bois, Paris, France
e-mail: cyril.allouche@atos.net

M. Baboulin
LRI and Université Paris-Sud, Orsay, France
e-mail: marc.baboulin@lri.fr

T. Goubault de Brugière (✉)
Atos-Bull, LRI and Université Paris-Sud, Orsay, France
e-mail: timothee.goubault@lri.fr

B. Valiron
LRI and CentraleSupélec, Orsay, France
e-mail: benoit.valiron@lri.fr

© Springer Nature Switzerland AG 2018
D. M. Kilgour et al. (eds.), *Recent Advances in Mathematical and Statistical Methods*, Springer Proceedings in Mathematics & Statistics 259,
https://doi.org/10.1007/978-3-319-99719-3_1

bit is formally a unit vector in $\mathbb{C}^2$ (modulo a phase factor) and represents a linear superposition of both states 0 and 1. Using the usual Dirac notation, the state $|\psi\rangle$ of one qubit is the vector

$$|\psi\rangle = \alpha\,|0\rangle + \beta\,|1\rangle = \begin{pmatrix} \alpha \\ \beta \end{pmatrix}. \tag{1}$$

We compose spaces of states for systems of several qubits by using the tensor product of the spaces of states of each qubit. Then a system of $n$ qubits is a unit vector that belongs to $\mathbb{C}^{2^n}$. With this formalism, quantum gates are unitary matrices, i.e matrices whose inverse are their own adjoint. Depending on the physical realization of the quantum memory, some unitary matrices might be easier to implement than others [11]: we refer to these gates as *elementary*. Among the elementary quantum gates usually considered, we can mention the gates presented in Table 1: the Pauli matrices $X$, $Y$ and $Z$, the Hadamard gate $H$, the $T$-gate and the two-qubit gates CNOT and SWAP.

A quantum circuit is then a series of elementary quantum gates operating on $n$ qubits for some $n > 0$. It represents a global quantum operator that corresponds to a matrix of $\mathcal{U}(2^n)$, where $\mathcal{U}(2^n)$ denotes the set of unitary matrices of size $2^n \times 2^n$ (see, e.g., [10] for a comprehensive introduction to quantum computing).

A quantum circuit can be represented as in Fig. 1. Each wire corresponds to a quantum bit and we read from left to right the gates that are applied to the system. In this case, we first apply a Hadamard gate on the first qubit (tensored with the identity on the second qubit), then the Pauli gate $X$ is applied to the second qubit, controlled by the first one. This means that if the first qubit was in state $|0\rangle$, the state is unchanged, and if it was in state $|1\rangle$ the gate $X$ is applied. One can check that the controlled-$X$ gate is equivalent to the CNOT gate. Finally, the overall operator $U$

**Table 1** Usual elementary unitary matrices

$$\begin{pmatrix} 0 & 1 \\ 1 & 0 \end{pmatrix} \qquad \begin{pmatrix} 0 & -i \\ i & 0 \end{pmatrix} \qquad \begin{pmatrix} 1 & 0 \\ 0 & -1 \end{pmatrix} \qquad \begin{pmatrix} 1 & 0 & 0 & 0 \\ 0 & 1 & 0 & 0 \\ 0 & 0 & 0 & 1 \\ 0 & 0 & 1 & 0 \end{pmatrix} \qquad \begin{pmatrix} 1 & 0 & 0 & 0 \\ 0 & 0 & 1 & 0 \\ 0 & 1 & 0 & 0 \\ 0 & 0 & 0 & 1 \end{pmatrix}$$

$$\quad X \qquad\qquad Y \qquad\qquad Z \qquad\qquad\qquad \text{CNOT} \qquad\qquad \text{SWAP}$$

$$\frac{1}{\sqrt{2}}\begin{pmatrix} 1 & 1 \\ 1 & -1 \end{pmatrix} \qquad \begin{pmatrix} 1 & 0 \\ 0 & e^{i\pi/4} \end{pmatrix}$$

$$\qquad H \qquad\qquad\quad T$$

**Fig. 1** Example of a quantum circuit

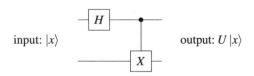

input: $|x\rangle$         output: $U\,|x\rangle$

applied to the system is the product

$$U = \Lambda(X) \times (H \otimes I_2), \tag{2}$$

where $\Lambda(X)$ denotes the fact that the gate $X$ is controlled by the first qubit.

A set of gates is said to be *universal* when any unitary can be implemented via a quantum circuit using these gates. Since the mid-1990s various universality results have been shown (see, e.g. [5]). For example the set composed of all the 1-qubit gates and the CNOT gate is sufficient to implement any operator. Another example is the set of H, T and CNOT gates which is also universal. In order to implement a general quantum operator on a concrete system, it is necessary to decompose it into elementary gates. If these elementary gates are chosen from a universal set, then it is theoretically possible to implement this operator.

Quantum computing yields several challenges. One of the problem is to actually generate a quantum circuit from a textual description. Several programming languages have been developed to address this issue [6, 15, 17]. Another problem is to optimize the generated quantum circuits by simplifying them as much as possible, for example by using rewrite rules in order to minimize the number of elementary gates [9]. Also many efforts have been made to provide software that simulates quantum circuits on classical computers in order to help researchers to make progress in view of a future quantum computer. In this case the optimization of circuits can be understood as minimizing the simulation time.

In this paper we are instead interested in the *synthesis of quantum circuits*. Contrary to the case where the circuit is explicitly described, here a unitary operator is provided as a matrix and the problem consists in finding a quantum circuit that implements it optimally.

We can impose various constraints on the solution circuit such as the choice of the considered elementary gates, the physical medium, the arrangement of qubits, the memory properties, etc. We can evaluate the optimality of the solution by measuring

- the number of elementary gates,
- the time to find the circuit,
- the time to classically simulate the circuit,
- the error between the targeted operator and the implemented operator (for example using the norm of the difference between the corresponding matrices).

Over the years more and more efficient methods have been developed to synthesize an arbitrary quantum operator [1, 8, 13, 16]. Most synthesis frameworks rely on linear algebra methods to decompose unitary matrices. The first methods aimed at decomposing the operator column by column [1, 8]. One can cite as example the QR method, via Givens rotations [16]. Other decomposition methods have also been proposed, for example the recent block-ZXZ decomposition [4], or the quantum Shannon decomposition [13] that relies on the use of the sine cosine decomposition of a unitary operator $U \in U(2^n)$:

$$U = \begin{pmatrix} A_1 & 0 \\ 0 & A_2 \end{pmatrix} \begin{pmatrix} C & -S \\ S & C \end{pmatrix} \begin{pmatrix} B_1 & 0 \\ 0 & B_2 \end{pmatrix} \tag{3}$$

where $A_1, A_2, B_1, B_2 \in U(2^{n-1})$ and $C, S$ are diagonal real matrices such that $C^2 + S^2 = I_{2^{n-1}}$. For an overview of the history and links between these various methods, refer to [12].

In this context, there exists a less typical method that focuses on a decomposition of the operator as a linear combination of other operators chosen from a given set. This method enables to reuse optimized circuits in order to implement more complex operators [7]. To our knowledge, this is the only method using such a technique. This method, which we informally call the *reuse method*, has been shown to be efficient on specific cases [7]. Our objective in this paper is to determine whether this method can be efficiently extended to a general framework for circuit synthesis.

The paper is organized as follows. In Sect. 2, we recall the main principles of the reuse method. In Sect. 3, we select the groups that can be used in synthesizing circuits via the reuse method. In Sect. 4, we study the potential group candidates. We conclude in Sect. 5.

## 2 The Reuse Method

The reuse method has emerged from the following motivation: if we know how to implement circuits (supposedly efficiently), can we directly reuse these circuits in order to implement new operators?

Based on this idea, Klappenecker and Rötteler replied in the affirmative [7]. Below is a simplified version of [7, Th. 6].

**Theorem 1** *Let $G \subset U(2^m)$ be a group of order $2^n$, and $T = (t_1, \ldots, t_n)$ be a transversal of $G$ (i.e any member $g$ of $G$ can be written as $g = t_1^{\alpha_1} \ldots t_n^{\alpha_n}$ with $\alpha_i \in \{0, 1\}$). Suppose*

$$A = \sum_{g \in G} \beta_g g \tag{4}$$

*with $A \in U(2^m)$ and define the coefficient matrix $C_A = (\beta_{g^{-1}h})_{g,h \in G}$. Then the coefficients $(\beta_g)_{g \in G}$ can be chosen such that $C_A$ is unitary and the operator $A$ can be implemented as depicted in Fig. 2.*

This remains a simplified version, sufficient for the rest of our study. An illustration of the method can be found in [7, Sect. 3], where there is an implementation of the Hartley transform via a linear combination of powers of the Fourier transform.

A key point in the use of this method is the distribution of information between the group and the matrix of coefficients. When the group contains sufficient information, such as the Fourier transform powers group, the coefficient matrix is easy to compute and the efficiency of the quantum Fourier transform synthesis is used to produce an efficient circuit on non trivial operators. An alternative would be to consider the

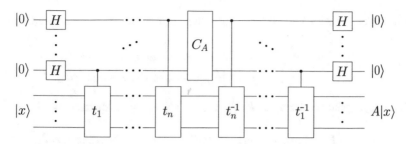

**Fig. 2** Quantum circuit implementing a linear combination of operators

problem in the other direction: the group is simple, contains little information but the matrix of coefficients—which now has a maximum of information—has a structure that makes its implementation effective.

For example, if the group is circulant then the matrix of coefficients will be circulant and diagonalizable in the Fourier basis. If the group is symmetric and its elements are involutive, then the matrix will be diagonalizable in the Hadamard base. In these cases, information can be predominantly contained in the coefficient matrix but the implementation of the coefficient matrix, although inevitably costly in terms of gates, is much simpler than for any generic operator (see the article by Bullock and Markov for the implementation of diagonal operators [2]).

However among all the possible matrix groups, some are more suitable than others for a generic synthesis method. In the next section we narrow our research by investigating the theoretical properties of "good" groups for general synthesis.

## 3 Characterization of Candidate Groups G

In this section we discuss under which conditions the reuse method can be used as a generic method for the synthesis of circuits.

We can already eliminate the case where the group $G$ is Abelian. Indeed, in this case the matrices of the group $G$ commute in pairs and are therefore simultaneously diagonalizable, just like any member of the span of $G$. One cannot reach all unitary matrix but only those diagonalizable in a specific basis.

Ideally, the group $G$ should be built easily for any number of qubits either with an adaptable construction for any $n$ or with a recursive approach. In fact, we can show how to construct a solution group $K$ and its matrix of coefficients for $n + m$ qubits from a solution group $G$ for $n$ qubits and a solution group $H$ for $m$ qubits.

We use can the properties of the tensor product to construct the group $K$. Indeed, by setting $K = G \otimes H$, provided that $U(2^n) \subseteq span(G)$ and $U(2^m) \subseteq span(H)$ then we have $U(2^{n+m}) \subseteq span(G \otimes H)$. Recall the identity

$$(g_1 \otimes g_2)(h_1 \otimes h_2) = (g_1 h_1) \otimes (g_2 h_2) \tag{5}$$

which is used to provide an expression of the coefficient matrix associated with $K$:

$$
\begin{aligned}
C_K = (\beta_{g^{-1}h})_{g,h\in G\otimes H} &= \left(\beta_{(g_1^{-1}\otimes h_1^{-1})^{-1}(g_2\otimes h_2)}\right)_{g_1,g_2\in G,h_1,h_1\in H} \\
&= \left(\beta_{(g_1^{-1}g_2)\otimes(h_1^{-1}h_2)}\right)_{g_1,g_2\in G,h_1,h_1\in H}.
\end{aligned}
\tag{6}
$$

With an appropriate ordering of $K$, the matrix $C_K$ can be expressed as

$$
C_K =
\begin{pmatrix}
\beta_{(g_1g_1,h_1h_1)} & \cdots & \beta_{(g_1g_n,h_1h_1)} & \beta_{(g_1g_1,h_1h_2)} & \cdots & \beta_{(g_1g_n,h_1h_2)} & \cdots \\
\vdots & & \vdots & \vdots & & \vdots & \\
\beta_{(g_ng_1,h_1h_1)} & \cdots & \beta_{(g_ng_n,h_1h_1)} & \beta_{(g_ng_1,h_1h_2)} & \cdots & \beta_{(g_ng_n,h_1h_2)} & \cdots \\
\beta_{(g_1g_1,h_2h_1)} & \cdots & \beta_{(g_1g_n,h_2h_1)} & \beta_{(g_1g_1,h_2h_2)} & \cdots & \beta_{(g_1g_n,h_2h_2)} & \cdots \\
\vdots & & \vdots & \vdots & & \vdots & \\
\beta_{(g_ng_1,h_2h_1)} & \cdots & \beta_{(g_ng_n,h_2h_1)} & \beta_{(g_ng_1,h_2h_2)} & \cdots & \beta_{(g_ng_n,h_2h_2)} & \cdots \\
& \vdots & & & \vdots & & \vdots
\end{pmatrix}.
\tag{7}
$$

Thus, if a series of operations $P$ factors $C_G$ and a series of operations Q factors $C_H$, then $(P \otimes I)$ block-factorizes $C_K$ and $(I \otimes Q)$ factorizes each block of $C_K$. Thus *a priori* $(P \otimes Q)$ factorizes $C_K$.

Therefore, if a solution for one qubit has been found, we can generate a solution for an arbitrary number of qubits by successive tensor products. Now, because the available memory is limited,[1] it is desired to minimize the number of auxiliary qubits by logical qubits especially if additional qubits are necessary for error correcting codes [14]. In our study the size of the group G has been fixed to a maximum of 8 elements so as to have only 3 auxiliary qubits per logic bit. This accounts for the fact that quantum memory is expensive.

Only a few potential groups then satisfy the above restrictions:

- the projective Pauli group,
- the dihedral group over 3 qubits,
- the quaternion group.

## 4   Study of the Candidates

The two 8-element groups – quaternion and dihedral group – are very similar: we only consider the latter. Indeed, the results on one of the two groups are immediately transposable to the other group.

---

[1] Simulating quantum computation on a conventional computer is known to be expensive [10] since a linear increase in the number of manipulated qubits yields an exponential increase in the size of the required memory.

This section analyzes first the base cases: the projective Pauli group and the dihedral group. In a second step, we discuss the behavior of the factorization mentioned in Sect. 3 for the case of two qubits in the context of the dihedral group.

### 4.1 The Projective Pauli Group

In the original publication, [7, Th. 6] has been extended to the case of projective groups in [7, Th. 7]. The particular projective group that we consider is

$$G = \{I, X, Z, XZ\}. \tag{8}$$

By setting $A = a_0 I + a_1 X + a_2 Z + a_3 XZ$ the associated coefficient matrix is

$$C_A = \begin{pmatrix} a_0 & a_1 & a_2 & a_3 \\ a_1 & a_0 & a_3 & a_2 \\ a_2 & -a_3 & a_0 & -a_1 \\ a_3 & -a_2 & a_1 & -a_0 \end{pmatrix}. \tag{9}$$

Klappenecker and Rötteler [7, Eq. 12] gave the factorization

$$CNOT \times CNOT^{(2,1)} \times (H \otimes I_2) \times C_A \times (H \otimes I_2) \times CNOT = A \otimes I_2 \tag{10}$$

with

$$CNOT^{(2,1)} = \begin{pmatrix} 1 & 0 & 0 & 0 \\ 0 & 0 & 0 & 1 \\ 0 & 0 & 1 & 0 \\ 0 & 1 & 0 & 0 \end{pmatrix}.$$

This shows that the synthesis of $C_A$ is as difficult as the synthesis of $A$. No improvement can therefore be achieved with this group.

### 4.2 The Dihedral Group

The idea is to get rid of the projective character of the Pauli group by adding matrices to the $G$ group, i.e with

$$G = \{I, -I, X, -X, Z, -Z, XZ, -XZ\}. \tag{11}$$

The coefficient matrix then becomes

$$
C_A = \begin{pmatrix}
a_0 & a_1 & a_2 & a_3 & a_4 & a_5 & a_6 & a_7 \\
a_1 & a_0 & a_3 & a_2 & a_5 & a_4 & a_7 & a_6 \\
a_2 & a_3 & a_0 & a_1 & a_7 & a_6 & a_5 & a_4 \\
a_3 & a_2 & a_1 & a_0 & a_6 & a_7 & a_4 & a_5 \\
a_4 & a_5 & a_6 & a_7 & a_0 & a_1 & a_2 & a_3 \\
a_5 & a_4 & a_7 & a_6 & a_1 & a_0 & a_3 & a_2 \\
a_7 & a_6 & a_5 & a_4 & a_2 & a_3 & a_0 & a_1 \\
a_6 & a_7 & a_4 & a_5 & a_3 & a_2 & a_1 & a_0
\end{pmatrix} . \tag{12}
$$

The best factorization that we have found is

$$
P \times C_A \times P^{\dagger} = \begin{pmatrix} I & & & \\ & U & & \\ & & I & \\ & & & U \end{pmatrix} = I \otimes \Lambda(U) \tag{13}
$$

where

$$
P = (SWAP \otimes I) \times (I \otimes SWAP) \times (\Lambda(Z) \otimes I) \times H^{\otimes 3} \tag{14}
$$

and where $U$ is some arbitrary $2 \times 2$ unitary matrix, a priori not simpler to synthesize than the matrix $A$.

We can then conclude that no improvement can neither be found for this group.

## 4.3 Factorization for Two Qubits

In this section, we highlight the fact that the factorization procedure envisioned in Sect. 3 is not so simple to use, and that it does not necessarily provide a usable decomposition.

Consider indeed an operator $A$ on 2 qubits. Using the dihedral group, the block factorization on $C_A$ would then lead to

$$
\begin{pmatrix} I & & & \\ & V & & \\ & & I & \\ & & & V \end{pmatrix} \tag{15}
$$

with $V$ a 2 by 2 block-matrix with blocks of size 8 by 8. Applying the same factorization on each block of $V$ gives a matrix of the shape

$$
\begin{pmatrix}
I & & & & 0 & & \\
& U_1 & & & & U_2 & \\
& & I & & & & 0 \\
& & & U_1 & & & U_2 \\
0 & & & & I & & \\
& U_3 & & & & U_4 & \\
& & 0 & & & & I \\
& & & U_3 & & & U_4
\end{pmatrix},
\tag{16}
$$

with $U_1$, $U_2$, $U_3$ and $U_4$ arbitrary matrices of size $2 \times 2$, such that $\begin{pmatrix} U_1 & U_2 \\ U_3 & U_4 \end{pmatrix}$ is unitary. Synthesizing $A$ therefore corresponds to synthesizing this matrix, which does not seem too less costly. This hints at the fact that extending the study to larger groups might not trivially help in getting a working solution.

## 5 Conclusion

We have recalled the fundamentals of the synthesis of quantum circuits. We started from an already existing method, aiming at implementing linear combinations of known circuits in order to attempt to derive a generic synthesis method. By clarifying how a generic synthesis method can be compositionally derived, we have illustrated the complexity of the problem. We presented the issues encountered when restricting the approach to small groups of one-qubit operators. This study calls for a more in-depth analysis of larger groups of two- or three-qubit operators.

## References

1. Barenco, A., Bennett, C.H., Cleve, R., DiVincenzo, D.P., Margolus, N., Shor, P., Sleator, T., Smolin, J.A., Weinfurter, H.: Elementary gates for quantum computation. Phys. Rev. A **52**(5), 3457 (1995)
2. Bullock, S.S., Markov, I.L.: Asymptotically optimal circuits for arbitrary n-qubit diagonal computations. Quant. Inf. Comput. **4**(1), 27–47 (2004)
3. Chi-Chih Yao, A.: Quantum circuit complexity. In: Proceedings of the 34th Annual Symposium on Foundations of Computer Science (SFCS'93), pp. 352–361. IEEE Computer Society, Washington, DC, USA (1993)
4. De Vos, A., De Baerdemacker, S.: Block-ZXZ synthesis of an arbitrary quantum circuit. Phys. Rev. A **94**(5), 052317 (2016)
5. Deutsch, D., Barenco, A., Ekert, A.: Universality in quantum computation. Proc. R. Soc. Lond. A **449**, 669–677 (1995)
6. JavadiAbhari, A., Patil, S., Kudrow, D., Heckey, J., Lvov, A., Chong, F.T., Martonosi, M.: ScaffCC: Scalable compilation and analysis of quantum programs. Parallel Comput. **45**, 2–17 (2015)
7. Klappenecker, A., Rötteler, M.: Quantum software reusability. Int. J. Found. Comput. Sci. **14**(05), 777–796 (2003)

8. Knill, E.: Approximation by quantum circuits. Technical Report LANL report LAUR-95-2225, Los Alamos National Laboratory (1995)
9. Maslov, D., Dueck, G.W., Miller, D.M., Negrevergne, C.: Quantum circuit simplification and level compaction. IEEE Trans. Comput.-Aided Des. Integr. Circ. Syst. **27**(3), 436–444 (2008)
10. Nielsen, M.A., Chuang, I.L.: Quantum Computation and Quantum Information. Cambridge University Press, Cambridge (2011)
11. Reck, M., Zeilinger, A., Bernstein, H.J., Bertani, P.: Experimental realization of any discrete unitary operator. Phys. Rev. Lett. **73**(1), 58 (1994)
12. Saeedi, M., Arabzadeh, M., Zamani, M.S., Sedighi, M.: Block-based quantum-logic synthesis. Quant. Inf. Comput. **11**(3), 262–277 (2011)
13. Shende, V.V., Bullock, S.S., Markov, I.L.: Synthesis of quantum-logic circuits. IEEE Trans. Comput.-Aided Des. Integr. Circ. Syst. **25**(6), 1000–1010 (2006)
14. Steane, A.M.: Error correcting codes in quantum theory. Phys. Rev. Lett. **77**(5), 793 (1996)
15. Valiron, B., Ross, N.J., Selinger, P., Alexander, D.S., Smith, J.M.: Programming the quantum future. Commun. ACM **58**(8), 52–61 (2015)
16. Vartiainen, J.J., Möttönen, M., Salomaa, M.M.: Efficient decomposition of quantum gates. Phys. Rev. Lett. **92**(17), 177,902 (2004)
17. Wecker, D., Svore, K.M.: LIQUi|⟩: A software design architecture and domain-specific language for quantum computing (2014). ArXiv:1402.4467

# Robust Reliable $H_\infty$ Control and Input-to-State Stabilization for Uncertain Hybrid Systems

Mohamad S. Alwan, Xinzhi Liu and Taghreed G. Sugati

**Abstract** The main objective of this paper to design a robust reliable $H_\infty$ control and a switching law for a class of uncertain switched systems under an average dwell time switching signal that guarantees ISS not only when all the actuators are operational, but also when some of them experience failure. The faulty actuator output is assumed to be nonzero, which is treated as a disturbance signal that is augmented with the system disturbance input. The input-to-state stability (ISS) property is analyzed by the multiple Lyapunov functions and comparison principle approach. A numerical example is introduced to illustrate the validity of the theoretical results.

**Keywords** Switched systems · ISS · Average dwell time · Reliable control
$H_\infty$ control

## 1 Introduction

There has been a growing interest in studying switched systems in the last three decades due to their widespread applications in different fields such as aircraft, automotive industry, robotics, control systems, biological, epidemic disease models; see [7, 8, 10] and the references therein. By a switched system we mean a special class of hybrid systems that consist of a family of continuous- or discrete-time dynamical subsystems (or modes), and a switching rule (or signal). The role of the switching signal is to govern the jump among the subsystems. The stability of switched systems has received much attention and has been studied using either the common Lyapunov function method [11], or the multiple Lyapunov function method [2]. It has been realized that it is more convenient to use multiple Lyapunov functions than

M. S. Alwan (✉) · X. Liu · T. G. Sugati
University of Waterloo, Waterloo, ON N2L 3G1, Canada
e-mail: malwan@uwaterloo.ca

X. Liu
e-mail: xzliu@uwaterloo.ca

T. G. Sugati
e-mail: tsugati@uwaterloo.ca

© Springer Nature Switzerland AG 2018
D. M. Kilgour et al. (eds.), *Recent Advances in Mathematical and Statistical Methods*, Springer Proceedings in Mathematics & Statistics 259,
https://doi.org/10.1007/978-3-319-99719-3_2

13

the common Lyapunov function since having only one Lyapunov function for all the modes under study is not practical and is difficult to construct.

The reliable control is the controller that tolerates actuator and/or sensor failures. In reality, the failure of control components is frequently encountered, yet the immediate repair may not be feasible, such as in the case of aerospace or submarine system, etc. Therefore, designing a reliable controller to guarantee an acceptable level of performance becomes crucial. The trend to design reliable controllers has been increased; see for instance [4, 12, 15, 16, 18]. In most of the available results about reliable control, the faulty actuators are modelled as outages i.e., the output is assumed to be zero. In [1, 9, 12, 16], the output signal is considered as a disturbance signal with bounded magnitude that is augmented with the system disturbance signal.

The $H_\infty$ control has received a great deal of attention in control theory [3, 17]. It is a useful measure used to guarantee the performance of the plant when dealing with control problems that involve robust design. However, in the event of control component failures, the stability or performance of the plant may not be achieved by such designs. Therefore, it would be advantageous if it is associated with a reliable control design to handle such failures when they occur. One may refer to [1, 9, 12, 18].

In practice, most of the real control systems are subject to some disturbance inputs. ISS notion, introduced in [13] which addresses the system response to a bounded disturbance when the unforced system is asymptotically stable, is an efficient tool to deal with these disturbances. As a result, it becomes important in the modern nonlinear control theory and design [1, 13, 14].

This paper is organized as follows. Section 2 involves the problem description, definitions, and a useful lemma. The main results and proofs are stated in Sect. 3. A numerical example with simulations is presented in Sect. 4. The conclusion is given in Sect. 5.

## 2 Problem Formulation and Preliminaries

Throughout this paper, $\mathbb{R}^n$ denotes the $n$-dimensional Euclidean space; $\mathbb{R}_+$ refers to the nonnegative real numbers; $\mathbb{R}^{n \times m}$ is the class of all $n \times m$ real matrices. A symmetric matrix $P$ is said to be positive definite if all its eigenvalues are positive. Moreover, If $P \in \mathbb{R}^{n \times n}$, denote by $\lambda_{max}(P)(\lambda_{min}(P))$ the maximum (minimum) eigenvalue of $P$. If $V(x) = x^T P x$, the following inequalities are always true

$$c_1 ||x||^2 \leq V(x) \leq c_2 ||x||^2, \tag{1}$$

where $c_1 = \lambda_{min}(P)$, $c_2 = \lambda_{max}(P)$. If $x \in \mathbb{R}^n$, then $||x||$ refers to the Euclidean vector norm of $x$. $L_2[t_0, \infty)$ is the space of square integrable vector-valued functions on $[t_0, \infty)$ and $|| \cdot ||_2$ denotes $L_2[t_0, \infty)$-norm (i.e., $w \in L_2[t_0, \infty)$ means $||w||_2^2 = \int_{t_0}^{\infty} ||w(t)||^2 dt < \infty$). Consider a class of uncertain switched systems given by

$$\begin{cases} \dot{x} = (A_{\rho(t)} + \Delta A_{\rho(t)})x + B_{\rho(t)}u + G_{\rho(t)}w + f_{\rho(t)}(x), \\ z = C_{\rho(t)}x + F_{\rho(t)}u, \quad x(t_0) = x_0, \end{cases} \quad (2)$$

where $x \in \mathbb{R}^n$ is the system state, $u \in \mathbb{R}^q$ is the control input, $w \in \mathbb{R}^p$ is an input disturbance, which is assumed to be bounded, and $z \in \mathbb{R}^r$ is the controlled output. $\rho$ is the switching law which is a piecewise constant function defined by $\rho : [t_0, \infty) \rightarrow \mathscr{S} = \{1, 2, \cdots, N\}$. The role of $\rho$ is to switch among the system modes. For each $i \in \mathscr{S}$, $A_i$ is a non Hurwitz matrix, $K_i \in \mathbb{R}^{q \times n}$ is the control gain matrix such that $u = K_i x$, where $(A_i, B_i)$ is assumed to be stabilizable, $f_i(x) \in \mathbb{R}^n$ is some nonlinearity, $A_i$, $B_i$, $G_i$, $C_i$ and $F_i$ are known real constant matrices, and $\Delta A_i$ is a deterministic piecewise continuous function of time $t$ which represents parameter uncertainty with bounded norm and it also gives the structure of the system uncertainty. For any $i \in \mathscr{S}$, the closed-loop system is

$$\begin{cases} \dot{x} = (A_i + \Delta A_i + B_i K_i)x + G_i w + f_i(x), \\ z = C_{ic}x, \quad x(t_0) = x_0, \quad \text{where } C_{ic} = C_i + F_i K_i. \end{cases} \quad (3)$$

To analyze the reliable stabilization with respect to actuator failures, the $q$ control actuators are divided into two sets. $\Sigma \subseteq \{1, 2, \ldots, q\}$ the set of actuators that are susceptible to failure, i.e., they may occasionally fail, and $\overline{\Sigma} \subseteq \{1, 2, \ldots, q\} - \Sigma$ the other set of actuators which are robust to failures and essential to stabilize the given system. The elements of $\Sigma$ are redundant in terms of the stabilization but necessary to improve the system performance, while the elements of $\overline{\Sigma}$ are required to stabilize the system and assumed that they never fail, i.e., the pair $(A_i, B_{i\overline{\Sigma}})$ is assumed to be stabilizable.

For $i \in \mathscr{S}$, consider the decomposition of the control matrix $B_i = B_{i\Sigma} + B_{i\overline{\Sigma}}$, where $B_{i\Sigma}$, $B_{i\overline{\Sigma}}$ are the control matrices associated with $\Sigma$, $\overline{\Sigma}$ respectively, and $B_{i\Sigma}$, $B_{i\overline{\Sigma}}$ are generated by zeroing out the columns corresponding to $\overline{\Sigma}$ and $\Sigma$, respectively. For a fixed $i \in \mathscr{S}$, let $\sigma \subseteq \Sigma$ corresponds to some of the actuators that experience failure, and assume that the output of faulty actuators is any arbitrary energy-bounded signal (or disturbance input) which belongs to $L_2[t_0, \infty)$. Then, the decomposition becomes $B_i = B_{i\sigma} + B_{i\overline{\sigma}}$, where $B_{i\sigma}$ and $B_{i\overline{\sigma}}$ have the same definition of $B_{i\Sigma}$ and $B_{i\overline{\Sigma}}$, respectively. Furthermore, the augmented disturbance input to the system becomes

$$w_\sigma^F = (w^T \ (u_\sigma^F)^T)^T,$$

where $u_\sigma^F \in \mathbb{R}^q$ is the failure vector whose elements corresponding to the set of faulty actuators $\sigma$, and $F$ here stands for "failure". Since the control input $u$ is applied to the system through the normal actuators, and the outputs of the faulty actuators are assumed to be arbitrary signals, the closed-loop system becomes

$$\begin{cases} \dot{x} = (A_i + \Delta A_i + B_{i\overline{\sigma}}K_i)x + G_{ic}w_\sigma^F + f_i(x), \quad i \in \mathscr{S} = \{1, 2, \ldots, N\}, \\ z = C_{ic}x, \quad x(t_0) = x_0, , \quad \text{where } G_{ic} = (G_i \ B_{i\sigma}). \end{cases} \quad (4)$$

**Definition 2.1** [6] (*Class-K function*)   A function $\rho : [0, r) \to [0, \infty)$ is said to belong to class $\mathcal{K}$ (i.e., $\rho \in \mathcal{K}$) if it is continuous, strictly increasing, and $\rho(0) = 0$.

**Definition 2.2** (*Input-to-State Stability*) System (3) is said to be robustly globally exponentially ISS if there exist positive constants $\lambda$, $\bar{\lambda}$ and a function $\rho \in \mathcal{K}$ such that, for any solution $x(t) = x(t, t_0, x_0)$,

$$||x|| \leq \bar{\lambda}||x_0||e^{-\lambda(t-t_0)} + \rho \left( \sup_{t_0 \leq \tau \leq t} ||w(\tau)|| \right), \quad \forall t \geq t_0.$$

**Definition 2.3** (*input-to-state stability with an $H_\infty$-norm (ISS-$H_\infty$)*) Given a constant $\gamma > 0$, system (3) is said to be ISS-$H_\infty$ if there exists a state feedback law $u(t) = K_i x(t)$, such that, for any admissible parameter uncertainties $\Delta A_i$, the closed loop system (3) is globally exponentially ISS, and the controlled output $z$ satisfies

$$||z||_2^2 = \int_{t_0}^{\infty} ||z||^2 \, dt \leq \gamma^2 ||w||_2^2 + m_0,$$

for some positive constant $m_0$.

**Assumption A** *For $i \in \mathcal{S}$, the admissible parameter uncertainties are defined by*

$$\Delta A_i(t) = D_i \mathcal{U}_i(t) H_i, \quad \forall t \in \mathbb{R}_+,$$

*with $D_i$, $H_i$ being known real matrices with appropriate dimensions that give the structure of the uncertainty, and $\mathcal{U}_i(t)$ being unknown real time-varying matrix representing the uncertain parameter and satisfying $||\mathcal{U}_i(t)|| \leq 1$.*

**Lemma 2.4** *For any arbitrary positive constants $\xi_1$, $\xi_2$ and $\xi_3$, and a positive definite matrix $P$, we have*

(i)   $2x^T P(\Delta A)x \leq x^T \left( \xi_1 PDD^T P + \frac{1}{\xi_1} H^T H \right) x.$

(ii)   $2x^T PGw \leq x^T \left( \xi_2 PGG^T P \right) x + \frac{1}{\xi_2} w^T w.$

(iii)   $2x^T Pf(x) \leq x^T \left( \xi_3 P^2 + \frac{1}{\xi_3} \delta I \right) x$ *such that $||f(x)||^2 \leq \delta ||x||^2$ with $\delta > 0$.*

*Proof* For (i), we have

$$0 \leq (\sqrt{\xi_1} x^T (PD\mathcal{U}) - \frac{1}{\sqrt{\xi_1}} x^T H^T)(\sqrt{\xi_1} x^T (PD\mathcal{U}) - \frac{1}{\sqrt{\xi_1}} x^T H^T)^T$$

$$= \xi_1 x^T PDD^T Px + \frac{1}{\xi_1} x^T H^T Hx - 2x^T (PD\mathcal{U}H)x,$$

which leads to $2x^T (PD\mathcal{U}H)x \leq x^T \left( \xi_1 PDD^T P + \frac{1}{\xi_1} H^T H \right) x$, which yields the desired result. The inequalities in (*ii*) and (*iii*) can be proved similarly.   $\square$

**Average Dwell Time Condition (ADTC)** [5]. The number of switches $N(t_0, t)$ in the interval $(t_0, t)$ for a finite $t$ satisfies $N(t_0, t) \leq N_0 + \frac{t-t_0}{\tau_a}$, where $N_0 > 0$ is the chatter bound, and $\tau_a$ is the average dwell time.

Here, by *dwell time* we mean the time between two consecutive switches, while the *chatter bound* is an upper bound for the number of switches in an interval of length smaller than $\tau_a$.

## 3 Main Results

**Theorem 3.1** *Let the controller gain $K_i$ and the constant $\gamma_i > 0$ be given, and assume that Assumption A holds. Then, the switched control system (3) is robustly globally exponentially ISS with an $H_\infty$-norm bound $\gamma$ if the ADTC holds, and there exist positive constants $\xi_{1i}$, $\xi_{2i}$, $\xi_{3i}$, and a positive definite matrix $P_i$ satisfying the Riccati-like equation*

$$(A_i + B_iK_i)^T P_i + P_i(A_i + B_iK_i) + \xi_{1i}P_iD_iD_i^T P_i + \frac{1}{\xi_{1i}}H_i^T H_i + C_{ic}^T C_{ic}$$

$$+ \xi_{2i}P_iG_iG_i^T P_i + \xi_{3i}P_i^2 + \frac{1}{\xi_{3i}}\delta_i I + \alpha_i P_i = 0, \tag{5}$$

*where $\delta_i > 0$ such that $||f_i(x)||^2 \leq \delta_i||x||^2$, and $\alpha_i > 0$ is the decay rate of mode i.*

*Proof* Let $x(t) = x(t, t_0, x_0)$ be the solution of system (3). For any $i \in \mathscr{S}$, define $V_i(x) = x^T P_i x$ as a Lyapunov function candidate for the *ith* mode. Then,

$$\dot{V}_i(x) = x^T[(A_i + B_iK_i)^T P_i + P_i(A_i + B_iK_i)]x + 2x^T P_i(\Delta A_i)x$$

$$+ 2x^T P_iG_iw + 2x^T P_i f_i(x)$$

$$\leq x^T[(A_i + B_iK_i)^T P_i + P_i(A_i + B_iK_i) + \xi_{1i}P_iD_iD_i^T P_i$$

$$+ \xi_{2i}P_iG_iG_i^T P_i + \frac{1}{\xi_{1i}}H_i^T H_i$$

$$+ \xi_{3i}P_i^2 + \frac{1}{\xi_{3i}}\delta_i I]x + \frac{1}{\xi_{2i}}w^T w = -\alpha_i V_i(x) + \frac{1}{\xi_{2i}}w^T w,$$

where we used $||f_i(x)||^2 \leq \delta_i||x||^2$ and Lemma 2.4 in the second bottom line, and condition (5) in the last line. Hence, for each subinterval $[t_{k-1}, t_k)$ we have, after adding-subtracting the term $\theta_i V_i(x)$,

$$\dot{V}_i(x) \leq -(\alpha_i - \theta_i)V_i(x) - \theta_i V_i(x) + w^T w/\xi_{2i}$$

$$\leq -\bar{\alpha}_i V_i(x) - \theta_i V_i(x) + w^T w/\xi_{2i},$$

where $\bar{\alpha}_i = \alpha_i - \theta_i$ for some $0 < \theta_i < \alpha_i$. The foregoing inequality implies that

$$\dot{V}_i(x) \leq -\overline{\alpha}_i V_i(x), \quad \text{for all } t \in [t_{k-1}, t_k),$$

provided that the sum $-\theta_i V_i(x) + w^T w/\xi_{2i} < 0$ or $V_i(x) > \frac{1}{\theta_i \xi_{2i}} ||w||^2$. By (1), $||x|| > \frac{||w||}{\sqrt{\theta_i c_2 \xi_{2i}}} =: \rho_i(||w||)$. Then, for all $t \in [t_{k-1}, t_k)$, $V_i(x(t)) \leq V_i(x(t_{k-1}))e^{-\overline{\alpha}_i(t-t_{k-1})}$ provided that $||x|| > \rho(||w||)$, where $\rho(||w||) = \max_{i \in \mathscr{S}}\{\rho_i(||w||)\}$. From (1), we have for any $i, j \in \mathscr{S}$

$$V_j(x(t)) \leq \mu V_i(x(t)), \quad \mu = c_2/c_1, \tag{6}$$

where $c_1 = \min_{i \in \mathscr{S}}\{\lambda_{min}(P_i)\}$ and $c_2 = \max_{i \in \mathscr{S}}\{\lambda_{max}(P_i)\}$. Then, for $i \in \mathscr{S}$ and $t \in [t_{k-1}, t_k)$, we have $V_i(x(t)) \leq \mu^{k-1}e^{-\overline{\alpha}_i(t-t_{k-1})}e^{-\overline{\alpha}_{i-1}(t_{k-1}-t_{k-2})}\cdots e^{-\overline{\alpha}_1(t_1-t_0)}V_1(x_0)$ provided that $||x|| > \rho(||w||)$. Letting $\alpha^* = \min\{\overline{\alpha}_i; i \in \mathscr{S}\}$, one may get

$$V_i(x(t)) \leq \mu^{k-1}e^{-\alpha^*(t-t_0)}V_1(x_0) = e^{(k-1)\ln\mu - \alpha^*(t-t_0)}V_1(x_0)$$

provided that $||x|| > \rho(||w||)$. Using the ADTC with $N_0 = \frac{\eta}{\ln\mu}$, $\tau_a = \frac{\ln\mu}{\alpha^*-\nu}$, ($\nu < \alpha^*$), for some arbitrary positive constant $\eta$, we get

$$V_i(x(t)) \leq e^{\eta - \nu(t-t_0)}V_1(x_0) \quad \text{provided that } ||x|| > \rho(||w||).$$

This implies that [6] $||x|| \leq b||x_0||e^{-\nu(t-t_0)/2} + \gamma(\sup_{t_0 \leq \tau \leq t}||w(\tau)||)$, $t \geq t_0$, where $b = \sqrt{e^{\eta}c_2/c_1}$, and $\gamma(s) = \sqrt{\frac{c_2}{c_1}}\rho(s)$, which completes the proof of exponential ISS.

To prove the upper bound on the output magnitude $||z||$, for any $i \in \mathscr{S}$, we introduce the performance function $J_i = \int_{t_0}^{\infty}(z^T z - \gamma_i^2 w^T w)dt$. Then,

$$\begin{aligned}
J_i &\leq \int_{t_0}^{\infty}(z^T z - \gamma_i^2 w^T w)\,dt + \int_{t_0}^{\infty}\dot{V}_i\,dt + V_i(x_0) \\
&\leq \int_{t_0}^{\infty}(z^T z - \gamma_i^2 w^T w)\,dt + V_i(x_0) + \int_{t_0}^{\infty}\{x^T[(A_i+B_iK_i)^T P_i + P_i(A_i+B_iK_i) \\
&\quad + \xi_{1i}P_iD_iD_i^T P_i + \frac{1}{\xi_{1i}}H_i^T H_i + \xi_{3i}P_i^2 + \frac{1}{\xi_{3i}}\delta_i I - \gamma_i^{-2}P_iG_iG_i^T P_i \\
&\quad + \gamma_i^{-2}P_iG_iG_i^T P_i]x + 2x^T P_iG_iw\}\,dt \\
&= V_i(x_0) + \int_{t_0}^{\infty}\{x^T[(A_i+B_iK_i)^T P_i + P_i(A_i+B_iK_i) + \xi_{1i}P_iD_iD_i^T P_i + \frac{1}{\xi_{1i}}H_i^T H_i \\
&\quad + \xi_{3i}P_i^2 + \frac{1}{\xi_{3i}}\delta_i I + \gamma_i^{-2}P_iG_iG_i^T P_i + C_{ic}^T C_{ic}]x\}\,dt \\
&\quad - \int_{t_0}^{\infty}\gamma_i^2(w - \gamma_i^{-2}G_i^T P_ix)^T(w - \gamma_i^{-2}G_i^T P_ix)\,dt.
\end{aligned}$$

The last term is strictly negative, so, using condition (5) with $\gamma_i^{-2} = \xi_{2i}$, we get $J_i \le V_i(x_0)$. Recalling the definition of $J_i$, we see that $||z||_2^2 \le \gamma^2||w||_2^2 + m_0$, where $m_0 = \max_{i \in \mathscr{S}}\{V_i(x_0)\}$, and $\gamma = \max_{i \in \mathscr{S}}\{\gamma_i\}$. This completes the proof. $\quad\square$

**Theorem 3.2** (Reliability) *Let the constant $\gamma_i > 0$ be given. Assume that Assumption A holds, the switched control system* (4) *is robustly globally exponentially ISS-$H_\infty$ if the ADTC holds, the controller gain $K_i = -\frac{1}{2}\varepsilon_i B_{i\overline{\sigma}}^T P_i$, for some constants $\varepsilon_i > 0$, and positive definite matrix $P_i$, and there exist positive constants $\xi_{1i}, \xi_{2i}, \xi_{3i}, \varepsilon_i$, and a positive definite matrix $P_i$ satisfying the Riccati-like equation*

$$A_i^T P_i + P_i A_i + P_i(\xi_{1i}D_iD_i^T + \xi_{2i}G_{ic}G_{ic}^T - \varepsilon_i B_{i\overline{\Sigma}}B_{i\overline{\Sigma}}^T + \xi_{3i}I)P_i$$
$$+ \frac{1}{\xi_{1i}}H_i^T H_i + C_{ic}^T C_{ic} + \frac{1}{\xi_{3i}}\delta_i I + \alpha_i P_i = 0, \tag{7}$$

*where $\delta_i$ is a positive constant such that $||f_i(x)||^2 \le \delta_i||x||^2$ holds.*

*Proof* Let $x(t) = x(t, t_0, x_0)$ be the solution of system (4). For any $i \in \mathscr{S}$, define $V_i(x) = x^T P_i x$ as a Lyapunov function candidate for the *i*th mode. Then,

$$\dot{V}_i(x)$$
$$= x^T[A_i^T P_i + P_i A_i + 2P_i(\Delta A_i) + (B_{i\overline{\sigma}}K_i)^T P_i + P_i B_{i\overline{\sigma}}K_i]x$$
$$+ 2x^T P_i G_{ic}w_\sigma^F + 2x^T P_i f_i(x)$$
$$= x^T[A_i^T P_i + P_i A_i + 2P_i(\Delta A_i) - \varepsilon_i P_i(B_{i\overline{\sigma}})(B_{i\overline{\sigma}})^T P_i]x$$
$$+ 2x^T P_i G_{ic}w_\sigma^F + 2x^T P_i f_i(x)$$
$$\le x^T[A_i^T P_i + P_i A_i + \xi_{1i}P_i D_i D_i^T P_i + \xi_{2i}P_i G_{ic}G_{ic}^T P_i$$
$$+ \frac{1}{\xi_{1i}}H_i^T H_i + \xi_{3i}P_i^2 + \frac{1}{\xi_{3i}}\delta_i I - \varepsilon_i P_i(B_{i\overline{\sigma}})(B_{i\overline{\sigma}})^T P_i]x + \frac{1}{\xi_{2i}}(w_\sigma^F)^T w_\sigma^F$$
$$\le x^T[A_i^T P_i + P_i A_i + P_i(\xi_{1i}D_iD_i^T + \xi_{2i}G_{ic}G_{ic}^T - \varepsilon_i B_{i\overline{\Sigma}}B_{i\overline{\Sigma}}^T$$
$$+ \xi_{3i}I)P_i + \frac{1}{\xi_{1i}}H_i^T H_i$$
$$+ \frac{1}{\xi_{3i}}\delta_i I]x + \frac{1}{\xi_{2i}}(w_\sigma^F)^T w_\sigma^F = -\alpha_i V_i(x) + \frac{1}{\xi_{2i}}(w_\sigma^F)^T w_\sigma^F,$$

where we used $||f_i(x)||^2 \le \delta_i||x||^2$ and Lemma 2.4 in the third bottom line, the fact that [12] $B_{i\overline{\Sigma}}(B_{i\overline{\Sigma}})^T \le B_{i\overline{\sigma}}(B_{i\overline{\sigma}})^T$, and condition (5) in the last line. Then, for all $t \in [t_{k-1}, t_k)$, we have

$$\dot{V}_i(x) \le -\overline{\alpha}_i V_i(x) - \theta_i V_i(x) + (w_\sigma^F)^T w_\sigma^F/\xi_{2i},$$

where $\overline{\alpha}_i = \alpha_i - \theta_i$ and $0 < \theta_i < \alpha_i$. This implies that $\dot{V}_i(x) \le -\overline{\alpha}_i V_i(x)$, for all $t \in [t_{k-1}, t_k)$ provided that $||x|| > \frac{||w_\sigma^F||}{\sqrt{\theta_i c_2 \xi_{2i}}} =: \rho_i(||w_\sigma^F||)$. As done in Theorem 3.1, one may get $V_i(x(t)) \le e^{\eta - \nu(t-t_0)}V_1(x_0)$ provided that $||x|| > \rho(||w||)$, where $\rho(||w||) = \max_{i \in \mathscr{S}}\{\rho_i(||w||)\}$. This also implies that [6]

$$\|x\| \le b\|x_0\|e^{-\nu(t-t_0)} + \gamma(\sup_{t_0 \le \tau \le t} \|w_\sigma^F(\tau)\|), \quad t \ge t_0,$$

where $b = \sqrt{e^\eta c_2/c_1}$, $\gamma(s) = \sqrt{\frac{c_2}{c_1}}\rho(s)$. As for the upper bound on $\|z\|$, we follow the same steps in Theorem 3.1, where $J_i = \int_{t_0}^\infty (z^T z - \gamma_i^2 (w_\sigma^F)^T w_\sigma^F)dt$, to obtain $\|z\|_2^2 \le \gamma^2 \|w_\sigma^F\|_2^2 + m_0$, where $m_0 = \max_{i \in \mathscr{S}}\{V_i(x_0)\}$, and $\gamma = \max_{i \in \mathscr{S}}\{\gamma_i\}$.        □

## 4  Numerical Example

*Example 1*  Consider system (3) where $\mathscr{S} = \{1, 2\}$,

$$A_1 = \begin{bmatrix} 0.2 & 0.1 \\ 0 & -6 \end{bmatrix}, B_1 = \begin{bmatrix} -7 & 1 \\ 0.1 & 0.2 \end{bmatrix}, C_1 = \begin{bmatrix} 2 & 0.1 \\ 0 & 2 \end{bmatrix}, F_1 = \begin{bmatrix} 0.1 & -2 \\ 0.1 & 0 \end{bmatrix},$$

$$D_1 = \begin{bmatrix} 1 \\ 0 \end{bmatrix}, H_1 = \begin{bmatrix} 0 & 1 \end{bmatrix}, G_1 = \begin{bmatrix} 1 & 0 \\ 0 & 1 \end{bmatrix}, f_1 = 0.01\begin{bmatrix} \sin(x_1) \\ \sin(x_2) \end{bmatrix}, \mathscr{U}_1 = \sin(t),$$

$\varepsilon_1 = 2$, $\xi_{11} = 0.2$, $\gamma_1 = 0.1$, $\alpha_1 = 2$, $\xi_{21} = \gamma_1^{-2}$, $\xi_{31} = 1$, and $\theta_1 = 1$ with $t_0 = 0$. From $\|f_i(x)\|^2 \le \delta_i \|x\|^2$, one may get $\delta_1 = 0.01$. As for the second mode, we take

$$A_2 = \begin{bmatrix} -9 & 0.2 \\ 0 & 0.1 \end{bmatrix}, B_2 = \begin{bmatrix} 0.1 & 0.5 \\ 0.1 & -8 \end{bmatrix}, C_2 = \begin{bmatrix} 1 & 0 \\ 0 & 0.5 \end{bmatrix}, F_2 = \begin{bmatrix} 0.1 & 0 \\ -3 & 0.1 \end{bmatrix},$$

$$D_2 = \begin{bmatrix} 0 \\ 1 \end{bmatrix}, H_2 = \begin{bmatrix} 1 & 0 \end{bmatrix}, G_2 = \begin{bmatrix} 1 & 0 \\ 0 & 1 \end{bmatrix}, f_2 = 0.01\begin{bmatrix} \sin(x_1) \\ \sin(x_2) \end{bmatrix}, \mathscr{U}_2 = \sin(t),$$

$\varepsilon_2 = 0.5$, $\xi_{12} = 0.3$, $\gamma_2 = 0.15$, $\alpha_2 = 2.5$, $\xi_{22} = \gamma_2^{-2}$, $\xi_{32} = 1$, and $\theta_2 = 1.5$. From $\|f_i(x)\|^2 \le \delta_i \|x\|^2$, one may get that $\delta_2 = 0.01$. Let the system input disturbance be defined by $w(t) = [\sin(t) \ \sin(t)]^T$.

**Case 1** (*All the actuators are operational*) When all the control actuators are operational, from Riccati-like equation,

$$P_1 = \begin{bmatrix} 1.6437 & 0.0149 \\ 0.0149 & 0.2499 \end{bmatrix}, P_2 = \begin{bmatrix} 0.1633 & 0.0859 \\ 0.0859 & 0.2724 \end{bmatrix},$$

with $c_{11} = \lambda_{min}(P_1) = 0.2498$, $c_{12} = \lambda_{max}(P_1) = 1.6439$, $c_{21} = \lambda_{min}(P_2) = 0.1161$, $c_{22} = \lambda_{max}(P_2) = 0.3197$, so, $c_1 = 0.1161$, $c_2 = 1.6439$, and

$$K_1 = \begin{bmatrix} 11.5047 & 0.0796 \\ -1.6467 & -0.0649 \end{bmatrix}, K_2 = \begin{bmatrix} -0.0062 & -0.0090 \\ 0.1514 & 0.5342 \end{bmatrix}.$$

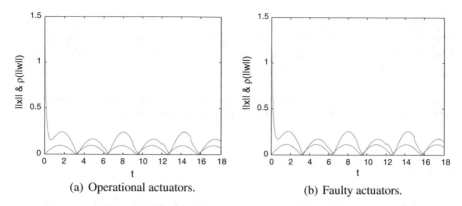

(a) Operational actuators.          (b) Faulty actuators.

**Fig. 1** Input-to-state stabilization

Thus, the matrices $A_1 + B_1 K_1$ and $A_2 + B_2 K_2$ are Hurwitz. The average dwell time is $\tau_a = \frac{\ln \mu}{\alpha^* - \nu} = 2.7898$, with $\nu = 0.05$.

Figure 1a shows the simulation results of $||x||$ (top) and $\gamma(||w||) = \sqrt{c_2/c_1} \rho(||w||)$ (bottom), where $\rho(s) = \max\{\rho_1(s), \rho_2(s)\}$ and $\rho_i(s) = s/\sqrt{c_2 \theta_i \xi_{2i}}$, and $\tau_a = 3$.

**Case 2** (*Failure in the second actuator in the first mode and first actuator in the second mode*) When there is a failure in the second actuator, i.e., $B_{1\Sigma} = \{2\}$ and $B_{1\overline{\Sigma}} = \begin{bmatrix} -7 & 0 \\ 0.1 & 0 \end{bmatrix}$, and $B_{2\Sigma} = \{1\}$ and $B_{2\overline{\Sigma}} = \begin{bmatrix} 0 & 0.5 \\ 0 & -8 \end{bmatrix}$, we have from Riccati-like equation,

$$P_1 = \begin{bmatrix} 1.1265 & -0.1913 \\ -0.1913 & 0.3110 \end{bmatrix}, \quad P_2 = \begin{bmatrix} 0.1676 & 0.0980 \\ 0.0980 & 0.2436 \end{bmatrix},$$

with $c_{11} = \lambda_{\min}(P_1) = 0.2683$, $c_{12} = \lambda_{\max}(P_1) = 1.1691$, $c_{21} = 0.1005$, $c_{22} = 0.3107$, so $c_1 = 0.1005$, $c_2 = 1.1691$, and the control gain matrices

$$K_1 = \begin{bmatrix} 7.9046 & -1.3703 \\ 0 & 0 \end{bmatrix}, \quad K_2 = \begin{bmatrix} 0 & 0 \\ 0.1751 & 0.4750 \end{bmatrix}.$$

Thus, the matrices $A_1 + B_1 K_1$ and $A_2 + B_2 K_2$ are Hurwitz, and $\tau_a = 2.5834$. Figure 1b shows the simulation results of $||x||$ (top) and $\gamma(||w||) = \sqrt{c_2/c_1} \rho(||w||)$ (bottom), where $\rho(s) = \max\{\rho_1(s), \rho_2(s)\}$ and $\rho_i(s) = s/\sqrt{c_2 \theta_i \xi_{2i}}$, $\tau_a = 3$.

## 5 Conclusion

We have considered a time-varying parameter uncertainty in the system state, an $L_2$ norm-bounded input disturbance, and a linearly bounded nonlinear term. The output of the faulty actuators has been treated as a disturbing signal that has been augmented with the system disturbance. We have shown that, using the average dwell time with multiple Lyapunov functions, the switched system is exponentially input-to-state stabilizable, when every individual mode is exponentially input-to-state stabilized by a reliable feedback controller.

**Acknowledgements** This work was partially supported by NSERC Canada. The third author acknowledges the sponsorship of King Abdulaziz University, Saudi Arabia.

# References

1. Alwan, M.S., Liu, X.Z., Xie, W.-C.: On design of robust reliable $H_\infty$ control and input-to-state stabilization of uncertain stochastic systems with state delay. Commun. Nonlinear Sci. Numer. Simul. **18**(4), 1047–1056 (2013)
2. Branicky, M.S.: Multiple Lyapunov functions and other analysis tools for switched hybrid systems. IEEE Trans. Autom. Control **43**(4), 475–482 (1998)
3. Chen, G., Xiang, Z.: Robust reliable $H_\infty$ control of switched stochastic systems with time delays under asynchronous switching. Adv. Differ. Equ. A SpringerOpen J. article(86) (2013)
4. Cheng, X.M., Gui, W.H., Gan, Z.J.: Robust reliable control for a class of time-varying uncertain impulsive systems. J. Central S. Univ. Technol. **12**(1), 199–202 (2005)
5. Hespanha, J.P., Morse, A.S.: Stability of switched systems with average dwell-time. In: Proceedings of the 38th IEEE Conference on Decision and Control, vol. 3, pp. 2655–2660 (1999)
6. Khalil, H.K.: Nonlinear Systems, 3rd edn. Prentice-Hall, Upper Saddle River (2002)
7. Liberzon, D.: Switching in Systems and Control. Birkhäuser, Boston (2003)
8. Liberzon, D., Morse, A.S.: Basic problems is stability and design of switched systems. IEEE Control Syst. Mag. **19**(5), 59–70 (1999)
9. Lu, J., Wu, Z.: Robust reliable $H_\infty$ control for uncertain switched linear systems with disturbances. In: Second International Conference (ICIECS). IEEE Xplore, Dec 2010
10. Morse, A.S. (ed.): Control Using Logic-Based Switching. Lecture Notes in Control and Information Sciences, vol. 222. Springer, New York (1997)
11. Narendra, K.S., Balakrishnan, J.: A common Lyapunov function for stable LTI systems with commuting A-matrices. IEEE Trans. Autom. Control **39**(12), 2469–2471 (1994)
12. Seo, C.J., Kim, B.K.: Robust and reliable $H_\infty$ control for linear systems with parameter uncertainty and actuator failure. Automatica **32**(3), 465–467 (1996)
13. Sontag, E.D.: Smooth stabilization implies coprime factorization. IEEE Trans. Autom. Control **34**(4), 435–443 (1989)
14. Teel, A.R., Moreau, L., Nešic, D.: A note on the robustness of ISS stability. In: Proceeding of the 40th IEEE on Decision and Control, pp. 875–880. Florida (2001)
15. Veillette, R.J.: Reliable state feedback and reliable observers. In: Proceedings of the 31st Conference on Decision and Control, pp. 2898–2903 (1992)
16. Veillette, R.J., Medanic, J.V., Perkins, W.R.: Design of reliable control systems. IEEE Trans. Autom. Control **37**(3), 290–304 (1992)
17. Xie, L., de Souza, C.E.: Robust $H_\infty$ control for linear systems with norm-bounded time-varying uncertainty. IEEE Trans. Autom. Control **37**(8), 1188–1191 (1992)
18. Yang, G.H., Wang, J.L., Soh, Y.C.: Reliable $H_\infty$ control design for linear systems. Automatica **37**(5), 717–725 (2001)

# Exact Coloring of Sparse Matrices

Shahadat Hossain and Ahamad I. Khan

**Abstract** Given the sparsity pattern of a sparse matrix, we consider the problem of partitioning its columns into fewest groups with the property that no two columns in the same group have nonzero entries in the same row position. Many efficient heuristic algorithms approximately solve the partitioning problem as coloring the vertices of a suitable graph associated with the matrix. In this paper we study exact methods for minimum partitioning (coloring) of columns based on a branch-and-bound approach. We propose efficient sparse data structures to implement the coloring methodology and present a new tie-breaking method for choosing columns to color at each branching step. Results from numerical experiments on standard test instances demonstrate the benefit of our approach with regard to computational efficiency and coloring quality.

**Keywords** Branch-and-bound · Column partitioning · Structural orthogonality
Data structures · Jacobian matrix

## 1 Introduction

Given an undirected graph $G = (V, E)$, the optimization version of vertex coloring problem (VCP) is to assign labels or colors to the vertices in $V$ such that vertices that are connected by an edge in $E$ have different colors while the number of colors is minimized. While VCP has many real-world applications it is also known to be computationally intractable [1]. In this paper we study the problem of minimum column partitioning of sparse matrices which is equivalent to coloring the vertices of the column intersection graph [2–4]. Given the sparsity pattern (location of nonzero entries) of a matrix $A \in \mathbb{R}^{m \times n}$ we consider partitioning $A$'s columns into groups with

S. Hossain (✉) · A. I. Khan
University of Lethbridge, Lethbridge, Canada
e-mail: shahadat.hossain@uleth.ca

A. I. Khan
e-mail: ai.khan@uleth.ca

© Springer Nature Switzerland AG 2018
D. M. Kilgour et al. (eds.), *Recent Advances in Mathematical
and Statistical Methods*, Springer Proceedings in Mathematics & Statistics 259,
https://doi.org/10.1007/978-3-319-99719-3_3

the property that no two columns in the same group have nonzero entries in the same row position. Formally, let $\Phi$ be a mapping defined as $\Phi : \{1, 2, \ldots, n\} \mapsto \{1, 2, \ldots, p\}$ such that $\Phi(j) = \Phi(l)$, $j \neq l \Rightarrow \nexists i$ for which $a_{ij} \neq 0$ and $a_{il} \neq 0$. In other words, each column receives a color (group) label from the set $\{1, 2, \ldots, p\}$ such that the columns receiving the same color label satisfy the property that they are "structurally orthogonal" [2]. The problem we want to solve is to find a mapping which minimizes the number of column groups or colors $p$. This problem and its many variants arise in computational optimization where first- and/or higher-order derivatives (gradients, Jacobians, Hessians) of some differentiable function need to be evaluated in an iterative scheme e.g., in Newton's method and is known to be NP-hard [2, 4].

Many efficient heuristics have been proposed in the literature to approximately solve large instances of VCP while there are only few exact methods and are usually limited to solving small instance sizes. To avoid difficulties due to symmetry classical integer linear program (ILP) formulations are usually strengthened with constraints to cut down many symmetric solutions. A recent approach to solving exact VCP is to apply a brach-and-price scheme on a set cover ILP formulation which allows an exponential number of decision variables. Implicit enumeration methods color the vertices successively and try to reuse the colors that have already been used. A widely known implicit algorithm called DSATUR (exact algorithm) due to Brélaz [5] is a modification of the original algorithm due to Brown [6]. For a recent survey of exact and heuristic graph coloring methods we refer to the paper [7].

In this paper we give an exact column partitioning scheme based on DSATUR algorithm and describe data structures that make the implementation computationally efficient. The main contributions of this paper are the following.

1. In [8] authors use two publicly available exact graph coloring software on a set of test matrix instances to obtain minimum partition. The column intersection graph associated with the sparse matrix is generated first which is then input to the coloring code. In our implementation the column intersection graph associated with the sparsity pattern of matrix $A$ which is isomorphic to the adjacency graph of $A^\top A$ is never explicitly formed. Instead, we store the sparsity pattern of $A$ and $A^\top$ as compressed matrices: compressed sparse row (CSR) and compressed sparse column (CSC). To the best of our knowledge this is the first implementation of a branch-and-bound exact algorithm for optimal column partitioning that avoids the generation of the graph associated with the potentially dense matrix $A^\top A$.
2. A maximal clique (a lower bound) is identified simply as columns in a row with maximum number of nonzero entries.
3. Our computer implementation utilizes expressive power of graph-theoretic concepts while exploiting the known sparsity of the matrix. We employ a special heap data structure, namely the bucket heap, to allow efficient calculation and update of saturation degree of columns. We also introduce a new tie-breaking strategy to choose the next column to branch.

The remainder of the paper is structured in the following way. In Sect. 2 we give a brief description of the DSATUR algorithm and introduce the main data structures.

The new tie-breaking strategy is then presented along with the ones by Sewell [9] and Segundo [10]. Section 3 contains results from numerical experiments on a standard set of test instances. The paper is concluded in Sect. 4 with directions on further research.

## 2 Data Structures and Algorithm

The sparsity pattern of sparse matrix $A$ is stored internally with compressed sparse vectors corresponding to rows and columns. Compressed Sparse Row (CSR) storage scheme is a popular data structure where the sparse row vectors are stored contiguously. A simple implementation of CSR can be provided using three arrays: *rowptr* array indexes into *colind* and *value* arrays, with *rowptr(i)* indicating the location (index) of the first element of row $i$ in the arrays *colind* and *value*. Thus, elements in row $i$ are accessed as

$$value(k) \text{ and are located in } (i, colind(k)), k = rowptr(i) \textbf{ to } rowptr(i+1) - 1.$$

*Compressed Sparse Column (CSC)* is simply the transposed matrix stored using the CSR. The array *value* is not needed if we are storing the sparsity pattern only. The software package DSJM [11] enables access to columns and rows by maintaining both CSR and CSC structures for a sparse matrix.

A frequently needed operation in our implementation is to identify the columns that are structurally dependent on (or neighbors of) a given column :

$$\mathcal{N}(A(:, j)) = \{l \mid A(:, j) \text{ is structurally dependent on } A(:, l)\}$$

which is easily obtained using the sparse data structure as $l = $ colind(indj) where indj = rowptr(i) **to** rowptr(i+1) - 1, i = rowind(indi), indi = colptr(j) **to** colptr(j+1) - 1.

The saturation degree of an uncolored column $j$ is the number of distinct colors assumed by its neighbors $\mathcal{N}(j)$. In our DSATUR-based exact coloring scheme, a maximal clique is identified by iterating over the CSR data structure row by row. The number of nonzeros in row $i$ is obtained as $\rho_i = rowptr(i+1) - rowptr(i)$ and $\rho_{max} = \max_i\{\rho_i\}$ is the size of a maximal clique such that the columns in a row with $\rho_{max}$ nonzeros determine a maximal clique which is used as a lower bound (*LB*) in the algorithm. The columns in the maximal clique are assigned color labels $1, \ldots, \rho_{max}$ and are never recolored thus obtaining a partial coloring of the columns of the sparse matrix. This forms the root node of the branch-and-bound tree (BBT). A leaf node in the BBT corresponds to a coloring of all $n$ columns of the matrix and the number of colors in the coloring defines an upper bound (*UB*). The algorithm works by selecting an uncolored column and sequentially trying each of the existing colors in the current coloring and if none can be applied creates a new color label to color the selected column and thus creating a new subproblem for each such feasible color. Each subproblem thus created invokes a new recursive call to the algorithm. A recursive call terminates under any one of the following conditions,

1. the call corresponds to a leaf node in BBT
2. the number of colors in the current partial coloring is equal to or greater than the current best coloring (*UB*)
3. the current best coloring (*UB*) is same as the lower bound (*LB*)

Figure 1 depicts our exact color algorithm EXACTCOLOR. Parameters NUM-COLUMN and NUM-COLOR denote, respectively, the number of colored columns and the number of colors in current partial coloring. At the root node of BBT we have NUM-COLOR = NUM-COLUMN = $\rho_{max}$. A variable named *maxSaturation* is maintained to update color information of uncolored columns and it is initialized to the value of $\rho_{max}$ at the root node. Lines 1 to 4 check the terminating conditions as described above.

Function getColumn on line 5 returns an uncolored column (*jcol*) to be colored next. The array *handled* keeps track of colored/uncolored status of columns. The **for**−loop on line 7 sequentially considers each of the feasible colors (using function

```
EXACTCOLOR(NUM-COLUMN,NUM-COLOR)
 1   if NUM-COLOR ≥ UB or NUM-COLUMN = N
 2       then return NUM-COLOR
 3   if UB = LB
 4       then return UB
 5   jcol ← getColumn()
 6   handled[jcol] ← TRUE
 7   for each color i from 1 to NUM-COLOR
 8       do
 9               if colorAvailable(jcol, i)
10                   then
11                           color[jcol] ← i
12                           deleteColumn(head, next, previous, satDeg[jcol], jcol)
13                           if i > maxSaturation
14                               then maxSaturation ← maxSaturation +1
15                                       createNewColorClass()
16                           IncSatDeg(jcol, color[jcol])
17                           NColor ← EXACTCOLOR(NUM-COLUMN + 1, NUM-COLOR)
18                           if NColor < UB
19                               then UB ← NColor
20                           decSatDeg(jcol, color[jcol])
21                           color[jcol] ← N
22                           addColumn(head, next, previous, satDeg[jcol], jcol)
23                           if UB ≤ NUM-COLOR
24                               then handled[jcol] ← FALSE
25                                       return UB
26   if NUM-COLOR + 1 < UB
27       then color[jcol] ← NUM-COLOR + 1
28           deleteColumn(head, next, previous, satDeg[jcol], jcol)
29           if NUM-COLOR + 1 > maxSaturation
30               then maxSaturation ← maxSaturation +1
31                       createNewColorClass()
32           incSatDeg(jcol, color[jcol])
33           NColor ← EXACTCOLOR(NUM-COLUMN + 1, NUM-COLOR + 1)
34           if NColor < UB
35               then UB ← NColor
36           decSatDeg(jcol, color[jcol])
37           color[jcol] ← N
38           addColumn(head, next, previous, satDeg[jcol], jcol)
39   handled[jcol] ← FALSE
40   return UB
```

**Fig. 1**   An exact algorithm for column partitioning

colorAvailable) in the current coloring to be assigned to the selected column. Function deleteColumn removes *jcol* from the list of uncolored columns. Once *jcol* is assigned a color the function incSatDeg updates (increases by at most 1) the saturation degree of the uncolored neighbors of *jcol*. A new subproblem gets created by making a recursive call on line 17. On return from the call the value of upper bound (*UB*) is updated if a better coloring was found. The steps from line 11 to line 15 must be undone (lines 20 to 25) to try a new color on *jcol*. Lines 26 to 39 handles the case when none of the existing colors is feasible for *jcol*. In this case the number of colors gets increased in the recursive call.

Two most frequently used sparse matrix operations in the implementation of algorithm in Fig. 1 are

1. an efficient tagging scheme to keep track of processed and unprocessed columns,
2. a bucket data structure (bucket heap) to efficiently find a column with maximal/minimal degree.

Due to space constraints we describe the bucket heap only briefly. A full description of the data structures is given in [12]. The bucket heap is implemented with three arrays of fixed size N: *head*, *previous*, and *next*. Each uncolored column belong to one and only one saturation degree list. The first element in a degree list is stored in *head* such that a nonzero value for *head*[*sd*] denotes the index of a column with saturation degree *sd*; a zero value indicates an empty degree list. The algorithm maintains the value of highest saturation degree in variable *maxSaturation*. To find a column with largest saturation degree a linear scan of *head* is performed starting at *maxSaturation*. Columns in the same saturation degree list are efficiently accessed via the arrays *next* and *previous* such that the next column of *jcol* in its list is *next*[*jcol*]; a value of zero means that *jcol* is the last column in its list. Similarly, the previous column of *jcol* in its list is *previous*[*jcol*]; a value of zero means that *jcol* is the first column in its list. This structure ensures that insertion and deletion of a column can be performed in amortized constant time [12].

We note that Healy and Ju [13] use an adjacency list representation of graphs (as opposed to adjacency matrix in [14]) and define a priority queue data structure to select the next vertex to be colored. In our implementation we work directly on the sparse representation of the matrix given in CSR and CSC as implemented in [11] and hence avoid the explicit construction or storage of the intersection graph.

## 2.1 Column Selection and Tie-breaking Strategies

The choice of the next uncolored column to be colored plays an important role in the computational efficiency of brach-and-bound exact algorithms. An uncolored column with maximum saturation degree [5] tends to minimize the number of branches in the BBT at a tree node. However, this column selection heuristic makes use of information gathered from only the immediate neighborhood of uncolored columns. If there are more than one column with maximum saturation degree, the column chosen is one that is structurally dependent on largest number of uncolored columns. On the other hand a better choice can be made for the next column to color by utilizing information from an extended neighborhood of uncolored columns. Below we describe two such strategies from the literature and a new tie-breaking rule.

Let $\mathscr{J}$ denote the set of uncolored columns with maximum saturation degree. Also let $F(j)$ denote the set of color labels that are feasible for column $j$ and define

$$F_{\mathscr{N}}(j) = \bigcup_{j' \in \mathscr{N}(j) \text{ and } j' \text{ is uncolored}} F(j')$$

### 2.1.1 Sewell's Rule [9] (*Sewel*)

Sewell's rule to break tie is to select a column which has the maximum number of common available colors in the neighborhood of uncolored columns:

$$\max_{j \in \mathscr{J}} F(j) \cap F_{\mathscr{N}}(j)$$

This tie-breaking strategy reduces the number of subproblems because to break tie a column is selected that has the maximum number of common available colors thus leaving fewer choices for the uncolored columns in the neighborhood.

### 2.1.2 PASS Rule [10] (*Segundo*)

This tie-breaking approach due to Pablo San Segundo [10] is computationally less expensive than Sewell's rule. Column $j$ is selected similarly as in Sewell's, but while calculating the common available colors it considers only the uncolored neighbors that have maximum saturation degree:

$$\max_{j \in \mathscr{J}} F(j) \cap F_{\mathscr{N}}(j), \text{ where } F_{\mathscr{N}}(j) = \bigcup_{j' \in \mathscr{N}(j) \text{ and } j' \neq j, j' \in \mathscr{J} \text{ and } j' \text{ is uncolored}} F(j')$$

### 2.1.3 A New Tie-breaking Strategy (*New*)

We propose a new tie-breaking rule. It is slightly different than Sewell's rule. Among the uncolored columns with maximum saturation degree the search neighborhood is restricted to columns with saturation degree of at least 1:

$$\max_{j \in \mathscr{J}} F(j) \cap F_{\mathscr{N}}(j), \text{ where } F_{\mathscr{N}}(j)$$

$$= \bigcup_{j' \in \mathscr{N}(j) \text{ and } j' \text{ is uncolored and has at least one colored neighbor}} F(j')$$

This rule cuts down the search space by not considering columns with saturation degree 0 since they do not contribute to the maximization criteria used to select the column to be colored.

## 3  Numerical Experiments

In this section, we provide results from numerical experiments on selected test instances. The data set for the experiments is obtained from The Matrix Market [15], University of Florida Sparse Matrix Collection [16], and DIMACS coloring benchmark problems. Our exact coloring implementation was done in C++ and the code was compiled using $-O2$ optimization flag with a g++ version 4.4.7 compiler. The experiments were performed using a PC with 3.4 GHz Intel Xeon CPU, 8 GB RAM, 32 KB L1, 256 KB L2 and 8 MB L3 cache running Linux.

We perform two types of experiments. The purpose of the first set of experiments, depicted in Tables 1, 2, and 3, is to assess the computational advantage of new data structures that are discussed in Sect. 2 (identified as $DSATUR_N$) as compared with a base implementation (identified as $DSATUR_B$) that uses adjacency matrix data structure (see [17]). In the second experiment, depicted in Table 4 we compare the effectiveness of tie-breaking strategies with $DSATUR_N$. Column labels $m, n, nnz, \chi$ denote number of rows, number of columns, number of nonzero entries, and the size of the minimum column partition (chromatic number of adjacency graph of $A^\top A$), respectively.

Each of $DSATUR_N$ and $DSATUR_B$ first finds a maximal clique and its size is used as a lower bound (listed in Tables 1, 2, and 3 under column labeled $LB$), assigns colors to the columns of the respective clique, and calls the exact color algorithm to assign colors to the remaining columns. Thus, larger maximal clique implies better computational efficiency, in general. $DSATUR_N$ identifies a maximal clique by a linear scan of sparse data structure (column indices of a row with maximum number of nonzero entries $\rho_{max}$) while $DSATUR_B$ runs an exact algorithm but explores only a fixed number of subproblems. For instances *lpireactor*, *robot24c1mat5*, and *robot24c1mat5* of Table 1 and *ash331GPIA*, *ash608GPIA* , *ash958GPIA* of Table 2 $DSATUR_B$ obtains larger maximal clique than $DSATUR_N$ ($\rho_{max}$ value is indicated within parentheses) while in Table 3 $\rho_{max}$ for instance named *GL6D9* is 28 and the maximal clique found by $DSATUR_B$ is of size 17. On all other instances $DSATUR_B$ and $DSATUR_N$ report identical maximal clique size.

Table 1 includes test instances for which optimal coloring is achieved by both $DSATUR_B$ and $DSATUR_N$. For each test instance the table depicts the clock time in seconds (*Time*) and the number of subproblems (*NSub*) explored to obtain the minimum partition. Time is rounded down to zero (0) if it is less than one-hundredth of a second. On 19 out of 20 instances $DSATUR_N$ is found to be faster than $DSATUR_B$ by an order of magnitude. Also, on a majority of instances $DSATUR_N$ explores fewer subproblems to confirm optimality. Instances on which one of the implementation terminates while the other does not within one hour of cpu time are reported in Table 2.

**Table 1** Running time and number of subproblems for instances that are solved by both the implementations

| Name | m | n | nnz | χ | LB | DSATUR_B | | DSATUR_N | |
|---|---|---|---|---|---|---|---|---|---|
| | | | | | | Time | NSub | Time | NSub |
| bcsstm07 | 485 | 485 | 1810 | 11 | 11 | 0.01 | 475 | 0 | 475 |
| dwt221 | 221 | 221 | 925 | 12 | 12 | 0 | 210 | 0 | 210 |
| dwt918 | 918 | 918 | 4151 | 13 | 13 | 0.08 | 906 | 0.26 | 115,457 |
| flower41 | 121 | 129 | 386 | 5 | 5 | 0 | 4837 | 0 | 127 |
| flower81 | 625 | 513 | 1538 | 5 | 5 | 0.02 | 1249 | 0 | 554 |
| gre512 | 512 | 512 | 2192 | 5 | 5 | 0.52 | 110,710 | 0.02 | 6414 |
| jagmesh5 | 1180 | 1180 | 4465 | 7 | 7(5) | 0.1 | 1174 | 0 | 1174 |
| lpireactor | 318 | 808 | 2591 | 78 | 78(66) | 0.02 | 731 | 0 | 90 |
| lunda | 147 | 147 | 1298 | 21 | 21 | 0 | 127 | 0 | 127 |
| mesh2e1 | 306 | 306 | 1162 | 10 | 10 | 0.01 | 297 | 0 | 297 |
| mk9b1 | 378 | 36 | 756 | 7 | 4 | 0 | 1399 | 0 | 209 |
| n4c5b10 | 120 | 630 | 1320 | 11 | 11 | 0.05 | 897 | 0 | 886 |
| nos3 | 960 | 960 | 8402 | 18 | 18 | 0.2 | 943 | 0 | 943 |
| nos6 | 675 | 675 | 1965 | 5 | 5 | 0.03 | 671 | 0 | 671 |
| robot24c1mat5 | 404 | 302 | 15,118 | 102 | 99(91) | 0.6 | 204 | 0.02 | 356 |
| west0655 | 655 | 655 | 2854 | 12 | 12 | 0.04 | 644 | 0 | 644 |
| will199GPIA | 6010 | 701 | 12,323 | 7 | 6 | 0.12 | 696 | 0 | 696 |

**Table 2** Running time and number of subproblems for instances that are solved by one and not by the other

| Name | $m$ | $n$ | $nnz$ | $LB$ | $DSATUR_B$ | | | | $DSATUR_N$ | | |
|---|---|---|---|---|---|---|---|---|---|---|---|
| | | | | | $UB/\chi$ | Time | $NSub$ | | $UB/\chi$ | Time | $NSub$ |
| ash331GPIA | 4185 | 662 | 8370 | 3(2) | 5* | – | 7.13E+08 | | 4 | 0 | 1332 |
| ash608GPIA | 7844 | 1216 | 15,688 | 3(2) | 5* | – | 3.77E+08 | | 4 | 0 | 1605 |
| ash958GPIA | 12,506 | 1916 | 25,012 | 3(2) | 5* | – | 2.43E+08 | | 4 | 0.01 | 3689 |
| dwt878 | 878 | 878 | 4136 | 10 | 12* | – | 5.29E+08 | | 10 | 0 | 869 |
| jagmesh1 | 936 | 936 | 3600 | 7 | 9* | – | 4.23E+08 | | 8 | 10.04 | 6.17E+06 |
| lnsp511 | 511 | 511 | 2796 | 11 | 12* | – | 8.23E+08 | | 11 | 0 | 501 |
| n3c5b6 | 120 | 210 | 840 | 7 | 7 | 0.6 | 412233 | | 9* | – | 3.56E+09 |
| nos5 | 468 | 468 | 2820 | 23 | 25* | – | 9.11E+08 | | 23 | 0.01 | 978 |
| poisson2D | 367 | 367 | 2417 | 9 | 10* | – | 1.18E+09 | | 9 | 0 | 362 |
| sherman1 | 1000 | 1000 | 2375 | 7 | 8* | – | 5.02E+08 | | 7 | 0.03 | 1945 |

**Table 3** Number of subproblems for instances that cannot be solved by either

| Name | | | | | $DSATUR_B$ | | $DSATUR_N$ | |
|------|------|------|---------|---------|--------|----------|--------|----------|
| | $m$ | $n$ | $nnz$ | $LB$ | $UB$ | $NSub$ | $UB$ | $NSub$ |
| abb313GPIA | 50,463 | 1557 | 101,857 | 6 | 10* | 2.76E+08 | 10* | 7.24E+08 |
| bcsstm07 | 420 | 420 | 3836 | 26 | 30* | 1.02E+09 | 28* | 1.14E+09 |
| GL6D9 | 340 | 545 | 4349 | 28(B17) | 30* | 7.72E+08 | 29* | 3.52E+08 |
| n3c5b5 | 210 | 252 | 1260 | 6 | 10* | 1.39E+09 | 10* | 3.46E+09 |
| plat1919 | 1919 | 1919 | 17159 | 19 | 24* | 2.24E+08 | 23* | 9.82E+08 |
| sphere3 | 258 | 258 | 1026 | 7 | 9* | 1.26E+09 | 9* | 2.65E+09 |
| steam1 | 240 | 240 | 3762 | 21 | 23* | 1.56E+09 | 22* | 1.27E+09 |

The column with label $UB/\chi$ displays the the size of optimal partition ($\chi$) or the best upper bound achieved ($UB$) on partition size (denoted by an asterisk *) within the allotted time for nonterminating instances. Out of 7 instances, $DSATUR_N$ terminates on 6 of them. Remarkably, on 4 of the terminating instances optimal partition is found very quickly by $DSATUR_N$ while exploring fewer than 2000 subproblems.

Table 3 displays test results for instances on which both $DSATUR_N$ and $DSATUR_B$ fail to terminate within one hour. While the best partition obtained in the allotted time is close ($DSATUR_N$ is never worse than $DSATUR_B$), the advantage of new sparse data structure is quite evident. On most of the instances, $DSATUR_N$ explores more subproblems than $DSATUR_B$.

Instances with suffix *GPIA* are taken from DIMACS coloring benchmark collection; they arise in optimal direct determination of sparse Jacobian matrices [18]. In the survey paper [7] authors use branch-and-price algorithm based on a set cover formulation with column generation [17] and a branch-and-cut algorithm to instance *ash958GPIA*. Neither of the algorithms could find optimal coloring (the chromatic number is reported to be unknown in the paper). In Table 2 we see that $DSATUR_N$ solves the instance optimally.

In our second experiment, we study the effect of different tie-breaking strategies with $DSATUR_N$ on a subset of instances. In Table 4 *Simple* denotes the strategy whence the column chosen to be colored next is $head[sd]$ where $sd$ is the maximum saturation degree while *Sewell*, *Segundo*, and *New*, denote respective tie-breaking strategies discussed in Sect. 2. For each test matrix, we report for each $UB$ value the time in seconds required and the number of subproblems explored to reach the $UB$. For example, on test instance *bcsstm07*, examining the first row of Table 4 we see that for *Simple* and *Sewell* the first $UB$ of 30 is achieved having explored 395 subproblems in less than one-hundredth of a second (indicated by a 0; the corresponding entry for each of *Segundo* and *New* is a dash (–) indicating that a better first $UB = 29$ ( shown in the second row) is achieved having explored the same number of subproblems. The second row corresponds to $UB$ value of 29 and we see that *Simple* explores 16105 subproblems in 0.03 seconds and *Sewell* explores 7.11E+05 subproblems in 5.7 seconds, and that the best $4UB$ for *Sewell* and *New* is 29; the asterisk (*) indicates

**Table 4** Effectiveness of Tie-breaking strategies in $DSATUR_N$

| Name | Simple | | | Sewell | | | Segundo | | | New | | |
|---|---|---|---|---|---|---|---|---|---|---|---|---|
| | UB | Time | NSub | UB | Time | NSub | UB | Time | NSub | UB | Time | NSub |
| bcsstm07 | 30 | 0 | 395 | 30 | 0 | 395 | – | – | – | – | – | – |
| | 29 | 0.03 | 16,105 | 29* | 5.7 | 7.11E+05 | 29 | 0 | 395 | 29* | 0.01 | 395 |
| dwt878 | 28* | 57.61 | 1.62E+07 | – | – | – | 28* | 0 | 481 | – | – | – |
| | 10 | 0 | 869 | 10 | 0 | 869 | 10 | 0 | 869 | 10 | 0 | 869 |
| flower41 | 5 | 0 | 161 | 5 | 0 | 172 | 5 | 0 | 282 | 5 | 0 | 127 |
| flower71 | 5 | 0 | 439 | 5 | 0 | 402 | 5 | 0 | 485 | 5 | 0 | 400 |
| jagmesh1 | 9 | 0 | 983 | 9* | 0.04 | 932 | 9* | 0.02 | 968 | 9* | 0.04 | 963 |
| | 8 | 10.04 | 6.17E+06 | – | – | – | – | – | – | – | – | – |
| jagmesh5 | 7 | 0 | 1174 | 7 | 0.11 | 1174 | 7 | 0.02 | 1174 | 7 | 0.12 | 1174 |
| lnsp511 | 12 | 0 | 501 | 12 | 0 | 501 | – | – | – | 12 | 0 | 501 |
| | 11 | 0 | 1005 | 11 | 0 | 920 | 11 | 0 | 501 | 11 | 0 | 595 |
| lunda | – | – | – | – | – | – | 22 | 0 | 127 | – | – | – |
| mk9b1 | 21 | 0 | 127 | 21 | 0 | 127 | 21 | 0 | 243 | 21 | 0 | 127 |
| | 7 | 0 | 414 | 7 | 0 | 209 | 7 | 0 | 197 | 7 | 0 | 209 |
| n3c5b5 | 12 | 0 | 247 | 12 | 0 | 247 | – | – | – | 12 | 0 | 247 |
| | 11 | 0 | 301 | 11 | 0 | 289 | 11 | 0 | 247 | 11 | 0 | 344 |
| | 10* | 14.22 | 1.36E+07 | 10* | 7.11 | 1.59E+06 | 10* | 0 | 2104 | 10* | 2.74 | 667,379 |
| n3c5b6 | – | – | – | – | – | – | – | – | – | 13 | 0 | 204 |
| | – | – | – | 12 | 0 | 204 | 12 | 0 | 204 | 12 | 0 | 245 |
| | 11 | 0 | 204 | 11 | 0 | 253 | 11 | 0 | 1347 | 11 | 0 | 323 |
| | 10 | 0 | 6738 | 10 | 1.55 | 398,017 | 10 | 0.17 | 69,813 | 10 | 3.12 | 809,260 |
| | 9* | 1225.99 | 1.22E+09 | 9* | 432.45 | 9.88E+07 | 9* | 3217.28 | 1.34E+09 | 9* | 16.28 | 3.74E+06 |

(continued)

**Table 4** (continued)

| Name | Simple | | | Sewell | | | Segundo | | | New | | |
|---|---|---|---|---|---|---|---|---|---|---|---|---|
| | UB | Time | NSub | UB | Time | NSub | UB | Time | NSub | UB | Time | NSub |
| nos3 | 20 | 0 | 943 | – | – | – | – | – | – | – | – | – |
| | 19 | 0.01 | 2406 | 19 | 0.01 | 943 | – | – | – | – | – | – |
| | 18 | 0.01 | 3266 | 18 | 0.2 | 1844 | 18 | 0 | 943 | 18 | 0.01 | 943 |
| nos5 | 24* | 6.2 | 2.37E+06 | 24* | 0 | 446 | 24 | 0 | 446 | 24* | 0.01 | 446 |
| | – | – | – | – | – | – | 23 | 0.01 | 978 | – | – | – |
| plat1919 | 24 | 0.01 | 1901 | – | – | – | 24 | 0.01 | 1901 | 24* | 0.03 | 1901 |
| | 23* | 0.02 | 3359 | – | – | – | 23* | 0.03 | 3871 | – | – | – |
| sphere3 | – | – | – | 11 | 0 | 338 | 11 | 0 | 252 | – | – | – |
| | 10 | 0 | 252 | 10 | 0.06 | 23,568 | 10 | 0 | 1197 | 10 | 0 | 252 |
| | 9* | 0.88 | 702048 | 9* | 0.6 | 176,461 | 9* | 6.6 | 2.69E+06 | 9* | 9.49 | 2.46E+06 |
| steam1 | – | – | 220 | 24* | 0.03 | 7813 | 24* | 0 | 220 | 24 | 0 | 0.01 |
| | 22* | 4.16 | 1.91E+06 | – | – | – | – | – | – | 23* | 0.01 | 537 |

that no improvement on *UB* could be achieved within one hour of total running time. On the other hand, the best *UB* for *Segundo* and *Simple* is 28. Interestingly, on *jagmesh1 Simple* finds optimal partition while the others do not terminate in the allotted time. A similar situation is observed for *Segundo* on *nos5*. While no general conclusion can be reached on the effectiveness of the four tie-breaking strategies, it is clear that the running time is directly proportional to the subproblems explored.

## 4  Concluding Remarks

In this paper we have proposed an efficient implementation of a branch-and-bound exact algorithm for coloring sparse matrices. We have presented results from numerical experiments on an extensive set of test instances to validate the computational effectiveness of our implementation as compared with a graph coloring implementation based on adjacency matrix representation. As an immediate application of the method presented in the paper, we refer to the work [19] where a small critical submatrix (subgraph) is colored exactly and the coloring is extended to the remaining columns. Another promising research direction is to incorporate improving lower bounds [20] as the algorithm progresses. Currently, a lower bound is computed at the root node of the branch-and-bound tree which is never updated.

**Acknowledgements** This research is supported in part by Natural Sciences and Engineering Research Council of Canada (NSERC) Discovery Grant (Individual). We thank the referees for many helpful remarks on the manuscript.

## References

1. Garey, M.R., Johnson, D.S.: Computers and Intractability: A Guide to the Theory of NP-Completeness. W. H. Freeman & Co., New York, NY, USA (1979)
2. Coleman, T.F., Moré, J.J.: Estimation of sparse Jacobian matrices and graph coloring problems. SIAM J. Numer. Anal. **20**(1), 187–209 (1983)
3. Gebremedhin, A.H., Manne, F., Pothen, A.: What color is your Jacobian? Graph coloring for computing derivatives. SIAM Rev. **47**(4), 629–705 (2005)
4. Hossain, S., Steihaug, T.: Optimal direct determination of sparse Jacobian matrices. Optim. Methods Softw. **28**(6), 1218–1232 (2013)
5. Brélaz, D.: New Methods to Color the Vertices of a Graph. Commun. ACM **22**(4), 251–256 (1979)
6. Brown, J.R.: Chromatic scheduling and the chromatic number problem. Manage. Sci. **19**(4-part-1), 456–463 (1972)
7. Malaguti, E., Toth, P.: A survey on vertex coloring problems. Int. Trans. Oper. Res. **17**(1), 1–34 (2010)
8. Hossain, S., Steihaug, T.: Graph coloring in the estimation of sparse derivative matrices: instances and applications. Discrete Appl. Math. **156**(2), 280–288 (2008)
9. Sewell, E.C.: An improved algorithm for exact graph coloring. DIMACS Ser. Discrete Math. Theor. Comput. Sci. **26**, 359–373 (1996)

10. Segundo, P.S.: A new DSATUR-based algorithm for exact vertex coloring. Comput. Oper. Res. **39**(7), 1724–1733 (2012)
11. Hasan, M., Hossain, S., Khan, A.I., Mithila, N.H., Suny, A.H.: DSJM: A Software Toolkit for Direct Determination of Sparse Jacobian Matrices, pp. 275–283. Springer, Cham (2016)
12. Khan, A.I.: Improved implementation of some coloring Algorithms for the determination of large and sparse Jacobian matrices. M.Sc. thesis, University of Lethbridge, Canada (2017)
13. Healy, P., Ju, A.: An Experimental Analysis of Vertex Coloring Algorithms on Sparse Random Graphs, pp. 174–186. Springer, Cham (2014)
14. Trick, M.A.: Easy code for graph coloring. http://mat.gsia.cmu.edu/COLOR/solvers/trick.c. Accessed: 2017-01-13
15. The matrix market collection. http://math.nist.gov/MatrixMarket/matrices.html. Accessed 13 Jan 2017
16. Davis, T.A., Hu, Y.: The University of Florida sparse matrix collection. ACM Trans. Math. Softw. **38**(1), 1:1–1:25 (2011)
17. Mehrotra, A., Trick, M.A.: A column generation approach For graph coloring. INFORMS J. Comput. **8**, 344–354 (1995)
18. Hossain, S.: Cseggraph: a graph colouring instance generator. Int. J. Comput. Math. **86**(10–11), 1956–1967 (2009)
19. Hossain, S., Suny, A.H.: Determination of large sparse derivative matrices: structural orthogonality and structural degeneracy. In: Proceedings of 15th Cologne-Twente Workshop on Graphs and Combinatorial Optimization 2017, pp. 83–87. Cologne, Germany (2017)
20. Gaur, D.R., Hossain, S., Saha, A.: Determining sparse Jacobian matrices using two-sided compression: an algorithm and lower bounds. In: Bélair, J., Frigaard, I.A., Kunze, H., Makarov, R., Melnik, R., Spiteri, R.J. (eds.) Mathematical and Computational Approaches in Advancing Modern Science and Engineering, pp. 425–434. Springer, Switzerland (2016)

# A General Method for Selection Function Optimization in Genetic Algorithms

**Nawar Ismail and Matthew Demers**

**Abstract** Genetic algorithms are often used as a mechanism to solve complicated problems in optimization. In the schemes that we are concerned with, a population of members, which are each defined by a set of parameters, are used with the desire to optimize some value called the *fitness*. The fitness of each member in a population is measured and used during a *selection* process which defines a likelihood for any member to carry on to the subsequent iteration (often called a *generation*) of the algorithm. *Mutations* are then stochastically applied to the population. This alters the parameters of the population members. Combining the effects of selection and mutation tends to increase the average fitness of a population. Our principal concern is in determining how to select members from one iteration to the next. Measuring how well a selection mechanism performs is computationally demanding, making its optimization difficult. We apply an additional genetic algorithm to a simplified model to give an approximate optimization for the selection mechanism. In this paper, we detail the general procedure for this optimization.

**Keywords** Genetic algorithms · Iterative methods · Optimization
Predictive models

## 1 Introduction

A genetic algorithm (GA) is, loosely, an iterative scheme designed with the purpose of finding an optimal solution to a potentially very difficult or complex problem. In general, large numbers of difficult evaluations impose time constraints. Many techniques have been developed to improve the utility of the algorithm, such as functional approximation and determining representative simulation run length which both reduce the difficulty of evaluation, and fitness estimation which can reduce

N. Ismail · M. Demers (✉)
University of Guelph, 50 Stone Rd E, Guelph, ON, Canada
e-mail: mdemers@uoguelph.ca

N. Ismail
e-mail: nismail@uoguelph.ca

© Springer Nature Switzerland AG 2018
D. M. Kilgour et al. (eds.), *Recent Advances in Mathematical
and Statistical Methods*, Springer Proceedings in Mathematics & Statistics 259,
https://doi.org/10.1007/978-3-319-99719-3_4

evaluation numbers [1–3]. Additionally, the operators used can be designed to produce improvements more efficiently [4]. Finally, the parameters used in the algorithm strongly influence the success of the output but the ideal values are often difficult to determine [5, 6]. In this paper, we are concerned with optimizing a particular parameter of these algorithms, the selection function (see Sect. 3) with a generally applicable technique.

There are many parameters in genetic algorithm to be chosen, such as the number of members in a population, mutation rates, selection probabilities (as well as application specific parameters). Often, these values are chosen through trial and error, or "experimentally" [6]. Finding optimal parameters is difficult due to number of possibilities and the generality of problems tackled by GAs [6]. This difficulty suggests the use of a GA to optimize the parameters of the original GA. However, directly applying a GA to the output of another GA would require an infeasible amount computation time. We propose that a model can instead be used to optimize the parameters of the algorithm.

We apply our investigation to a particular optimization problem; however, we maintain that the procedures presented here are generally applicable. The goal of our optimization problem is to obtain configurations of so-called "creatures" that maximize their displacement on a flat planar surface by the end of a fixed time. These sets of mechanical components operate in a physically simulated environment. Many similar optimizations involving virtual creatures have been studied [7].

## 2  Optimization Setup

### 2.1  Creatures

In our framework, we define a creature as a set of mechanical components and how they are connected. There are three possible component types in any creature: pistons, rigid bars, and contact spheres, which will be referred to as *muscles*, *bones*, and *nodes* respectively to remain consistent with the biological naming associated with *genetic* algorithms.

The nodes act as anchors for the connecting muscles and bones, and are the source of environment interaction. The bones will maintain a fixed length, while the muscles oscillate their length sinusoidally with time, at different rates. With these components, each creature will travel a deterministic displacement at the end of a time, $t = t_{max}$. The projection of this displacement on the plane is what we take to be the creature's *fitness*,[1]

$$f = \sqrt{x_{com}(t_{max})^2 + y_{com}(t_{max})^2}, \tag{1}$$

---

[1]The goal is to travel across the plane. The height of a creature plays no (direct) role in this. So only the displacement in the x-y plane is considered.

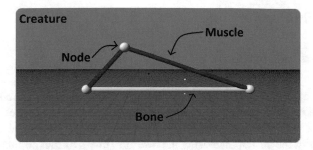

**Fig. 1** A creature consists of three components: muscles (red) which provide a potential driving force, bones (white) which provide structure, and nodes which interact with the environment. These define a sufficient set of components that allows a creature to move, provided its configuration allows it. A 2D creature is shown for simplicity, but simulations are run in 3D

where $x_{com}$ and $y_{com}$ are the center of mass coordinates. This fitness is the objective function that we would like to maximize. For simplicity, the muscles and bones are massless, making the nodes the only massive component (Fig. 1).

## 2.2 Evaluating Fitness

The are six forces responsible for the net force on each node are gravity, muscle forces, bone forces, surface collision, ground friction and drag.

The net force on a node is then the sum of these six forces; namely:

$$\mathbf{F}_{node} = \mathbf{F}_g + \mathbf{F}_m + \mathbf{F}_b + \mathbf{F}_c + \mathbf{F}_f + \mathbf{F}_d. \tag{2}$$

From $\mathbf{F} = m\ddot{\mathbf{r}}$, we get that

$$\mathbf{r}_j(t) = \frac{1}{m_j} \int \int \sum_{forces} \mathbf{F}_{node,j}(t, \mathbf{r}_1, \mathbf{r}_2, ..., \mathbf{r}_{max}) dt^2, \tag{3}$$

where $\mathbf{r}_j$ is the position of node $j$, and $\mathbf{F}_{node,j}$ is the net force acting on that node. This coupled with Eq. 1 defines the mathematical function we are trying to optimize.

We simulate the movement of each node by iteratively evaluating this equation numerically. At the end of each simulation (consisting of 9000 unit time step iterations), the displacement in the plane of the creature's center of mass is recorded as the creature's fitness.

# 3 Algorithm

## 3.1 Genetic Algorithm

Our genetic algorithm begins with an initial population of $N$ members.[2] In our scheme, each member of the population is a creature as defined in Sect. 2.1. *Genetic operators* are then iteratively applied to the population. These operators act on a population with the aim of increasing the average fitness of that population [8]. The operators used are the selection function, and the mutations (see Sect. 3.2). An outline of the algorithm used can be found in Algorithm 1.1. The algorithm can terminate on many different end conditions. We mainly end our simulations when improvements become negligible or at the end of a fixed number of generations.

---

**Algorithm 1.1** Genetic Algorithm

---

$P \leftarrow$ INITIATEPOPULATION( )                     ▷ with creatures
**while** end condition not met **do**
    EVALUATEFITNESSES($P$)
    $P \leftarrow$ SELECT($P$)
    $P \leftarrow$ MUTATE($P$)
**end while**

---

## 3.2 Genetic Operators

### 3.2.1 Selection Function

*Selection functions* act on a population to select creatures from one iteration of the algorithm to the next [8]. There are several types of selection functions [8]. We specifically investigated a type of rank selection. After fitness evaluation, creatures in the current generation are ordered from highest to lowest fitness. The creature with the greatest fitness would have rank 0, the creature with the second greatest would have rank 1, and so on. We could also consider a rank percentage which is bounded by 0 and 1, regardless of population size.

We must balance the variance of the selection function with how strongly we select for the best creatures. With too little variation, the probability of being trapped at or near a local maximum would be very high [8]. Conversely, selecting uniformly (without regard for fitness) would be a pointless exercise. Determining how to distribute this balance in our selection function is our principal concern.

---

[2]Values of $N$ between 100, and 1000 are typically used. This was determined through trial and error. Future work may determine an ideal value through the techniques described here.

### 3.2.2 Mutations

At the conclusion of each generation, all creatures may undergo one or more *mutations*. Mutations alter the properties of a creature, which ultimately affects its fitness. There are three mutation types in our scheme:

1. **Modify Characteristic**: Changes a property of a component. Examples include: random node locations, modifying node mass, and modifying muscle contraction rate.
2. **Add Component**: Add a node, muscle, or bone. Adding a node may generate additional connections.
3. **Remove Component**: Remove a node, muscle, or bone. Removing a node will also remove connected muscles and bones.

These essentially span the set of simple alterations, and provide a mechanism to explore other creature configurations [8]. These are applied to creatures with some small probability. Our simulations indicate that most mutations will decrease performance, but a handful will cause improvements. Coupling mutations with the selection function means that previously successful creatures are being modified, causing improvements in their design over time.

## 4 Methods

### 4.1 Overview

To optimize the form of the selection function, it must be assigned a fitness. We use the average fitness of the creatures produced after 300 generations to represent the ability of a selection function.[3]

A statistical model of our creatures will be used to reduce the computational cost required to evaluate the fitness of many selection functions. This model is implemented by replacing creatures with their most representative statistic: their fitness. The model will therefore deal with floating point numbers instead of a complicated structure whose fitness is computationally expensive to measure. This is a sort of *functional approximation*, where we use an alternate expression for the fitness [3].

The selection function acts identically except it considers fitnesses rather than creatures (which would have those *associated* fitnesses). The mutation operator however, is intimately tied to the physical design of a creature. So reducing its structure to a single value requires some careful considerations.

---

[3]This must be evaluated several times to obtain a proper statistic, which can be demanding.

## 4.2   *Estimating Impact*

To emulate the mutation operator, we look at the distribution of how the mutations
tend to affect the creature's fitness. It is straightforward to see that the change in
fitness after a creature is mutated (or *impact*), correlates to the fitness of the creature.
For example, creatures with a greater fitness would be likely to suffer negative effects
when a mutation occurs due to disruptions in their more specialized structures.

Combining the fact that each creature has its own distribution, with the fact that
these distributions depends on fitness, we conclude that each fitness has its own
distribution. To properly mimic it, we collect a sample of genomes with various
associated fitnesses, and apply this sampled distribution to our model.

We start by collecting a list of impact statistics. To do this, we first determine a set
of fitness levels that span the range of fitnesses typically seen. The genetic algorithm
is run until it produces a creature with a fitness within some margin of a desired
level. Mutations are applied to several copies of this creature. Measuring the change
in fitness for each creature provides us with a sample of impact statistics. If we
sample these impacts from many different creatures at each fitness level, we obtain
a reasonable sample of impact statistics grouped by fitness level.[4] This is outlined in
Algorithm 1.3 and gives us the required statistics for our model.

The fitnesses of the creatures typically range from 0-400. Based on our available
computational time, we chose our levels to be at $5 * 1.25^i$ for $i = 0, \ldots, 20$. 1000
impact statistics were collected from each of over 1800 creatures spanning these
fitness levels, providing us with nearly two million impact statistics.

---

**Algorithm 1.2** Obtaining Impact Statistics

---

**for all** Fitness levels **do**
    **for** $M$ creatures found at this level **do**
        *Population* ← $N$ copies of creature
        $f_0$ ← initial creature's fitness
        **for all** $N$ creatures **do**
            apply round of mutations
            $f$ ← new fitness
            record impact statistic as $f_0 - f$
        **end for**
    **end for**
**end for**

---

[4]Care should be taken as to not sample multiple creatures from the same instance of the algorithm.
Otherwise they will not be independent.

## 4.3 Model

Our model aims to approximate the fitnesses produced by the genetic algorithm that simulates creatures, without actually simulating them. The utility of this is not creature optimization (at least not directly), since we remove any concept of creature, but instead to greatly decrease the computational cost associated with measuring the fitness of a selection function.[5] In our model, when the mutation operator is called on a population of fitnesses, the fitness of each member is looked up and a random impact corresponding to that fitness is applied to their fitness. Since the distribution of impacts is contained in our sampling, this approximates the true nature of impacts.[6] These changes to Algorithm 1.1 are shown in Algorithm 1.3.

---

**Algorithm 1.3** Model Genetic Algorithm

---

**function** IMPACTMODEL($f$)
   *impacts* $\leftarrow$ dataset with fitness closest to $f$
   **return** uniformly selected value from *impacts*
**end function**


$P \leftarrow$ INITIATEPOPULATION( )         ▷ with fitnesses sampled from initial populations of creatures
**while** end condition not met **do**
   $P \leftarrow$ SELECT($P$)
   **for all** population members **do**
      $f \leftarrow f +$ IMPACTMODEL($f$)
   **end for**
**end while**

---

To demonstrate the validity of our model, we run both algorithms (the one which simulates creatures, and the one which only considers their fitness) and measure the fitness of the selection function (as described in Sect. 4.1). This is done for a selection function of the form,

$$P(x) = (1 - x)^p \sin(\pi x) \qquad (4)$$

for several different values of $p$. This function was based on our intuition for how the mass of the selection function should be distributed - essentially a reasonable guess at a good selection function. As can be seen in Fig. 2, our simplified model follows the general trend obtained by the algorithm which actually simulates the creatures. Since the trends are similar, the maxima in both the real simulation and our model would likely occur for similar selection functions.

---

[5]This decreased cost will then be used to optimize the selection function, which in turn improves the creature optimization.

[6]More advanced statistics or added corrections can be implemented to improve the quality of our model. As a basic implementation this will suit our purposes.

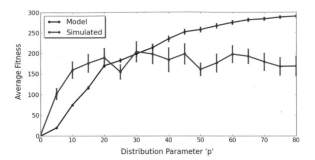

**Fig. 2** A comparison between the actual data obtained from simulating the creatures (red) and the models predictions (black) for a selection function of the form, $P(x) = (1 - x)^p \sin(\pi x)$. Each point corresponds to the particular selection function's fitness. Notice the relatively large fluctuations found in the simulated data. This results not only from a large variance at each point, but also demonstrates a limitation in acquiring large data sets due to the high computation cost that we aim to eliminate. Under the considerations that our model **greatly** simplifies the problem (by eliminating the creature), the two graphs follow a similar trend and so we validate it as an approximation to the actual selection function fitness

## 4.4 Selection Function Optimization

We can now approximate the fitness of a selection function in a feasible time scale which allows us to optimize the selection function. To avoid assuming the form of the ideal selection function, we define the function,

$$\sigma_n(a_1, a_2, \ldots a_n) = \frac{n}{\sum a_i} \cdot \sum_{i=0}^{n} \begin{cases} a_i & \frac{i}{n} < x < \frac{i+1}{n} \\ 0 & else \end{cases}, \tag{5}$$

which corresponds to a normalized set of $n$ columns of height $a_i n / \sum a_i$ that are equally spaced on the domain [0, 1]. With sufficiently large $n$, this function can be used to approximate any function we would be concerned with, and so it is used as our selection function.

We use a third genetic algorithm to determine the parameters, $a_i$ of the selection function $\sigma_n$, to optimize our model of the fitness of a selection function.[7] We fill our population with 300 members. Each member has a set of $n$ numbers corresponding to $a_i$ in 5. The selection function used in this third algorithm is $P(x) = (1 - x)^{27} \sin(\pi x)$, since we have seen its validity when optimizing creatures.[8] Mutations consist of potentially reassigning some numbers with new random values. With this, everything needed to optimize the selection function is set in place.

---

[7]The other two being: (1) the one used in creature optimization, and (2) the one used in our model.
[8]One could consider optimizing *this* selection function as well. However, they would find themselves optimizing endlessly. At some point an educated guess must be made.

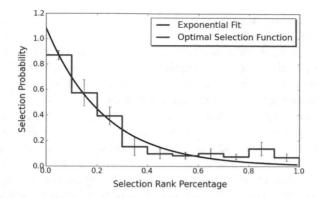

**Fig. 3** The average $\sigma_n$ function outputted by the selection function optimization procedure (red). The least squares exponential fit $P(r_p) = 1.08e^{-4.44r_p}$ was fitted to the $\sigma$ function (black). Here, $P(r_p)$ is the probability of a creature with rank percentage $r_p$ to be selected. We chose $n = 10$, but higher values of $n$ can be used, although this may make the optimization more difficult. Either the $\sigma$ function or the fitted curve can be taken to be an optimal selection function

## 5  Results

Our model aimed to approximate the fitnesses produced by the optimization of creatures. It was able to generate trends similar to those that resulted from actually simulating the creatures. This is shown in Fig. 2.

Taking our model to be a reasonable predictor of a selection function's fitness, it was used in an additional genetic algorithm. This genetic algorithm optimized the parameters in the selection function defined by Eq. 5. The optimal selection function that was produced was fitted to the exponential seen in Fig. 3. When this selection function was used to optimize creatures, the selection function's fitness was $230 \pm 10$. Although this is likely not the highest possible fitness, it does surpass all other tested selection functions. The best of those selection functions produced a fitness of $200 \pm 20$. This means that the fitness of our optimized selection function increased by $(15 \pm 2)\%$.

## 6  Discussion and Conclusion

Our primary concern was optimizing the selection function used in our optimization of creatures. To overcome the excessive computational cost associated with this, we developed a model capable of approximating selection function fitness. Our model removed the need to simulate creatures by only considering their best representative estimator, their fitness. To allow for this simplification, the mutation operator was approximated by using a sample of impacts at various fitness levels. With this, our model matched the general trend obtained when actually simulating the creatures, validating our model as an approximation.

The model was used to optimize a selection function with a general form. An ideal solution was found to be an exponential decay and produced $15 \pm 2\%$ higher creature fitness on average after 300 generations than other tested functions. The generality of our method, would allow it to be applied in many different optimization problems.

The determination of the selection function form would be an unaccessible task without similar considerations to those presented here. Brute force optimizations can still be done, but may be limited to considering a handful of values [9]. The most computationally demanding task in our technique is the acquisition of a sufficient sample of creatures. Collecting the ~2000 creatures used here required around 10 days of computation (on a single machine). However, we observed similar results with ~200 creatures, implying some robustness with regard to quantity. In addition, the collecting of genomes - which amounts to recording the solutions to the problem - has other uses like analysing solution behaviours and their characteristics, and can be collected passively as the problem is studied. It does not have to be the focus of the optimization, and can this technique can be applied after a sufficient set is collected.

Future work could relate to improving the statistical methods applied to our model, the simplicity of which amounts to our largest source of error. One could also consider extensions such as: if and how the selection function should change as the algorithm iterates, optimization of population size, or ideal mutation rates, as considered in [6].

# References

1. Sun, C., Zeng, J., Pan, J., Xue, S., Jin, Y.: A new fitness estimation strategy for particle swarm optimization (2013)
2. Branke, J., Asafuddoula, M., Bhattacharjee, K.S., Ray, T.: Efficient use of partially converged simulations in evolutionary. Optimization (2017). https://doi.org/10.1109/TEVC.2016.2569018
3. Regis, R., Shoemaker, C.: Local function approximation in evolutionary algorithms for the optimization of costly functions. IEEE Trans. Evol. Comput. **8**, 490–505 (2004). https://doi.org/10.1109/TEVC.2004.835247
4. Rasheed, K., Hirsh, H.: Informed operators: speeding up genetic-algorithm-based design optimization using reduced models (2000)
5. Eiben, A.E., Smit, S.K.: In Autonomous Search, p. 1536. Springer, Torino (2011)
6. Aine, S., Kumar, R., Chakrabarti, P.P.: Adaptive parameter control of evolutionary algorithms to improve quality-time trade-off (2009)
7. Lehman, J., et al.: The surprising creativity of digital evolution: a collection of anecdotes from the evolutionary computation and artificial life research communities (2018)
8. Kumar, R.: Blending roulette wheel selection and rank selection in genetic algorithms. Int. J. Mach. Learn, Comput (2012)
9. Pongcharoen, P., Hicks, C., Braiden, P., Stewardson, D.: Determining optimum genetic algorithm parameters for scheduling the manufacturing and assembly of complex products. Int. J. Prod. Econ. **78**, 311 (2002)

# Exploring the Method of Colour Stealing for Contractive Iterated Function Systems

**Eva Kasanda and Matthew Demers**

**Abstract** Plotting fractals generated by an Iterated Function System (IFS) can be challenging and computationally intensive, so an algorithm referred to as the *chaos game* is employed. Here, given a seed point, IFS mappings are chosen at random in sequence, with each subsequent point mapped from the one before it through the new mapping. Utilizing this approach, we may plot attractors accurately and quickly. Attractors may be coloured in many ways, but of interest is the method of *colour stealing* (Barnsley, Superfractals. Academic Press, London [1]; Barnsley, Theory and Application of Fractal Tops, Fractals in Engineering, Tours. Springer, France [2]; Kunze et al., Maple Conference 2006 Proceedings [3]). Complications to the existing scheme arise in implementation, particularly when considering assigning colour values to pixels. These lead us to explore some slight modifications of the original framework, making use of the notions of *finite code space* and a metric for use in practical computation. Further, we explore an extension of the notion of the fractal top by defining a general projection function and showcase some resulting attractors.

**Keywords** Fractal · Colour stealing · Chaos game · MATLAB · Code space Fractal bottom

## 1 Introduction

The goal of this work is first to recall the technique of colour stealing, due to Barnsley [1, 2]. Then, we generalise this method by considering a slightly modified formulation, and create a related framework for practical implementation when creating

E. Kasanda (✉) · M. Demers
University of Guelph, Guelph, ON, Canada
e-mail: ekasanda@uoguelph.ca

M. Demers
e-mail: mdemers@uoguelph.ca

© Springer Nature Switzerland AG 2018
D. M. Kilgour et al. (eds.), *Recent Advances in Mathematical and Statistical Methods*, Springer Proceedings in Mathematics & Statistics 259,
https://doi.org/10.1007/978-3-319-99719-3_5

these pictures using a computer. Similar implementations have been explored by Barnsley in the past [4–7].

In order to talk about iterated function systems, we first need to discuss some crucial definitions. Consider a metric, $d$, acting on a space $\mathbf{X}$. A function $f : \mathbf{X} \to \mathbf{X}$ on a complete metric space $(\mathbf{X}, d)$ is said to be contractive if there exists a contraction factor $0 \leq k < 1$ such that

$$d(f(x), f(y)) \leq k \cdot d(x, y) \quad \forall x, y \in \mathbf{X}. \tag{1}$$

We denote the set of all contraction mappings on $\mathbf{X}$ as $Con(\mathbf{X})$.

Banach's fixed point theorem [1, 3] states that for a contraction mapping $w \in Con(\mathbf{X})$, there is a unique globally attractive fixed point, $\bar{x} \in \mathbf{X}$, such that

$$\begin{aligned} w(\bar{x}) &= \bar{x} \\ \lim_{n \to \infty} d(w^{on}(x), \bar{x}) &= 0 \quad \forall x \in \mathbf{X}. \end{aligned} \tag{2}$$

This theorem allows us to approximate a fixed point of a contraction mapping with arbitrary precision. For a contraction mapping $w \in Con(\mathbf{X})$ on the complete metric space $(\mathbb{X}, d)$, we define a corresponding set-valued mapping as

$$\hat{w}(\mathbf{S}) = \{w(x) \mid x \in \mathbf{S}\}, \quad \mathbf{S} \subseteq \mathbf{X} \tag{3}$$

Given $N$ set-valued contraction mappings, $\hat{w}_1(\mathbf{X}), \hat{w}_2(\mathbf{X}), \ldots \hat{w}_N(\mathbf{X})$, we define $\hat{W}(\mathbf{X})$ as

$$\hat{W}(\mathbf{X}) = \bigcup_{i=1}^{N} \hat{w}_i(\mathbf{X}). \tag{4}$$

This union of $N$ set-valued contraction mappings is called an N-map iterated function system, or IFS. It can be shown that an IFS defined in this way is itself a contraction mapping on $\mathcal{H}(\mathbf{X})$, the space of non-empty compact subsets of $\mathbf{X}$ under the Hausdorff metric. For more details, see [8].

Banach's Fixed Point Theorem tells us that the IFS, $\hat{W}$, has a fixed point in $\mathcal{H}(\mathbf{X})$, and that this fixed point can be approached by iteratively applying $\hat{W}$ to any initial point in $\mathbf{X}$. However, since $\mathcal{H}(\mathbf{X})$ is a space of sets, the fixed point for a set-valued contraction mapping will be not a single point, but a set of points called the attractor of the IFS.

## 2 The Chaos Game

The attractor of a given IFS may be efficiently plotted by using a method which we shall refer to as the Chaos game. The Chaos game is an algorithm which relies on random selection of IFS mappings, one at a time in a sequence, and is carried out as

**(a)**          **(b)**          **(c)**          **(d)**

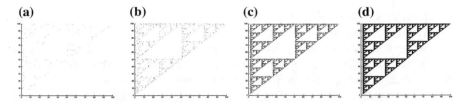

**Fig. 1** Attractor of the Sierpinski Triangle IFS (see Sect. 6), produced using **a** 100, **b** 1000, **c** 10,000, and **d** 100,000 iterations of the Chaos Game (see Sect. 6 for IFS mappings)

follows. First, a probability $p$ is assigned to each mapping, $\hat{w}_i$, of the IFS such that

$$\sum_{i=1}^{N} p_i = 1, \tag{5}$$

and we select a single initial point, $x_0$, to be our starting point for drawing the attractor. A mapping $w_{\sigma_i}$ is randomly selected according to the associated probabilities. We then define the next point in the iteration to be $x_{i+1} = w_{\sigma_i}(x_i)$. We continue to select random mappings and apply them to the previously obtained point until a satisfactory image is obtained. The $n$th point plotted can be written as

$$x_n = w_{\sigma_n}(w_{\sigma_{n-1}}(w_{\sigma_{n-2}}(\ldots w_{\sigma_2}(w_{\sigma_1}(x_0))))) \tag{6}$$

where $\sigma_i$ is a randomly selected integer from 1 to $N$.

It can be proven [3] that a sequence of points obtained through using this method densely approaches the attractor for almost every semi-infinite random sequence of mappings chosen. Thus, we can obtain a good approximation of the attractor with a tremendously reduced computational cost. The probabilities $p_i$ are selected based on the point density achieved by each mapping selection in order to reduce the time to obtain a dense approximation to the attractor (see Sect. 6). For more details on this method, see [1], for example. With the Chaos Game, the exponential increase in points resulting from iterative applications of the entire IFS to a set of points is avoided as only one point needs be stored at a time. Figure 1 illustrates the resulting attractor when using increasing numbers of iterations for the chaos game. For most of the images obtained in this project, 100,000 points were used.

## 3   Colour Stealing

The concept of using an image to colour an attractor has been explored in previous work [1–3, 5]. M. Barnsley had the idea of using the dynamics of another IFS in order to colour a fractal such that the colours mimic a natural pattern. It was our goal to first replicate this technique (called colour stealing) for ourselves and then to expand on it in interesting ways. This drawing technique involves keeping track of the mappings chosen at each iteration of the chaos game. In doing so, we obtain a "history" that tells us exactly how each point was obtained. Each point is thus associated with a sequence of integers that acts as an address for that point. We call these sequences *codes*, which help to form what we call a *code space*.

The code space $\Omega_N$ for a given integer, $N$, is the space of all semi-infinite strings whose elements are integers from 1 to $N$. $\Omega_N$ represents the set of all possible codes for an N-map IFS. In general, a code $\sigma$ in a code space $\Omega_N$ is given by

$$\sigma = \lim_{n \to \infty} \sigma_n \, \sigma_{n-1} \, \sigma_{n-2} \, \sigma_{n-3} \, \ldots \, \sigma_3 \, \sigma_2 \, \sigma_1 \quad \{1 \le \sigma_i \le N \mid \sigma_i \in \mathbb{N} \; \forall \; i\}. \tag{7}$$

Note that the elements are numbered from right to left. This convention is chosen in order to better convey the fact that the leftmost element of the code, the one corresponding to the most recent iteration, is the most influential with regards to the position of the resulting point. An example of a code in the space $\Omega_4$ might be

$$\sigma = \ldots 1\,4\,3\,1\,1\,2\,4\,3\,2\,2\,2\,3 \tag{8}$$

Note that since we are dealing with a finite number of points, and thus a finite number of mappings, in practice we do not consider semi-infinite strings. Instead, for practical implementation, we present a modified definition of code space to consider finite strings. Given an N-map IFS $W$, an initial point $x_0 \in \mathbf{X}$, and a code $\sigma = \sigma_n \, \sigma_{n-1} \, \ldots \, \sigma_2 \, \sigma_1 \in \Omega_N$, we define an address map $\phi_W : \Omega_N \to \mathbb{X}$ as

$$\phi_W(\sigma) = w_{\sigma_n}(w_{\sigma_{n-1}}(w_{\sigma_{n-2}}(\ldots w_{\sigma_2}(w_{\sigma_1}(x_0))))). \tag{9}$$

Iterating the chaos game $n$ times will always generate $n$ distinct codes for $n$ not necessarily distinct points. The point generated by the $i$th iteration of the chaos game will have a corresponding code of length $i$. Note that the address map $\phi_W(\sigma)$ is surjective but not injective, and so many distinct codes may lead to the same point in $\mathbf{X}$.

When dealing with images produced by a computer display, we must consider that images differ from Cartesian plots in that they are formed of a finite grid of discrete pixels, rather than an uncountably infinite number of points. In order to steal colours from an image with finite resolution, we consider an image with a discrete number of pixels, $P_{tot}$. We can think of each pixel as a box-shaped collection of points. Any given set of pixels must form a partition for $\mathbf{X}$.

The chaos game can yield points which are arbitrarily close or even directly on top of each other. When drawing an image of the resulting attractor, each pixel containing at least one point will be coloured. In other words, the pixel $P_j$ is coloured as long as $\phi_W(\sigma) \in P_{jk}$ for at least one code $\sigma$ generated by the chaos game. To use the previously discussed technique of colour stealing, we consider $\mathbf{X} = [0, 1]^2$ and an image function, $I_Q(\mathbf{P})$, which maps a set of pixels, $\mathbf{P}$, to a set of $3 \times 1$ vectors representing the RGB triplets which define the colour of each pixel in the image $Q$.

We also define a pixel mapping function, $P_Q(x)$, which maps a point $x \in \mathbf{X} = [0, 1]^2$ to the pixel $(j, k)$ in which it is located. For a square image with square pixels, that function can be written explicitly as

$$P_Q(x, y)$$
$$= \left\{ (j, k) \Big| j + p_x \leq \frac{x - x_{min}}{\rho} < j + 1 + p_x, k + p_y \leq \frac{y - y_{min}}{\rho} < k + 1 + p_y \right\}$$
(10)

where $p_x$ and $p_y$ are pixel offsets, and $x_{min}$ and $y_{min}$ are the leftmost and lowermost values of $x$ and $y$, respectively, of all the plotted points on the attractor. Similarly, $x_{max}$ and $y_{max}$ are respectively the rightmost and uppermost values of $x$ and $y$. Together, these six values serve to normalize and center the attractor on the square image. The pixel size, $\rho$, is defined as

$$\rho = \frac{1}{D} max\{(x_{max} - x_{min}), (y_{max} - y_{min})\}$$
(11)

with D being the number of pixels in one dimension of the colouring image, $Q$. For example, a $300 \times 300$ pixel image will have $D = 300$. For the sake of simplicity, only square images with an equal number of pixels in each dimension were used. The pixel offsets required to center the image are calculated such that the attractor will fill the square image in the dimension in which it is largest, but will create black bars on either side of the attractor in the other dimension to ensure that the attractor remains appropriately scaled and centered on the square image.

To implement the aforementioned method of colour stealing, we first select a square image, $Q_V$, and map the pixels in the image to $\mathbf{X} = [0, 1]^2$ such that $D^2$ pixels of size $\rho$ will completely fill $\mathbf{X}$ without overlapping. Next, we require two N-map IFSs: $\hat{V}$ and $\hat{W}$ with probabilities, $p_i$ associated with each mapping. Starting from a single seed point, $x_0$, we simultaneously play two chaos games using the same random sequence of map selections for both. With the codes generated by the randomly selected mappings, we plot the attractor for $W$, the "drawing IFS" as before, except that it is now drawn as an image $Q_W$ with pixel dimensions $D^2$. We add colour to this attractor using $V$, the aptly named "colouring IFS". For each point $\phi_W(\sigma)$, the corresponding point $\phi_V(\sigma)$ is mapped to a pixel $(j, k) \in \mathbf{P}$ in $Q_V$. The image mapping function $I_{Q_V}(j, k)$ outputs the RGB triplet, corresponding to the colour of the pixel $(j, k)$ in $Q_V$. This is the pixel colour corresponding to the code $\sigma$.

Finally, we paint each pixel $P_Q(\phi_W(\sigma))$ on $Q_W$ with the RGB triplet corresponding to $\sigma$, which is given by $I_{Q_V}(P_Q(\phi_V(\sigma)))$ as described above. The new image, $Q_W$ will display the geometric shape of the attractor of the drawing IFS, $W$, but uses the colours of the image $Q_V$. It should be noted that $Q_W$ is drawn such that it has the same pixel dimensions as $Q_V$ and thus the same pixel mapping function, $P_Q$ can be used for both images. The effect is this: As we execute the chaos game using a single code, two (typically different) IFSs generate two (typically different) sets of points. Points

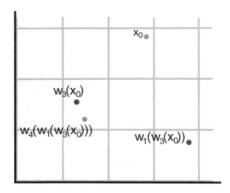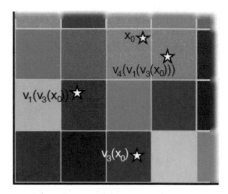

**Fig. 2** Illustration of the way the colours are stolen from an image $Q_V$ and applied to the points generated by the chaos game. Note the two points located in the same pixel of $Q_W$ which are causing a conflict. How can we decide whether this pixel should be coloured blue or green?

visited by the "drawing" IFS, $W$, are plotted, but shaded with the colours overlying the current point generated by the "colouring" IFS, $V$. In this way, the colours of the attractor for $W$ are "stolen" from whatever image is chosen to overlay the attractor for $V$.

Figure 2 illustrates this process with a small-scale example.

The example described above illustrates a key problem encountered in this method. As mentioned previously, the chaos game can generate multiple codes which all lead to points within a single pixel.

Thus, after completing the chaos game, each pixel $(j, k)$ will, in general, be associated with a set of codes, denoted $\hat{\sigma}_{jk}$, that map to that pixel. As we require only one colour to shade the pixel with, a single choice must be made from among this set.

We first define the size of a code. Based around the concept of a norm, the size of a code is defined to be

$$S(\sigma) = \sum_{i=0}^{n-1} \frac{\sigma_{n-i} - 1}{N^i} \tag{12}$$

Recall that the first element of a code is the rightmost number. Therefore, the size of a code $\sigma = 1\ 2\ 2\ 1\ 1\ 2$ in $\Omega_2$ would be

$$S(1\ 2\ 2\ 1\ 1\ 2) = \frac{0}{2^0} + \frac{1}{2^1} + \frac{1}{2^2} + \frac{0}{2^3} + \frac{0}{2^4} + \frac{1}{2^5} \tag{13}$$
$$= 0.78125$$

As mentioned previously, the choice to represent codes as having the leftmost element represent the mapping number corresponding to the most recent transformation is rooted in the fact that the most recent mapping selection is most influential with regards to the position of the resulting point. Thus, our notation convention parallels that of a base-N number, having the most significant digit on the left and the least significant digit on the right. Now that we have a means for comparing the sizes of codes, we can introduce the fractal top [1, 2]:

$$\bar{\tau}_\phi(j, k) = \left\{ \max_{S(\sigma \in \Omega_N)} \left| P(\phi(\sigma)) = (j, k) \right\} \right. \tag{14}$$

In words, the fractal top of a pixel $(j, k)$ is the largest code which is mapped to a point within that pixel. The fractal top gives us the means to select a unique code as we required earlier; however, the decision to select the largest code is not necessary, and other methods of code discrimination could be explored. We generalize this notion by instead using a function $\tau(\hat{\sigma}_{jk})$, which acts as a projection of the set of codes $\hat{\sigma}_{jk}$ to a single code $\sigma_{jk}$ within that set.

Finally putting this all together, we can define our new image as

$$Q_W(P_{jk}) = I_{Q_V} \circ P_Q \circ \phi_V \circ \tau \circ \hat{\sigma}_j. \tag{15}$$

In this equation, $\hat{\sigma}_{jk}$ gives us the set of all codes which satisfy $\phi_W(\sigma) \in P_{jk}$, or the set of all codes which the drawing IFS, $W$, maps to points within the pixel $P_j$. $\tau$ selects a single code from this set, and $\phi_V$ maps that code to a point in $\mathbf{X}$ using the colouring IFS, $V$. $P_Q$ determines the pixel in which said point belongs, and $I_{Q_V}$ gives the colour of the overlaid image, $Q_V$, at that pixel. Some images obtained using colour stealing, with the previously described "fractal top" used as our code projection function, $\tau$, are illustrated in Fig. 3.

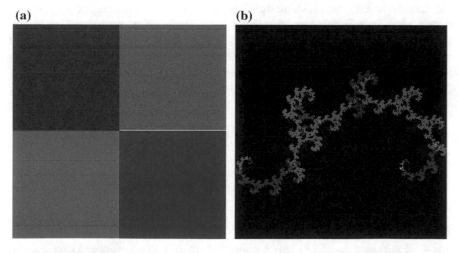

**(a)**          **(b)**

**Fig. 3** Example of colour stealing. Image **a** depicts the colouring image, $I$, image **b** shows the end result, $Q_W$, using the Golden Dragon IFS as a drawing IFS and the Twin Dragon IFS as a colouring IFS (see Sect. 6)

# 4  Discussion

It should be emphasized that using a different colouring attractor can yield a completely different colour scheme, as illustrated in Fig. 4b, c.

We now test some variations of the standard colour stealing technique. The first variation we attempted was to set $\phi_W$ and $\phi_V$ to the same IFS. In this case, any given code will result in the same point on both the drawing and colouring attractors. Thus, the resulting image is simply a cutout of $Q_V$, as if shape of the the drawing/colouring attractor has been applied as a mask to $Q_V$. This is illustrated in Fig. 4d.

Given any sequence of mappings chosen during the chaos game, the same points will be visited in the same order using both the "drawing" and "coloring" IFS. The result is outlined in [3].

Suppose now we consider a drawing IFS $W$ and a colouring IFS $V$ but employ the colour stealing application twice; the first time choosing the projection function to be the fractal top as described before, and the second time choosing it to be defined as follows:

$$\tau_\phi(j, k) = \left\{ \min_{S(\sigma \in \Omega_N)} \left| P(\phi(\sigma)) = (j, k) \right. \right\}. \tag{16}$$

We call this projection function the 'fractal bottom', as we are now selecting the smallest code in the set. In Fig. 5, we compare the result of colour stealing using the fractal top and using the fractal bottom.

Notice that while there is a distinct difference, not all the points change colour. The colour will stay the same if the colour corresponding to the fractal top is equal to that of the fractal bottom. This occurs in two cases: The first occurs when the top and bottom codes coincidentally map to the same RGB colour. The second case occurs when there is only one code that maps to that pixel. For a general projection function, the colour of a given pixel will stay the same if all points within that pixel are mapped to the same RGB colour. It would be interesting to explore the relation between the number of points which change colour and the fractal dimension, since

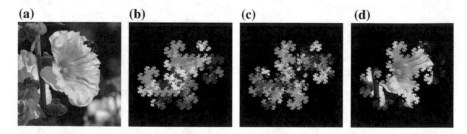

**(a)**            **(b)**            **(c)**            **(d)**

**Fig. 4** Illustration of the effect of the colouring IFS selection on the resulting image. Image **a** depicts the colouring image, $I$, image **b** shows the result of colour stealing using the Golden Dragon as a colouring IFS, while image **c** shows the result of colour stealing using the Levy Dragon as a colouring IFS **d** shows the result of colour stealing using the Twin Dragon as a colouring IFS. All images use the Twin Dragon as a drawing IFS (see Sect. 6)

**(a)**                          **(b)**                          **(c)**

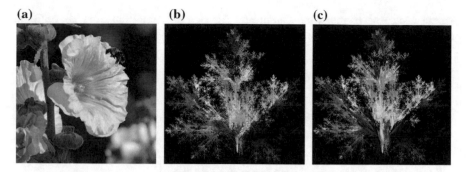

**Fig. 5** Comparison of images obtained using **b** the fractal top **c** the fractal bottom with the Maple Leaf attractor. Both images were obtained using the square fractal attractor as a colouring IFS (see Sect. 6). Image **a** shows the colouring image, $Q_V$

they are both related to the density of the points on the attractor. A more detailed discussion of the colour distribution obtained through colour stealing can be found in Barnsley's work [1, 2, 4–7].

# 5   Conclusion

The goal of this project was to explore Barnsley's colour stealing technique and its properties. In doing so, we made use of a generalised projection function in place of the previously defined fractal top. Additionally, we defined a finite code space and a way of comparing these finite codes for practical implementation. The results showed that different choices of the projection function can lead to differences in the final pictures. Another topic explored was the use of same IFS colour-stealing. The images obtained using these techniques were very interesting and required further examination in order to better understand their properties.

# 6   Appendix

Listed below are some of the IFSs used to obtain the images above. The IFS is presented as a matrix of the form

$$
\begin{bmatrix}
a_1 & b_1 & c_1 & d_1 & e_1 & f_1 & p_1 \\
a_2 & b_2 & c_2 & d_2 & e_2 & f_2 & p_2 \\
\vdots & \vdots & \vdots & \vdots & \vdots & \vdots & \vdots \\
a_n & b_n & c_n & d_n & e_n & f_n & p_n
\end{bmatrix}
\tag{17}
$$

where each row contains the parameters for one mapping, and first six columns contain the parameters for a set-valued mapping of the form

$$\hat{w}_i(\mathbf{X}) = \begin{bmatrix} a & b \\ c & d \end{bmatrix} \mathbf{X} + \begin{bmatrix} e \\ f \end{bmatrix}. \tag{18}$$

and $p_i$ is the probability associated with the mapping $\hat{w}_i(\mathbf{X})$.

$$\text{Sierpinski Triangle IFS} = \begin{bmatrix} 0.5 & 0 & 0 & 0.5 & 1 & 1 & 0.33 \\ 0.5 & 0 & 0 & 0.5 & 1 & 50 & 0.33 \\ 0.5 & 0 & 0 & 0.5 & 50 & 50 & 0.34 \end{bmatrix}$$

$$\text{Fern IFS} = \begin{bmatrix} 0 & 0 & 0 & 0.16 & 0 & 0 & 0.01 \\ 0.85 & 0.04 & -0.04 & 0.85 & 0 & 1.6 & 0.85 \\ 0.2 & -0.26 & 0.23 & 0.22 & 0 & 1.6 & 0.07 \\ -0.15 & 0.28 & 0.26 & 0.24 & 0 & 0.44 & 0.07 \end{bmatrix}$$

$$\text{Maple Leaf IFS} = \begin{bmatrix} 0.14 & 0.01 & 0 & 0.51 & -0.08 & -1.31 & 0.25 \\ 0.43 & 0.52 & -0.45 & 0.5 & 1.49 & -0.75 & 0.25 \\ 0.45 & -0.49 & 0.47 & 0.47 & -1.62 & -0.74 & 0.25 \\ 0.49 & 0 & 0 & 0.51 & 0.02 & 1.62 & 0.25 \end{bmatrix}$$

$$\text{Square IFS} = \begin{bmatrix} 0.5 & 0 & 0 & 0.5 & 1 & 1 & 0.25 \\ 0.5 & 0 & 0 & 0.5 & 50 & 1 & 0.25 \\ 0.5 & 0 & 0 & 0.5 & 1 & 50 & 0.25 \\ 0.5 & 0 & 0 & 0.5 & 50 & 50 & 0.25 \end{bmatrix}$$

$$\text{Golden Dragon IFS} = \begin{bmatrix} 0.62327 & -0.40337 & 0.40337 & 0.62367 & 0 & 0 & 0.5 \\ -0.37633 & -0.40337 & 0.40337 & -0.37633 & 1 & 0 & 0.5 \end{bmatrix}$$

$$\text{Levy Dragon} = \begin{bmatrix} 0.5 & -0.5 & 0.5 & 0.5 & 0 & 0 & 0.5 \\ 0.5 & 0.5 & -0.5 & 0.5 & 0.5 & 0.5 & 0.5 \end{bmatrix}$$

$$\text{Twin Dragon} = \begin{bmatrix} 0.5 & -0.5 & 0.5 & 0.5 & 0 & 0 & 0.5 \\ 0.5 & -0.5 & 0.5 & 0.5 & 0.5 & -0.5 & 0.5 \end{bmatrix}$$

# References

1. Barnsley, M.: Superfractals. Academic Press, London (2006)
2. Barnsley, M.: Theory and Application of Fractal Tops, Fractals in Engineering, Tours. Springer, France (2005)
3. Kunze, H., Demers, M., Levere, K.: Fractal tops and colour stealing. In Maple Conference 2006 Proceedings (2006)
4. Barnsley, M.: Transformations between self-referential sets. Am. Math. Mon. **116**(4), 291–304 (2009)
5. Barnsley, M., Harding, B., Igudesman, K.: How to transform and filter images using iterated function Systems. SIAM J. Imaging Sci. **4**(4), 1001–1028 (2011)

6. Barnsley, M., Vince, A.: The chaos game on a general iterated function. Ergodic Theory Dyn. Syst. **31**(4), 1073–1079 (2011)
7. Barnsley, M., Harding, B.: Three-dimensional fractal homeomorphisms. In: Benoit Mandelbrot: A Life in Many Dimensions, pp. 117–143 (2015)
8. Hutchinson, J.: Fractals and self-similarity. Indiana Univ. Math. J. **30**, 713–747 (1981)

# Infinite Products Involving Binary Digit Sums

**Samin Riasat**

**Abstract**  Let $(u_n)_{n\geq 0}$ denote the Thue-Morse sequence with values $\pm 1$. The Woods-Robbins identity below and several of its generalisations are well-known in the literature

$$\prod_{n=0}^{\infty} \left(\frac{2n+1}{2n+2}\right)^{u_n} = \frac{1}{\sqrt{2}}.$$

No other such product involving a rational function in $n$ and the sequence $u_n$ seems to be known in closed form. To understand these products in detail we study the function

$$f(b,c) = \prod_{n=1}^{\infty} \left(\frac{n+b}{n+c}\right)^{u_n}.$$

We prove some analytical properties of $f$. We also obtain some new identities similar to the Woods-Robbins product.

**Keywords**  Prouhet-Thue-Morse sequence · Woods and Robbins product
Closed formulas for infinite products

## 1  Introduction

Let $s_k(n)$ denote the sum of the digits in the base-$k$ expansion of the non-negative integer $n$. Although we only consider $k = 2$, our results can be easily extended to all integers $k \geq 2$. Put $u_n = (-1)^{s_2(n)}$. In other words, $u_n$ is equal to 1 if the binary expansion of $n$ has an even number of 1's, and is equal to $-1$ otherwise. This is the so-called Thue-Morse sequence with values $\pm 1$. We study infinite products of the form

S. Riasat (✉)
University of Waterloo, Waterloo, ON, Canada
e-mail: sriasat@uwaterloo.ca

© Springer Nature Switzerland AG 2018
D. M. Kilgour et al. (eds.), *Recent Advances in Mathematical
and Statistical Methods*, Springer Proceedings in Mathematics & Statistics 259,
https://doi.org/10.1007/978-3-319-99719-3_6

$$f(b, c) := \prod_{n=1}^{\infty} \left( \frac{n+b}{n+c} \right)^{u_n}.$$

The only known non-trivial value of $f$ (up to the relations $f(b, b) = 1$ and $f(b, c) = 1/f(c, b)$) seems to be

$$f\left( \frac{1}{2}, 1 \right) = \sqrt{2},$$

which is the famous Woods-Robbins identity [7, 8]. Several infinite products inspired by this identity were discovered afterwards (see, e.g., [5, 6]), but none of them involve the sequence $u_n$. In this paper we compute another value of $f$, namely,

$$f\left( \frac{1}{4}, \frac{3}{4} \right) = \frac{3}{2}.$$

In Sect. 2 we look at properties of the function $f$ and introduce a related function $h$. In Sect. 3 we study the analytical properties of $h$. In Sect. 4 we try to find infinite products of the form $\prod R(n)^{u_n}$ admitting a closed form value, with $R$ a rational function.

This paper forms the basis for the paper [3]. While the purpose of [3] is to compute new products of the forms $\prod R(n)^{u_n}$ and $\prod R(n)^{t_n}$, $t_n$ being the Thue-Morse sequence with values 0, 1, we restrict ourselves in this paper to studying products of the form $\prod R(n)^{u_n}$ in greater depth.

## 2 General Properties of $f$ and a New Function $h$

We start with the following result on convergence.

**Lemma 1** *Let $R \in \mathbb{C}(x)$ be a rational function such that the values $R(n)$ are defined and non-zero for integers $n \geq 1$. Then, the infinite product $\prod_n R(n)^{u_n}$ converges if and only if the numerator and the denominator of $R$ have same degree and same leading coefficient.*

*Proof* See [3], Lemma 2.1.

Hence $f(b, c)$ converges for any $b, c \in \mathbb{C} \setminus \{-1, -2, -3, \dots\}$. Using the definition of $u_n$ we see that $f$ satisfies the following properties.

**Lemma 2** *For any $b, c, d \in \mathbb{C} \setminus \{-1, -2, -3, \dots\}$,*

1. $f(b, b) = 1$,
2. $f(b, c)f(c, d) = f(b, d)$,
3. $f(b, c) = \left( \frac{c+1}{b+1} \right) f\left( \frac{b}{2}, \frac{c}{2} \right) f\left( \frac{c+1}{2}, \frac{b+1}{2} \right)$.

*Proof* The only non-trivial claim is part 3. To see why it is true, note that $u_{2n} = u_n$ and $u_{2n+1} = -u_n$, so that

$$f(b, c) = \prod_{n=1}^{\infty} \left( \frac{n+b}{n+c} \right)^{u_n}$$

$$= \left( \frac{1+c}{1+b} \right) \prod_{n=1}^{\infty} \left( \frac{2n+b}{2n+c} \right)^{u_n} \prod_{n=1}^{\infty} \left( \frac{2n+1+c}{2n+1+b} \right)^{u_n}$$

$$= \left( \frac{1+c}{1+b} \right) \prod_{n=1}^{\infty} \left( \frac{n+\frac{b}{2}}{n+\frac{c}{2}} \right)^{u_n} \prod_{n=1}^{\infty} \left( \frac{n+\frac{c+1}{2}}{n+\frac{b+1}{2}} \right)^{u_n}$$

$$= \left( \frac{c+1}{b+1} \right) f \left( \frac{b}{2}, \frac{c}{2} \right) f \left( \frac{c+1}{2}, \frac{b+1}{2} \right)$$

as desired.

One can ask the natural question: is $f$ the unique function satisfying these properties? What if we impose some continuity/analyticity conditions?

Using the first two parts of Lemma 2 we get

$$f(b, c) f(d, e) = \frac{f(b, c) f(c, d) f(d, e) f(d, c)}{f(c, d) f(d, c)} = \frac{f(b, e) f(d, c)}{f(c, c)} = f(b, e) f(d, c).$$

Hence the third part may be re-written as

$$f(b, c) = \frac{f \left( \frac{b}{2}, \frac{b+1}{2} \right)}{b+1} \bigg/ \frac{f \left( \frac{c}{2}, \frac{c+1}{2} \right)}{c+1}. \tag{1}$$

This motivates the following definition.

**Definition 1** Define the function

$$h(x) := f \left( \frac{x}{2}, \frac{x+1}{2} \right). \tag{2}$$

Then Eqs. (1) and (2) give the following result.

**Lemma 3** *For any* $b, c \in \mathbb{C} \setminus \{-1, -2, -3, \dots\}$,

$$f(b, c) = \frac{c+1}{b+1} \cdot \frac{h(b)}{h(c)}. \tag{3}$$

So understanding $f$ is equivalent to understanding $h$, in the sense that each function can be completely evaluated in terms of the other. Moreover, taking $c = b + \frac{1}{2}$ in Eq. (3) and then using Eq. (2) gives the following result.

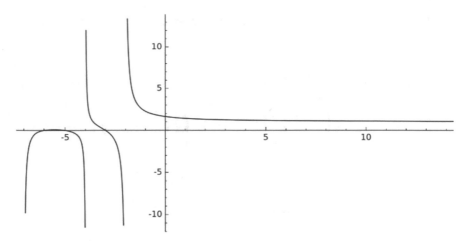

**Fig. 1**  Approximate plot of $h(x)$

**Lemma 4**  *The function h defined by Eq.* (2) *satisfies the functional equation*

$$h(x) = \frac{x+1}{x+\frac{3}{2}} h\left(x + \frac{1}{2}\right) h(2x). \tag{4}$$

Again one may ask: is $h$ the unique solution to Eq. (4)? What about monotonic/continuous/smooth solutions?

An approximate plot of $h$ is given in Fig. 1 with the infinite product truncated at $n = 100$.

## 3  Analytical Properties of *h*

The following lemma forms the basis for the results in this section.

**Lemma 5**  *For* $b, c \in (-1, \infty)$,

1. *if* $b = c$, *then* $f(b, c) = 1$.
2. *if* $b > c$, *then*

$$\left(\frac{c+1}{b+1}\right)^2 < f(b, c) < 1.$$

3. *if* $b < c$, *then*

$$1 < f(b, c) < \left(\frac{c+1}{b+1}\right)^2.$$

*Proof*  Using Lemma 2 it suffices to prove the second statement.

Let $b > c > -1$ and put

$$a_n = \log\left(\frac{n+b}{n+c}\right), \quad S_N = \sum_{n=1}^{N} a_n u_n, \quad U_N = \sum_{n=1}^{N} u_n. \tag{5}$$

Note that $a_n$ is positive and strictly decreasing to 0. Using $s_2(2n) + s_2(2n+1) \equiv 1$ (mod 2) it follows that $U_n \in \{-2, -1, 0\}$ and $U_n \equiv n$ (mod 2) for each $n$. Using summation by parts,

$$S_N = a_{N+1} U_N + \sum_{n=1}^{N} U_n(a_n - a_{n+1}).$$

So $-2a_1 < S_N < 0$ for large $N$. Exponentiating and taking $N \to \infty$ gives the desired result.

Lemmas 3–5 immediately imply the following results.

**Theorem 1** $h(x)/(x+1)$ *is strictly decreasing on* $(-1, \infty)$ *and* $h(x)(x+1)$ *is strictly increasing on* $(-1, \infty)$.

**Theorem 2** *For* $b, c \in (-1, \infty)$, $f(b, c)$ *is strictly decreasing in* $b$ *and strictly increasing in* $c$.

**Theorem 3** *For* $x \in (-2, \infty)$,

$$1 < h(x) < \left(\frac{x+3}{x+2}\right)^2.$$

We now give some results on differentiability.

**Theorem 4** $h(x)$ *is smooth on* $(-2, \infty)$.

*Proof* Recall the definition of $h$:

$$h(x) = \prod_{n=1}^{\infty} \left(\frac{2n+x}{2n+1+x}\right)^{u_n}.$$

Then taking $b = x/2$ and $c = (x+1)/2$ in Eq. (5) shows that the sequence $S_n$ of smooth functions on $(-2, \infty)$ converges pointwise to $\log h$.

Differentiating with respect to $x$ gives

$$S_N' = \sum_{n=1}^{N} \frac{u_n}{(2n+x)(2n+1+x)} = \sum_{n=1}^{N} u_n \left(\frac{1}{2n+x} - \frac{1}{2n+1+x}\right).$$

Hence

$$\left| S_N' - S_M' \right| \leq \sum_{n=M+1}^{N} \left( \frac{1}{2n+x} - \frac{1}{2n+1+x} \right)$$

$$\leq \sum_{n=M+1}^{N} \left( \frac{1}{2n-1+x} - \frac{1}{2n+1+x} \right)$$

$$= \frac{1}{2M+1+x} - \frac{1}{2N+1+x}$$

$$< \frac{1}{2M-1} \to 0$$

as $M \to \infty$, for any $x \in (-2, \infty)$ and $N > M$. Thus $S_n'$ converges uniformly on $(-2, \infty)$, which shows that $\log h$, hence $h$, is differentiable on $(-2, \infty)$.

Now suppose that derivatives of $h$ up to order $k$ exist for some $k \geq 1$. Note that

$$S_N^{(k+1)} = (-1)^k k! \sum_{n=1}^{N} u_n \left( \frac{1}{(2n+x)^{k+1}} - \frac{1}{(2n+1+x)^{k+1}} \right).$$

As before,

$$\left| S_N^{(k+1)} - S_M^{(k+1)} \right| \leq k! \sum_{n=M+1}^{N} \left( \frac{1}{(2n+x)^{k+1}} - \frac{1}{(2n+1+x)^{k+1}} \right)$$

$$\leq k! \sum_{n=M+1}^{N} \left( \frac{1}{(2n-1+x)^{k+1}} - \frac{1}{(2n+1+x)^{k+1}} \right)$$

$$= \frac{k!}{(2M+1+x)^{k+1}} - \frac{k!}{(2N+1+x)^{k+1}}$$

$$< \frac{k!}{(2M-1)^{k+1}} \to 0$$

as $M \to \infty$, for any $x \in (-2, \infty)$ and $N > M$. Hence $S_n^{(k+1)}$ converges uniformly on $(-2, \infty)$, i.e., $h^{(k)}$ is differentiable on $(-2, \infty)$.

Therefore, by induction, $h$ has derivatives of all orders on $(-2, \infty)$.

**Theorem 5** *Let $a \geq 0$. Then*

$$\log h(x) = \log h(a) + \sum_{k=1}^{\infty} \frac{(-1)^{k-1}}{k} \left( \sum_{n=2}^{\infty} \frac{u_n}{(n+a)^k} \right) (x-a)^k$$

*for $x \in [a-1, a+1]$.*

*Proof* Let $H(x) = \log h(x)$. By Theorem 4,

$$H^{(k+1)}(x) = (-1)^k k! \sum_{n=2}^{\infty} \frac{u_n}{(n+x)^{k+1}}.$$

Hence

$$|H^{(k+1)}(x)| \leq k! \sum_{n=2}^{\infty} \frac{1}{|n+x|^{k+1}} \leq k! \sum_{n=2}^{\infty} \frac{1}{(n+a-1)^{k+1}}$$

for $x \in [a-1, a+1]$. So by Taylor's inequality, the remainder for the Taylor polynomial for $H(x)$ of degree $k$ is absolutely bounded above by

$$\frac{1}{k+1} \left( \sum_{n=2}^{\infty} \frac{1}{(n+a-1)^{k+1}} \right) |x-a|^{k+1}$$

which tends to 0 as $k \to \infty$, since $a \geq 0$ and $|x - a| \leq 1$. Therefore $H(x)$ equals its Taylor expansion about $a$ for $x$ in the given range.

## 4  Infinite Products

Recall that

$$f(b, c) = \prod_{n=1}^{\infty} \left( \frac{n+b}{n+c} \right)^{u_n}.$$

From Lemma 2 we see that

$$\prod_{n=1}^{\infty} \left( \frac{(n+b)(n+\frac{b+1}{2})(n+\frac{c}{2})}{(n+c)(n+\frac{c+1}{2})(n+\frac{b}{2})} \right)^{u_n} = \frac{c+1}{b+1} \tag{6}$$

for any $b, c \neq -1, -2, -3, \ldots$, and if $b, c \neq 0, -1, -2, \ldots$, then

$$\prod_{n=0}^{\infty} \left( \frac{(n+b)(n+\frac{b+1}{2})(n+\frac{c}{2})}{(n+c)(n+\frac{c+1}{2})(n+\frac{b}{2})} \right)^{u_n} = 1. \tag{7}$$

Some interesting identities can be obtained from Eqs. (6) and (7). For example, in Eq. (6), taking $c = (b+1)/2$ gives

$$\prod_{n=1}^{\infty} \left( \frac{(n+b)(n+\frac{b+1}{4})}{(n+\frac{b+3}{4})(n+\frac{b}{2})} \right)^{u_n} = \frac{b+3}{2(b+1)} \tag{8}$$

while taking $b = 0$ gives

$$\prod_{n=1}^{\infty} \left( \frac{(n + \frac{1}{2})(n + \frac{c}{2})}{(n + c)(n + \frac{c+1}{2})} \right)^{u_n} = c + 1 \tag{9}$$

for any $b, c \neq -1, -2, -3, \ldots$.

We now turn our attention to the functional Eq. (4). Recall that it reads

$$h(x) = \frac{x+1}{x+\frac{3}{2}} h\left(x + \frac{1}{2}\right) h(2x).$$

Taking $x = 0$ gives

$$h(0) = \frac{2}{3} h\left(\frac{1}{2}\right) h(0).$$

Since $1 < h(0) < 9/4$ by Theorem 3, cancelling $h(0)$ from both sides gives $h(1/2) = 3/2$. This shows that

$$\prod_{n=0}^{\infty} \left( \frac{4n+3}{4n+1} \right)^{u_n} = 2. \tag{10}$$

Next, taking $x = 1/2$ in Eq. (4) gives

$$h\left(\frac{1}{2}\right) = \frac{3}{4} h(1)^2$$

hence $h(1) = \sqrt{2}$ (since $1 < h(1) < 16/9$ by Theorem 3) and we recover the Woods-Robbins product

$$\prod_{n=0}^{\infty} \left( \frac{2n+2}{2n+1} \right)^{u_n} = \sqrt{2}. \tag{11}$$

Similarly, taking $x = -1/2$ in Eq. (4) gives

$$h\left(-\frac{1}{2}\right) = \frac{1}{2} h(0) h(-1) = \frac{1}{2} f\left(0, \frac{1}{2}\right) f\left(-\frac{1}{2}, 0\right) = \frac{1}{2} f\left(-\frac{1}{2}, \frac{1}{2}\right),$$

i.e.,

$$\prod_{n=1}^{\infty} \left( \frac{(4n-1)(2n+1)}{(4n+1)(2n-1)} \right)^{u_n} = \frac{1}{2}. \tag{12}$$

Taking $x = 1$ in Eq. (4) gives

$$h(1) = \frac{4}{5} h\left(\frac{3}{2}\right) h(2)$$

hence $h(3/2)h(2) = 5\sqrt{2}/4$ and this gives

$$\prod_{n=0}^{\infty} \left( \frac{(4n+3)(2n+2)}{(4n+5)(2n+3)} \right)^{u_n} = \frac{1}{\sqrt{2}}. \tag{13}$$

Taking $x = 3/2$ in Eq. (4) and using the previous result gives

$$h(2)^2 h(3) = \frac{3}{\sqrt{2}}$$

which is equivalent to

$$\prod_{n=0}^{\infty} \left( \frac{(2n+2)(n+1)}{(2n+3)(n+2)} \right)^{u_n} = \frac{1}{\sqrt{2}}. \tag{14}$$

Equations (10)–(14) can also be combined in pairs to obtain other identities.

## 5   Concluding Remarks

The quantity $h(0) \approx 1.62,816$ appears to be of interest [1, 4]. It is not known whether its value is irrational or transcendental. We give the following explanation as to why $h(0)$ might behave specially in a sense.

Note that the only way non-trivial cancellation occurs in the functional equation Eq. (4) is when $b = 0$. Likewise, non-trivial cancellation occurs in Eq. (1) or property 3 in Lemma 2 only for $(b, c) = (0, 1/2)$ and $(1/2, 0)$. That is, the victim of any such cancellation is always $h(0)$ or $h(0)^{-1}$. So one must look for other ways to understand $h(0)$.

Using the only two known values $h(1/2) = 3/2$ and $h(1) = \sqrt{2}$, the following expressions for $h(0)$ can be obtained from Theorem 5.

- By taking $x = 0$ and $a = 1$,

$$h(0) = \sqrt{2} \exp \left( -\sum_{k=1}^{\infty} \frac{1}{k} \sum_{n=2}^{\infty} \frac{u_n}{(n+1)^k} \right).$$

- By taking $x = 1$ and $a = 0$,

$$h(0) = \sqrt{2} \exp \left( \sum_{k=1}^{\infty} \frac{(-1)^k}{k} \sum_{n=2}^{\infty} \frac{u_n}{n^k} \right).$$

- By taking $x = 0$ and $a = 1/2$,

$$h(0) = \frac{3}{2} \exp\left(\sum_{k=1}^{\infty} \frac{1}{k} \sum_{n=2}^{\infty} \frac{u_{2n+1}}{(2n+1)^k}\right).$$

- By taking $x = 1/2$ and $a = 0$,

$$h(0) = \frac{3}{2} \exp\left(\sum_{k=1}^{\infty} \frac{(-1)^k}{k} \sum_{n=2}^{\infty} \frac{u_{2n}}{(2n)^k}\right).$$

The Dirichlet series

$$\sum_{n=0}^{\infty} \frac{u_n}{(n+1)^k} \quad \text{and} \quad \sum_{n=1}^{\infty} \frac{u_n}{n^k}$$

appearing in the above expressions were studied by Allouche and Cohen [2].

**Acknowledgements** This work is part of a larger joint work [3] with Professors Jean-Paul Allouche and Jeffrey Shallit. I thank the professors for helpful discussions and comments. I also thank the anonymous referees for their feedback.

# References

1. Allouche, J.-P.: Thue, Combinatorics on words, and conjectures inspired by the Thue-Morse sequence. J. de Théorie des Nombres de Bordeaux **27**(2), 375–388 (2015)
2. Allouche, J.-P., Cohen, H.: Dirichlet series and curious infinite products. Bull. Lond. Math. Soc. **17**, 531–538 (1985)
3. Allouche, J.-P., Riasat, S., Shallit, J.: More infinite products: Thue-Morse and the gamma function. Ramanujan J. (2018). https://doi.org/10.1007/s11139-017-9981-7
4. Allouche, J.-P., Shallit, J.: The ubiquitous Prouhet-Thue-Morse sequence. Sequences and Their Applications: Proceedings of SETA'98, pp. 1–16 (1999)
5. Allouche, J.-P., Shallit, J.: Infinite products associated with counting blocks in binary strings. J. Lond. Math. Soc. **39**, 193–204 (1989)
6. Allouche, J.-P., Sondow, J.: Infinite products with strongly $B$-multiplicative exponents. Ann. Univ. Sci. Budapest. Sect. Comput. **28**, 35–53 (2008) [Errata: Ann. Univ. Sci. Budapest. Sect. Comput. **32**, 253 (2010)]
7. Robbins, D.: Solution to problem E 2692. Amer. Math. Monthly **86**, 394–395 (1979)
8. Woods, D.R.: Elementary problem proposal E 2692. Amer. Math. Monthly **85**, 48 (1978)

# Part II
# Analytical and Computational Methods in Inverse Problems

# Image-Driven Two-Point Boundary Value Inverse Problems: A Case Study

Victoria Brott and Herb Kunze

**Abstract** The collage method for treating boundary value inverse problems, given observational data values across the domain, is well-established in the literature. Here, instead, we formulate an inverse problem where the information about the dependent variable is given in the form of a greyscale image. The image gives no actual values, but does give some comparative information across the domain. In this paper, for the Sturm-Liouville two-point boundary value problem

$$(k(x)u'(x))' + q(x)u(x) = f(x)$$
$$u(0) = u_0$$
$$u(L) = u_L,$$

we consider the inverse problem:

> Given $f(x), q(x),$ the BCs, and a 256-grayscale image of the level values of $u(x)$, recover an estimate of $k(x)$.

For context, we can think of the greyscale image as representing the isotherms of the steady-state heat distribution, concentrations in a chemical system, or population densities. After summarizing the mathematical framework, we focus on a particular example, considering several scenarios for which we can solve this inverse problem and exploring the impact of observation noise and image resolution on the recovered approximation.

**Keywords** Inverse problems · Sturm-Liouville two-point boundary value problems · Image-driven · Collage theorem

V. Brott (✉) · H. Kunze
Department of Mathematics and Statistics, University of Guelph, Guelph, Canada
e-mail: vbrott@uoguelph.ca

H. Kunze
e-mail: hkunze@uoguelph.ca

© Springer Nature Switzerland AG 2018
D. M. Kilgour et al. (eds.), *Recent Advances in Mathematical and Statistical Methods*, Springer Proceedings in Mathematics & Statistics 259,
https://doi.org/10.1007/978-3-319-99719-3_7

# 1  Introduction

In a typical differential equations inverse problem, one seeks to estimate parameters
in the model equation from observational data of the dependent variable. A fundamental inverse problem for the Sturm-Liouville two-point boundary value problem
(BVP) [1],

$$(k(x)u'(x))' + q(x)u(x) = f(x) \tag{1}$$
$$u(0) = u_0 \tag{2}$$
$$u(L) = u_L, \tag{3}$$

is:

> *Given $f(x)$, $q(x)$, the BCs, and the measurements of $u(x)$,*      $(p')$
>
> $0 \le x \le L$, *recover an estimate of $k(x)$.*

for $N \ge 1$ most practical methods of solving this inverse problem begin with the
weak form of problem $(P')$ obtained by integrating both sides with respect to elements of a suitable set of basis functions. In one-dimension, for example, we use
the finite element "hat basis" functions. The integration process yields a linear system of equations in the coefficients $\lambda_i$ of $k(x)$ with respect to this basis. Instead of
solving this system directly, one typical solves a minimization problem involving an
appropriate least squares function. Often, an addition penalty function is added for
the purpose of regularization. The process is described pleasantly in the book [2],
indeed for this specific problem. In [3–5], we illustrate that the collage method can
be used to solve problem $(P')$. In fact, we demonstrate that the collage method gives
results that compare well with other computationally more-expensive methods.

In this paper, we instead assume that the given information about the dependent
variable comes in the form of a greyscale image produced from level values of the
dependent variable and seek to solve the inverse problem.

> *Given $f(x)$, $q(x)$, the BCs, and a 256-greyscale image of the*      $(P)$
>
> *level values of $u(x)$, recover an estimate of $k(x)$.*

(One motivation for studying this problem is the idea of extending the work to two
spatial dimensions, where the greyscale image could be a biomedical scan or a spatial
population density profile.)

In the next brief section, we present a summary of the collage method in the
context of two-point BVPs. The resulting minimization problem for the objective
function of the parameters $\lambda_i$, called the squared collage distance, is stated in (5). We
discuss problem $(P)$ in the final section, illustrating via example how the solution
method plays out. The key question becomes: is it possible to shift from the greyscale
image values to $u$-values (and then use the collage method)?

## 1.1 The Collage Method for Two-Point BVPs

We state Banach's fixed point theorem.

**Theorem 1** (Banach) *Let $(X, d)$ be a complete metric space and $T : X \to X$ be a contraction map:*

$$\exists c \in [0, 1) \text{ such that } d(Tu, Tv) \leq c \, d(u, v) \text{ for all } u, v \in X.$$

*Then there exists a unique fixed point $\bar{u} \in X$ of $T$ such that $T\bar{u} = \bar{u}$. Furthermore, $d(T^{\circ n}u, \bar{u}) \to 0$ as $n \to \infty$.*

Many inverse problems can be recast in terms of approximating a target element $u \in X$ by a fixed point $\bar{u}$ of some contraction map $T$: find $T$ such $d(u, \bar{u})$ is sufficiently small. A simple consequence of Banach's fixed point theorem is the collage theorem, the key result in fractal imaging [6, 7]. The collage theorem allows us to shift to a different minimization problem.

**Theorem 2** (Collage) *Let $(X, d)$ be a complete metric space and $T : X \to X$ be a contraction map with contraction factor $c \in [0, 1)$. Then*

$$d(u, \bar{u}) \leq \frac{1}{1 - c} d(u, Tu)$$

*where $\bar{u}$ is the fixed point of $T$.*

The collage theorem allows us to bound the fixed point approximation error $d(u, \bar{u})$ by the factor $\frac{1}{1-c}$ times the "collage distance" $d(u, Tu)$. In a practical problem, the candidate contraction maps are typically selected from a family defined in terms of some parameters, say $T_\lambda$ for $\lambda \in \Lambda$, each with fixed point $u_\lambda$ and contractivity factor $c_\lambda \in [0, 1)$. So we can minimize the penalized objective function

$$\min_{\lambda \in \Lambda} d\left(u_{target}, T_\lambda u_{target}\right) + \gamma_1 \max\{0, -c_\lambda\} + \gamma_2 \max\{0, c_\lambda - 1\},$$

where $u_{target}$ is the target element in $X$, $\gamma_1$ and $\gamma_2$ are two positive parameters, and the minimization in $\lambda$ may be done over a suitable subset of $\Lambda$. The final two terms in the objective function add a positive penalty when $c_\lambda$ lies outside of [0,1]. Note that the regularity of the objective function depends strictly on the first term. In practice, we often just solve

$$\min_{\lambda \in \Lambda} d\left(u_{target}, T_\lambda u_{target}\right).$$

In the case of Sturm-Liouville two-point BVPs, following [3], the role of $T$ is played by a Picard integral operator with an adjustment to replace the second boundary condition (at $x = L$) with a condition at the other endpoint ($x = 0$). Integrate (1), divide by $k(x) \neq 0$ for all $x$, and integrate again. Reversing the order of integration on the integral leads to the the definition of the Picard operator of interest:

$$(Tu)(x) = u_0 + u_0'(x - 0) - \int_0^x (x - s) \left[ \frac{-f(s) + q(s)u(s) + k'(s)u'(s)}{k(s)} \right] ds \quad (4)$$

Note that a fixed point $u$ of $T$ satisfies $u(0) = 0$ and $u'(0) = u'(0)$. In order for this $u$ to satisfy boundary condition at $x = L$, we impose that $(Tu)(L) = u_L$; this equation can be solved for $u'(0)$,

$$u_0' = \frac{1}{L} \left( u_L - u_0 + \int_0^L (L - s) \left[ \frac{-f(s) + q(s)u(s) + k'(s)u'(s)}{k(s)} \right] ds \right),$$

and plugged back into (4) to give a Picard operator that depends on $u_L$ instead. For our inverse problem, with $k$ determined in terms of some parameters $\lambda$, we solve

$$\min_{\lambda \in \Lambda} \Delta^2 = \min_{\lambda \in \Lambda} d_2^2 \left( u_{target}, T_\lambda u_{target} \right) = \min_{\lambda \in \Lambda} \int_0^L \left( u_{target}(x) - \left( T_\lambda u_{target} \right)(x) \right)^2 dx,$$
$$(5)$$

setting $\gamma_1$ and $\gamma_2$ to 0. In [3], the contractivity of $T$ on the interval $[0, \delta]$, $\delta$ small, is established. As we work on $[0, L]$ here, with $L$ imposed, we note that we can break the larger interval up into perhaps many pieces each of small enough width for the earlier result and then use some inequalities to return to a minimization problem for the operator on the full interval. That is, let $T_i$ be the Picard operator defined on the interval $[(i - 1)\delta, i\delta]$, $i = 1, \ldots, N$, with $\delta = \frac{1}{N}$; then we have theoretical justification for minimizing the collage distance on each interval, but this is undesirable since we do not want a piecewise defined differential equation. Instead we note

$$\min_{\lambda \in \Lambda} d_2^2 (u, Tu) = \min_{\lambda \in \Lambda} \left( \sum_{i=1}^N d_2^2 (u, T_i u) \right) \geq \sum_{i=1}^N \min_{\lambda \in \Lambda} d_2^2 (u, T_i u),$$

and so we can minimize the collage distance on the entire interval to control the sum of the errors on the individual intervals.

We mention that the occurrence of $k(x)$ in both the numerator and denominator of the integrand in (4) complicates the minimization of the squared collage distance. In our work, we use Particle Swarm Ant Colony Optimization (PSACO) [8] to find the minimizing parameter values.

## 1.2 A Case Study of the Inverse Problem

In order to set the stage for our academic study, we first choose "true" values for the parameters in (1)–(3). In what follows, similar to the examples in [4, 5, 9, 10], we set $k_{true}(x) = 1 + 3x$. In addition we always use $q(x) = 0$, $L = 5$, $u_0 = 0$, and $u_L = 100$. We will consider two values for $f(x)$. In all cases, we solve the BVP numerically, sample the solution at $N$ uniformly distributed data points (including the two endpoints), add Gaussian (relative) noise with low amplitude $\varepsilon$, and, finally, produce an $N \times 1$ pixel greyscale image from the noised sample values. The color black is assigned to the pixel with the highest sample value and the color white is assigned to the pixel with the lowest sample value; all other pixels are coloured with the appropriate shade of grey. In our work, we use $N$ values of 128, 256, 512, and 1024. (When we display these images in a figure, we duplicate each pixel vertically so that the shading is easier to see.) The generated image is the key input to the updated inverse problem $(P)$:

*Given $f(x)$, $q(x)$, the BCs, and a 256-greyscale image of the level values   $(P)$*
*of $u(x)$, recover an estimate of $k(x)$ in the form $k(x) = \lambda_1 + \lambda_2 x$.*

Our goal is to define a target function $u_{Target}(x)$ from the input image and then minimize the collage distance in (5). Of course, the amount of noise in the input image (corresponding to $\varepsilon$) induces a corresponding level of imprecision in $u_{Target}(x)$, and in addition there are natural cases to consider.

Case 1: $u_0 \neq u_L$, with min $u = u_0$ and max $u = u_L$, or vice-versa.
In this setting, we are able to approximate the change in $u$ corresponding to a change of one greyscale level: $\frac{|u_L - u_0|}{256}$. As a result, we are able to produce an approximation of the measured and noised $u$ values. Interpolating these values produces $u_{target}(x)$.

Case 2: $u_0 \neq u_L$, not in Case 1.
We remain able to approximate the change in $u$ corresponding to a change of one greyscale level: $\frac{|u_L - u_0|}{|grey(0) - grey(N)|}$, where $grey(p)$ gives the greyscale value of pixel $p$. We are able to produce an approximation of the measured and noised $u$ values. Interpolating these values produces $u_{target}(x)$.

As a case study, we set $f(x) = x(1 - 3x)$. For sake of illustration, in Fig. 1, we show plots of the data values for $u$ recovered from the input image, along with the original (unknown to the inverse problem) numerical solution, for two of the settings. For Cases 1 and 2, we present in Figs. 2 and 3, respectively, the 256-greyscale images obtained as input for the inverse problem, at each resolution and with different levels of relative noise. Striations are present in all of the noised images, but are far more visible in Fig. 3.

Tables 1 and 2 present the results for Cases 1 and 2, respectively, for each value of $N$ and the three values of relative noise. We can make some general observations. In either case, for a fixed noise setting, increasing the value of $N$ (which corresponds to the number of data measurements and, hence, the image resolution) improves the recovery. Also, for a fixed value of $N$, increasing the noise level worsens the results.

We also wish to observe that the magnitude of $f(x)$ plays a significant role in the quality of results. If we instead use $f(x) = 10x(1 - 3x)$, enlarging the range of $f$ values by a factor of 10 compared to the earlier case study, we find the $u$ values, of course, enjoy a similar effect. As a result, the ability to approximate the change in $u$

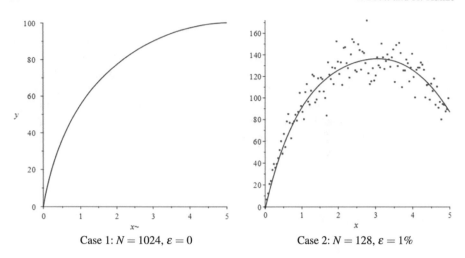

Case 1: $N = 1024$, $\varepsilon = 0$                 Case 2: $N = 128$, $\varepsilon = 1\%$

**Fig. 1** Data values for $u$ recovered from the 256-greyscale image for two settings

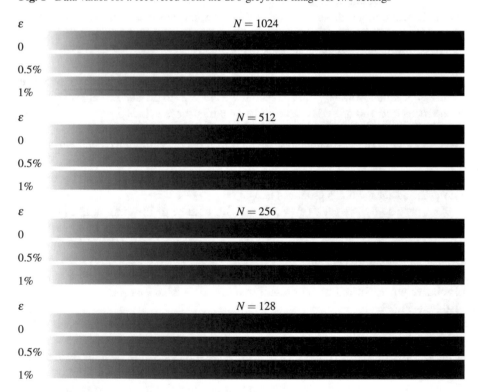

**Fig. 2** Input 256-greyscale isotherm images for case 1

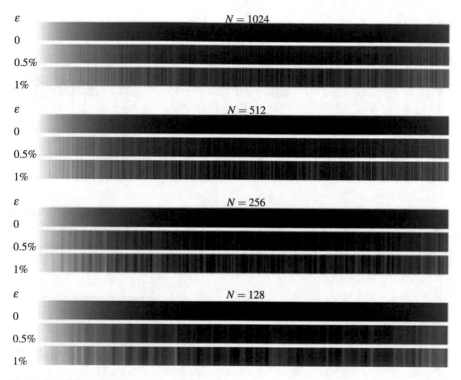

**Fig. 3** Input 256-greyscale isotherm images for case 2

**Table 1** Recovered parameter values for Case 1. True values are $(\lambda_1, \lambda_2) = (1, 3)$

| $\varepsilon = 0$ | | | | $\varepsilon = 0.5\%$ | | | | $\varepsilon = 1\%$ | | | |
|---|---|---|---|---|---|---|---|---|---|---|---|
| $N$ | $\lambda_1$ | $\lambda_2$ | $\Delta^2$ | $N$ | $\lambda_1$ | $\lambda_2$ | $\Delta^2$ | $N$ | $\lambda_1$ | $\lambda_2$ | $\Delta^2$ |
| 1024 | 1.00 | 2.91 | 0.835 | 1024 | 1.01 | 2.95 | 0.839 | 1024 | 1.03 | 3.00 | 0.847 |
| 512 | 1.01 | 2.87 | 0.863 | 512 | 1.02 | 2.89 | 0.865 | 512 | 1.03 | 2.95 | 0.883 |
| 256 | 1.01 | 2.76 | 1.010 | 256 | 1.03 | 2.79 | 1.017 | 256 | 1.04 | 2.85 | 1.045 |
| 128 | 1.05 | 2.59 | 1.540 | 128 | 1.05 | 2.61 | 1.552 | 128 | 1.06 | 2.63 | 1.554 |

corresponding to a change of one grey-scale worsens, and the potential error in the target function grows. In general, the error in our recovered parameters increases. In addition, we can consider the following case.

Case 3: $u_0 = u_L$.

We are not able to approximate the change in $u$ corresponding to a change of one greyscale level. We need one additional bit of information.

**Table 2**  Recovered parameter values for Case 2. True values are $(\lambda_1, \lambda_2) = (1, 3)$

| | $\varepsilon = 0$ | | | | $\varepsilon = 0.5\%$ | | | | $\varepsilon = 1\%$ | | |
|---|---|---|---|---|---|---|---|---|---|---|---|
| $N$ | $\lambda_1$ | $\lambda_2$ | $\Delta^2$ | $N$ | $\lambda_1$ | $\lambda_2$ | $\Delta^2$ | $N$ | $\lambda_1$ | $\lambda_2$ | $\Delta^2$ |
| 1024 | 1.03 | 3.00 | 1.588 | 1024 | 1.03 | 2.96 | 1.656 | 1024 | 1.03 | 2.91 | 2.009 |
| 512 | 1.05 | 2.98 | 1.640 | 512 | 1.02 | 2.89 | 1.975 | 512 | 1.01 | 2.90 | 2.217 |
| 256 | 1.08 | 2.95 | 1.920 | 256 | 1.10 | 3.24 | 2.802 | 256 | 1.12 | 3.59 | 4.091 |
| 128 | 1.17 | 2.88 | 2.930 | 128 | 1.25 | 3.41 | 5.724 | 128 | 1.35 | 3.97 | 9.044 |

In both Case 3 and the setting of an $f$ with a large range, we benefit from the ability to "run the experiment again" and gather new observations using a different $f$. For these cases, we are exploring whether any theoretical tools and results for PDEs can be helpful.

## 1.3  Conclusion

We have performed preliminary exploration of image-driven two-point inverse BVPs using the collage method, with some success. We focused on an academic example similar to those in the existing literature. In the case of different greyscale values at the image endpoints, we demonstrated some reasonable outcomes for problem $(P)$: the larger the resolution of the input image, the better the recovered approximation of $k(x)$; the lower the amplitude $\varepsilon$ of the relative noise in the input image, the better the approximation of $k(x)$; and the approximation of $k(x)$ is reasonable in the case of small $\varepsilon$.

**Acknowledgements**  This research was partially supported by Natural Sciences and Engineering Research Council of Canada (NSERC) in the form of Discovery Grants (HK).

## References

1. Keller, H.: Numerical Methods For Two-Point Boundary-Value Problems. Dover, New York (1992)
2. Vogel, C.R.: Computational Methods for Inverse Problems. SIAM, Philadelphia (2002)
3. Kunze, H., Murdock, S.: Solving inverse two-point boundary value problems using collage coding. Inverse Prob. **22**, 1179–1190 (2006)
4. Levere, K., Kunze, H.: Using the collage method to solve 1-D two-point boundary value inverse problems at steady state. Nonlinear Anal.: Theory Methods Appl. **12**(71), e1487–e1495 (2009)
5. Yodzis, M., Kunze, H.: Collage-based approaches for elliptic partial differential equations inverse problems. In: AIP Conference Proceedings, p. 020176 (2017)

6. Barnsley, M., Ervin, V., Hardin, D., Lancaster, J.: Solution of an inverse problem for fractals and other sets. Proc. Natl. Acad. Sci. **83**, 1975–1977 (1985)
7. Barnsley, M.: Fractals Everywhere. Academic Press, New York (1988)
8. Shelokar, P.S., Siarry, P., Jayaraman, V.K., Kulkarni, B.D.: Particle swarm and ant colony algorithms hybridized for improved continuous optimization. Appl. Math. Comput. **188**(1), 129–142 (2007)
9. Hasanov, A.: An inverse polynomial method for the identication of the leading coecient in the SturmLiouville operator from boundary measurements. Appl. Math. Comput. **140**, 501–515 (2003)
10. Kunze, H., Mendivil, F., La Torre, D., Vrscay, E.: Fractal-Based Methods in Analysis. Springer (2012). ISBN 1461418909

# Circle Inversion IFS

**Maxwell Fitzsimmons and Herb Kunze**

**Abstract** Suppose $C$ is a circle in $\mathbb{R}^2$ with radius $r > 0$ and centre $\tilde{o}$. We can represent $\tilde{x} \in \mathbb{R}^2$ as $\tilde{x} = ar(\cos(\theta), \sin(\theta)) + \tilde{o}$, where $\theta$ is measured from any fixed ray originating from $\tilde{o}$ and $a \geq 0$. The circle inversion map $\tau$ with respect to $C$ is given by

$$\tau(\tilde{x}) = \frac{1}{a}r(\cos(\theta), \sin(\theta)) + \tilde{o},$$

for $x \in \mathbb{R}^2 \setminus \{\tilde{o}\}$. Consider $N$ circles and $N$ associated circle inversion maps. In the literature a modified version of the chaos game is played with these maps to generate pictures [1, 2]. In this work we establish rigorously that there exists an attractor to the iterated function system consisting of modified circle inversion maps, and that the regular chaos game will generate the attractor. We do this by proving that the iterated function systems consisting of certain compositions of these modified, non-expansive circle inversion maps, are contractive.

**Keywords** Fractals · Iterated function systems · Chaos game · Circle inversion

## 1 Introduction

A common algorithm to generate fractals is to use the chaos game with an iterated function system (IFS). Typical IFS theory states [3]

**Theorem 1** *Let $(X, d)$ be a complete metric space and for $i = 1, 2, \ldots, N$ let $f_i : X \to X$ be contraction maps. Then there exists a non-empty compact subset $A$ of $X$ satisfying*

M. Fitzsimmons (✉) · H. Kunze
University of Guelph, 50 Stone Rd E, Guelph, ON, Canada
e-mail: mfitzsim@uoguelph.ca

H. Kunze
e-mail: hkunze@uoguelph.ca

© Springer Nature Switzerland AG 2018
D. M. Kilgour et al. (eds.), *Recent Advances in Mathematical and Statistical Methods*, Springer Proceedings in Mathematics & Statistics 259,
https://doi.org/10.1007/978-3-319-99719-3_8

$$A = \bigcup_{i=1}^{N} f_i(A).$$

*We call A the attractor of the IFS.*

We shall refer to the hypothesis of Theorem 1 as the "finite contractive IFS" hypothesis. The typical way to "draw" an attractor is to play the chaos game.

**Theorem 2** (Chaos Game Theorem) *Let the hypothesis of Theorem 1 hold. Let $\{i_n\}_{n=1}^{\infty}$ be a sequence of numbers such that $i_n \in \{1, 2, \ldots, N\}$ for all $n \in \mathbb{N}$ and for all $n \in \mathbb{N}$ $i_n = k$ with probability $p_k > 0$, where $\Sigma_{k=1}^{N} p_k = 1$. Let A be the attractor of the IFS and let $x_0 \in X$. Then the sequence $\{x_n\}_{n=1}^{\infty}$ defined by $x_n = f_{i_n}(x_{n-1})$ satisfies $\lim_{m \to \infty} d_H(\overline{\{x_n\}_{n=m}^{\infty}}, A) = 0$, where $d_H$ is the Hausdorff metric induced by $(X, d)$. Furthermore if $x_0 \in A$ then $\overline{\{x_n\}_{n=1}^{\infty}} = A$.*

Theorems 1 and 2 are very well known and there has been large amount of research in this area. For example see [4, 5] for some relevant material.

Let $C_i = \{\tilde{x} \in \mathbb{R}^2 | d(\tilde{o}_i, \tilde{x}) \leq r_i\}$ be a closed circle in $\mathbb{R}^2$ with radius $r_i > 0$ and centre $\tilde{o}_i$, where $d$ is the Euclidean metric. Let $[N] = \{n \in \mathbb{N} : n \leq N\}$. Now let $X = \cup_{i \in [N]} C_i$. Then $(X, d)$ is a complete metric space. Let $\tilde{x} \in \mathbb{R}^2 \setminus \{\tilde{o}_i\}$. Then $\forall i \in [N]$, $\tilde{x} = a_i r_i \tilde{\omega}(\theta_i) + \tilde{o}_i$ where $\tilde{\omega}(\theta_i) = (\cos(\theta_i), \sin(\theta_i))$ and $\theta_i \in [0, 2\pi)$ is measured from some fixed ray starting at $\tilde{o}_i$. We call $a_i \geq 0$ the radial scaling factor of $\tilde{x}$ with respect to $C_i$.

**Definition 1** The circle inversion map with respect to $C_i$ is defined by

$$\tau_i(\tilde{x}) = \frac{1}{a_i} r_i \tilde{\omega}(\theta_i) + \tilde{o}_i \, , \, \forall \tilde{x} \in \mathbb{R}^2 \setminus \{\tilde{o}_i\}$$

Previous work concerning these circle inversion maps claim that use of the chaos game will produce a non-random picture of mathematical relevance [1, 2]; see Figs. 1 and 2 for an example of a circle inversion fractal. The authors of [1, 2] briefly justify the use of the chaos game stating the maps are contractive, which they are not (with respect to the Euclidean metric). In fact every point on $\partial C_i$ is a fixed point of $\tau_i$ violating the uniqueness of fixed points of contraction maps. Regardless, the authors suggest the following modification to the chaos game.

Let $x_m \in C_i$ for some $i \in [N]$, where $x_m$ is the last point generated so far by playing the chaos game. If the random number generator picks $i$, pick a new number $j$ until $x_m \notin C_j$ and let $x_{m+1} = \tau_j(x_m)$. This modification prevents the maps from being used where they would be expansive. Using this insight we define the map

**Definition 2** For $\tilde{x} \in X$, define

$$T_i(\tilde{x}) = \begin{cases} \tilde{x} & \tilde{x} \in C_i \\ \dfrac{1}{a_i} r_i \tilde{\omega}(\theta_i) + \tilde{o}_i & \tilde{x} \notin C_i \end{cases}$$

**Fig. 1** Example of a circle
inversion fractal

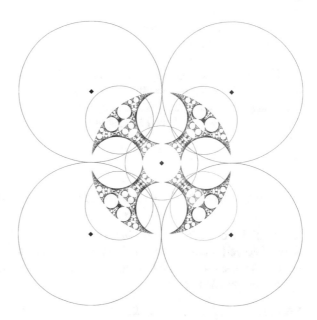

**Fig. 2** Figure 1 without the
inverting circles

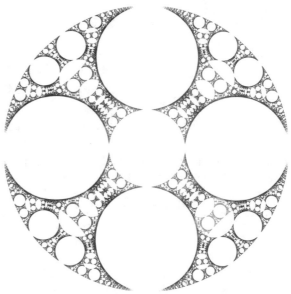

Henceforth the reader should assume the term "circle inversion map" refers to these $T_i$ maps not the $\tau_i$ maps.

One can see that playing the (unmodified) chaos game with these $T_i$ maps is equivalent to playing the modified chaos game outlined above by noticing $T_i \circ T_i = T_i$. Using the $T_i$ maps we will prove that there is a non-empty compact set $A \subseteq X$ that satisfies $A = \bigcup_{i=1}^{N} T_i(A)$ and show that the chaos game played with the $T_i$ maps will "draw" $A$.

## 2  Contractivity of Compositions of Circle Inversion Maps

Contractivity of an IFS is very important in the proof of Theorem 2. So it makes sense that we try to recover this property in some way. As we will see the $T_i$ maps are not contractive, however certain compositions are. To see this we need a series of intermediate results.

**Proposition 1** *For all $\tilde{x}, \tilde{y} \in X$, where $\tilde{x} = a_i \tilde{\omega}(\alpha_i) + \tilde{o}_i$ and $\tilde{y} = b_i r_i \tilde{\omega}(\beta_i) + \tilde{o}_i$, we have*

$$d(T_i(\tilde{x}), T_i(\tilde{y})) \leq w_i(\tilde{x}, \tilde{y}) d(\tilde{x}, \tilde{y}),$$

*where*

$$w_i(\tilde{x}, \tilde{y}) = \begin{cases} 1 & \tilde{x}, \tilde{y} \in C_i \\ \frac{1}{a_i} & \tilde{x} \notin C_i, \tilde{y} \in C_i \\ \frac{1}{b_i} & \tilde{x} \in C_i, \tilde{y} \notin C_i \\ \min\{\frac{1}{a_i}, \frac{1}{b_i}\} & \tilde{x}, \tilde{y} \notin C_i \end{cases}$$

*Proof* It is easy to show that $\tilde{x} \in C_i$ if and only if $a_i \leq 1$. Let $\tilde{x}, \tilde{y} \in X$ be as in the statement of the Proposition. Then we have

$$\begin{aligned} d^2(\tilde{x}, \tilde{y}) &= ||\tilde{x} - \tilde{y}||^2 \\ &= ||(\tilde{x} - \tilde{o}_i) - (\tilde{y} - \tilde{o}_i)||^2 \\ &= r_i^2(a_i^2 + b_i^2 - 2a_i b_i \cos(\alpha_i - \beta_i)). \end{aligned}$$

Suppose $\tilde{x}, \tilde{y} \in C_i$ then $T_i(\tilde{x}) = \tilde{x}$ and $T_i(\tilde{y}) = \tilde{y}$ so $d(T_i(\tilde{x}), T_i(\tilde{y})) = d(\tilde{x}, \tilde{y})$. Without loss of generality let $\tilde{x} \notin C_i$ and $\tilde{y} \in C_i$. Then

$$\begin{aligned} d^2(T_i(\tilde{x}), T_i(\tilde{y})) &= r_i^2\left(\frac{1}{a_i^2} + b_i^2 - 2\frac{1}{a_i}b_i \cos(\alpha_i - \beta_i)\right) \\ &= r_i^2 \frac{1}{a_i^2}\left(1 + a_i^2 b_i^2 - 2a_i b_i \cos(\alpha_i - \beta_i)\right). \end{aligned}$$

If $1 + a_i^2 b_i^2 \leq a_i^2 + b_i^2$ we have our result. Indeed

$$1 + a_i^2 b_i^2 - a_i^2 - b_i^2 = (a_i^2 - 1)(b_i^2 - 1) \leq 0$$

as $a_i^2 \in (1, \infty)$ and $b_i^2 \in [0, 1]$. Thus

$$d^2(T_i(\tilde{x}), T_i(\tilde{y})) \leq r_i^2 \frac{1}{a_i^2}\left(a_i^2 + b_i^2 - 2a_i b_i \cos(\alpha_i - \beta_i)\right) = \frac{1}{a_i^2} d^2(\tilde{x}, \tilde{y}).$$

Now suppose $\tilde{x}, \tilde{y} \notin C_i$ then

$$\begin{aligned}
d^2(T_i(\tilde{x}), T_i(\tilde{y})) &= r_i^2 \left(\frac{1}{a_i^2} + \frac{1}{b_i^2} - 2\frac{1}{a_i b_i} \cos(\alpha_i - \beta_i)\right) \\
&= \frac{1}{a_i^2 b_i^2} r_i^2 \left(b_i^2 + a_i^2 - 2a_i b_i \cos(\alpha_i - \beta_i)\right) \\
&= \frac{1}{a_i^2 b_i^2} d^2(\tilde{x}, \tilde{y}).
\end{aligned}$$

Thus $d(T_i(\tilde{x}), T_i(\tilde{y})) = \frac{1}{a_i b_i} d(\tilde{x}, \tilde{y})$. Since $\frac{1}{a_i}, \frac{1}{b_i} < 1$ their product must be less than either term. $\qquad \square$

We can see that the maps satisfy $d(T_i(\tilde{x}), T_i(\tilde{y})) \leq d(\tilde{x}, \tilde{y})$. We say functions with this property are non-expansive.

The following properties of the $w_i$ functions are not difficult to prove.

**Proposition 2** *For all $\tilde{x}, \tilde{y} \in X$*

1. *$w_i(\tilde{x}, \tilde{y})$ is continuous on $X \times X$*
2. *$w_i(\tilde{x}, \tilde{y}) = 1 \iff \tilde{x}, \tilde{y} \in C_i$*
3. *$w_i(\tilde{x}, \tilde{y}) \leq 1$*

We will now be working exclusively with compositions of the $T_i$ maps, so it is convenient to define a notation for them.

**Definition 3** Let $\Sigma_N^M$ be the set of sequences of length $M$ of numbers from 1 to $N$. That is $\Sigma_N^M = \{\sigma = \sigma_M \sigma_{M-1} \ldots \sigma_1 : \sigma_i \in [N], i \in [M]\}$.

**Definition 4** For $\sigma \in \Sigma_N^M$ and for functions $T_i, i \in [N]$, define

$$T_\sigma = T_{\sigma_M} \circ T_{\sigma_{M-1}} \circ \cdots \circ T_{\sigma_1}.$$

For example, let $\sigma \in \Sigma_3^2$ be $\sigma = 13$. Then $T_{13} = T_1 \circ T_3$.

Contractivity of the composition maps will be a consequence of the following lemma.

**Lemma 1** *Let $\sigma \in \Sigma_N^M$, $\sigma = \sigma_M \sigma_{M-1} \ldots \sigma_1$ and $\tilde{x}, \tilde{y} \in X$. Define $\tilde{x}_{\sigma_i} = T_{\sigma_i}(\tilde{x}_{\sigma_{i-1}})$, $\tilde{x}_{\sigma_0} = \tilde{x}$ and $\tilde{y}_{\sigma_i} = T_{\sigma_i}(\tilde{y}_{\sigma_{i-1}})$, $\tilde{y}_{\sigma_0} = \tilde{y}$. Let*

$$w_\sigma(\tilde{x}, \tilde{y}) = \prod_{i=1}^{M} w_{\sigma_i}(\tilde{x}_{\sigma_{i-1}}, \tilde{y}_{\sigma_{i-1}}).$$

*Then*

1. $d(T_\sigma(\tilde{x}), T_\sigma(\tilde{y})) \le w_\sigma(\tilde{x}, \tilde{y}) d(\tilde{x}, \tilde{y})$,
2. $w_\sigma(\tilde{x}, \tilde{y}) = 1 \iff \tilde{x}, \tilde{y} \in \bigcap_{i=1}^{M} C_{\sigma_i}$.

*Proof* 1. Can be shown by repeated application of Proposition 1.
2. ($\Leftarrow$) If $\tilde{x}, \tilde{y} \in \bigcap_{i=1}^{M} C_{\sigma_i}$ then $T_{\sigma_i}(\tilde{x}) = \tilde{x}$ for all $i \in [M]$. The same results holds
for $\tilde{y}$. By item 2 of Proposition 2 we have $w_{\sigma_i}(x_{\sigma_{i-1}}, y_{\sigma_{i-1}}) = w_{\sigma_i}(\tilde{x}, \tilde{y}) = 1$ for all
$i \in [M]$. Thus $w_\sigma(\tilde{x}, \tilde{y}) = 1$.
($\Rightarrow$) By item 3 of Proposition 2 we can see that if $w_\sigma(\tilde{x}, \tilde{y}) = 1$ then for all $i \in [M]$
we have $w_{\sigma_i}(\tilde{x}_{\sigma_{i-1}}, \tilde{y}_{\sigma_{i-1}}) = 1$. Then by item 2 of Proposition 2 we have for all $i \in$
$[M]$ $\tilde{x}_{\sigma_{i-1}}, \tilde{y}_{\sigma_{i-1}} \in C_{\sigma_i}$. So for all $i \in [M]$ $\tilde{x}_{\sigma_i} = T_{\sigma_i}(\tilde{x}_{\sigma_{i-1}}) = \tilde{x}_{\sigma_{i-1}}$ and we conclude
$\tilde{x}_{\sigma_i} = \tilde{x}_{\sigma_0} = \tilde{x}$. This means $\tilde{x}_{\sigma_{i-1}} = \tilde{x} \in C_{\sigma_i}$ for all $i \in [M]$. We can make the same
argument for $\tilde{y}$ and thus we conclude $\tilde{x}, \tilde{y} \in \cap_{i=1}^{M} C_{\sigma_i}$. $\qquad\square$

It is now finally possible to establish contractivity of appropriate compositions of
the circle inversion maps.

**Theorem 3** *Let $X = \cup_{i=1}^{N} C_i$ and let $\sigma \in \Sigma_N^M$. If $\cap_{i=1}^{M} C_{\sigma_i} = \emptyset$ then $T_\sigma$ is a contraction map on $X$.*

*Proof* By item 2 of Lemma 1 and $\cap_{i=1}^{M} C_{\sigma_i} = \emptyset$, $w_\sigma(\tilde{x}, \tilde{y}) \ne 1$. Furthermore $w_\sigma(\tilde{x}, \tilde{y})$
is the product of numbers $\le 1$ so $w_\sigma(\tilde{x}, \tilde{y}) \le 1$. Thus $w_\sigma(\tilde{x}, \tilde{y}) < 1$ for all $\tilde{x}, \tilde{y} \in X$
because $w_\sigma$ is continuous on $X \times X$ and hence achieves its maximum on $X \times X$.
Let $c_\sigma = \max_{\tilde{x}, \tilde{y} \in X} w_\sigma(\tilde{x}, \tilde{y})$ and we can conclude that $c_\sigma < 1$. By item 1 of Lemma
1 we have $d(T_\sigma(\tilde{x}), T_\sigma(\tilde{y})) \le c_\sigma d(\tilde{x}, \tilde{y})$. Therefore $T_\sigma$ is contractive. $\qquad\square$

It should be noted that the converse of the above theorem holds but is omitted due
to space constraints.
To avoid confusion, one should note that $\cap_{i=1}^{N} C_i = \emptyset$ does not imply that there
there is $i, j \in [N]$ such that $C_i \cap C_j = \emptyset$.

## 3 Infinite IFS and the Chaos Game with Circle Inversion Maps

Now, if we assume that $\cap_{i=1}^{N} C_i = \emptyset$, we have contraction maps of appropriate compositions of circle inversion maps. For notational convenience we introduce a definition.

**Definition 5** Let $M, N \in \mathbb{N}$ and $X = \cup_{i=1}^{N} C_i$. Then define

$$E_N^M = \{\sigma \in \Sigma_N^M : T_\sigma \text{ such that } \cap_{i=1}^{M} C_{\sigma_i} = \emptyset\}.$$

We can see that $\sigma \in E_N^M \implies T_\sigma$ is contractive by Theorem 3. We could apply finite contractive IFS theory to say: for any $M \in \mathbb{N}$ with $M \geq N$, there is a compact non-empty set $A_M \subseteq X$ that satisfies

$$A_M = \bigcup_{\sigma \in E_N^M} T_\sigma(A_M).$$

And we could play the chaos game with the composition maps in order to draw $A_M$. However we wish to play the chaos game with the the individual $T_i$ maps. One can show that if $\{\tilde{x}_i\}_{i \in \mathbb{N}}$ is the set of points made by the chaos game (with initial point starting on the attractor) then $\overline{\{\tilde{x}_i\}_{i \in \mathbb{N}}} \supseteq A_M$. In order to get $\{\tilde{x}_i\}_{i \in \mathbb{N}} \subseteq A_M$ we must have the result that for all $i \in [N]$, $T_i(A_M) \subseteq A_M$. We do not believe this result holds (for general $X$ with $\cap_{i=1}^N C_i = \emptyset$) for any $M$).

Thus we appeal to infinite IFS theory, particularly [6]. But first we need the following result.

**Lemma 2** *Let $X = \cup_{i=1}^N C_i$ with $\cap_{i=1}^N C_i = \emptyset$. Let the set of contraction factors of the $T_\sigma$ maps be*

$$\mathscr{C} = \left\{ c_\sigma : \exists M \in \mathbb{N}, \ \sigma \in E_N^M, \ c_\sigma = \max_{\tilde{x}, \tilde{y} \in X} w_\sigma(\tilde{x}, \tilde{y}) \right\}.$$

*Then $1 \notin \overline{\mathscr{C}}$.*

*Proof* Aside: Let $B \subseteq X$ then for all $x \in X$ define $d(x, B) = \inf_{b \in B} d(x, b)$. Suppose otherwise. Then there is a sequence of contraction factors $\{c_{\sigma^n}\}_{n \in \mathbb{N}} \to 1$ where each $\sigma^n \in E_N^{M_n}$ for some $M_n \in \mathbb{N}$. Recall that each $c_{\sigma^n} = \max_{\tilde{x}, \tilde{y} \in X} w_{\sigma^n}(\tilde{x}, \tilde{y})$. Since $X$ is compact, the max is achieved on $X$. For $n \in \mathbb{N}$ let $c_{\sigma^n} = w_{\sigma^n}(\tilde{x}_n, \tilde{y}_n)$. Also recall for all $i \in [M_n]$

$$w_{\sigma^n}(\tilde{x}_n, \tilde{y}_n) = \prod_{j=1}^{M_n} w_{\sigma_j^n}(\tilde{x}_{\sigma_{j-1}^n}, \tilde{y}_{\sigma_{j-1}^n}) \leq w_{\sigma_i^n}(\tilde{x}_{\sigma_{i-1}^n}, \tilde{y}_{\sigma_{i-1}^n}) \tag{1}$$

where $\tilde{x}_{\sigma_j^n} = T_{\sigma_j^n}(\tilde{x}_{\sigma_{j-1}^n})$ for $j \in [M_n]$ and $\tilde{x}_{\sigma_0^n} = \tilde{x}_n$. Make the analogous definition for the $\tilde{y}_{\sigma_j^n}$.

We claim that $\forall \delta > 0 \ \exists K \in \mathbb{N}$ such that $\forall n \geq K \ \forall i \in [M_n] \ d(\tilde{x}_{\sigma_{i-1}^n}, C_{\sigma_i^n}) < \delta$ and $d(\tilde{y}_{\sigma_{i-1}^n}, C_{\sigma_i^n}) < \delta$. By assumption we have for all $\varepsilon > 0$ there is a $K \in \mathbb{N}$ such that for all $n \geq K$ and for all $i \in [M_n]$

$$|1 - w_{\sigma^n}(\tilde{x}_n, \tilde{y}_n)| < \varepsilon$$
$$1 - w_{\sigma^n}(\tilde{x}_n, \tilde{y}_n) < \varepsilon$$
$$1 - \varepsilon < w_{\sigma^n}(\tilde{x}_n, \tilde{y}_n) \leq w_{\sigma_i^n}(\tilde{x}_{\sigma_{i-1}^n}, \tilde{y}_{\sigma_{i-1}^n}) \qquad \text{using (1)}$$
$$1 - \varepsilon < w_{\sigma_i^n}(\tilde{x}_{\sigma_{i-1}^n}, \tilde{y}_{\sigma_{i-1}^n}) \tag{2}$$

Let $\delta > 0$. Pick $\varepsilon = \min\left\{\frac{\delta}{a_{\max}}, \frac{\delta}{r_{\max}a_{\max}}\right\}$ and $a_{\max} = \max_{j \in [N]} \max_{\tilde{z} \in X} e_j$ and $e_j$, where is the radial scaling factor of $\tilde{z}$ with respect to $C_j$ and $r_{\max} = \max_{j \in [N]} r_j$. Let $a_{\sigma_i^n}$ be the radial scaling factor of $\tilde{x}_{\sigma_{i-1}^n}$ with respect to circle $C_{\sigma_i^n}$; similarly, let $b_{\sigma_i^n}$ be the radial scaling factor of $\tilde{y}_{\sigma_{i-1}^n}$ with respect to circle $C_{\sigma_i^n}$.

Case 1: $\tilde{x}_{\sigma_{i-1}^n}, \tilde{y}_{\sigma_{i-1}^n} \in C_{\sigma_i}$. Then $d(\tilde{x}_{\sigma_{i-1}^n}, C_{\sigma_i^n}) = 0$ and $d(\tilde{y}_{\sigma_{i-1}^n}, C_{\sigma_i^n}) = 0$. And we are done.

Case 2: $\tilde{y}_{\sigma_{i-1}^n} \in C_{\sigma_i}$ and $\tilde{x}_{\sigma_{i-1}^n} \notin C_{\sigma_i}$. Then $d(\tilde{y}_{\sigma_{i-1}^n}, C_{\sigma_i^n}) = 0$ and $w_{\sigma_i^n}(\tilde{x}_{\sigma_{i-1}^n}, \tilde{y}_{\sigma_{i-1}^n}) = \frac{1}{a_{\sigma_i^n}}$. By (2) we have $1 - \varepsilon < \frac{1}{a_{\sigma_i^n}}$, so we can say that $|1 - a_{\sigma_i^n}| < \varepsilon a_{\sigma_i^n} < \delta$. Let $\tilde{x}' = \frac{\tilde{x}_{\sigma_{i-1}^n} - \tilde{o}_{\sigma_i^n}}{a_{\sigma_i^n}} + \tilde{o}_{\sigma_i^n}$. Then $\tilde{x}' \in C_{\sigma_i}$ and $d(\tilde{x}_{\sigma_{i-1}^n}, \tilde{x}') = |1 - a_{\sigma_i^n}|r_{\sigma_i^n} < \varepsilon\, r_{\max}a_{\max} < \delta$. Thus $d(\tilde{x}_{\sigma_{i-1}^n}, C_{\sigma_i}) < \delta$.

Case 3: $\tilde{x}_{\sigma_{i-1}^n}, \tilde{y}_{\sigma_{i-1}^n} \notin C_{\sigma_i}$. Notice that

$$w_{\sigma_i^n}(\tilde{x}_{\sigma_{i-1}^n}, \tilde{y}_{\sigma_{i-1}^n}) \leq \min\left\{\frac{1}{a_{\sigma_i^n}}, \frac{1}{b_{\sigma_i^n}}\right\} \leq \max\left\{\frac{1}{a_{\sigma_i^n}}, \frac{1}{b_{\sigma_i^n}}\right\}.$$

From here the proof is identical to case 2.

Thus the claim is proved.

Now the sequence $\{\tilde{x}_n\}_{n \in \mathbb{N}}$ has a convergent subsequence by compactness, say $\{\tilde{x}_{n_k}\}_{k \in \mathbb{N}} \to \tilde{x}^*$. Since $\cap_{j \in [N]} C_j = \emptyset$ there is an $i \in [N]$ such that $\tilde{x}^* \notin C_i$. Let $0 < q = \min_{j \in [N]} {}_{\tilde{x}^* \notin C_j}\, d(\tilde{x}^*, C_j)$ and pick $\delta < \frac{q}{2}$. Then there is a $K \in \mathbb{N}$ such that for all $k \geq K$ we have $d(\tilde{x}^*, \tilde{x}_{n_k}) < \delta$ and for all $j \in [N]$ $d(\tilde{x}_{\sigma_j^{n_k}}, C_{\sigma_j^{n_k}}) < \delta$. Fix $k$ and pick $j \in [M_n]$ such that it is the least such $j$ with $T_{\sigma_j^{n_k}}(\tilde{x}^*) \neq \tilde{x}^*$, implying $T_{\sigma_{j-1}^{n_k}\sigma_{j-2}^{n_k}...\sigma_1^{n_k}}(\tilde{x}^*) = \tilde{x}^*$. Then we can see that

$$d(x^*, \tilde{x}_{\sigma_{j-1}^{n_k}}) = d(T_{\sigma_{j-1}^{n_k}\sigma_{j-2}^{n_k}...\sigma_1^{n_k}}(\tilde{x}^*), T_{\sigma_{j-1}^{n_k}\sigma_{j-2}^{n_k}...\sigma_1^{n_k}}(\tilde{x}_{n_k})) \leq d(\tilde{x}^*, \tilde{x}_{n_k}) < \delta.$$

Now consider $q \leq d(\tilde{x}^*, C_{\sigma_j^{n_k}}) \leq d(\tilde{x}^*, \tilde{x}_{\sigma_{j-1}^{n_k}}) + d(\tilde{x}_{\sigma_{j-1}^{n_k}}, C_{\sigma_j^{n_k}}) < 2\delta < q$. This is a contradiction.

Thus there is no such sequence of contraction factors and we conclude that $1 \notin \overline{\mathscr{C}}$. $\qquad \square$

Lemma 2 gives us this immediate result.

**Lemma 3** *Let* $X = \cup_{i=1}^{N} C_i$ *with* $\cap_{i=1}^{N} C_i = \emptyset$. *Then for all* $\sigma \in \bigcup_{M=N}^{\infty} E_N^M$ *there is a* $c \in [0, 1)$ *for all* $\tilde{x}, \tilde{y} \in X$ *such that*

$$d(T_\sigma(\tilde{x}), T_\sigma(\tilde{y})) \leq cd(\tilde{x}, \tilde{y}).$$

*Proof* By Lemma 2 we know that $c^* = \sup_{c \in \mathscr{C}} c < 1$. This means that $c^*$ is the largest contraction factor of any contractive composition map. And the result follows. $\quad\square$

Lemma 3 allows us to apply Theorem 1 of [6].

**Theorem 4** *Let* $X = \cup_{i=1}^{N} C_i$ *with* $\cap_{i=1}^{N} C_i = \emptyset$. *Then there exists a non-empty set* $A \subseteq X$ *satisfying*

$$A = \bigcup_{i=N}^{\infty} \bigcup_{\sigma \in E_N^i} T_\sigma(A).$$

*Proof* There are countably many maps $T_\sigma$ in the union. And by Lemma 3 we satisfy the hypothesis of Theorem 1 from [6]. As $X$ is bounded we trivially satisfy (i) of Theorem 1. Thus from (iv) of Theorem 1, we have the result. $\quad\square$

**Theorem 5** *Let* $X = \cup_{i=1}^{N} C_i$ *with* $\cap_{i=1}^{N} C_i = \emptyset$. *Then A as described in Theorem 4 satisfies the following:*

$$1. \ \forall i \in [N] \ T_i(A) \subseteq A$$
$$2. \ A = \bigcup_{i=1}^{N} T_i(A).$$

*Proof* 1. Let $i \in [N]$. By Theorem 3.3, $T_i(A) = \bigcup_{k=N}^{\infty} \bigcup_{\sigma \in E_N^k} T_i \circ T_\sigma(A)$. For $\sigma \in E_N^k$ for some $k$ then we must have $i\sigma = i\sigma_k\sigma_{k-1}\ldots\sigma_1 \in E_N^{k+1}$ as the composition of a non-expansive map with a contractive map is a contractive map. Thus we can see that

$$T_i(A) \subseteq \bigcup_{k=N+1}^{\infty} \bigcup_{\sigma \in E_N^k} T_\sigma(A) \subseteq \bigcup_{k=N}^{\infty} \bigcup_{\sigma \in E_N^k} T_\sigma(A) \subseteq A$$

2. $\bigcup_{i=1}^{N} T_i(A) \subseteq A$ follows immediately from item 1. Let $i \in [N]$, $j \in \mathbb{N}$ and $\gamma \in \Sigma_N^j$. From item 1 it is easy to show that $T_\gamma(A) \subseteq A$. Applying $T_i$ to both sides yields $T_{i\gamma}(A) \subseteq T_i(A)$. By picking $j$ and $\gamma$ carefully we can make $i\gamma$ be any sequence $\sigma$ of $E_N^k$, for any $k \in \mathbb{N}$, so long as $\sigma$ ends with $i$. Thus we can say

$$\bigcup_{k=N}^{\infty} \bigcup_{\sigma \in E_N^k} T_\sigma(A) = A \subseteq \bigcup_{i=1}^{N} T_i(A).$$

Therefore $A = \bigcup_{i=1}^{N} T_i(A)$. $\quad\square$

Item 2 of Theorem 5 is an identity we usually see with finite contractive IFS as in Theorem 1. It is a useful and conceptually pleasing result to have. As discussed earlier, item 1 of Theorem 5 is of immediate importance, since it is very useful in regards to the chaos game.

**Theorem 6** *Let $X = \cup_{i=1}^N C_i$ with $\cap_{i=1}^N C_i = \emptyset$, let $A$ be as described in Theorem 4 and let $\{\tilde{x}_n\}_{n=1}^\infty$ be the sequence of points generated by the chaos game played with the individual maps $T_i$, $i \in [N]$, with initial point $\tilde{x}_0 \in A$. Then $\overline{\{\tilde{x}_n\}_{n=1}^\infty} = \overline{A}$.*

*Proof* Let $\{i_n\}_{n=1}^\infty$ be the sequence of random numbers from 1 to N, with each number from 1 to N picked with probability greater than zero, such that for all $n \geq 1$ $\tilde{x}_n = T_{i_n}(\tilde{x}_{n-1})$. We show that $\{\tilde{x}_n\}_{n=1}^\infty$ is dense on $A$. Let $\tilde{a}_0 \in A$. Then there is $j_1 \in \mathbb{N}$, $j_1 \geq N$, $\sigma^1 \in E_N^{j_1}$ and $\tilde{a}_1 \in A$ such that $\tilde{a}_0 = T_{\sigma^1}(\tilde{a}_1)$. Since $\tilde{a}_1 \in A$ we do this again. Suppose we did this $k \in \mathbb{N}$ times. Thus there is a sequence of contraction maps $T_{\sigma^\ell}$ satisfying $\tilde{a}_0 = T_{\sigma^1} \circ T_{\sigma^2} \circ \cdots \circ T_{\sigma^k}(\tilde{a}_k)$. The map $T_{\sigma^1} \circ T_{\sigma^2} \circ \cdots \circ T_{\sigma^k}$ is just some composition of individual $T_i$ maps, $i \in [N]$. Thus there is an $M \in \mathbb{N}$ and a $\gamma \in \Sigma_N^M$ such that $T_{\sigma^1} \circ T_{\sigma^2} \circ \cdots \circ T_{\sigma^k} = T_\gamma$. A property of $\{i_n\}_{n=1}^\infty$ is that, with probability 1, it will contain any finite sequence of the numbers 1 to N infinitely often (this is sometimes referred to as the Infinite Monkey Theorem). Thus there are $m_1, m_2 \in \mathbb{N}$ with $m_1 \leq m_2$ such that $\tilde{x}_{m_2} = T_\gamma(\tilde{x}_{m_1})$. So

$$
\begin{aligned}
d(\tilde{x}_{m_2}, \tilde{a}_0) &= d(T_\gamma(\tilde{x}_{m_1}), T_\gamma(\tilde{a}_k)) \\
&= d(T_{\sigma^1} \circ T_{\sigma^2} \circ \cdots \circ T_{\sigma^k}(\tilde{x}_{m_1}), T_{\sigma^1} \circ T_{\sigma^2} \circ \cdots \circ T_{\sigma^k}(\tilde{a}_k)) \\
&\leq c^k d(\tilde{x}_{m_1}, \tilde{a}_k) \\
&\leq c^k diam(A),
\end{aligned}
$$

where $diam(A)$ is the diameter of $A$ and $c \in [0, 1)$ is the contraction factor from Lemma 3. Thus $\overline{\{\tilde{x}_n\}_{n=1}^\infty} \supseteq \overline{A}$. By item 1 of Theorem 5 $T_i(A) \subseteq A$. Since $x_0 \in A$ it follows that $\{\tilde{x}_n\}_{n=1}^\infty \subseteq A$. Therefore $\overline{\{\tilde{x}_n\}_{n=1}^\infty} = \overline{A}$. $\qquad \square$

The above Theorem can be extended to include a result involving the starting point $x_0 \in X$ where $x_0$ is not necessarily in $A$.

**Corollary 1** *Let $X = \cup_{i=1}^N C_i$ with $\cap_{i=1}^N C_i = \emptyset$, $A$ be as described in Theorem 4, and $\{\tilde{x}_n\}_{n=1}^\infty$ be the sequence of points generated by the chaos game played with the individual maps $T_i, i \in [N]$, with initial point $\tilde{x}_0 \in X$. Then*

$$
\lim_{m \to \infty} d_H(\overline{\{\tilde{x}_n\}_{n=m}^\infty}, \overline{A}) = 0.
$$

This result follows by playing the chaos game twice with the one random infinite string and two initial points $x_0 \in X$ and $a_0 \in A$ then recalling the $T_i$ maps are non-expansive.

# 4 Conclusions

It can be seen now that the use of the modified chaos game in [1, 2] is justified. We have shown that for $X = \cup_{i=1}^{N} C_i$ with $\cap_{i=1}^{N} C_i = \emptyset$ there exists a non-empty set $A$ satisfying $A = \cup_{i=1}^{N} T_i(A)$ and that playing the chaos game with the $T_i$ maps will produce $\overline{A}$.

**Acknowledgements** This research was partially supported by the Natural Sciences and Engineering Research Council of Canada (NSERC) in the form of a Discovery Grant (HK).

# References

1. Clancy, C., Frame, M.: Fractal geometry of restricted sets of circle inversions. Fractals **3**(4) (1995)
2. Frame, M., Cogevina, T.: An infinite circle inversion limit set fractal. Comput. Graph. **24**(5) (2000)
3. Hutchinson, J.E.: Fractals and self similarity. Indiana Univ. Math. J. **30**(5), 713–747 (1981)
4. Mauldin, R.D., Urbański, M.: Graph Directed Markov Systems. Cambridge University Press (2003)
5. Boreland, B., Kunze, H.: Function representation with circle inversion map systems. In: AIP Conference Proceedings, vol. 1798, No. 1, p. 020179. AIP Publishing (2017)
6. Gwóźdź-Lukawska G., Jachymski J.: The Hutchinson-Barnsley theory for infinite iterated function systems. Bull. Aust. Math. Soc. **72**(3) (2005) https://doi.org/10.1017/S0004972700035267

# Inverse Problems and Total Variation Minimization for Iterated Function Systems on Maps

Herb Kunze and Davide La Torre

**Abstract** We consider the inverse problem associated with iterated function system with greyscale maps (IFSM): Given a target function $f$, find an IFSM, such that its fixed point $\bar{f}$ is sufficiently close to $f$ in the $L^p$ distance. In this paper, we extend the collage-based method by adding a total variation term to the collage distance, with the notion that the solution to this modified minimization problem turns out to be less noisy than the one without this term. Numerical experiments are provided.

**Keywords** Iterated function systems on maps · Total variation · Inverse problem

## 1 Introduction

In fractal image coding based on Generalized Fractal Transforms (GFT), one seeks to approximate a target image or signal by the fixed point of a contractive fractal transform operator (see [9] and the references therein).

The usual formulation involves a fixed set of geometric contraction maps along with a corresponding set of greyscale maps. The inverse problem, which involves the determination of the best greyscale map parameters for a given target image, is based on the so-called "collage theorem," a simple consequence of Banach's fixed point theorem.

H. Kunze (✉)
Department of Mathematics and Statistics, University of Guelph, N1G 2W1 Guelph, Canada
e-mail: hkunze@uoguelph.ca

D. La Torre
Department of Economics, Management and Quantitative Methods,
University of Milan, 20122 Milan, Italy
e-mail: davide.latorre@unimi.it

D. La Torre
Dubai Business School, University of Dubai, 14143 Dubai, UAE
e-mail: dlatorre@ud.ac.ae

© Springer Nature Switzerland AG 2018
D. M. Kilgour et al. (eds.), *Recent Advances in Mathematical and Statistical Methods*, Springer Proceedings in Mathematics & Statistics 259,
https://doi.org/10.1007/978-3-319-99719-3_9

Another consequence of Banach's fixed point result is that the approximation of the target image or signal can be generated by iteration of the fractal transform. In [3] and [4], the authors showed that one can find an iterated function system on greyscale maps to approximate any target signal or image with arbitrary precision, and they provided a suboptimal but systematic approach for doing so.

In [10] the authors extend the approach developed in [3] along two different directions: first they search for a set of maps and greyscale map parameters that not only minimizes the collage error but also maximizes the entropy of the parameter set and, second, they try to maximize the sparsity of the set of greyscale parameters. In their formulation, the minimization of the collage error is studied as a multi-criteria problem. Three different and conflicting criteria are considered, namely collage error, entropy and sparsity, and the problem is reduced to a single-criterion model by means of a scalarization that combines all objective functions with different trade-off weights.

In [12] the authors show that under certain hypotheses, an IFSM is a contraction on the complete space of functions of bounded variation (BV). It then possesses a unique attractor of BV. The authors also present some BV-based inverse problems based on the collage theorem for contraction maps.

The notions of total variation (TV) or bounded variation have had several applications in image analysis and, in particular, in noise removal. The main justification of this comes from the fact signals with spurious detail have high total variation (see [16]). The process of reducing the total variation of the signal removes unwanted detail whilst preserving important details such as edges. Several definitions of total variation are available in the literature, one can see [5, 13] for an overview of many of the most recently used ones and lengthy reference lists. In the classical approach (see, for example, [2, 14], the total variation of a differentiable greyscale image $f : \mathbb{R}^n \to \mathbb{R}$ is defined as follows,

$$\|f\|_{TV} = \int_X \|\nabla f(x)\|_2 \, dx, \tag{1}$$

that is, the integral of the $\| \cdot \|_2$ norm of the gradient.

A typical TV-based denoising problem will have the following form: Given a noisy image (function) $f^*$, solve the following optimization problem,

$$\min_{f \in \mathscr{F}} d_Y(f^*, f) + \lambda \|f\|_{TV}$$

where $\mathscr{F}$ denotes an appropriate space of functions representing the images. The first term in the objective function is the the so-called *data fitting* term, which imposes the condition that the denoised image $f$ should be close to the noisy data $f^*$. The second term is the TV regularization term – higher values of the regularization parameter $\lambda > 0$ will, in general, yield solutions $f(\lambda)$ with lower TV.

In this paper, we examine the idea of TV-based denoising applied to the inverse problem for iterated function systems on gresycale maps. In other words, the above space $\mathscr{F}$ turns out to be the space of all fractal fixed point solutions to an IFSM operator. Because in general the solution to a fixed point equation involving the IFSM operator are non-differentiable in nature, it makes no sense to calculate a TV-norm. Instead we replace the TV norm with the distance from a ideally denoised function: For our purposes we consider a flat and constant function $\tilde{f}$ that is equal to the average of the target $f^*$ over $X$, that is

$$\tilde{f} = \frac{1}{\mu_L(X)} \int_X f^*(x) d\mu_L$$

where $\mu_L$ is the Lebesgue measure on $X$. The above TV-norm is then replaced by the following term

$$d_Y(f, \tilde{f})$$

and the inverse problem with total variation minimization problem takes the form

$$\min_{f \in \mathscr{F}} d_Y(f^*, f) + \lambda d_Y(f, \tilde{f})$$

## 2   Iterated Function Systems on Maps

The action of a GFT $T : X \rightarrow X$ on an element $u$ of the complete metric space $(X, d)$ can be summarized in the following steps. It produces a set of $N$ spatially-contracted copies of $u$ and then it modifies the values of these copies by means of a suitable range-mapping. Finally, it recombines them using an appropriate operator in order to get the element $v \in X$, $v = Tu$ [1, 6, 9, 11].

In all these cases, under appropriate conditions, the fractal transform $T$ is a contraction and thus Banach's fixed point theorem guarantees the existence of a unique fixed point $\bar{u} = T\bar{u}$.

The inverse problem is a key factor for applications: given a "target" element $v \in X$, we look for a point-to-point contraction mapping $T$ with fixed point $\bar{u}$ such that $d(v, \bar{u})$ is as small as possible. In practical applications, however, it is difficult to construct solutions to this problem and one relies on the following simple consequence of Banach's fixed point theorem, known in the fractal coding literature as the *collage theorem*, which states that

$$d(v, \bar{u}) \leq \frac{1}{1 - c} d(v, Tv) \tag{2}$$

($c$ is the contractivity factor of $T$). Instead of trying to minimize the error $d(v, \bar{u})$, one looks for a contraction mapping $T$ that minimizes the *collage error $d(v, Tv)$*.

In this section we focus on the method of iterated function systems on greyscale maps, as formulated in [3]. IFSMs extend the classical notion of iterated function systems (IFS) [9] and can be used to generate integrable "fractal" functions (see [7], [8]). An IFSM can be used to approximate a given element $u$ of $L^2([0, 1])$. We consider the case in which $u : [0, 1] \to [0, 1]$ and the space

$$X = \left\{ u : [0, 1] \to [0, 1], u \in L^2[0, 1] \right\}. \tag{3}$$

The ingredients of an $N$-map IFSM on $X$ are

1. a set of $N$ contractive maps $w = \{w_1, w_2, \ldots, w_N\}$, $w_i(x) : [0, 1] \to [0, 1]$, most often affine in form:

$$w_i(x) = s_i x + a_i, \quad 0 \le s_i < 1, \quad i = 1, 2, \ldots, N; \tag{4}$$

2. a set of associated functions—the greyscale maps— $\phi = \{\phi_1, \phi_2, \ldots, \phi_N\}$, $\phi_i : R \to R$. Affine maps are usually employed:

$$\phi_i(t) = \alpha_i t + \beta_i, \tag{5}$$

with the conditions

$$\alpha_i, \beta_i \in [0, 1] \tag{6}$$

and

$$0 \le \sum_{i=1}^{N} \alpha_i + \beta_i < 1. \tag{7}$$

Associated with the $N$-map IFSM $(w, \phi)$ is the *fractal transform* operator $T$, the action of which on a function $u \in X$ is given by

$$(Tu)(x) = \sum_{i=1}^{N}{}' \phi_i(u(w_i^{-1}(x))), \tag{8}$$

where the prime means that the sum operates on all those terms for which $w_i^{-1}$ is defined.

**Theorem 1** [3] $T : X \to X$ *and for any* $u, v \in X$ *we have*

$$d_2(Tu, Tv) \le C d_2(u, v) \tag{9}$$

*where*

$$C = \sum_{i=1}^{N} s_i^{\frac{1}{2}} \alpha_i \tag{10}$$

*and $d_2$ is the $L^2$ metric,*

$$d_2(u, v) = \left( \int_0^1 (u(x) - v(x))^2 \, dx \right)^{\frac{1}{2}}. \tag{11}$$

When $C < 1$, then $T$ is contractive on $X$, implying the existence of a unique fixed point $\bar{u} \in X$ such that $\bar{u} = T\bar{u}$.

The inverse problem associated with IFSM can, in principle, be solved to arbitrary accuracy, using a procedure defined in Forte and Vrscay [3]. The squared collage distance function associated with an $N$-map IFSM may be written as a quadratic form,

$$\Delta_N^2(z) = z^T A z + b^T z + c, \tag{12}$$

where $z = (\alpha_1, \ldots, \alpha_N, \beta_1, \ldots, \beta_N)$. The maps $w_k$ are chosen from an infinite set $W$ of fixed affine contraction maps on $[0, 1]$ which satisfy the following properties.

**Definition 1** We say that $W$ generates an $m$-dense and nonoverlapping family $A$ of subsets of $I$ if for every $\epsilon > 0$ and every $B \subset I$ there exists a finite set of integers $i_k, i_k \geq 1, 1 \leq k \leq N$, such that

1. $A = \cup_{k=1}^N w_{i_k}(I) \subset B$,
2. $m(B \backslash A) < \epsilon$, and
3. $m(w_{i_k}(I) \cap w_{i_l}(I)) = 0$ if $k \neq l$,

where $m$ denotes Lebesgue measure.

Let

$$W^N = \{w_1, \ldots w_N\} \tag{13}$$

be the $N$ truncations of $w$. Let $\Phi^N = \{\phi_1, \ldots, \phi_N\}$ be the $N$-vector of affine greyscale maps. Let $\Omega$ be a compact subset of set $R^{2N}$ which describes the set of all possible constraints and let $z_N$ be the solution of the previous quadratic optimization problem over $\Omega$. Let $\Delta_{N,min}^2 = \Delta_N^2(z_N)$. In Forte and Vrscay [3], the following result was proved.

**Theorem 2** [3]

$$\Delta_{N,min}^2 \to 0 \text{ as } N \to \infty.$$

Using the collage theorem, the inverse problem may be solved to arbitrary accuracy. A practical choice for the contraction maps $w$ on $X = [0, 1]$ is

$$w_{ij}(x) = 2^{-i}(x + j - 1), \quad i = 1, 2, \ldots, M, \quad j = 1, 2, \ldots, 2^i, \tag{14}$$

where

$$N = \sum_{i=1}^M 2^i.$$

## 3  Iterated Function Systems on Functions of Bounded Variation

In this section we show that, under some hypotheses, an IFSM operator is a contraction with respect to the usual norm introduced into the space of functions of bounded variation.

**Definition 2** The *total variation* of a function $f : [a, b] \to \mathbb{R}$ is defined as

$$V_a^b(f) = \sup_{P \in \mathscr{P}} \sum_{j=0}^{n} |f(x_{j+1}) - f(x_j)|, \tag{15}$$

where the supremum is taken over the set of all partitions of $[a, b]$,

$$\mathscr{P} = \{P = \{x_0, \dots, x_n\} | P \text{ is a partition of } [a, b], x_0 = a, x_n = b\} .$$

If $f : [a, b] \to \mathbb{R}$ is differentiable and its derivative is Riemann-integrable, its total variation is given by

$$V_a^b(f) = \int_a^b |f'(x)| \, dx . \tag{16}$$

**Definition 3** A real-valued function $f : [a, b] \to \mathbb{R}$ is said to be of *bounded variation* (or a "BV function") on $[a, b]$ if its total variation is finite, i.e. $V_a^b(f) < +\infty$. Let us denote by $BV([a, b])$ the space of functions of bounded variation on $[a, b]$.

**Theorem 3** [15] *The functional $f \to |f(a)| + V_a^b f$ is a norm over $BV([a, b])$. We shall denote this norm as $\|f\|_{BV}$. The normed space $(BV([a, b]), \|f\|_{BV})$ is complete.*

In addition, the following covering condition on the $w_i$ is assumed:

$$[a, b] = \bigcup_{i=1}^{N} w_i([a, b]) . \tag{17}$$

Associated with the IFSM $(\mathbf{w}, \Phi)$ is a so-called *IFSM operator* or *fractal transform* on the space of $L^p$ integrable functions on $[a, b]$ via the action

$$Tf(x) = \sum_{i=1}^{N} \phi_i(f(w_i^{-1}(x))), \tag{18}$$

where the sum operates on all those terms for which $w_i^{-1}(x)$ is defined.

For the remainder of this paper, we assume that the IFS maps $w_i : [a, b] \rightarrow [a, b]$ and associated maps $\phi_i : \mathbb{R} \rightarrow \mathbb{R}$ are affine, i.e.,

$$w_i(x) = s_i x + a_i \quad \text{and} \quad \phi_i(t) = \alpha_i t + \beta_i \quad \text{so that} \quad K_i = |\alpha_i|. \tag{19}$$

**Theorem 4** [12] *The operator $T$ defined in* Eq. (18) *maps* $BV([a, b])$ *into itself.*

**Theorem 5** [12] *For $f, g \in BV([a, b])$,*

$$\|Tf - Tg\|_{BV} \leq K\|f - g\|_{BV} \quad \text{where} \quad K = \sum_{i=1}^{N} K_i. \tag{20}$$

**Theorem 6** [12] *If $K$ in* Eq. (20) *satisfies $K < 1$, then the IFSM operator $T$ possesses a unique fixed point $\bar{f} \in BV([a, b])$. Moreover, for all $f_0 \in BV([a, b])$, the sequence $T^n f_0$ converges to $\bar{f}$ when $n \rightarrow +\infty$. Finally, the following estimate holds*

$$\|f\|_{BV} \leq \frac{\sum_{i=1}^{N} |\beta_i|}{1 - K}. \tag{21}$$

Note that the condition $K < 1$ implies that $\bar{f} \in L^\infty([a, b])$, as expected.

**Theorem 7** [12] *If (i) the maps $w_i$ are non-overlapping, (ii) $K = \sum_{i=1}^{N} K_i > 1$, and (iii) $\sum_{i=1}^{N} c_i^{1/p} K_i < 1$, then $T$ possesses a unique fixed point $\bar{f} \in L^p[a, b]$. If, in addition, $\bar{f}$ is not constant then $\bar{f} \notin BV([a, b])$.*

## 4  Total Variation Minimization

The inverse problem for IFSM with total variation minimization can be formulated as follows

$$\min_{f \in \mathscr{F}} \ d_Y(f^*, f) + \lambda d_Y(f, \tilde{f}) \tag{22}$$

As a reminder from the introduction, the novelty or idea of this work is to combine the two competing objectives: the first term in the objective function represents the true error in approximating a target element $f^*$ by an element $f$, and the second term in the objective function represents the total variation of $f$ from the mean value $\tilde{f}$. Of course, we will use the collage theorem in (2) to switch to the minimization problem

$$\min_{f \in \mathscr{F}} \ d_Y(Tf, f) + \lambda d_Y(f, \tilde{f}) \tag{23}$$

where $T$ is the appropriate fractal transform, $d_Y(Tf, f)$ is the collage distance, and where the contractivity condition arising from Theorems 1 and 6 are satisfied. We wish to see how the two objectives interact as we adjust the value of the nonnegative constant $\lambda$.

To show how the method works, let us proceed with some numerical examples. We consider the target function $u(x) = 0.8x^2 + 0.1$ on $[0, 1]$. We divide the interval $[0, 1]$ into $N = 16$ subintervals $I_i = \left[\frac{i-1}{N}, \frac{i}{N}\right], i = 1, \ldots, N$, and introduce the IFS maps and corresponding greyscale maps

$$w_i(x) = s_i x + b_i = \frac{1}{N}x + \frac{i}{N} \text{ and } \phi(t) = \alpha_i t + \beta_i, \ i = 1, \ldots, N.$$

The maps induce the fractal transform

$$(Tu)(x) = \phi_i(u(w_i^{-1}(x))), \ x \in I_i, \ i = 1, \ldots, N.$$

To ensure that $Tu$ has range inside $[0, 1]$, we require

$$0 \leq \beta_i \leq 1 \text{ and } 0 \leq \alpha_i + \beta_i \leq 1, \ i = 1, \ldots, N, \tag{24}$$

and to guarantee contractivity of $T$ with respect to the $L^2$ and $TV$ norms (as per Theorems 1 and 6) we also require respectively that

$$\sum_{i=1}^{N} |s_i|^{\frac{1}{2}} |\alpha_i| \leq 1 \text{ and } \sum_{i=1}^{N} |\alpha_i| \leq 1. \tag{25}$$

Let

$$u^* = \int_0^1 u(x)\, dx,$$

and let $l_{collage}$ and $l_{TV}$ be in $[0, 1]$ satisfying $l_{collage} + l_{TV} = 1$. Then we seek to solve

$$\min_{\alpha_i, \beta_i} \Delta = l_{collage} \|Tu - u\|_2^2 + l_{TV} \|Tu^* - u^*\|_{TV} \text{ subject to (24) and (25)},$$

where we use the squared collage distance for convenience.

Table 1 reports the results for $N = 16$ and a selection of values for $l_{collage}$ and $l_{TV}$. The table reports the values of each norm and the total variation of $\bar{u}$, the fixed point of $T$. We see that the total variation of $\bar{u}$ decreases as we increase the value of $l_{TV}$, that is, as we increase the impact of the total variation norm $\|Tu^* - u^*\|_{TV}$.

Figure 1 presents the graphs of the target function $u$ and the approximation of $\bar{u}$ produced after ten iterations of $T$ on the zero function.

Table 2 presents the results for $N = 64$. We see a similar impact on the total variation of the fixed point of $T$.

Figure 2 presents the graphs of $u$ and $\bar{u}$

**Table 1**  Results for 16 subintervals

| $l_{collage}$ | $l_{TV}$ | $\|Tu - u\|_2^2$ | $\|Tu^* - u^*\|_{TV}$ | $\|\bar{u}\|_{TV}$ |
|---|---|---|---|---|
| 1.00 | 0.00 | 0.0039616055 | 1.0156250000 | 0.8087506835 |
| 0.98 | 0.02 | 0.0399564088 | 0.5650510193 | 0.7460404293 |
| 0.95 | 0.05 | 0.0836060280 | 0.4113486842 | 0.7196455886 |
| 0.90 | 0.10 | 0.1492181030 | 0.2204860257 | 0.4997316128 |
| 0.85 | 0.15 | 0.2194616346 | 0.0444335170 | 0.0869439131 |
| 0.80 | 0.20 | 0.2379638705 | 0.0000000000 | 0.0000000000 |

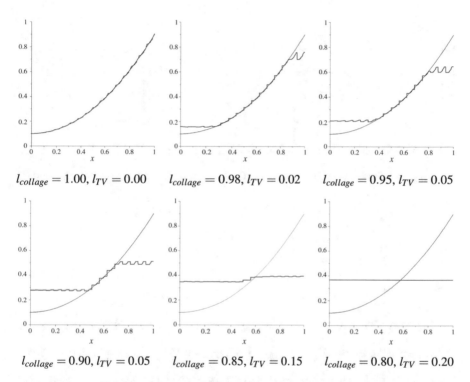

$l_{collage} = 1.00, l_{TV} = 0.00$ $\qquad$ $l_{collage} = 0.98, l_{TV} = 0.02$ $\qquad$ $l_{collage} = 0.95, l_{TV} = 0.05$

$l_{collage} = 0.90, l_{TV} = 0.05$ $\qquad$ $l_{collage} = 0.85, l_{TV} = 0.15$ $\qquad$ $l_{collage} = 0.80, l_{TV} = 0.20$

**Fig. 1**  Results for 16 subintervals: from left to right, top to bottom, we increase the weight given to the total variation minimization. The target curve is drawn in black, and the approximation of the attractor is drawn in red

## 4.1  Conclusions

We introduced the notion of combining the two objectives of minimizing the collage distance involving a map $T$ (which controls the fixed point approximation error via the collage theorem) and minimizing the total variation. In general, unless the target function is flat, these objectives are in competition with each other. In the numerical

**Table 2** Results for 64 subintervals

| $l_{collage}$ | $l_{TV}$ | $\|Tu - u\|_2^2$ | $\|Tu^* - u^*\|_{TV}$ | $\|\bar{u}\|_{TV}$ |
|---|---|---|---|---|
| 1.00 | 0.00 | 0.0008700454 | 0.7875000000 | 0.7979003906 |
| 0.98 | 0.02 | 0.0407576429 | 0.5653117029 | 0.8360723869 |
| 0.95 | 0.05 | 0.0843533008 | 0.4112823848 | 0.7138321759 |
| 0.90 | 0.10 | 0.1493716297 | 0.2217555758 | 0.5255290848 |
| 0.85 | 0.15 | 0.2126053455 | 0.0612094378 | 0.1486163983 |
| 0.80 | 0.20 | 0.2384791094 | 0.0000000000 | 0.0000000000 |

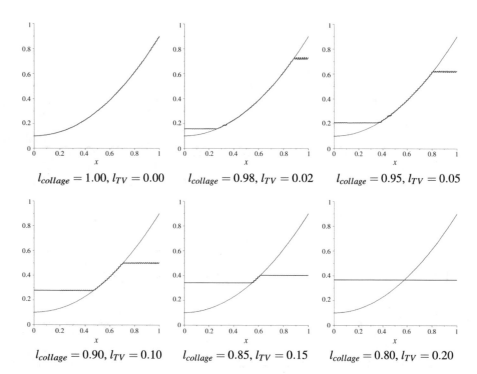

**Fig. 2** Results for 64 subintervals: from left to right, top to bottom, we increase the weight given to the total variation minimization. The target curve is drawn in black, and the approximation of the attractor is drawn in red

examples, we saw that total variation of the the fixed point of $T$ decreases as we give the total variation more weight in the combined objective function.

**Acknowledgements** This research was partially supported by Natural Sciences and Engineering Research Council of Canada (NSERC) in the form of a Discovery Grant (HK).

# References

1. Barnsley, M.F.: Fractals Everywhere. Academic Press, New York (1989)
2. Chan, T.F., Golub, G.H., Mulet, P.: A nonlinear primal-dual method for total variation-based image restoration. SIAM J. Sci. Comput. **20**(6), 19641977 (1999)
3. Forte, B., Vrscay, E.R.: Solving the inverse problem for function and image approximation using iterated function systems. Dyn. Contin. Discret. Impuls. Syst. **1**(2), 177–232 (1995)
4. Forte, B., Vrscay, E.R.: Theory of generalized fractal transforms. In: Fisher, Y. (Ed.) Fractal Image Encoding and Analysis, NATO ASI Series F 159:14568. New York, Springer (1998)
5. Goldluecke, B., Strekalovskiy, E., Cremers, D.: The natural vectorial total variation which arises from geometric measure theory. SIAM J. Imaging Sci. **5**(2), 537–563 (2012)
6. Hutchinson, J.: Fractals and self-similarity. Indiana Univ. J. Math. **30**, 713–747 (1981)
7. Iacus, S., La Torre, D.: A comparative simulation study on the IFS distribution function estimator. Nonlinear Anal. Real World Appl. **6**(5), 858–873 (2005)
8. Iacus, S., La Torre, D.: Approximating distribution functions by iterated function systems. J. Appl. Math. and Decision Sci. **1**, 33–46 (2005)
9. Kunze, H., La Torre, D., Mendivil, F., Vrscay, E.R.: Fractal-Based Methods in Analysis. Springer, New York (2012)
10. Kunze, H., La Torre, D., Vrscay, E.R.: Collage-based inverse problems for IFSM with entropy maximation and sparsity constraints. Image Anal. Stereol. **32**(3), 183–188 (2013)
11. La Torre, D., Vrscay, E.R., Ebrahimi, M., Barnsley, M.: Measure-valued images, associated fractal transforms and the affine self-similarity of images. SIAM J. Imaging Sci. **2**(2), 470–507 (2009)
12. La Torre, D., Mendivil, F., Vrscay, E.R.: Iterated function systems on functions of bounded variations. Fractals **24**(2), 1650019 (2016)
13. Li, M., Han, C., Wang, R., Guo, T.: Shrinking gradient descent algorithms for total variation regularized image denoising. Comput. Optim. Appl. **68**(3), 643–660 (2017)
14. Rudin, L., Osher, S., Fatemi, E.: Nonlinear total variation based oise removal algorithms. Phys. D **60**, 259–268 (1992)
15. Rudin, W.: Real and Complex Analysis. McGraw Hill, New York (1974)
16. Strong, D., Chan, T.: Edge-preserving and scale-dependent properties of total variation regularization. Inverse Prob. **19**, 165–187 (2003)

# Using the Collage Method to Solve Inverse Problems for Vector-Valued Variational Problems on a Perforated Domain in Reflexive Banach Spaces

Herb Kunze, Davide La Torre and Manuel Ruiz Galán

**Abstract** Recent work establishes that the solution of the parameter estimation on a perforated domain can be approximated by instead solving the inverse problem on the much easier to work with associated solid domain. In this work, we consider vector-valued variational problems on a perforated domain and show that the inverse problems on the perforated and associated solid domains can be similarly connected. The approach relies on a "generalized collage theorem" built from the vector-valued Lax-Milgram Theorem in reflexive Banach spaces. The method will be demonstrated on a numerical example.

**Keywords** Collage theorem · Inverse problem · Perforated domain

## 1 Introduction

The inverse problem literature is rich with problems considering the estimation of unknown parameters in a proposed governing model of a phenomenon of interest. Many such problems can be cast in terms of the approximation of a target element in a complete metric space by the fixed point of a contraction map. A simple consequence of Banach's Fixed Point Theorem called the Collage Theorem can be employed to

H. Kunze (✉)
Department of Mathematics and Statistics, University of Guelph, Guelph N1G 2W1, Canada
e-mail: hkunze@uoguelph.ca

D. La Torre
Department of Economics, Management and Quantitative Methods, University of Milan, Milan 20122, Italy
e-mail: davide.latorre@unimi.it

D. La Torre
Dubai Business School, University of Dubai, Dubai 14143, UAE
e-mail: dlatorre@ud.ac.ae

M. Ruiz Galán
Department of Applied Mathematics, University of Granada, Granada 18071, Spain
e-mail: mruizg@ugr.es

© Springer Nature Switzerland AG 2018
D. M. Kilgour et al. (eds.), *Recent Advances in Mathematical and Statistical Methods*, Springer Proceedings in Mathematics & Statistics 259, https://doi.org/10.1007/978-3-319-99719-3_10

shift from the problem of directly minimizing the fixed point approximation error to instead minimizing a simpler quantity referred to as the "collage distance" (because of its roots in fractal imaging) (see [1]). This approach and general philosophy has been used to establish "generalized collage theorem" in various settings. Very recently, in [2], it was shown that the vector-valued Lax-Milgram Theorem could be used to generate such a result useful for solving related inverse problems.

In other recent work, we have considered inverse problems for partial differential equations on perforated or porous domains [3–5]. A porous medium or perforated domain is a material characterized by a partitioning of the total volume into a solid portion often called the "matrix" and a pore space, usually referred to as "holes," that can be either materials different from that of the matrix or real physical holes. When formulating differential equations over porous media, the term "porous" implies that the state equation is written in the matrix only, while boundary conditions should be imposed on the whole boundary of the matrix, including the boundary of the holes. Porous media can be found in many areas of applied sciences and engineering including petroleum engineering, chemical engineering, civil engineering, aerospace engineering, soil science, geology, material science, and many more areas.

Since porosity in materials can take different forms and appear in varying degrees, solving differential equations over porous media is often a complicated task and the holes' size and their distribution play an important role in its characterization. Furthermore, numerical simulations over perforated domains need a very fine discretization mesh which often requires a significant computational time. The mathematical theory of differential equations on perforated domains is usually based on the theory of "homogenization" in which heterogeneous material is replaced by a fictitious homogeneous one. Of course this implies the need of convergence results linking together the model on a perforated domain and on the associated homogeneous one. In the case of porous media, or heterogeneous media in general, characterizing the properties of the material is a tricky process and can be done on different levels, mainly the microscopic and macroscopic scales, where the microscopic scale describes the heterogeneities and the macroscopic scale describes the global behavior of the composite.

The approach is to consider two related problems for steady-state reaction-diffusion, problem $(P_\varepsilon)$ on a perforated domain $\Omega_\varepsilon$ and problem $(P)$ on the related solid domain $\Omega$:

$$\begin{cases} \nabla \cdot (K^\lambda(x, y)\nabla u(x, y)) = f^\lambda(x, y), & \text{in } \Omega_\varepsilon, \\ u(x, y) = 0, & \text{on } \partial\Omega_\varepsilon, \end{cases} \qquad (P_\varepsilon)$$

and

$$\begin{cases} \nabla \cdot (K^\lambda(x, y)\nabla u(x, y)) = f^\lambda(x, y), & \text{in } \Omega, \\ u(x, y) = 0, & \text{on } \partial\Omega. \end{cases} \qquad (P)$$

The inverse problem of interest for $(P_\varepsilon)$ is to estimate $\lambda$ given observational data for a solution. The earlier work establishes a relationship between parameter values $\lambda$

in the two problems: one can use the data from the solution to $(P_\varepsilon)$ in the inverse problem for $(P)$ to estimate $\lambda$, with the connection strengthening as $\varepsilon$ decreases.

Our formulation of the inverse problem uses the (generalized) collage theorem, based on the Lax-Milgram theorem, with derivatives being taken in the weak sense, leading to a minimization problem for a function of the parameters $\lambda$ one desires to estimate. Letting $u$ denote the observed solution, perhaps an interpolation of observational data values, we must solve

$$\min_{\lambda \in \Lambda} F(u, \lambda).$$

Other recent works used the vector-valued Lax-Milgram Theorem to generate a version of a generalized collage theorem useful for solving inverse problems for variational equations [6, 7] and related systems [2]. In other earlier works, in various settings, it has been illustrated that the collage method compares quite favorably to other inverse problem solution methods. The approach is typically far less computationally intensive, and, in any case, can be used as a first approach for methods that require a good initial guess of parameter values.

The goal of this paper is to explore the extension of these ideas further by considering inverse problems for a system of boundary value problems on a perforated domain in the reflexive Banach space setting.

In the next section, we briefly present the theory and machinery for inverse boundary value problems in reflexive Banach spaces. In the third section, we present an example that shows that our methods can be extended to the more complicated setting mentioned earlier.

## 2 Inverse Boundary Value Problems in Reflexive Banach Spaces

The first result we mention is the following vector-valued version of the Lax-Milgram theorem. Given a real normed space $G$, we write $G^*$ for its topological dual space. The proofs and more details about these results can be found in [2].

**Theorem 1** *Suppose that $E$ is a real reflexive Banach space, $N \geq 1$, $F_1, \ldots, F_N$ are real Banach spaces and that $a_1 : E \times F_1 \longrightarrow \mathbb{R}, \ldots, a_N : E \times F_N \longrightarrow \mathbb{R}$ are continuous bilinear forms. Then, for all $\phi_1^* \in F_1^*, \ldots, \phi_N^* \in F_N^*$ there exists a unique $x_0 \in E$ such that*

$$\begin{cases} \phi_1^* = a_1(x_0, \cdot) \\ \quad \cdots \\ \phi_N^* = a_N(x_0, \cdot) \end{cases}$$

*if, and only if,*

$$\left.\begin{array}{c} \phi_1^* = a_1(x_0, \cdot) \\ \cdots \\ \phi_N^* = a_N(x_0, \cdot) \end{array}\right\} \Rightarrow x = 0$$

*and there exists $\rho > 0$ satisfying*

$$(\phi_1, \ldots, \phi_N) \in F_1 \times \cdots \times F_N \Rightarrow \rho \sum_{k=1}^N \|\phi_k\| \le \left\| \sum_{k=1}^N a_k(\cdot, \phi_k) \right\|.$$

*Moreover, if these equivalent conditions hold and $x_0 \in E$ is the unique solution, then*

$$\|x_0\| \le \frac{1}{\rho} \max_{k=1,\ldots,N} \|\phi_k^*\|.$$

As a consequence, we derive this generalized collage theorem:

**Corollary 1** *Let $E$ be a real reflexive Banach space, let $N \ge 1$, let $F_1, \ldots, F_N$ be real Banach spaces, let $\phi_1^* \in F_1^*, \ldots, \phi_N^* \in F_N^*$ and let $\Lambda$ be a nonempty set such that for all $\lambda \in \Lambda$ there exist $N$ continuous bilinear forms $a_{1\lambda} : E \times F_1 \longrightarrow \mathbb{R}, \ldots, a_{N\lambda} : E \times F_N \longrightarrow \mathbb{R}$ and $\rho_\lambda > 0$ with*

$$\left.\begin{array}{c} \phi_1^* = a_{1\lambda}(x_0, \cdot) \\ \cdots \\ \phi_N^* = a_{N\lambda}(x_0, \cdot) \end{array}\right\} \Rightarrow x = 0$$

*and*

$$(\phi_1, \ldots, \phi_N) \in F_1 \times \cdots \times F_N \Rightarrow \rho_\lambda \sum_{k=1}^N \|y_k\| \le \left\| \sum_{k=1}^N a_{k\lambda}(\cdot, \phi_k) \right\|.$$

*Let us also suppose that for all $\lambda \in \Lambda$, $x_\lambda \in E$ is the unique solution of the variational system*

$$x \in E \text{ and } \left\{\begin{array}{c} \phi_1^* = a_{1\lambda}(x, \cdot) \\ \cdots \\ \phi_N^* = a_{N\lambda}(x, \cdot) \end{array}\right. .$$

*Then for each $x_0 \in E$ and for all $\lambda \in \Lambda$ the inequality*

$$\|x_\lambda - x_0\| \le \frac{1}{\rho_\lambda} \max_{k=1,\ldots,N} \|\phi_k^* - a_{k\lambda}(x_0, \cdot)\|$$

*is valid.*

If one wants to approximate the solution $x_0$ in the sense of the collage distance, that is, minimize $\{\|x_\lambda - x_0\| : \lambda \in \Lambda\}$, according to Corollary 1, it suffices to minimize

$$\left\{ \frac{1}{\rho_\lambda} \max_{k=1,\ldots,N} \|\phi_k^* - a_{k\lambda}(x_0, \cdot)\| : \lambda \in \Lambda \right\},$$

although if

$$\rho := \inf_{\lambda \in \Lambda} \rho_\lambda > 0,$$

then we only need to minimize

$$\left\{ \max_{k=1,\ldots,N} \|\phi_k^* - a_{k\lambda}(x_0, \cdot)\| : \lambda \in \Lambda \right\}.$$

Under such an assumption, $\rho > 0$, we also suppose that each space $F_k$, $(k = 1, \ldots, N)$ has a Schauder basis $\{\Upsilon_{ki}\}_{i \geq 1}$, in such a way that if $\{\Upsilon_{ki}^*\}_{i \geq 1}$ denotes its sequence of biorthogonal functionals, then the non-restrictive condition

$$M := \max_{k=1,\ldots,N} \sup_{i \geq 1} \|\Upsilon_{ki}^*\| < \infty$$

holds. In order to discretize our optimization problem, let us also assume that $E$ admits a Schauder basis $\{\Theta_i\}_{i \geq 1}$ and define, for each $n \geq 1$ and $k = 1, \ldots, N$

$$E_n := \text{span}\{\Theta_1, \ldots, \Theta_n\}, \qquad F_{kn} := \text{span}\{\Upsilon_{k1}, \ldots, \Upsilon_{kn}\}$$

and let $\Pi_n$ be the $n^{\text{th}}$-projection of $E$ onto $E_n$, that is, for all $x \in E$,

$$\Pi_n x := \sum_{i=1}^{n} \Theta_i^*(x)\Theta_i.$$

We also suppose that for all $\lambda \in \Lambda$, $k = 1, \ldots, N$ and $n \geq 1$

$$x \in E_n \text{ and } \begin{cases} 0 = a_{1\lambda}(x, \cdot) \\ \quad \cdots \\ 0 = a_{N\lambda}(x, \cdot) \end{cases} \Rightarrow x = 0,$$

and there exists $\rho_\lambda^n > 0$ such that

$$(\phi_1, \ldots, \phi_N) \in F_{1n} \times \cdots \times F_{Nn} \Rightarrow \rho_\lambda^n \sum_{k=1}^{N} \|\phi_k\| \leq \left\| \sum_{k=1}^{N} a_{k\lambda}(\cdot, \phi_k) \right\|.$$

Then, Theorem 1 guarantees the existence of a unique $x_j^n \in E_n$ such that

$$(\phi_1, \ldots, \phi_N) \in F_{1n} \times F_{nN} \Rightarrow \begin{cases} \phi_1^*(\phi_1) = a_1(x_j^n, \phi_1) \\ \quad \cdots \\ \phi_N^*(\phi_N) = a_N(x_j^n, \phi_N) \end{cases}$$

When we apply Corollary 1 to this vector-valued variational problem, we get

$$\|x_\lambda^n - \Pi_n x_0\| \leq \frac{M}{\rho_\lambda^n} \max_{k=1,\ldots,N} \sum_{i=1}^n |\phi_0^*(\Upsilon_{ki}) - a_{k\lambda}(\Pi_n x_0, \Upsilon_{ki})|,$$

and if

$$\gamma := \sup_{\lambda \in \Lambda,\, n \geq 1} \rho_\lambda^n > 0,$$

then it is enough to minimize

$$\varphi_n(j) := \max_{k=1,\ldots,N} \sum_{i=1}^n |\phi_0^*(\Upsilon_{ki}) - a_{k\lambda}(\Pi_n x_0, \Upsilon_{ki})|,$$

or equivalently, the discrete objective function

$$F_n(j) := \sum_{k=1}^N \sum_{i=1}^n (\phi_0^*(\Upsilon_{ki}) - a_{k\lambda}(\Pi_n x_0, \Upsilon_{ki}))^2, \tag{1}$$

which is quadratic and then easier to minimize.

## 3  Inverse Problems on Perforated Domains: An Example

Given a compact and convex set $\Omega$, we denote by $\Omega_B$ the collection of holes $\cup_{j=1}^m B(x_j, \varepsilon_j)$ where $x_j \in \Omega$, $\varepsilon_j > 0$, and the holes $B(x_j, \varepsilon_j)$ are nonoverlapping and lie strictly in the interior of $\Omega$. We let $\varepsilon = \max_j \varepsilon_j$. If the holes are not circles but compact and convex subsets of $\Omega$, we can always embed these sets in circles with $\varepsilon$ being the largest diameter of them. We denote by $\Omega_\varepsilon$ the closure of the set $\Omega \backslash \Omega_B$. As an example, we consider the 2D linear system

$$-\nabla \cdot (\kappa(x, y)\nabla u) + Au = f, \ (x, y) \in \Omega_\varepsilon \tag{2}$$

$$u(x, y) = 0 \text{ on } \partial\Omega_\varepsilon \tag{3}$$

with

$$\kappa(x, y) = 1 + x + \frac{y}{2}, \ A = \begin{bmatrix} 0 & 1 \\ \frac{7}{10} & 0 \end{bmatrix}, \ u = \begin{bmatrix} u_1 \\ u_2 \end{bmatrix}, \ f(x, y) = \begin{bmatrix} 2x^2 + y^2 \\ x^{-\frac{3}{5}} \end{bmatrix}, \tag{4}$$

and $\Omega_\varepsilon$ is $\Omega = [0, 1]^2$ with 12 diamond-shaped holes (see Fig. 1a). We note that this academic example has (at least) three interesting features: the system is strongly coupled by the matrix $A$, we've chosen a hole shape other than a circle, and the

(a)                              (b)                              (c)

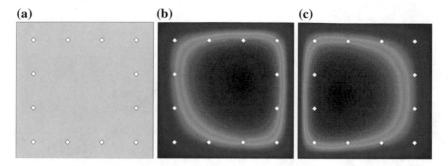

**Fig. 1** **a** The region $\Omega_\varepsilon$, **b** Isotherms of the solution $u_1(x, y)$, and **c** Isotherms of the solution $u_2(x, y)$

second entry in $f$, $f_2$, is an interesting function. Indeed, $f_2(x, y) = x^{-\frac{3}{5}}$ satisfies

$$\int_0^1 \int_0^1 (f_2)^2 \, dxdy = \infty, \quad \text{while} \quad \int_0^1 \int_0^1 (f_2)^{\frac{3}{2}} \, dxdy = 10,$$

so $f_2$ is not in the Hilbert space $L^2([0, 1]^2)$ but is in the space $L^{\frac{3}{2}}([0, 1]^2)$. The isotherms of the components of the solution $u(x, y)$ are presented in Fig. 1b and c.

We sample each solution component at an array of uniformly-distributed data points in $\Omega$. If a sample point lies inside a hole, we discard it. We fit an 8th-degree polynomial to each of the data sets to produce target functions $u_1(x, y)$ and $u_2(x, y)$.

We consider the inverse problem: Given the target $u$, $A$, and $f(x, y)$, approximate $\kappa(x, y) = \lambda_1 + \lambda_2 x + \lambda_3 y$ such that the resulting system admits $u$ as an approximate solution.

Multiplying component $i$ of (2) with a test function $(v_k)_i(x, y)$, integrating over $\Omega$, and using Green's second identity, we arrive at, for $i = 1, 2$,

$$a_1(u_1, (v_k)_1) = \iint_\Omega (\kappa \nabla u_1 \cdot \nabla(v_k)_1 + u_2(v_k)_1) \, dA$$

$$a_2(u_2, (v_k)_2) = \iint_\Omega (\kappa \nabla u_2 \cdot \nabla(v_k)_2 + 0.7u_1(v_k)_2) \, dA$$

$$\phi_i((v_k)_i) = \iint_\Omega f_i(v_k)_i \, dA.$$

Using the collage method, we construct

$$F_n(\lambda) = \sum_{k=1}^N \sum_{i=1}^2 (\phi_i((v_k)_i) - a_i(u_i, (v_k)_i))^2, \tag{5}$$

where $N$ is the number of basis functions we use. We see that using a highly refined

**(a)**

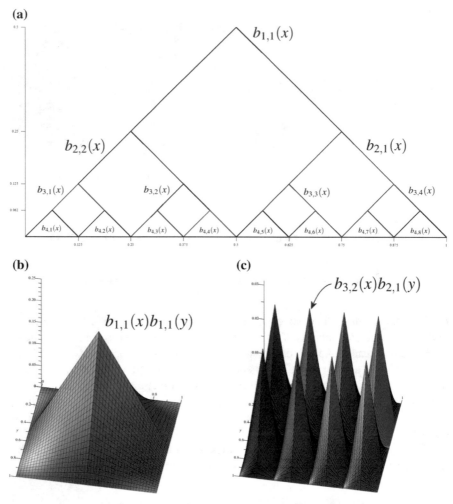

**Fig. 2** Schauder basis elements of **a** $L^{\frac{3}{2}}([0, 1])$ and **b** and **c** $L^{\frac{3}{2}}([0, 1]^2)$

The Banach space $L^{\frac{3}{2}}([0, 1])$ admits the Schauder basis $\{b_{p,q}\}$, with the first few elements illustrated in Fig. 2a. The Schauder basis for the Banach space $L^{\frac{3}{2}}([0, 1]^2)$ consists of the functions $b_{p,q}(x)b_{r,s}(y)$. In a Hilbert space setting, one typically works with a finite element basis characterized by basis functions $\xi_i$ that are piecewise linear, have value 1 at node $i$ of the mesh, and have value 0 at all other nodes; this structure produces the "hat basis" in one dimension, and a basis of hexagonally-based pyramids in two dimensions. As a result, it is of interest to illustrate typical Schauder basis elements for contrast. Figure 2b and c presents some Schauder basis elements.

Table 1 presents results for several values of $N$. We see that the results are quite good in the case $N = 5$, remain good for $N = 21$, but worsen significantly for

**Table 1** Recovered parameter values. True values are $\lambda = \left(1, 1, \frac{1}{2}\right)$

| $N$ | $b_{i,j}(x)b_{k,l}(y)$ | Recovered $\lambda$ |
|---|---|---|
| 5 | $i, k = 1, \ j, l = 1$<br>$i, k = 2, \ j, l \in \{1, 2\}$ | $(1.0435, 0.8295, 0.5404)$ |
| 21 | $i, k = 1, \ j, l = 1$<br>$i, k = 2, \ j, l \in \{1, 2\}$<br>$i, k = 3, \ j, l \in \{1, 2, 3, 4\}$ | $(1.0909, 0.7984, 0.4297)$ |
| 85 | $i, k = 1, \ j, l = 1$<br>$i, k = 2, \ j, l \in \{1, 2\}$<br>$i, k = 3, \ j, l \in \{1, 2, 3, 4\}$<br>$i, k = 4, \ j, l \in \{1, \ldots, 8\}$ | $(1.2298, 0.7006, 0.1549)$ |

$N = 85$. This outcome makes sense when one considers that the finer basis corresponding to large $N$ values will include elements that are supported on a domain that is coincident with a hole. Indeed, shrinking the holes dramatically makes the results improve for all $N$, as the impact of the perforations is marginalized and our earlier work on unperforated domains takes hold. Alternatively, given knowledge of the hole sizes and distributions, one could discard the basis functions that interact with the holes, also improving results in the case that the pore space is small compared to the matrix. We can also note that using the collage theorem that is appropriate in a Hilbert space setting leads to incredibly poor results, since this example problem does not live in such a space.

## 4  Conclusions

We have extended the use of the generalized collage theorem arising from the vector-valued Lax-Milgram Theorem to vector-valued variational problems on perforated domains in a Banach space setting. We presented a seemingly simple example that is nonetheless very challenging due to several complexities. The example illustrates that the method works. A priori knowledge of the hole sizes and distribution helps improve results

**Acknowledgements** This research was partially supported by Natural Sciences and Engineering Research Council of Canada (NSERC) in the form of a Discovery Grant (HK) and by project MTM2016-80676-P (AEI/FEDER, UE).

# References

1. Kunze, H., Mendivil, F., La Torre, D., Vrscay, E.: Fractal-Based Methods in Analysis. Springer-Verlag (2012). ISBN 1461418909
2. Kunze, H., La Torre, D., Levere, K., Ruiz Galán, M.: Inverse Problems via the "Generalized Collage Theorem" for Vector-valued Lax-Milgram-Based Variational Problems. Mathematical Problems in Engineering (2015)
3. Kunze, H., La Torre, D.: Collage-type approach to inverse problems for elliptic PDEs on perforated domains. Electron. J. Differen. Equat. **48**, 1–11 (2015)
4. Kunze, H., La Torre, D.: An inverse problem for a system of steady-state reaction-diffusion equations acting on a perforated domain. AIP Conference Proc. **1798**, 020089 (2017)
5. Marchenko, V.A., Khruslov, E.Y.: Homogenization of Partial Differential Equations. Birkhauser, Boston (2006)
6. Berenguer, M.I., Kunze, H., La Torre, D., Ruiz, Galán M.: Galerkin schemes and inverse boundary value problems in reflexive banach spaces. J. Comput. Appl. Math. **275**, 1–8 (2015)
7. Kunze, H., La Torre, D., Vrscay, E.R.: A generalized collage method based upon the Lax-Milgram functional for solving boundary value inverse problems. Nonlinear Anal. **71**(12), 1337–1343 (2009)

# Inverse Problems Using Iterated Function Systems with Place-Dependent Probabilities

Davide La Torre, Erik A. Maki, Franklin Mendivil and Edward R. Vrscay

**Abstract** We are concerned with the approximation of probability measures on a compact metric space $(X, d)$ by invariant measures of Iterated Function Systems with Place-Dependent Probabilities (IFSPDP). Using the Collage Theorem, we formulate the corresponding inverse problem and look for an IFSPDPs which map a target measure $\nu$ as close as possible to itself in terms of an appropriate metric on $\mathscr{M}(X)$, the space of probability measures on $X$.

**Keywords** Iterated function systems · Place-dependent probabilities · Inverse problem of measure approximation · Collage theorem · Moments of measures

## 1 Introduction

In this paper we are concerned with the problem of approximating probability measures on a compact metric space $(X, d)$ with invariant measures of iterated function systems (IFS) with place-dependent probabilities (IFSPDP): systems of

D. La Torre (✉)
Department of Economics, Management and Quantitative Methods,
University of Milan, 20122 Milan, Italy
email: davide.latorre@unimi.it

D. La Torre
Dubai Business School, University of Dubai, Dubai 14143, UAE
e-mail: dlatorre@ud.ac.ae

E. A. Maki · E. R. Vrscay
Department of Applied Mathematics, University of Waterloo, Waterloo, ON, Canada
e-mail: emaki@uwaterloo.ca

E. R. Vrscay
e-mail: ervrscay@uwaterloo.ca

F. Mendivil
Department of Mathematics and Statistics, Acadia University, Wolfville, NS, Canada
e-mail: franklin.mendivil@acadiau.ca

© Springer Nature Switzerland AG 2018 115
D. M. Kilgour et al. (eds.), *Recent Advances in Mathematical
and Statistical Methods*, Springer Proceedings in Mathematics & Statistics 259,
https://doi.org/10.1007/978-3-319-99719-3_11

contraction mappings on $X$, $\mathbf{w} = \{w_1, w_2, \ldots, w_N\}$ with associated probabilities $\mathbf{p} = \{p_1, p_2, \ldots, p_N\}$, the latter of which are place-dependent, i.e., $p_i : X \to \mathbb{R}$. (This is in contrast to the case of IFS with constant probabilities which has usually been assumed in the literature.) We consider the special case $X = [0, 1]$ with affine IFS maps and probabilities, i.e.,

$$w_i(x) = a_i x + b_i \,, \quad p_i(x) = \alpha_i x + \beta_i \,, \quad 1 \le i \le N. \tag{1}$$

The ideas and methods developed here can, at least in principle, be extended to the general case $[0, 1]^n$. This paper may be considered to be a place-dependent extension of [2], in which the inverse problem of measure approximation using IFS with constant probabilities was treated.

The paper is organized as follows: Sect. 2 recalls the classical definition of IFS with constant probabilities, Sect. 3 presents the definition of IFS with place-dependent probabilities, and Sect. 4 deals with the inverse problem in terms of the Collage Theorem.

## 2   IFS with Constant Probabilities

In what follows, we let $(X, d)$ denote a compact metric space. An $N$-map *Iterated Function System* (IFS) on $X$, $\mathbf{w} = \{w_1, \ldots, w_N\}$, is a set of $N$ contraction mappings on $X$, i.e., $w_i : X \to X$, $i = 1, \ldots, N$, with contraction factors $c_i \in [0, 1)$. (See [1, 4, 6].) Associated with an $N$-map IFS is the following set-valued mapping $\hat{\mathbf{w}}$ on the space $\mathscr{H}([a, b])$ of nonempty compact subsets of $X$:

$$\hat{\mathbf{w}}(S) := \bigcup_{i=1}^{N} w_i(S) \,, \quad S \in \mathscr{H}([a, b]). \tag{2}$$

**Theorem 1** [4] *For $A, B \in \mathscr{H}(X)$,*

$$h(\hat{\mathbf{w}}(A), \hat{\mathbf{w}}(B)) \le c H(A, B) \quad \text{where} \quad c = \max_{1 \le i \le N} c_i < 1 \tag{3}$$

*and $h$ denotes the Hausdorff metric on $\mathscr{H}(X)$.*

**Corollary 1** [4] *There exists a unique set $A \in \mathscr{H}([a, b])$, the attractor of the IFS* $\mathbf{w}$, *such that*

$$A = \hat{\mathbf{w}}(A) = \bigcup_{i=1}^{N} w_i(A). \tag{4}$$

*Moreover, for any $B \in \mathscr{H}([a, b])$, $h(A, \hat{\mathbf{w}}^n B) \to 0$ as $n \to \infty$.*

An $N$-map *Iterated Function System with (constant) Probabilities (IFSP)* $(\mathbf{w}, \mathbf{p})$ is an $N$-map IFS $\mathbf{w}$ with associated probabilities $\mathbf{p} = \{p_1, \ldots, p_N\}$, $\sum_{i=1}^{N} p_i = 1$. Let $\mathcal{M}(X)$ denote the set of probability measures on (Borel subsets of) $X$ and $d_{MK}$ the Monge-Kantorovich distance on this space: For $\mu, \nu \in \mathcal{M}(X)$, with Monge-Kantorovich metric,

$$d_{MK}(\mu, \nu) = \sup_{f \in Lip_1(X)} \left[ \int f \, d\mu - \int f \, d\nu \right]. \tag{5}$$

where $Lip_1(X) = \{f : X \to \mathbb{R} \mid |f(x) - f(y)| \leq d(x, y)\}$. The metric space $(\mathcal{M}(X), d_{MK})$ is complete [1, 4].

Associated with an $N$-map IFSP is a mapping $M : \mathcal{M} \to \mathcal{M}$, often referred to as the *Markov operator*, defined as follows. Let $\nu = M\mu$ for any $\mu \in \mathcal{M}(X)$. Then for any measurable set $S \subset X$,

$$\nu(S) = (M\mu)(S) = \sum_{i=1}^{N} p_i \, \mu(w_i^{-1}(S)). \tag{6}$$

**Theorem 2** [4] *For $\mu, \nu \in \mathcal{M}(X)$,*

$$d_{MK}(M\mu, M\nu) \leq c \, d_{MK}(\mu, \nu). \tag{7}$$

**Corollary 2** [4] *There exists a unique measure $\bar{\nu} \in \mathcal{M}(X)$, the* invariant measure *of the IFSP $(\mathbf{w}, \mathbf{p})$, such that*

$$\bar{\mu}(S) = (M\bar{\mu})(S) = \sum_{i=1}^{N} p_i \bar{\mu}(w_i^{-1}(S)). \tag{8}$$

*Moreover, for any $\nu \in \mathcal{M}(X)$, $d_{MK}(\bar{\mu}, M^n \nu) \to 0$ as $n \to \infty$.*

**Theorem 3** [4] *The support of the invariant measure $\bar{\mu}$ of an $N$-map IFSP $(\mathbf{w}, \mathbf{p})$ is the attractor $A$ of the IFS $\mathbf{w}$, i.e.,*

$$supp \, \bar{\mu} = A. \tag{9}$$

*Example 1* The following two-map IFS on $X = [0, 1]$,

$$w_1(x) = \frac{1}{2}x, \quad w_2(x) = \frac{1}{2}x + \frac{1}{2}, \tag{10}$$

with attractor $A = [0, 1]$. We now consider two IFSP having these IFS maps. These examples will be helpful for an understanding of IFS with place-dependent maps.

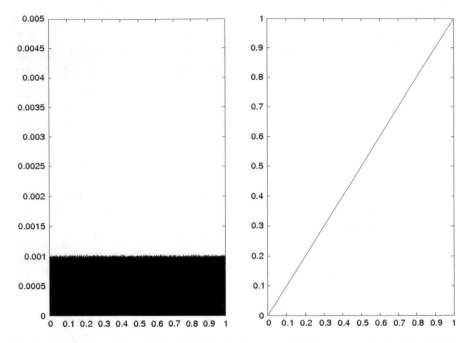

**Fig. 1** Left: Histogram approximation of invariant measure $\bar{\mu}$ (Lebesgue measure) of the IFSP in Example 1, Case 1. Right: Approximation to cumulative distribution function $F(x)$ of $\bar{\mu}$

1. **Case 1**: $p_1 = p_2 = \dfrac{1}{2}$. It is well known that the invariant measure $\bar{\mu}$ of this IFSP is (uniform) Lebesgue measure on [0,1]. A histogram approximation to this measure, obtained by using the "Chaos Game" [1], is shown in the left plot of Fig. 1. (In all histogram approximations presented in this paper, $10^8$ iterates were generated and placed into 1000 nonoverlapping bins on [0, 1].) The histogram approximation may be used to generate an approximation to the cumulative distribution function (CDF) for this measure, defined on $X = [0, 1]$ as follows,

$$F(x) = \int_0^x d\bar{\mu}. \tag{11}$$

   In this case, $F(x) = x$. The approximation to the CDF is shown in the right plot of Fig. 1.

2. **Case 2**: $p_1 = \dfrac{2}{5}$, $p_2 = \dfrac{3}{5}$. A histogram approximation to the invariant measure $\bar{\mu}$ of this IFSP is shown in the left plot of Fig. 2. Since $p_1 < p_2$, it follows that $\bar{\mu}([0, 1/2]) < \bar{\mu}([1/2, 1])$. This asymmetry is then propagated in a self-similar manner over smaller dyadic subintervals of [0,1]. The approximation to the CDF of this invariant measure generated by the histogram is shown in the right plot of the figure.

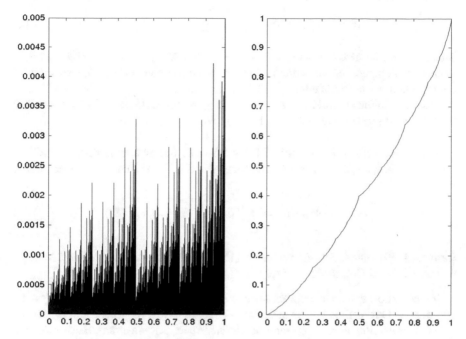

**Fig. 2** Left: Histogram approximation of invariant measure $\bar{\mu}$ (Lebesgue measure) of the IFSP in Example 1, Case 2. Right: Approximation to cumulative distribution function $F(x)$ of $\bar{\mu}$

## 3   IFS with Place-Dependent Probabilities

We now consider the case in which the probabilities, $p_i$, $1 \leq i \leq N$, associated with an $N$-map IFS **w** are place-dependent, i.e., $p_i : X \to \mathbb{R}$ such that

$$\sum_{i=1}^{N} p_i(x) = 1 , \quad \text{for all } x \in X. \tag{12}$$

The result is an $N$-map *Iterated Function Systems with Place-Dependent Probabilities* (IFSPDP) [1].

In the special case $X \subset \mathbb{R}$ and affine probabilities $p_i$ as given in Eq. (1), substitution into (12) along with the fact that the functions $x$ and 1 are linearly independent over [0,1] yields the following conditions on the $\alpha_i$ and $\beta_i$,

$$\sum_{i=1}^{N} \alpha_i = 0, \quad \sum_{i=1}^{N} \beta_i = 1. \tag{13}$$

Two other conditions must be imposed, namely, (i) $0 \leq p_i(0) \leq 1$ and $0 \geq p_i(1) \leq 1$ for $1 \leq i \leq N$, which lead to the following additional constraints,

$$0 \le \beta_i \le 1, \quad 0 \le \alpha_i + \beta_i \le 1, \quad 1 \le i \le N. \tag{14}$$

These constraints also imply that $-1 \le \alpha_i \le 1$. For $N \ge 1$, we shall let $\Sigma^N \subset \mathbb{R}^{2N}$ denote the compact region defined by all of the above constraints. This region will be important in our treatment of the inverse problem.

Note that in the special case $\alpha_i = 0$, $1 \le i \le N$, the IFSPDP reduces to an IFSP with constant probabilities $p_i = \beta_i$, $1 \le i \le N$.

Associated with an $N$-map IFSPDP, $(\mathbf{w}, \mathbf{p})$, is a Markov operator $M : \mathcal{M}(X) \to \mathcal{M}(X)$, defined as follows. Let $\nu = M\mu$ for any $\mu \in \mathcal{M}(X)$. Then for any measurable set $S \subset X$,

$$\nu(S) = (M\mu)(S) = \sum_{i=1}^{N} (p_i \circ w_i^{-1})(S)\mu(w_i^{-1}(S)). \tag{15}$$

**Lemma 1** [9] *Given $M$ as defined in* Eq. (15)*, then $M$ maps $\mathcal{M}(X)$ to itself. In other words, if $\mu \in \mathcal{M}(X)$, then $\nu = M\mu \in \mathcal{M}(X)$.*

We now show that under appropriate conditions, the above Markov operator can be contractive. Our method begins in the same manner as that of Hutchinson [4] for the constant probability case. Some modifications are necessary in order to accommodate the place-dependency of the probabilities. The following Lemma, which is easily proved using a change-of-variable approach, will be useful. Its proof, which can be found in [9], is omitted here.

**Lemma 2** *Let $\mu \in \mathcal{M}(X)$ and $\nu = M\mu$. Then for any $f$ continuous function $f : X \to \mathbb{R}$,*

$$\int_X f(x)\,d\nu(x) = \int_X f(x)\,d(M\mu)(x)$$
$$= \sum_{i=1}^{N} \int_X p_i(x) \cdot (f \circ w_i)(x)\,d\mu(x). \tag{16}$$

We shall also need the following Lemma.

**Lemma 3** [9] *Let $(X, d)$ be a compact metric space and let $f : X \to \mathbb{R}$ be Lipschitz on $X$ with Lipschitz constant $K \ge 0$. If $f(y_0) = 0$ for some $y_0 \in X$, then $|f(x)| \le K\,diam(X)$ for all $x \in X$.*

**Theorem 4** [9] *Let $(X, d)$ be a compact metric space and $(\mathbf{w}, \mathbf{p})$ an $N$-map IFSPDF with IFS maps $w_i : X \to X$ with contraction factors $c_i \in [0, 1)$. Furthermore, assume that the probabilities $p_i : X \to \mathbb{R}$ are Lipschitz functions, with Lipschitz constants $K_i \ge 0$. Let $M : \mathcal{M}(X) \to \mathcal{M}(X)$ be the Markov operator associated with this IFSPDP, as defined in (15). Then for any $\mu, \nu \in \mathcal{M}(X)$,*

$$d_{MK}(M\mu, M\nu) \le (c + KDN)d_{MK}(\mu, \nu),\tag{17}$$

where $c = \max\limits_i c_i$, $K = \max\limits_i K_i$ and $D = diam(X) < \infty$.

**Theorem 5** *The support of the invariant measure $\bar{\mu}$ of an N-map IFSPDP* $(\mathbf{w}, \mathbf{p})$ *is the attractor A of the IFS* $\mathbf{w}$, *i.e.,*

$$supp\, \bar{\mu} = A.\tag{18}$$

*Example 2* We return to the two-map IFS on $X = [0, 1]$ of Example 1,

$$w_1(x) = \frac{1}{2}x, \quad w_2(x) = \frac{1}{2}x + \frac{1}{2},\tag{19}$$

and consider two two-map IFSPDP maps which are perturbations of the equal-probability IFSP of Case 1 above, where $\bar{\mu}$ = uniform Lebesgue measure.

1 **Case 1:** $p_1(x) = -\frac{1}{10}x + \frac{1}{2}$, $p_2(x) = \frac{1}{10}x + \frac{1}{2}$. Note that $p_1(0) = p_2(0) = \frac{1}{2}$. For $x \in (0, 1]$, $p_2(x) - p_1(x) = \frac{1}{5}x > 0$, i.e., the asymmetry in the probabilities increases from 0 to its maximum value $\frac{1}{5}$ at $x = 1$. As such, we expect that there will be an asymmetry of the invariant measure $\bar{\mu}$, weighted toward $x = 1$ at all scales. However, the asymmetry will be less "drastic" as compared to the constant probability case $p_1 = \frac{2}{5}$, $p_2 = \frac{3}{5}$.

   A histogram approximation to this measure, obtained by using a place-dependent version of the "Chaos Game," is shown in the left plot of Fig. 3. The approximation to the CDF $F(x)$ of $\bar{\mu}$ yielded by this histogram is shown in the right plot of the figure.

2 **Case 2:** $p_1(x) = \frac{1}{10}x + \frac{1}{2}$, $p_2(x) = -\frac{1}{10}x + \frac{1}{2}$. Once again, $p_1(0) = p_2(0) = \frac{1}{2}$. For $x \in (0, 1]$, $p_1(x) - p_2(x) = \frac{1}{5}x > 0$, i.e., the asymmetry in the probabilities is reversed from Case 1. We therefore expect that the asymmetry in the invariant measure $\bar{\mu}$ will be weighted toward $x = 0$.

   A histogram approximation to this measure is shown in the left plot of Fig. 4. The approximation to the CDF $F(x)$ of $\bar{\mu}$ yielded by this histogram is shown in the right plot of the figure.

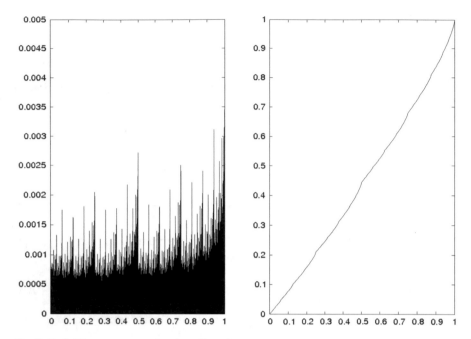

**Fig. 3** Left: Histogram approximation of invariant measure $\bar{\mu}$ of the two-map IFSPDP in Example 2, Case 1. Right: Approximation to cumulative distribution function $F(x)$ of $\bar{\mu}$

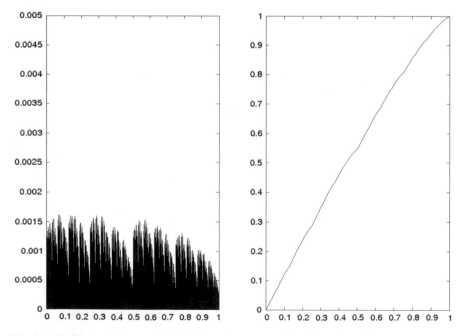

**Fig. 4** Left: Histogram approximation of invariant measure $\bar{\mu}$ of the IFSPDP in Example 2, Case 2. Right: Approximation to cumulative distribution function $F(x)$ of $\bar{\mu}$

## 4   Inverse Problem of Measure Approximation Using IFSPDP

The formal inverse problem of measure approximation using IFSPDP may be posed as follows: Given a target measure $v \in \mathcal{M}(X)$ and an $\epsilon > 0$, find an IFSPSP $(\mathbf{w}, \mathbf{p})$ with invariant measure $\bar{\mu}$ such that $d_{MK}(\bar{\mu}, v) < \epsilon$. Such inverse problems involving fractal transforms are generally intractable so we consider a reformulated problem based on the *Collage Theorem*, a simple consequence of Banach's Fixed Point Theorem.

**Theorem 6** *(Collage Theorem)* [1] *Let $(Y, d_y)$ be a complete metric space and $T$ : $Y \to Y$ a contraction mapping with contraction factor $c_T \in [0, 1)$ and fixed point $\bar{y}$. Then for any $y \in Y$,*

$$d_y(y, \bar{y}) \leq \frac{1}{1 - c_T} d(y, Ty). \tag{20}$$

From the Collage Theorem, we now consider the following modified inverse problem: Given a target measure $v \in \mathcal{M}(X)$ and a $\delta > 0$, find an IFSPDP $(\mathbf{w}, \mathbf{p})$ with associated (contractive) Markov operator $M : \mathcal{M}(X) \to \mathcal{M}(X)$ such that $d_{MK}(Mv, v) < \delta$. Then, from the Collage Theorem, it follows that $d_{MK}(\bar{\mu}, v) < \delta(1 - c)^{-1}$.

As in [2], our strategy is to work with fixed sets of affine IFS maps $w_i : X \to X$, $1 \leq i \leq N$, optimizing over the unknown probability functions $p_i(x)$, $1 \leq i \leq N$. The IFS maps will be chosen from an infinite set of contraction maps on $X$ which satisfies the following refinement condition:

**Definition 1** Let $(X, d)$ be a compact metric space. An infinite set of contraction maps, $\mathcal{W} = \{w_1, w_2, \ldots\}$ is said to satisfy an $\epsilon$-contractivity condition on $X$ if for each $x \in X$, and any $\epsilon > 0$, there exists an $i^* \in \{1, 2, \ldots\}$ such that $w_{i^*}(X) \subset N_\epsilon(x)$, where $N_\epsilon(x) = \{y \in X \mid d(x, y) < \epsilon\}$ denotes the $\epsilon$-neighbourhood of $x$.

If $\mathcal{W}$ satisfies the $\epsilon$-contractivity condition on $X$, then $\inf_{i \geq 1} c_i = 0$, where $c_i$ is the contractivity factor of $w_i$. A useful set of affine maps on $X = [0, 1]$ which satisfies the $\epsilon$-contractivity condition is given by the following wavelet-type functions (here it is convenient to use two indices),

$$w_{ij}(x) = \frac{1}{2^j}[x + j - 1], \quad i = 1, 2, \ldots, \quad 1 \leq j \leq 2^i. \tag{21}$$

The following result, proved in Theorem 3.9 of [2], provides the existence of a solution to the inverse problem for measure approximation using IFSP, i.e., IFS with constant probabilities (see also [5] and [7]).

**Theorem 7** [2] *Let $(X, d)$ be a compact metric space and $\mu \in \mathcal{M}(X)$ be a target measure. Furthermore, let $\mathcal{W}$ be an infinite set of contraction maps on $X$ and $\mathbf{w}^N = \{w_1, w_2, \ldots, w_N\}$, $N \geq 1$ denote an $N$-map IFS selected from $\mathcal{W}$. We now consider the $N$-map IFSP $(\mathbf{w}^N, \mathbf{p}^N)$ defined over the following compact region in $\mathbb{R}^N$,*

$$\Sigma^N = \left\{ (p_1^N, p_2^N, \dots, p_N^N) \in \mathbb{R}^N \;\middle|\; p_i^N \geq 0, 1 \leq i \leq N \text{ and } \sum_{i=1}^{N} p_i^N = 1 \right\}, \quad (22)$$

*and let $M^N$ denote its associated Markov operator. Let $\mathbf{q}^N \in \Sigma^N$ be a point at which the collage distance $d_{MK}(\mu, M^N \mu)$ is minimized and let this minimum value be denoted as $\Delta_{\min}^N$. Then*

$$\lim_{N \to \infty} \Delta_{\min}^N = 0. \quad (23)$$

The solution to the inverse problem for IFSPDP with affine probability functions follows almost trivially from the above result. We replace the IFSP associated with an $N$-map IFS, $\mathbf{w}^N$, selected from the infinite set $\mathscr{W}$ by an $N$-map IFSPDP $(\mathbf{w}^N, \alpha^N, \beta^N)$ defined over the following compact region $\Sigma^N \subset \mathbb{R}^{2N}$. Since the special case $\alpha_1 = \alpha_2 = \dots = \alpha_N = 0$ corresponds to the $N$-map IFSP considered in Theorem 3.5 of [2], with $p_i = \beta_i$, $1 \leq i \leq N$, it follows that the (non-negative) minimum collage distance achieved on $\Sigma^N \supset \Pi^N$, which we denote as $\overline{\Delta}_{\min}^N$, must satisfy the inequality,

$$\overline{\Delta}_{\min}^N \leq \Delta_{\min}^N, \quad N \geq 1. \quad (24)$$

From (23), it follows that

$$\lim_{N \to \infty} \overline{\Delta}_{\min}^N = 0, \quad (25)$$

thus proving the existence of a solution to the inverse problem for measure approximation for affine IFSPDP on $X$ (for more details see [8]).

## 5 Conclusion

The new results of this paper are concerned with the problem of approximating probability measures on a compact metric space $(X, d)$ with invariant measures of iterated function systems with place-dependent probabilities. This paper may be considered to be a place-dependent extension of [2], in which the inverse problem of measure approximation using iterated function systems with constant probabilities was treated.

**Acknowledgements** This research was partially supported by Natural Sciences and Engineering Research Council of Canada (NSERC) in the form of Discovery Grants (FM and ERV). Support from the Department of Applied Mathematics and the Faculty of Mathematics, University of Waterloo, in the form of research and teaching assistantships (EAM), is also gratefully acknowledged.

# References

1. Barnsley, M.F.: Fractals Everywhere. Academic Press, New York (1989)
2. Forte, B., Vrscay, E.R.: Solving the inverse problem for measures using iterated function systems: a new approach. Adv. Appl. Prob. **27**, 800–820 (1995)
3. Forte, B., Vrscay, E.R.: Inverse problem methods for generalized fractal transforms. In: Fisher, Y. (Ed.) Fractal Image Coding and Analysis, NATO ASI Series F, vol. 159. Springer, Berlin (1998)
4. Hutchinson, J.: Fractals and self-similarity. Indiana Univ. J. Math. **30**, 713–747 (1981)
5. Iacus, S., La Torre, D.: A comparative simulation study on the IFS distribution function estimator. Nonlinear Anal. Real World Appl. **6**(5), 858–873 (2005)
6. Kunze, H., La Torre, D., Mendivil, F., Vrscay, E.R.: Fractal-Based Methods in Analysis. Springer, New York (2012)
7. La Torre, D., Vrscay, E.R.: Fractal-based measure approximation with entropy maximization and sparsity constraints. AIP Conf. Proc. **1443**, 63–71 (2012)
8. La Torre, D., Maki, E., Mendivil, F., Vrscay, E.R.: Iterated function systems with place-dependent probabilities and the inverse problem of measure approximation using moments, Fractals, in press. https://doi.org/10.1142/S0218348X18500767 (2018)
9. Maki, E.A.: Iterated function systems with place-dependent probabilities and the inverse problem of measure approximation using moments. M. Math. Thesis, Department of Applied Mathematics, University of Waterloo (2015)

# Solving Inverse Problems for Fractional ODEs via the Collage Theorem

Kimberly M. Levere and Brent Van De Walker

**Abstract** In this paper, we consider an inverse problem for a general class of fractional ordinary differential equations. Using the collage theorem, a consequence of Banach's classical Fixed Point Theorem, we establish a "collage method" for solving this inverse problem under certain restrictions. We apply this method to some model fractional ordinary differential equations in which we only use solution data (perhaps adding relative noise to simulate experimental error) to recover other parameters present in the model.

**Keywords** Fractional calculus · Fractional ordinary differential equations
Inverse problems · Applied analysis · Collage theorem · Numerical analysis

## 1 Introduction

A common goal of many methods for solving inverse problems is to minimize the approximation error; the distance between the true solution $y$ and the solution reached when using parameters that have been found inversely, $y_\lambda$. Computational expense and the difficulty of expressing $y_\lambda$ in terms of the parameters of the problem make this a challenging task. One technique for tackling this challenge is a "collage method" that bounds the approximation error above by the collage distance, $\|y - Ty\|$. Here $T$ is an operator that depends on the parameters of the problem. A number of such "collage methods" exist in the literature, see for instance, [7, 8].

In this paper we develop a collage-based method for solving inverse problems for fractional ordinary differential equations (FODEs). We begin in Sect. 2 with some required background knowledge, so that we can discuss and develop a collage

K. M. Levere (✉) · B. Van De Walker
University of Guelph, 50 Stone Road East, Guelph, ON N1G 2W1, Canada
e-mail: klevere@uoguelph.ca

B. Van De Walker
e-mail: bvandewa@uoguelph.ca

© Springer Nature Switzerland AG 2018
D. M. Kilgour et al. (eds.), *Recent Advances in Mathematical
and Statistical Methods*, Springer Proceedings in Mathematics & Statistics 259,
https://doi.org/10.1007/978-3-319-99719-3_12

method for FODEs in Sect. 3. In Sect. 4 we present some examples of this theory in practice with closing remarks in Sect. 5.

## 2  Mathematical Preliminaries and Scope

In this paper, we will focus on scalar $q$th order FODEs of the form

$$^{C}D_a^q y(x) = f(x, y(x)) \tag{1}$$

$$y^{(k)}(a) = y_0^{(k)}, \tag{2}$$

where $f$ is a bounded and Lipschitz in its second argument and $(x, y)$ are in the space $\Omega = [0, \beta] \times [y_0^{(0)} - \alpha, y_0^{(0)} + \alpha]$, for $\alpha, \beta > 0$. Here we make use of a $q$th order Caputo fractional derivative, defined by

$$^{C}D_a^q f(x) = \frac{1}{\Gamma(n - q)} \int_a^x (x - t)^{n-q-1} f^{(n)}(t),$$

for $n - 1 < q \le n$ which results in physically meaningful initial conditions.

By appealing to a result from [10], we know that if $f$ is continuous, then (1)–(2) is equivalent to the nonlinear Volterra-type equation

$$y(x) = \sum_{k=0}^{n-1} \frac{x^k}{k!} y^{(k)}(a) + \frac{1}{\Gamma(q)} \int_0^x (x - t)^{q-1} f(t, y(t)) \, dt. \tag{3}$$

for $n - 1 < q \le n$. The following result establishes existence and uniqueness of solutions to (1)–(2).

**Theorem 1**  *Let* $\Omega = [0, \beta] \times [y_0^{(0)} - \alpha, y_0^{(0)} + \alpha]$, *for* $\alpha, \beta > 0$ *and* $f : \Omega \to \mathbb{R}$ *be K-Lipschitz in its second argument. If* $\|f\|_\infty \le \dfrac{\alpha \Gamma(q + 1)}{\beta^q}$, *then there exists at most one function* $y(x)$ *solving the initial value problem* (1)–(2).

One way to prove Theorem 1 is using Banach's Fixed Point Theorem, which we state for completeness.

**Theorem 2**  (Banach's Fixed Point Theorem) *Let* $(X, \| \cdot \|_X)$ *be a Banach space and let* $T : X \to X$ *be a contractive operator with contraction factor* $c \in [0, 1)$. *Then there exists a unique fixed point* $\bar{x} \in X$ *such that* $A\bar{x} = \bar{x}$. *Moreover, for any* $x \in X$, $\|A^{\circ s} x - \bar{x}\|_X \to 0$ *as* $s \to \infty$.

Recall that an operator $T : X \to Y$ is contractive if for any $x_1, x_2 \in X$

$$\|Tx_1 - Tx_2\|_Y \le c\|x_1 - x_2\|_X,$$

for some $c \in [0, 1)$.

Note: The assumption of $0 < q < 1$ has been found to be the most useful in practical applications (see [2], for instance).

*Proof* (of Theorem 1) Without loss of generality, we shift the initial conditions to the origin, that is $(a, y_0^{(k)}) \to (0, 0))$. We also assume that $0 < q < 1$ as it has been found to be the most useful in practical applications (see [2], for instance). In light of Banach's Fixed Point Theorem and with these considerations in mind, we can prove Theorem 1 by first defining a Picard-like operator $T$ to be equal to the right-hand side of (3) when $0 < q < 1$. That is,

$$(Ty)(x) = \frac{1}{\Gamma(q)} \int_0^x (x - t)^{q-1} f(t, y(t)) \, dt. \tag{4}$$

We must show that the hypotheses of Banach's Fixed Point Theorem are satisfied for this choice of $T$. That is,

1. $(X, \| \cdot \|_X)$ is a Banach space;
2. $T : X \to X$; and
3. $T$ is contractive with contraction factor $c \in [0, 1)$.

We begin by defining the set $X = \{y \in C[0, \beta] : \|y\|_\infty \le \alpha\}$, for $\alpha, \beta \ge 0$. This set is non-empty as it contains $y_0^{(0)} = 0$, and is a closed subset of $C[0, \beta]$. Equipped with the sup norm, $\| \cdot \|_\infty$, it is well known that $(X, \| \cdot \|_\infty)$ is a Banach space.

To show that $T : X \to X$, we let $y \in X$, and exhibit that $\|Ty\|_\infty \le \alpha$ (thus proving that $Ty$ is also an element of $X$).

$$
\begin{aligned}
\|Ty\|_\infty &= \frac{1}{\Gamma(q)} \sup_{x \in [0,\beta]} \left| \int_0^x (x - t)^{q-1} f(t, y(t)) \, dt \right| \\
&\le \frac{\|f\|_\infty}{\Gamma(q)} \sup_{x \in [0,\beta]} \left| \int_0^x (x - t)^{q-1} \, dt \right| \\
&= \frac{\|f\|_\infty}{\Gamma(q+1)} \sup_{x \in [0,\beta]} x^q \\
&\le \frac{\|f\|_\infty}{\Gamma(q+1)} \beta^q
\end{aligned}
$$

Utilizing the hypothesis that bounds $f$, $\|f\|_\infty \le \dfrac{\alpha \Gamma(q+1)}{\beta^q}$, we get

$$
\begin{aligned}
\|Ty\|_\infty &\le \frac{\|f\|_\infty}{\Gamma(q+1)} \beta^q \\
&\le \frac{\frac{\alpha \Gamma(q+1)}{\beta^q}}{\Gamma(q+1)} \beta^q \\
&= \alpha.
\end{aligned}
$$

Thus, if $y \in X$ then $Ty \in X$, so we have shown that $T : X \to X$.

Finally, to show that the operator $T$ is contractive, we must find a $c \in [0, 1)$ such that for $u, v \in X$, $\|Tu - Tv\|_\infty \leq c\|u - v\|_\infty$.

$$
\begin{aligned}
\|Tu - Tv\|_\infty &= \frac{1}{\Gamma(q)} \sup_{x \in [0,\beta]} \left| \int_0^x (x - t)^{q-1} (f(t, u(t)) - f(t, v(t)) \, dt \right| \\
&\leq \frac{1}{\Gamma(q)} \left( \sup_{x \in [0,\beta]} \int_0^x |(x - t)^{q-1}| \, dt \right) \left( \sup_{x \in [0,\beta]} \int_0^x |f(t, u(t)) - f(t, v(t))| \, dt \right) \\
&\leq \frac{K\|u - v\|_\infty}{q\Gamma(q)} \sup_{x \in [0,\beta]} x^q \\
&\leq \frac{K\beta^q}{\Gamma(q + 1)} \|u - v\|_\infty.
\end{aligned}
$$

Defining $c := \dfrac{K\beta^q}{\Gamma(q + 1)}$, we can either restrict our choices of $f$ or the space $\Omega$ so that $\beta^q$ is such that $c \in [0, 1)$.

Having established all of the hypotheses of Banach's Fixed Point Theorem, we must have that $T$ has a unique fixed point $\bar{y}$ such that $T\bar{y} = \bar{y}$. This unique fixed point serves as the unique solution to (1)–(2).

Diethelm and Ford present a similar, but more general result for existence and uniqueness for this case in [2].


## 3   Inverse Problems via Collage Coding

We now concern ourselves with developing a method for solving an inverse problem for the general FODE (1)–(2) discussed in Sect. 2. Recall the form of this FODE

$$
\begin{aligned}
^C D_a^q y(x) &= f(x, y(x)) \\
y^{(k)}(a) &= y_0^{(k)},
\end{aligned}
$$

for $n - 1 < q \leq n$. Suppose now that $f$ depends on a set of unknown parameters, $\lambda \in \mathbb{R}^{\dim \lambda}$. The goal of such an inverse problem is to find these unknown parameter values such that the approximation error, $\|y - \bar{y}\|_\infty$, is minimized. That is, parameter values $\lambda$ are chosen so that the solution to the FODE (1–2) is sufficiently close to the fixed point of the operator $T$. A number of classical methods exist for solving such problems, including regularization techniques and iteration schemes (see, for instance, [3]). The collage coding method introduced in [7] and explored in several different settings (see [5, 6, 8], for instance) takes a slightly different approach. Since in practice, representing the fixed point $\bar{y}$ in terms of the parameters $\lambda$ can be a difficult task in practical problems, the collage coding approach bounds the approximation error $\|y - \bar{y}\|_\infty$ above by a more readily minimizable distance. This method gets its name from "the Collage Theorem", a simple consequence of Banach's Fixed Point Theorem, that exactly builds this upperbound on the approximation error.

**Theorem 3** (Collage Theorem) *Let* $(X, \|\cdot\|_X)$ *be a Banach space and* $T : X \to X$ *be a contractive operator with contraction factor* $c \in [0, 1)$ *and unique fixed point* $\bar{y} \in X$. *Then*

$$\|y - \bar{y}\|_X \leq \frac{1}{1 - c}\|y - Ty\|_X.$$

For a proof of Theorem 3, see [1]. Appropriately, we call the distance $\|y - Ty\|_X$ the collage distance.

The Collage Theorem says that by minimizing the collage distance, provided that $c$ is bounded away from 1, we can guarantee that that approximation error is also controlled. While the collage method does provide a novel and robust method for solving inverse problems, the collage distance is a suboptimal bound on the approximation error, as the following theorem from [4] indicates.

**Theorem 4** (Suboptimality of the collage theorem) *Let* $(X, \|\cdot\|_X)$ *be Banach space, and let* $y \in X$ *be a target function. Further, let* $\lambda_{min} = argmin_\lambda \|y - Ty\|_X$ *be the parameter values that minimize the collage distance, with corresponding fixed point* $\bar{y}$ *of the contractive map* $T$. *Let* $\bar{y}_{\lambda_{opt}}$ *be the optimal fixed point that minimizes the approximation error* $\|y - \bar{y}\|_X$; *that is,* $\bar{y}_{\lambda_{opt}}$ *satisfies* $\|\bar{y}_{\lambda_{opt}} - y\|_X \leq \|w - y\|_X$ *for all* $w$ *satisfying* $Tw = w$ *and some parameters* $\lambda$. *Then*

$$\|y_{\lambda_{opt}} - \bar{y}\|_X \leq \frac{2}{1 - c_{\lambda_{min}}}\|y - Ty\|_X,$$

*where* $c_{\lambda_{min}}$ *is the contraction factor of* $T$.

In practice, the collage distance is more easily minimized than the approximation error as the parameters $\lambda$ are imbedded in the operator $T$ and thus we no longer need to worry about finding ways to express the fixed point $\bar{y}$ in terms of these parameters. Depending on the complexity of the problem, a variety of techniques may be required to execute this minimization.

Having shown the operator $T$ given in (4) for the FODE (1)–(2) satisfies the conditions of Banach's Fixed Point Theorem, and thus also those of the Collage Theorem, we may apply this methodology to an inverse problem for a FODE of this form.

## 4 Examples

*Example 1* In an effort to connect to existing literature, the first simulation of the collage method for FODEs comes from [2]

$$D^{0.5}y(x) = -y(x) + x^2 + \frac{2x^{1.5}}{\Gamma(2.5)} \tag{5}$$

$$y(0) = 0, \tag{6}$$

where $x \in [0, 1]$. One can easily show that the closed form solution to (5)–(6) is $y = x^2$.

For the inverse problem, we will use only sample data of this solution (as it is unlikely that we would be afforded a closed-form solution) and assume that some of the coefficients in the fully determined FODE (5)–(6) are unknown. We will attempt to recover the constants $\lambda_0$, $\lambda_1$, and $\lambda_2$ present in the related FODE

$$D^{0.5}y(x) = y(x) + \lambda_1 x^2 + \frac{\lambda_2 x^{1.5}}{\Gamma(2.5)} \tag{7}$$

$$y(0) = \lambda_0. \tag{8}$$

We begin by simulating $N$ solution data values on the interval $[0, 1]$ (perhaps adding relative Gaussian noise to simulate experimental error). We then fit a polynomial of desired degree $M$ to our simulated data and use this polynomial fit as our target solution, $y_{target}(x)$.

Note that while we only display the results for target solutions of degree 2, simulations with varying target polynomial degrees were run and produced comparable results for degrees higher than 2 (as unnecessary degrees were identified by the minimization technique as zeros). When using a degree of 1, the simulation returned less than desirable results, but we reason that a researcher seeing such a weak fit would not deem it satisfactory and would attempt to improve the fit before proceeding with the inverse problem.

Our Picard-like operator as in (4) has the form

$$Ty(x) = \lambda_0 + \frac{1}{\Gamma(0.5)} \int_0^x (x-t)^{-0.5} \left( y(t) + \lambda_1 t^2 + \frac{\lambda_2 t^{1.5}}{\Gamma(2.5)} \right) dt$$

We recall that Banach's fixed point theorem (and also the collage theorem) requires that we work on a Banach space. As we are working with the space of continuous functions, it would stand to reason then that we would use the sup norm, $\| \cdot \|_\infty$. However, this norm is computationally cumbersome in practice so instead we will work with the $\mathscr{L}^2$ norm. This is not cause for concern as the space of continuous functions is a subset of the space of $\mathscr{L}^2$ functions. Thus our squared collage distance is given by

$$\Delta^2 = \int_0^1 (y_{target}(x) - Ty(x))^2 \, dx$$

$$= \int_0^1 \left( y_{target}(x) - \lambda_0 - \frac{1}{\Gamma(0.5)} \int_0^x (x-t)^{-0.5} \left( y(t) + \lambda_1 t^2 + \frac{\lambda_2 t^{1.5}}{\Gamma(2.5)} \right) dt \right)^2 dx$$

**Table 1** Parameter estimates for Example 1 for various levels of relative noise, $\epsilon$ and data values, $N$

| N | $\epsilon$ | $\lambda_0 (\lambda_0)_{true} = 0$ | $\lambda_1 (\lambda_1)_{true} = 1$ | $\lambda_2 (\lambda_2)_{true} = 2$ | $\Delta$ |
|---|---|---|---|---|---|
| 10 | 0 | $-3.9447 \times 10^{-39}$ | 1.000 | 2.000 | $1.8439 \times 10^{-21}$ |
| | 0.01 | $0.3479 \times 10^{-3}$ | 0.7020 | 1.4447 | $0.8167 \times 10^{-4}$ |
| | 0.02 | $0.6958 \times 10^{-3}$ | 0.4040 | 0.8894 | $0.1633 \times 10^{-2}$ |
| 20 | 0 | $-4.3817 \times 10^{-39}$ | 1.000 | 2.000 | $0.1 \times 10^{-20}$ |
| | 0.01 | $0.2770 \times 10^{-3}$ | 0.8898 | 1.8051 | $0.6848 \times 10^{-6}$ |
| | 0.02 | $0.5541 \times 10^{-3}$ | 0.7796 | 1.6102 | $0.1370 \times 10^{-4}$ |
| 30 | 0 | $-3.9447 \times 10^{-39}$ | 1.000 | 2.000 | $2.9155 \times 10^{-21}$ |
| | 0.01 | $0.2416 \times 10^{-3}$ | 0.9492 | 1.9164 | $0.6125 \times 10^{-8}$ |
| | 0.02 | $0.4832 \times 10^{-3}$ | 0.8985 | 1.8327 | $0.1225 \times 10^{-4}$ |
| 50 | 0 | $-3.9447 \times 10^{-39}$ | 1.0000 | 2.0000 | $4.4721 \times 10^{-21}$ |
| | 0.01 | $0.2062 \times 10^{-3}$ | 0.9857 | 1.9817 | $0.5468 \times 10^{-10}$ |
| | 0.02 | $0.4124 \times 10^{-3}$ | 0.9714 | 1.9634 | $0.1094 \times 10^{-7}$ |

We arrive at estimates of the parameters $\lambda_i$, $i = 0, 1, 2$ using least squares minimization on $\Delta^2$. For more involved problems more exotic minimization techniques may be necessary. The results of a number of simulations with various levels of Gaussian noise applied to various numbers of data values are given in Table 1.

The results agree with our mathematical intuition; the more data we have, the better our estimates are. The more noisy the data is, the less accurate our results are. Even at 2% relative noise, our results strongly agree with the true parameter values. Fifty digits were preserved in calculations of these values, so some accuracy may have been lost due to this numerical choice as well.

In our next example, we explore a more difficult problem with a solution that is trigonometric rather than polynomial. This gives rise to a much more complicated forcing function and thus more exotic numerical methods will be necessary to solve this inverse problem. It also begins to exhibit the robustness of this inverse problem method.

*Example 2* In this slightly more difficult example, we explore a FODE of the form

$$D^{\frac{1}{2}} y(x) + 3y(x) + 2 = f(x) \tag{9}$$
$$y(0) = 0, \tag{10}$$

for $x \in [0, 1]$, where

$$f(x) = \sqrt{2} \cos(x) C \left( \sqrt{\frac{2x}{\pi}} \right) + \sqrt{2} \sin(x) S \left( \sqrt{\frac{2x}{\pi}} \right)$$

and

$$C(x) = \int_0^x \cos(t^2)\, dt \qquad \text{and} \qquad S(x) = \int_0^x \sin(t^2)\, dt$$

are the Fresnal cosine and sine integrals, respectively. This example recognizes that many fractional problems contain particularly complicated forcing functions $f(x)$ or solution functions. It also exhibits the robustness of the method to non-polynomial solutions as the solution to this FODE is $y(x) = \sin(x)$.

Our goal in this example will be to recover the unknown constants $\lambda_0$, $\lambda_1$ and $\lambda_2$ present in the related FODE

$$D^{\frac{1}{2}} y(x) + \lambda_1 y(x) + \lambda_2 = f(x)$$
$$y(0) = \lambda_0,$$

In this case, our Picard-like operator takes the form

$$Ty(x) = \lambda_0 + \frac{1}{\Gamma\left(\frac{1}{2}\right)} \int_0^x (x - t)^{-\frac{1}{2}} \left( f(t) - \lambda_1 y_{target}(t) - \lambda_2 \right) dt$$

As the true solution is not a polynomial and thus by fitting our data using a polynomial target there will be some approximation error present (independent of experimental or observational error). It will be of interest to investigate if a higher degree polynomial for the target solution improves our results (as we would expect). Further, the complexity of the right-hand side makes the integration and minimization needed to solve this problem far more difficult than in previous examples. Since the collage distance is a nonlinear function of the parameters, $\lambda_i$, the integration needed for the computation of the collage distance is approximated using a midpoint Riemann sum. We also note that we use a polynomial of degree 10 to fit our solution data. The results of these simulations are listed in Table 2.

While the results in this example aren't quite as good as what we saw in the previous example, we note that given the complexity of the problem that our results actually compare quite favourably. Upon experimenting with different numerical integration techniques (such as Simpson, Trapezoid and Newton-Cotes) we see comparable results. It also appears that an increase in the degree of the target polynomial used to fit the solution data has only a small effect on our results as the number of data values used increases. Finally, the use of least squares and gradient descent minimization schemes were both employed and we found little difference in the results that were reached. Increasing the number of data values sampled, $N$, continued to improve our results (as was the trend in Table 2) with a negligible increase in computing time.

**Table 2** Parameter estimates for Example 3 for various levels of relative noise, $\epsilon$ and data values, $N$

| $N$ | $\epsilon$ | $\lambda_0 (\lambda_0)_{true} = 0$ | $\lambda_1 (\lambda_1)_{true} = 3$ | $\lambda_2 (\lambda_2)_{true} = 2$ | $\Delta$ |
|---|---|---|---|---|---|
| 10 | 0 | $-0.1650 \times 10^{-3}$ | 2.9672 | 1.9107 | $0.1673 \times 10^{-3}$ |
| | 0.01 | $-0.1590 \times 10^{-2}$ | 2.7849 | 1.8821 | $0.1678 \times 10^{-2}$ |
| | 0.02 | $-0.1525 \times 10^{-1}$ | 2.5409 | 1.8273 | $0.1710 \times 10^{-1}$ |
| 20 | 0 | $-0.5154 \times 10^{-3}$ | 2.9760 | 1.9581 | $0.8277 \times 10^{-3}$ |
| | 0.01 | $0.2284 \times 10^{-1}$ | 2.8442 | 1.9045 | $0.1534 \times 10^{-2}$ |
| | 0.02 | $0.7658 \times 10^{-1}$ | 2.6825 | 1.8476 | $0.2972 \times 10^{-1}$ |
| 30 | 0 | $-0.1645 \times 10^{-4}$ | 2.9942 | 1.9687 | $0.5518 \times 10^{-4}$ |
| | 0.01 | $-0.5523 \times 10^{-2}$ | 2.9827 | 1.9248 | $0.3085 \times 10^{-3}$ |
| | 0.02 | $-0.9274 \times 10^{-1}$ | 2.9660 | 1.8761 | $0.6415 \times 10^{-2}$ |
| 50 | 0 | $-0.2494 \times 10^{-5}$ | 3.0041 | 2.0311 | $0.3311 \times 10^{-6}$ |
| | 0.01 | $-0.4168 \times 10^{-3}$ | 2.9660 | 1.9615 | $0.9131 \times 10^{-4}$ |
| | 0.02 | $0.6664 \times 10^{-2}$ | 3.0609 | 1.8914 | $0.1808 \times 10^{-3}$ |

## 5 Conclusions

We have derived and implemented a novel inverse problem method for treating some fractional ordinary differential equations. With existence and uniqueness proven via classical techniques, we have used Picard-like operators to build a collage distance that we minimized in order to guarantee that the approximation error was controlled. While this is a suboptimal method, we have exhibited the robustness of the method to a few different complexities, including the presence of a (classical) derivative in the collage distance, as well as a more complex forcing function, $f(x)$. Through these simulations, we have shown that the method performs strongly even when facing such complexities. Certainly experimental error challenges this technique, as it does not perform quite as well when the target solution is not exact. However, increasing the number of data values sampled certainly decreases this effect, as we would expect. More exotic numerical methods for integration and minimization can certainly assist this technique in successfully finding solutions. Perhaps further investigation into other such techniques might improve these results further.

## References

1. Barnsley, M.F., Ervin, V., Hardin, D., Lancaster, J.: Solution of an inverse problem for fractals and other sets. Proc. Natl. Acad. Sci. USA **83**, 1975–1977 (1995)
2. Diethelm, K., Ford, N.J.: Analysis of fractional differential equations. J. Math. Anal. Appl. **265**, 229–248 (2002)
3. Groetsch, C.W.: Inverse Problems in the Mathematical Sciences. Vieweg, Wiesbaden (1993)
4. Kunze, H.E., Hicken, J.E., Vrscay, E.R.: Inverse problems for ODEs using contraction mappings and suboptimality of the 'collage method'. Inverse Probl. **20**, 977–991 (2004)

5. Kunze, H.E., La Torre, D., Levere, K.M., Vrscay, E.R.: Solving inverse problems for deterministic and random delay integral equations using the collage method. Int. J. Math. Stat. (IJMS), **11**(1) (2012)
6. Kunze, H.E., Vasiliadis, S.: Using the collage method to solve ODEs inverse problems with multiple data sets. Theory Methods Appl. Nonlinear Anal. (2009)
7. Kunze, H.E., Vrscay, E.R.: Solving inverse problems for ordinary differential equations using the Picard contraction mapping. Inverse Probl. **15**, 745–770 (1999)
8. Levere, K.: A Collage-Based Approach to Inverse Problems for Systems of Nonlinear Partial Differential Equations. Ph.D. thesis, University of Guelph, Guelph, Ontario (2012)
9. Podlubny, I.: Fractional Differential Equations: An Introduction to Fractional Derivatives, Fractional Differential Equations, to Methods of Their Solution and Some of Their Applications. Academic Press, San Diego (1999)
10. Samko, S.G., Kilbas, A.A., Marichev, O.I.: Fractional Integrals and Derivatives: Theory and Applications. Gordon and Breach Science Publishers, Switzerland (1993)

# Part III
# Computational Methods and Modelling in Engineering and Mechanics

# Characterization of Fluid Dynamics in Capillary Vessels: Applications for Drug Delivery

Seraphin C. Abou

**Abstract** The delivery of a sufficient dose of pharmaceutical composite in microvessels as to safely achieve its desired therapeutic care poses severe risks. Yet, no theory is sufficiently expanded to portray the observed viscoelastic phenomena in variety of fluid flow conditions in capillaries. In this study, the dynamics of non-Newtonian pharmaceutical composite flow is explored by mapping its pathway as directly related to lymph flow in live cells. We hypothesize descriptors of the pharmaceutical composite flow can be elaborated at isobaric-isothermal non-Newtonian flow conditions to acquire constitutive equations. Then, the mechanism and energetics associated with such flow states, and the rheology effects due to the plasma-rich zones that form near the wall in capillaries are numerically characterized. The model portrays blood flow properties at the mesoscopic level and enables a computational framework at microvessel levels for prediction of the rheology of pharmaceutical composite that does not follow Newtonian dynamics but is compatible to that of the blood at different velocity profiles under both the normal and the pathological conditions.

**Keywords** Microsystems · Non-Newtonian · Rheology · Modeling and simulation

## 1 Introduction

Classical fluid mechanics, which stands on the application of the Navier-Stokes equations, including the continuum equations of motion cannot elaborate many important flow problems of practical significance. In this paper, the concept of non-Newtonian fluid flow is applied to clinical settings for drug delivery. By no means, does the analysis cover the dilution or solubility of pharmaceutical composite in live cells, but it expounds upon inherent details of the particulate nature of non-Newtonian drug

S. C. Abou (✉)
Mechanical Engineering Department, W.V.S. Tubman University,
PO Box. 3570, Harper, Maryland County, Republic of Liberia
e-mail: sabou@tubmanu.edu.lr; serchally@gmail.com

© Springer Nature Switzerland AG 2018
D. M. Kilgour et al. (eds.), *Recent Advances in Mathematical
and Statistical Methods*, Springer Proceedings in Mathematics & Statistics 259,
https://doi.org/10.1007/978-3-319-99719-3_13

139

composite modeling and blood cell characteristics in a mathematical representation of blood rheology features that might be considered to safely achieve desired therapeutic care and quality of life under both the normal and the pathological conditions.

We derive generic expressions of Non-Newtonian flow which integrate a variety of fluid mechanics phenomena. Although quantitative analysis has been performed for understanding attributes of blood flow resistance in vitro based on basic ideas of fluid flow, the simplifying assumptions as related to viscoelastic models have restricted ourselves to the tenets that model fluids' flow in ideal conditions – those that do not exhibit any frictional properties or describe strain rate dependence of viscosity and normal stress phenomena. Examples of prominent linear models are: The Bernoulli equation which considers the forces present in moving fluid while the friction due to viscous forces are neglected Eq. (1); The Jeffreys, and Maxwell models, respectively Eqs. (2), and (3), which are not valid to satisfy the principle of frame invariance, including models that obey the Newton law of viscosity, Eq. (4), to name a few:

$$\Delta p + \gamma \Delta z + \rho \frac{\bar{v}^2}{2} = 0 \tag{1}$$

$$\tau + \alpha_1 \frac{\partial \tau}{\partial t} = \mu_0 \left( \dot{\gamma} + \alpha_2 \frac{\partial \dot{\gamma}}{\partial t} \right) \tag{2}$$

$$\tau + \alpha_1 \frac{\partial \tau}{\partial t} = \mu_0 \dot{\gamma} \tag{3}$$

$$\left. \begin{array}{l} \rho \left( \frac{\partial u}{\partial t} + u.\nabla u + \alpha_1 \right) = -\nabla \rho + \mu \Delta u + f \\ \nabla . u = 0 \end{array} \right\} \tag{4}$$

where $\Delta p$- is pressure loss, $\bar{v}$- is the mean velocity, $\Delta z$- is the head loss; $\rho$- is the fluid density; $\alpha_1$ and $\alpha_2$- are relaxation and retardation time respectively; $\mu$- is constant fluid viscosity; $\dot{\gamma}$- is rate of strain tensor; $\tau$- is the stress; $u$- is fluid velocity; $\nabla u$- is velocity gradient; $p$- is pressure; and $f$- is external body force.

The higher the strain rate, the shorter the time at which the critical strain's departure from linear regime is reached, [3, 13, 14]. At the capillaries level, blood cell membranes deform due to hematocrit properties – the volume fraction of the red blood cells (RBCs) to the total blood volume [6, 15]. We come to the fact that neither the basic idea of the fluid flow, nor the knowledge of the bulk material properties of blood cells provide insights to express blood flow through narrow cylindrical tubes. Thus, reduction of viscosity decreases with decreasing tube size – Fahraeus-Lindqvist effects, [7].

In this framework, to account for blood flow resistance observed in-vivo, we argue that network modeling approach appears to be more realistic to modeling non-Newtonian pharmaceutical composite flow in capillaries. Yet, these considerations are still unable to account for all effective complexities and to make precise determination to the extent we can predict with high accuracy the flow conditions. However, to advance clinical care applications, the *Biot number* $= hL/k_s$ may be approximated to be small enough such that lumped capacitance model is applied to small sized droplet fluid. Of particular interest is to find what kind of descriptors can be used to acquire constitutive equations, and to analytically solve in safe manner capillary fluid flow problems. Therefore, to balance the body fluids transport phenomena, we examine the physical properties of the fluids within the body and pay detailed attention to effects of the extracellular and transcellular fluids although we are dealing with intracellular flow. Then, we emphasize on the characterization of non-Newtonian rheology effects due to the plasma-rich zone that forms near the wall in capillaries.

The physiological and the deformability properties of blood cells are factored to map the non-Newtonian fluid flow models analogous to those in mechanistic behaviors. This enables to relate physical-mechanical properties to those of leaf spring properties. Excluding the characteristic time dependence of at least one parameter that accounts for the fluid memory, the constitutive equations in real space coordinates which satisfy the Oldroyd's admissibility criteria, [3, 10–12], is expressed. One of the rationales which support this approach is that, when fluid suffers significant deformation in time, comparable to the relaxation time of the fluid, elastic effects become important to account for change of coordinate system and value invariant under rheological descriptors of neighboring fluid including extracellular and transcellular elements. These parameters are strongly influenced by the geometry of vessels.

## 2  Physical-Rheological Considerations

The resistance to fluid flow within Microvessel channels depends on the physical structure of the microvascular network and the rheological properties of the fluid. We illustrate diverse ranges of the behavior involved in both, the nature and the health care technology applications to deepen the analysis where most of the variables influence the fluid motion, including the versatile nature of the non-Newtonian pharmaceutical composite. Evidence indicates that physics of the flow that does not explicitly accounts for frictional properties or describe strain rate dependence of viscosity and normal stress phenomena, would merely depict the complexities of non-Newtonian fluids. As a result, we determine the pharmaceutical composite flow across the capillary membranes by Starling forces – hydrostatic and the oncotic forces which have been measured at well-defined steady states. But, yet, the molecular identity of capillary channels remains unknown [15]. Figure 1 depicts the capillary membrane pressure distributions.

The variance between capillary oncotic pressure and interstitial oncotic pressure determines the osmotic pressure gradient. It hastily induces decreasing apparent viscosity along with decreasing capillaries diameter which obeys the Fahraeus-Linqvist effect. Hence, flow resistance through capillaries is affected in many pathological conditions, making quantitative approach mere indicators to characterize the complex rheological properties of blood where apparent viscosity and relative viscosity relate

**Fig. 1** Capillary membrane
pressure distribution
$d \leq 9 \times 10^{-6}$ m

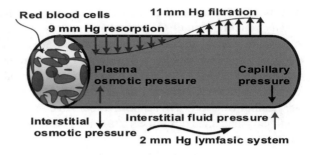

blood flow to the Newtonian fluid – the plasma. However, for Newtonian laminar flow, the Hagen-Poiseuille solution is satisfied to describe the viscosity:

$$\Delta p_L = \frac{8\mu Q}{\pi r^4} \Rightarrow \mu = \frac{\Delta p_L r^2}{2v_a} \tag{5}$$

where $\Delta p_L$ is the pressure drop per unit of length; $r$ is the radius of the tube;
$v_a$ is the average velocity

Figure 2 indicates that fluid viscosity is explicitly related to the number of the red cells concentration – hematocrit. Under physiological conditions, blood viscosity appears to be about three times higher than the viscosity of water, [16, 18].

The dynamics of the pharmaceutical fluid flow within capillaries is compatible to that of the blood. The fluid moves along with the blood from the bloodstream into the body's tissues and exhibits complex properties. Though, these states are referred to those of non-Newtonian fluids in general, the fluid may exhibit antihypertensive drug atenolol properties, attempt to stay within the blood and surrounding cells' interstitial space, [9]. Due to the deformation in microcirculation, the two-phase nature of blood results in non-Newtonian dynamics where vessel dimensions become comparable to cell diameter and the interactions between blood cells. Therefore, the nonlinear increase of viscosity with increasing hematocrit, as in Fig. 2, and the variation of the shear rate would impact to a great magnitude the interpretation of physiological and pathological behavior of the flow within microvessels.

**Fig. 2** Fluid Viscosity
related to hematocrit

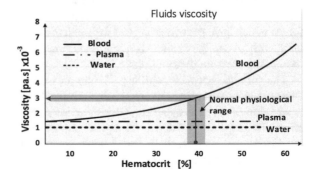

## 2.1   Factors Influencing Viscosity

The literature review illustrates that blood is non-Newtonian fluid, [2, 9]. In most of these references, however, the use of a capillary viscometer, has practical limitations that make it difficult to express values of the viscosity of the pharmaceutical composite over the lower ranges of shear rate. Moreover, the variation in shear rate is not linear as the radius of the tube changes. Also, the admission of the compatibility of the lymph to the pharmaceutical composite flow in capillaries adheres to the notion that the viscosity is anomalous and the Poiseuille law may not be directly applied to the conditions of the flow in the capillary circulation. The model of the pharmaceutical composite flow is schematically depicted in Fig. 3, showing that the flow of the pharmaceutical composite is explicitly influenced by blood and plasma viscosities, as well as the rheological properties of blood cells (e.g., deformability and aggregation of red blood cells in pathological conditions), including the disease processes and extreme physiological conditions. Hence, considerations for advanced factors which contribute to the variation of the viscosity of the flow in the capillaries include the following:

(1) The discontinuity in pressure at a given point of an interface of vessels. This results in product of the local value of surface tension, and twice the mean values of the curvature at the interface. It is known as the Young-Laplace law.
(2) The macromolecules of the blood on the inner endothelial surface which obstruct the pharmaceutical composite fluid flow in near-wall regions of microvessels either by increasing the local viscosity or by temporally sticking to passing blood cells, Fig. 3.
(3) The inner vessel contour which is irregular and may infer distortion of the red blood cells and resistance to fluid flow. Though, each local branch point leads to energy dissipation and perturbation of the velocity and concentration profiles in the downstream vessels.

Due to clinical applications, the use of the network approach might have a prognostic significance indicating more accurate profile of the pharmaceutical composite

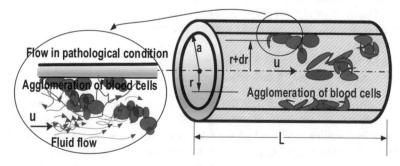

**Fig. 3**  Capillary fluid flow

flow within capillaries. Thus, specific patterns of the flow exhibit non-Newtonian behavior – time, spatial, and frictional force properties dependence of the viscosity, including isobaric-isothermal and steady boundary conditions.

Consider the velocity, $u$- of the fluid layer at a distance, $r$- from the center line of the capillary, the layer $r + dr$, the velocity gradient-$\vartheta$, Fig. 3, can be expressed as:

$$\vartheta = -\frac{du}{dr} \tag{6}$$

Eq. (6) gives the tangential stress -$\tau_s$ along the capillary wall and the viscous force $f_s$

$$\left.\begin{array}{l} \tau_s = \eta\vartheta \\ f_s = 2\pi\tau_s rL \end{array}\right\} \tag{7}$$

where L and r - are the length and the radius of the capillary, respectively.


# 3   Distorted Velocity Profile

Jean-Marie Poiseuille conducted experimental studies and determined the capillary flow resistance as function of the geometry of the blood vessels network is directly proportional to both the viscosity of blood and the length of the capillary segment, and inversely proportional to the fourth power of the vessel radius [1, 7]. However, this cannot be exhaustively sustained due to the strong influence of cellular pathology theory. In line with these observations, notice that intensified red blood cells (RBC) aggregation (i.e. erythrocyte) increases capillaries flow resistance (i.e. viscosity) under low shear forces. Also, cellular content of blood varies over a wide range at different levels of circulatory system. Scientists ignored the role of blood viscosity in flow through a given vascular network for various reasons:

(1) The medical diagnoses using fixed tissues, static, and microscopic observations of dead tissues have less basis to support blood viscosity factors, and the pharmaceutical fluid attributes
(2) The viscosity factor was considered as constant, rather than variable as reported in the Poiseuille equation and may not adhere to pharmaceutical fluid flow in capillaries
(3) The fourth power factor of the blood vessel radius was negligible and less important than the viscosity factor of first power.

These observations concur with the analysis portrayed in Fig. 4 and demonstrate that, increasing the length of the capillaries, the fluid velocity profile approaches to parabolic (Poiseuille) profile while the flow characteristics are laminar. Hence, the derivation of the law related to network modeling may be used to expand the analysis over specific aspects of local geometry of capillaries' curves and surfaces.

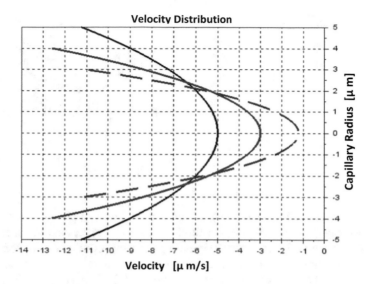

**Fig. 4** Fluid velocity distribution

Equations which describe the unsteadily incompressible flow through capillaries provide new insights to better understand the dynamic behavior of biological fluids composite dependence on flow conditions through capillaries. These equations, while solved in both temporal and spatial domains, suggest that, erythrocytes (i.e. red blood cells) aggregate in a special way forming rouleaux, and reduce the pharmaceutical composite fluid flow. However, in pathological conditions, it may not always be possible to determine the extent to which changes in rheological parameters effect the flow in the disease process. We argue that the fundamental governing one-dimensional equation of the flow can be described first, and then solved using the method of characteristics.

## 4   Model Description

Pharmaceutical composites flow at disparate scales across the capillary walls, through junctions between endothelial cells or through larger leaks in microvessel walls. We can illustrate the fluid motion without portraying in-depth the flow representation through interconnected lattices at a great degree of accuracy and physiological realm, Fig. 5. Upon the flow characteristics and the configuration of the capillaries, we idealized capillary wall for the flow patterns description based on the network modeling approach. The method has several advantages, namely, reasonable accuracy for solving highly complex free surface flow conditions.

Notice that strong pressure gradients may occur and may cause the pharmaceutical fluid break up. The liquid break-up process awaits future investigation. Neither the

**Fig. 5** The capillary
networks

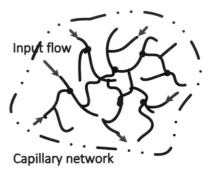

vascular system is geometrically challenged nor the breakup phenomenon is dealt
with in this paper. The rheological constitutive equation for pharmaceutical composite has not yet been fully explored. The main parameters considered are defined as:
$\mu_o$, and $\mu_b$- are the dynamic viscosities of pharmaceutical composite and the lymph,
respectively; $\rho_o$, and $\rho_b$- are the densities of fluid and the lymph, respectively; $u$- is
the mean fluid velocity; r - is the capillary radius at arbitrary time t; $\sigma_o$- is the surface
tension coefficient at the fluid-capillary interface.

The following assumption can be alleviated when a better rheological model is
formulated making the problem computationally more practical and verifiable:

(1) The pharmaceutical composite is non-Newtonian and possesses elastic and
    thixotropic properties;
(2) The fluid layer is uniform throughout the capillary length;
(3) Surfactants of the fluid are evenly distributed throughout the interface. Therefore,
    the Gibbs–Marangoni flow effects are not considered;
(4) The yield-stress values are properties of the fluid induced by various capillary
    shape factors, [8, 17]. In addition, the fluid conductance pathway depends on
    both the fluid and the geometry of the network of capillaries if less than 6 μm
    as shown in Fig. 5.

We derived equations that relate surface tension to surfactant concentration. Surface tension $\sigma$ has the units of energy over area and may be thought of as a negative
surface pressure, or as a line tension acting in all directions parallel to the capillary
surface. Thus, to map the gravitational assisted flow, the Bond number expresses the
ratio of capillary forces to gravitation force and accounts for the dominance of the
viscous forces over capillary forces. It is defined as:

$$B_o = \frac{\Delta \rho_o g R^2}{\sigma_o} \tag{8}$$

where R is the radius of the capillary; g is gravitational acceleration.

More importantly, we account for the curvature, the viscosity, the density of the
fluid, and the length of the capillary. Due to the aggregation of the red blood cells

on the capillary walls, a straightforward dimensional analysis yields that the average radius of the fluid $r_o \ll R$ depends upon time and six dimensionless parameters:

$$\frac{R_0}{R} = f\left(Re_o, \frac{x}{L}, \frac{\mu_o}{\mu_b}, C_a, \frac{tu}{R}, \frac{\rho_o}{\rho_b}, \frac{r_o}{R}\right) \tag{9}$$

where $Re_0$ is the Reynolds number for fluid flow; $R_0$ is the radius of the curvature of the capillary; and $C_a$ is the capillary number

$$C_a = k\left(\frac{\mu_b U}{\sigma_0}\right)^\varepsilon \tag{10}$$

where k is the curvature coefficient of the fluid interface.

Besides the special hemodynamic mechanisms affecting the pharmaceutical composite flow, the body autoregulation based on vascular control mechanisms further complicates the dimensional analysis, Eq. (9), where the capillary number is defined as the ratio of hydrodynamic shear forces to surface tension at a liquid–capillary and agglomerated red interface. Notice that pressure gradient $\Delta p$ of the fluid is not an independent parameter, [4], as it is related to the blood mean velocity - U.

## 4.1 Pathophysiological Consequence

As depicted in Fig. 3 we are submitting that the fluid zone closest to the capillary wall has the greatest contribution to flow resistance, as the frictional energy loss in this region is maximal. These conditions, in turn, affect the properties of the pharmaceutical composite flow. While the agglomeration of red blood cells at a low rate and the related drop in viscosity results in decreased local hydrodynamic resistance affecting, the general hydrodynamic resistance in the capillary system, the pathophysiological influences remain debatable because of the experimentally concluded variance between in-vivo and ex-vivo rheological behaviors of blood tissue, [5, 7]. In healthy conditions, the phenomenological properties are invariable for a healthy body where the hematocrit ratio is 45%, Fig. 2. Therefore, we may disregard changes in the density ratio, and the viscosity ratio in Eq. (9), which results in:

$$\frac{R_0}{R} = f\left(Re_o, \frac{x}{L}, \frac{tu}{R}, \frac{r_o}{R}, C_a\right) \tag{11}$$

Hence the relative viscosity given by so called Fahraeus-Lindqvist effects based on the tube diameter D is presented as:

$$\mu_{0.45} = 220e^{-1.3D} - 2.44e^{-0.06D^{0.645}} + 3.2 \tag{12}$$

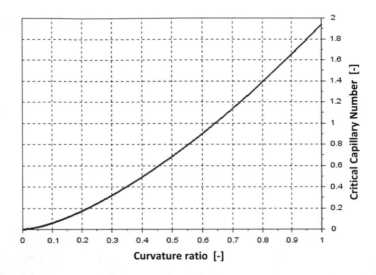

**Fig. 6** Critical Capillary number

To account for relevant source of measurement errors, although the Eq. (12) has been of great importance to ground knowledge about the flow characteristics, we deduce the agglomeration of the red blood cells concentrated in the central flow zone, while side branches from the main capillary line are fed by the plasma-rich zone. This concentration has lower hematocrit values as shown in Fig. 3. As a result, the manifestation of Eq. (11) implies the dependence of critical capillary number $C_{a, cr}$ upon the ratio of the capillary curvature and its diameter, $\frac{R_0}{R}$ as follows:

$$C_{a, cr} = k \left( \frac{R_0}{R} \right)^{\varepsilon} = 1.94 \left( \frac{R_0}{R} \right)^{3/2} \tag{13}$$

Figure 6 depicts the capillary number of the fluid as function of the curvature ratio. The collective knowledge portrayed by Fig. 5, indicates that, while we strongly adhere to the physical sense of the shear-rate dependence viscosity of the fluid, Eq. (13) supports that the variation of the pharmaceutical fluid rheological law is more obvious than those of the viscosity error law.

## 5 Discussion

Due to limited data, the analytical expression of the capillary ratio cannot provide a systemic dependence of parameters affecting the pharmaceutical composite flow distribution and the absorption rate through tissues. Further numerical and analytical investigation on curved, finite thin films, blood rheology is required to fully understand the effects of phenomenological coefficients on the flow, for example the curvature coefficient. Neither the vascular system geometrical challenges, nor the break-up phenomena are dealt with in this paper. In addition, in pathological conditions, due the distance traveled, the absorption rate and non-neglectable quantity of the volume may be dissipated before change of the direction occurs due to curvature orientation. In this case, the fate of the Non-Newtonian flow must be re-evaluated accounting for variable initial conditions.

# 6 Conclusion

Characterization of non-Newtonian rheology effects due to the plasma-rich zone that forms near the wall in capillaries has been studied with the help of a network model. Of particular interest this framework was to determine what kind of the flow descriptors can be elaborated to acquire constitutive equation and analytically solve in safe manner capillary fluid flow. For realistic predictions of the rheology of the fluid that does not follow Newtonian dynamics, the model portrayed blood flow descriptors at the mesoscopic level. The approach is capable to a greater extent of predicting the trend of the fluid flow dynamics complexity. The fluid flow methodology shows an appropriate step towards the generation of well-defined velocity profiles under both the normal and the pathological conditions. In the future, the present study can be improved by optimized numerics with inclusion of the absorption rate of the fluid to predict the fluid transfer in more realistic live cell situation.

# References

1. Baskurt, O.K., Meiselman, H.J.: Blood rheology and hemodynamics. Semin Throm Hemost. **29**(5), 435–450 (2003)
2. Bayliss, L.E.: The axial drift of the red cells when blood flows in a narrow tube. J. Physiol. **149**(3), 593–613 (1959)
3. Bird, R.B., Armstrong, C.: Dynamics of Polymeric Liquids, $2^{nd}$ ed., vol. 1. J. Wiley (1987)
4. Carreau, P.J., De Kee, D.: Rheology of Polymeric Systems. Hanser Publishers (1997)
5. Fahraeus, R., Lindqvist, T.: The viscosity of the blood in narrow capillary tubes. Am. J. Physiol. **96**, 562–568 (1931)
6. Fahraeus, R.: The influence of the rouleau formation of the erythrocytes on the rheology of the blood. Acta Med. Scand. **161**(2), 151–165 (1958)
7. Fahraeus, R.: The Suspension Stability of the Blood. Physiol. Rev. **9**, 241–274 (1929)
8. Fedosov, D.A., Peltomaeki, M., et al.: Deformation and dynamics of red blood cells in flow through cylindrical microchannels. Soft Matter **10**(24), 4258–4267 (2014)
9. Larson, R.G.: Constitutive Equations for Polymer Melts. Butterworth Publishers (1988)
10. Larson, R.G.: The Structure and Rheology of Complex Fluids. Oxford University Press, Oxford (1999)
11. Morais, A.F., Seybold, H.: Non-newtonian fluid flow through three-dimensional disordered porous media. Phys. Rev. Lett. **103**(19), 194–502 (2009)
12. Phan-Thien, N., Khan, M.K.: Flow of an Oldroyd-type fluid through a sinusoidally corrugated tube. J. Non-Newton. Fluid Mech. **24**(2), 203–220 (1987)

13. Popel, A.S.: Microcirculation and hemorheology. Ann. Rev. Fluid Mech. **37**, 43–69 (2005)
14. Sasd Han, K.-H., Frazier, A.B.: J. Appl. Phys. **96**(10), 57–97 (2004)
15. Sutera, S.P., Seshadri, V., Croce, P.A.: Capillary blood flow: II. Deformable model cells in tube flow. Microvasc. Res. **2**, 420–433 (1970)
16. Sochi, T.: Non-Newtonian flow in porous media. J. Poly., pp. 5007–5023 (2010)
17. Wells, R. E., Merrill, E. W.: Influence of flow properties of blood upon viscosity-hematocrit relationships. J. Clin. Invest **41**(8), 1591–1598 (1962)
18. Whittaker, S.R.F., et al.: The apparent viscosity of blood in the isolated hind limb of the dog and its variation with corpuscular concentration. J. Physiol., pp. 339–368 (1933)

# Large Eddy Simulation of Turbulent Flow Over a Hill Using a Canopy Stress Model

Md. Abdus Samad Bhuiyan and Jahrul M. Alam

**Abstract** Mathematical modelling of a turbulent flow over hilly terrains is an important topic in both mesoscale weather prediction and boundary layer meteorology. In comparison to the classical terrain-following coordinate approach, the immersed boundary technique on a Cartesian grid simplifies the implementation of the boundary condition on the surface of the hill, and this approach also mitigates discretization errors which would occur due to the terrain-following coordinate transformation. In the present research, we have extended a canopy stress model to formulate the boundary condition on the surface of a hill and considered the large eddy simulation method to predict the interaction between the near-surface coherent structures and a smooth hill. In addition to the canopy stress model, the turbulent stress has also been varied dynamically as the surface is approached, where the canopy stress model is derived based on the experimental observation that the drag coefficient becomes independent of the Reynolds number ($Re$) when $Re$ is sufficiently large. The proposed model has been tested by simulating a neutrally stratified atmospheric boundary layer over a periodic array of smooth hills. The agreement among the results of the present simulation, a dynamically similar experiment, and an equivalent numerical model suggests the potential benefits of the proposed method of simulating turbulent flow over hilly terrains.

**Keywords** Large eddy simulation · Turbulence · Canopy stress model · Hilly Terrian

Md. A. S. Bhuiyan (✉) · J. M. Alam
Memorial University of Newfoundland, St. John's, Canada
e-mail: masb80@mun.ca

J. M. Alam
e-mail: alamj@mun.ca

© Springer Nature Switzerland AG 2018                                     151
D. M. Kilgour et al. (eds.), *Recent Advances in Mathematical
and Statistical Methods*, Springer Proceedings in Mathematics & Statistics 259,
https://doi.org/10.1007/978-3-319-99719-3_14

# 1   Introduction

An accurate mathematical modelling of subgrid-scale turbulence for Atmospheric Boundary Layer (ABL) flows over a complex terrain is an important research topic. Atmospheric modelling areas, such as mesoscale weather prediction, boundary layer meteorology, exchange of energy between the surface and the atmosphere are influenced by complex terrains (i.e. a hilly surface). To improve our understanding of terrain-induced turbulence, a widely used Computational Fluid Dynamics (CFD) technique is the large eddy simulation (LES) methodology in which the large eddies are computed directly, and the subgrid scale (SGS) eddies are modelled. However, in the presence of a complex terrain, LES must be supplemented with an accurate stress boundary condition on the surface of hills, without which an extremely refined mesh is necessary to capture the viscous layer over the hilly surface [10]. In this article, we investigate the canopy stress method for modelling the subgrid-scale effects of surface topography and validate results of LES for the ABL flow over a hill using wind tunnel measurements. In LES the eddy-viscosity $\nu_\tau$ is obtained from the resolved rate of strain, which is known as the Smagorinsky model. A better result may be obtained by dynamically adapting $\nu_\tau$ to the distance from the terrain (e.g. [12]). Since turbulent eddies are affected by the length scale of uneven surface topography, an implementation of the standard Dynamic Smagorinsky model for ABL flows over a complex terrain is a challenging endeavour (see [7, 10]). In [12], $\nu_\tau$ was obtained from both the rate of strain and the rate of rotation. In other words, the Smagorinsky model can be modified by considering the rate of rotation. This approach – known as the wall adaptive eddy viscosity (WALE) model – adapts $\nu_\tau$ dynamically with the local distance from the surface topography (e.g. see [12] for details). One of our arguments in this research is that neither the Dynamics Smagorinsky model nor the WALE model correctly accounts for the terrain-induced SGS stress experienced by eddies passing over a complex terrain. In this article, we consider the LES of a turbulent flow over a hill in which a canopy stress method accounts for the terrain-induced SGS stress in addition to the standard SGS stress computed by the WALE model. To validate the results of such an LES, we consider experimental data from a reference (e.g. [8]) providing wind tunnel measurements of a flow over a smooth hill, which is an important aspect of this article.

Canopy stress methods for LES of forest canopies can be found in [2]. However, in Ref. [5] the canopy stress formulation of the pressure drag was examined to simulate the flow over ridges of varying heights. Reference [1] considered the canopy formulation of the viscous stress experienced by mesoscale eddies passing over an Agnesi hill. In the present work, a canopy stress formulation of both the viscous stress and the pressure drag has been verified along with the WALE model, where $\nu_\tau$ is dynamically adjusted to the vertical distance from the hill. As discuss by [5], a goal of the canopy stress method is to bypass the computational workload of the terrain following mesh that would resolve the viscous layer (see also [6, 7, 9]). For a complex terrain, resolving the viscous layer by an adaptive mesh produces inaccurate turbulence statistics [7]. Reference [11] illustrates that such errors are due to the terrain following mesh, and the error deteriorates if the mesh is refined in order to resolve the terrain. Such errors may be minimized with immersed boundary method [10] or by employing a mixed model based on an explicitly filtered LES. Nevertheless, the present validation of the canopy stress method against wind tunnel measurement is a significant improvement of the LES methodology for complex terrain.

The governing equations for LES, subgrid-scale WALE model, and the canopy stress method are discussed in Sect. 2. Numerical methods are briefly outlined in Sect. 3. The LES results and verification with wind tunnel measurements are outlined in Sect. 4, where the LES results have also been compared with that of another reference numerical model.

## 2 Mathematical Model

To simulate a neutrally stratified atmospheric boundary layer over a smooth hill, we solve the filtered Navier-Stokes equations (e.g. [7]),

$$\frac{\partial u_i}{\partial x_i} = 0,  \tag{1}$$

$$\frac{\partial u_i}{\partial t} + \frac{\partial (u_i u_j)}{\partial x_j} = -\frac{\partial p}{\partial x_i} - \frac{\partial \tau_{ij}}{\partial x_j} + f_s,  \tag{2}$$

where $\tau_{ij}$ is the usual SGS stress (force per unit area divided by density), which can be calculated by the WALE model and $f_s$ denotes the divergence of SGS stress exerted by the hill, which can be calculated by the canopy stress method.

Here, $u_i$ is the filtered velocity in the $x_i$ direction, $p$ is the pressure (divided by density), $\xi(x, y, z, t)$ is an indicator function representing the terrain.

### 2.1 Canopy Stress Parameterization

To parameterize the stress experienced by the hill, we assume that the hill can be modelled as a porous canopy. In (2), the canopy stress term $f_s$ vanishes on all grid points which are not in the canopy region (or hill). Thus, we define an indicator function such that $\xi(x, y, z) = 1$ if the point $(x, y, z)$ is inside the canopy, and $\xi(x, y, z) = 0$ if $(x, y, z)$ is outside the canopy. Let us consider

$$f_s = f_{ds}\xi(x, y, z)\,u_i + f_{df}\xi(x, y, z)\,|u_i|u_i,  \tag{3}$$

where on the right-hand side of (3), the first term represents the viscous stress experienced by an eddy passing over a hill [1], and the second term represents the pressure loss experienced by an eddy passing through a porous canopy [2]. There are several empirical methods to determine the coefficients $f_{ds}$ and $f_{df}$.

### 2.1.1  Skin Friction Drag

The skin friction drag is generated in the viscous boundary layer, which develops due to the viscous stress as the air flows over a solid body. To parameterize the viscous stress, let us model the porous canopy as a collection of smooth spheres of radii $d$ and the void fraction $\varepsilon$. Similar to the model considered in Refs. [3, 4], a mathematical formulation of the viscous stress in (3) is

$$f_{ds} = -\frac{150 \, \nu \, (1 - \varepsilon)^2}{d^2 \, \varepsilon^3}. \tag{4}$$

Using $\varepsilon = 0.02, d = \frac{\Delta x}{2} = 4.5\,\text{m}$, and the kinematic viscosity $\nu = 0.06345\,\text{m}^2\,\text{s}^{-1}$, we get $f_{ds} = -1128.5\,\text{s}^{-1}$.

### 2.1.2  Pressure Drag

A detailed discussion of the pressure drag associated with a forest canopy is given by [2]. Here, we model the hill as a canopy of spheres and consider the formulation of $f_{df}$ that is applied for a forest canopy. Based on the canopy region formed by spheres,

$$f_{df} = -\frac{1.75(1 - \varepsilon)}{d \, \varepsilon^3}, \tag{5}$$

which takes a value of $\rho f_{df} = 47{,}638.89\,\text{m}^{-1}$ for $\varepsilon = 0.02, d = \frac{\Delta x}{2} = 4.5\,\text{m}$.

For clarity, the canopy stress parameterization of the last term in (2) can be written as

$$f_s = -\frac{150 \, \nu \, (1 - \varepsilon)^2}{d^2 \, \varepsilon^3} \xi \, (x, y, z, t) \, u_i - \frac{1.75(1 - \varepsilon)}{d \, \varepsilon^3} \xi \, (x, y, z, t) \, |u_i| u_i. \tag{6}$$

In addition to modelling a component of the SGS stress by (6), the WALE formulation of the SGS stress $\tau_{ij}$ is examined in the present work.

## 2.2  Subgrid Scale Model for $\tau_{ij}$

In LES the Smagorinsky model filters all eddies of a scale that is smaller than the grid size such that

$$\tau_{ij} - \frac{1}{3}\tau_{kk}\delta_{ij} = 2\nu_\tau S_{ij} \quad \text{and} \quad \nu_\tau = (C_s\Delta)^2|S|,$$

where $C_s$ is the Smagorinsky constant, $\Delta = (\Delta x \Delta y \Delta z)^{1/3}$ is the LES filter width, $|S| = \sqrt{2S_{ij}S_{ij}}$, and the strain rate tensor is

$$S_{ij} = \frac{1}{2}\left(\frac{\partial u_i}{\partial x_j} + \frac{\partial u_j}{\partial x_i}\right).$$

Note that the velocity gradient tensor is

$$\frac{\partial u_i}{\partial x_j} = S_{ij} + \frac{1}{2}\left(\frac{\partial u_i}{\partial x_j} - \frac{\partial u_j}{\partial x_i}\right)$$

and the rate of rotation tensor $\frac{1}{2}\left(\frac{\partial u_i}{\partial x_j} - \frac{\partial u_j}{\partial x_i}\right)$ is not considered by the Smagorinsky model. In Ref. [12], it was shown that the inaccurate near-wall scaling of SGS dissipation with respect to classical Smagorinsky model can be improved by the WALE formulation of the eddy viscosity

$$\nu_\tau = (C_s\Delta)^2 = \frac{(S_{ij}^d S_{ij}^d)^{3/2}}{(S_{ij}^d S_{ij}^d)^{5/4} + (S_{ij}S_{ij})^{5/2}}$$

where we engage both the rate of strain and the rate of rotation through the velocity gradient tensor such that

$$S_{ij}^d = \frac{1}{2}\left[\left(\frac{\partial u_i}{\partial x_j}\right)^2 + \left(\frac{\partial u_j}{\partial x_i}\right)^2\right] - \frac{1}{3}\delta_{ij}\left(\frac{\partial u_k}{\partial x_k}\right)^2.$$

Based on numerical tests with the WALE model, $C_s = 0.325$ was adopted for the simulations reported in this article.

# 3 Computational Methods

An implementation of the canopy stress method is given by [1]. In the present work, the canopy stress method has been implemented within the Open source Field Operation and Manipulation (OpenFOAM) code, which is an object-oriented C++ library for solving the Navier-Stokes equation. A finite volume discretization of LES equations (1–2) has been implemented through the OpenFOAM library. OpenFOAM is released with a Navier-Stokes solver, `buoyantBoussinesqPimpleFoam`, which has been modified into a new solver, `topographyFOAM` for the purpose of testing the canopy stress method presented in this article. Our implementation of the canopy stress method has been tested with OpenFOAM 3.0.x and OpenFOAM

4.x. We have compared the results with two methods of time integration, such as the Crank-Nicolson method and the second order backward Euler method. Results obtained by the backward Euler method has been reported. For coupling the pressure with the velocity, i.e. for solving the continuity equation (1), we have adopted the 'Pressure Implicit with a Splitting of Operators (PISO)' algorithm. It is worth mentioning that the mesh is decomposed among multiple processors based on the message passing interface (MPI) routines implemented through the OpenFOAM library.

The boundary conditions in both horizontal directions are periodic, which mimics a simulation for a periodic array of hills. In the vertical direction, a standard wall boundary condition is considered at $z = 0$, and the boundary at $z = z_{max}$ is considered a plane of symmetry, where the vertical gradient of all quantities are zero.

## 4 Verification

We have considered two sets reference data for the validation of modelling a turbulent flow past a hill based on the canopy stress method. One of them is the result of a wind tunnel measurement conducted by [8] and the other is the result of another LES conducted by [9].

### 4.1 Periodic Array of a Smooth Hill

To mimic the Large Eddy Simulation of a neutrally stratified boundary layer flow over a periodic array of a smooth hill, let us consider the surface with a Gaussian shape defined by (7); i.e.

$$z_s = h \exp\left(-\frac{(x - c_1)^2}{L^2} - \frac{(y - c_2)^2}{L^2}\right), \tag{7}$$

where $(c_1, c_2)$ is the centre of the hill.

Using $h = 30$ m and $L = 50$ m in (7), the hill height is 30 m and the hill half-length (the distance from the centre to a point whose height is half the hill height) is 42 m. The computational domain is given by $L_x \times L_y \times L_z = 600$ m $\times$ 600 m $\times$ 510 m, and the mesh contains $N_x \times N_y \times N_z = 64 \times 64 \times 88$ finite volume cells, where $N_x$, $N_y$, and $N_z$ denote the number of cells in $x$, $y$, and $z$ directions, respectively. Note that the cells are of uniform size, $\Delta x = \Delta y = 9.375$ m, in the horizontal directions, but stretched in the vertical direction with $\Delta z_{min} = 0.96$ m near the boundary at $z = 0$, which is increased gradually to $\Delta z_{max} = 10.625$ m until half the model height is reached, and is left constant in the top half of the domain. A vertical cross section of the mesh is shown in Fig. 1 (left). The shapes of the hills defined by (7) and that considered in Ref. [9] have been compared in Fig. 1 (right), where the shape is normalized by hill height $h$ in both cases.

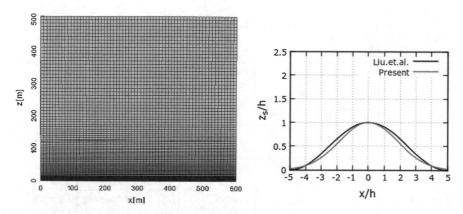

**Fig. 1** (left) Vertical slice of the grid is shown. (right) The vertical cross-section of the hill that compared with the Fig. 6 of [9]. Two hill equations are scaled by the vertical height of the hill and the shapes are similar

The flow is driven by a pressure gradient $\frac{dp}{dx}$ that is adjusted dynamically so that the mean velocity in the stream-wise direction is about 7 ms$^{-1}$. The kinematic viscosity is varied from $\nu = 5 \times 10^{-2}$ ms$^{-2}$ to $\nu = 10^{-5}$ ms$^{-2}$ for testing the result. Note that the time step $\Delta t = 0.01$ s, in our simulation, is larger than the time step $\Delta t = 0.0001$ s considered in the LES of Ref. [9].

A comparison for the vertical distribution of the stream-wise velocity $u(z)/u_r$ that is obtained from the present LES with that was obtained by the wind-tunnel measurement of [8] is presented in the bottom panel of Table 1 (experimental). Similarly, a comparison with respect to the LES results of [9] is presented in the top panel of Table 1 (numerical). We can see an excellent agreement between our LES results with the results of wind-tunnel measurements, and similarly for the reference LES. The relative errors reported in Table 1 indicate that the hill can be modelled accurately if the canopy stress method is incorporated in LES. The large error at the point (10, 10, 1.04) for the experimental case in Table 1 is due to the fact that the size of the hill in the wind-tunnel measurement was $O$(mm), which is $O$(10 m) in our simulation. With such a scale gap, the LES resolution need be high enough to capture the scales that are equivalent to what was captured in the experiment.

A graphical comparisons of the mean velocity distribution $u(z)/u_r$ along five vertical lines located at five stream-wise positions are presented in Fig. 2a. The standard deviation $\sigma(z)/u_r$ of the time averaged stream-wise velocity is presented in Fig. 2b. Figure 3 presents a time series of the turbulent kinetic energy (TKE), where TKE is the sum of the variances of stream-wise, span-wise, and vertical velocities.

**Table 1** Velocity differences at the different locations of the three-dimensional hill (Eq. 7) along with the absolute and relative differences in the numerical [9] and experimental [8]) analysis

| Location | | | | Velocity | | Difference | |
|---|---|---|---|---|---|---|---|
| Numerical | $x/h$ | $y/h$ | $z/h$ | Present $(u/u_r)$ | [9] $(u/u_r)$ | Absolute | Relative (%) |
| | 10 | 10 | 1.04 | 0.4183 | 0.3842 | 0.0296 | 8.49 |
| | 10 | 10 | 1.2020 | 1.0304 | 0.8445 | 0.1919 | 20.53 |
| | 10 | 10 | 1.5455 | 1.0045 | 0.8617 | 0.1424 | 14.85 |
| | 10 | 10 | 2.2323 | 0.9800 | 0.8596 | 0.1204 | 13.08 |
| | 10 | 10 | 3.0909 | 0.9697 | 0.8813 | 0.0884 | 9.55 |
| | 10 | 10 | 4.00 | 0.9719 | 0.9026 | 0.0693 | 7.39 |
| Experimental | $x/h$ | $y/h$ | $z/h$ | Present $(u/u_r)$ | [8] $(u/u_r)$ | Absolute | Relative (%) |
| | 10 | 10 | 1.04 | 0.4183 | 0.8449 | 0.4226 | 67.54 |
| | 10 | 10 | 1.2020 | 1.0304 | 0.8449 | 0.1859 | 19.83 |
| | 10 | 10 | 1.5455 | 1.0045 | 0.8678 | 0.1367 | 14.60 |
| | 10 | 10 | 2.2323 | 0.9800 | 0.8657 | 0.1143 | 12.38 |
| | 10 | 10 | 3.0909 | 0.9697 | 0.8755 | 0.0942 | 10.21 |
| | 10 | 10 | 4.00 | 0.9719 | 0.9210 | 0.0509 | 5.37 |

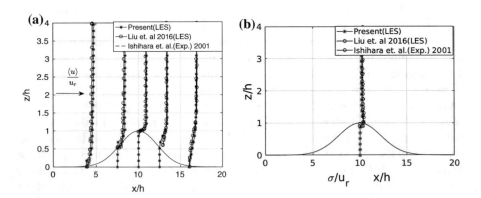

**Fig. 2** Comparison with the previous researches of the LES simulations of a different turbulent stress model of [9] and experimental results of [8] for (left) normalized mean velocity and (right) normalized standard deviations $\sigma$

## 5 Conclusions

A goal of the research is to validate a mathematical model of representing mountains/hills in LES. As mentioned in the introduction, LES aims to employ a relatively coarse mesh to capture the large eddies, where small eddies can be filtered with an SGS model, such as the Smagorinsky model or the WALE model. Due to such a criterion of LES, accurately capturing the effects of mountains is a challenging endeavour.

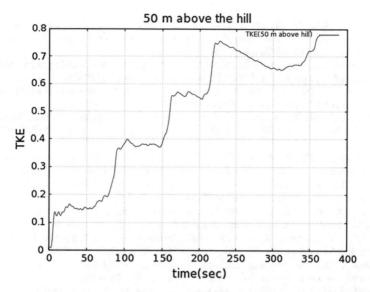

**Fig. 3** A time series of the turbulent kinetic energy (TKE) which represents the strength of eddies passing a fixed point above the hill

In this investigation, we show that the canopy stress method is an accurate model for representing a hill without requiring a complex mesh around the hill. However, the accuracy of our methodology as it is reported in this article must be interpreted carefully. The agreement between the LES results and the experimental results encourage further investigations in this direction. In particular, there is a gap in the literature dealing with the LES of atmospheric boundary layer flows over mountains or complex terrain. There is a growing interest in the canopy stress method [1, 2, 5] and similar methods dealing with complex terrains [9, 10]. Our results encourage further investigation of the canopy stress method for simulating atmospheric turbulence over complex terrain. Such work is currently underway.

**Acknowledgements** The authors acknowledge the computational facilities provided by SHAR-CNET, the regional High-Performance Computing Consortium (HPC) for universities in Ontario Canada, Industrial Research. Jahrul M. Alam acknowledges funding from NSERC (National Science and Engineering Research Council) in the form of a discovery grant; Md. Abdus Samad Bhuiyan acknowledges funding from Memorial University in the form of a President's award.

# References

1. Alam, J.M.: Toward a multiscale approach for computational atmospheric modeling. Mon. Weather Rev. **139**(12), 3906–3922 (2011)
2. Belcher, S., Finnigan, J., Harman, I.: Flows through forest canopies in complex terrain. Ecol. Appl. **18**(6), 1436–1453 (2008)

3. Bhuiyan, M.A.S., Hossain, M.A., Alam, J.M.: A computational model of temperature monitoring at a leakage in a leak detection system of a pipeline. In: Proceedings of the 25th Canadian Congress of Applied Mechanics, pp. 643–647 (2015)
4. Bhuiyan, M.A.S., Hossain, M.A., Alam, J.M.: A computational model of thermal monitoring at a leakage in pipelines. Int. J. Heat Mass Transf. **92**, 330–338 (2016)
5. Brown, A.R., Hobson, J., Wood, N.: Large-eddy simulation of neutral turbulent flow over rough sinusoidal ridges. Bound.-Layer Meteorol. **98**(3), 411–441 (2001)
6. Dupont, S., Brunet, Y., Finnigan, J.: Large-eddy simulation of turbulent flow over a forested hill: validation and coherent structure identification. Q. J. R. Meteorol. Soc. **134**(636), 1911–1929 (2008)
7. Goodfriend, E., Chow, F.K., Vanella, M., Balaras, E.: Large-eddy simulation of flow through an array of cubes with local grid refinement. Bound.-layer Meteorol. **159**(2), 285–303 (2016)
8. Ishihara, T., Fujino, Y., Hibi, K.: A wind tunnel study of separated flow over a two-dimensional ridge and a circular hill. J. Wind. Eng. **89**, 573–576 (2001)
9. Liu, Z., Ishihara, T., Tanaka, T., He, X.: Les study of turbulent flow fields over a smooth 3-d hill and a smooth 2-d ridge. J. Wind Eng. Ind. Aerodyn. **153**, 1–12 (2016)
10. Lundquist, K.A., Chow, F.K., Lundquist, J.K.: An immersed boundary method for the weather research and forecasting model. Mon. Weather Rev. **138**(3), 796–817 (2010)
11. Mahrer, Y.: An improved numerical approximation of the horizontal gradients in a terrain-following coordinate system. Mon. Weather Rev. **112**(5), 918–922 (1984)
12. Nicoud, F., Ducros, F.: Subgrid-scale stress modelling based on the square of the velocity gradient tensor. Flow Turbul. Combust. **62**(3), 183–200 (1999)

# A Computational Model for Adjusting Surface Tension Coefficient in Pseudo-potential Lattice Boltzmann Method

**Mahmud Ashrafizaadeh and Seyyed Meysam Khatoonabadi**

**Abstract** In the present study, an adjustable coefficient is introduced in order to make the pseudo-potential multiphase model more flexible for the simulation of a wide range of surface tensions. This coefficient can be utilized for different density ratios without any limitation. First, the effect of this coefficient is evaluated by the Laplace test. Then, density and pressure profiles along the interface are plotted which indicate that the major influence of the surface tension coefficient is localized along the interface. In other words, no negative influence is observed either for the density of two phases or for their pressures elsewhere. Hence, using the proposed surface tension coefficient, it is now possible to adjust the surface tension in multiphase Lattice Boltzmann flow simulations in a wider range. However, as the surface tension coefficient increases to increase the value of the fluid surface tension, the maximum spurious velocity might increase.

**Keywords** Surface tension coefficient · Pseudo potential · Lattice Boltzmann method

## 1 Introduction

The Lattice Boltzmann method (LBM) has attracted a lot of attentions in recent years due to its various capabilities and merits. In particular, it has gained a popularity in simulating complex flows such as multi-component and multiphase flows as well as flows through porous media in a wide range of scales from macro to micro. Despite the rapid adoption of LBM for simulating complex flows, it still has some drawbacks and deficiencies, specially when dealing with practical applications [1].

M. Ashrafizaadeh (✉) · S. M. Khatoonabadi
Department of Mechanical Engineering, Isfahan University of Technology, Isfahan, Iran
e-mail: mahmud@cc.iut.ac.ir

S. M. Khatoonabadi
e-mail: m.khatoonabadi@me.iut.ac.ir

© Springer Nature Switzerland AG 2018
D. M. Kilgour et al. (eds.), *Recent Advances in Mathematical and Statistical Methods*, Springer Proceedings in Mathematics & Statistics 259,
https://doi.org/10.1007/978-3-319-99719-3_15

The pseudo-potential model is the most prevalent model due to its efficiency in terms of being easy to employ and less computational costs [2]. Originally, Shan and Chen [3] introduced a model that had the capability of simulating multiphase and multicomponent flows. Nonetheless, the original model was not applicable to real physical problems. This limitation was due to a rather small achievable density ratio, thermodynamic inconsistency, and large spurious currents. Later, Yuan and Schaefer [4] incorporated several real equations of state (EOS) into the pseudo-potential function in order to reduce these limitations. Although the developed pseudo-potential model had numerous advantages, its application for real problems still had some limitations since some parameters like surface tension, density ratio, and temperature were tightly coupled to each other. To solve this problem some approaches have been suggested. Sbragaglia et al. [5] proposed a multi-range approach to adjust the surface tension and density ratio independently, but their model could not handle cases with density ratios over 100. Force schemes were also taken into account by some researchers. The most widely used one is the exact difference method (EDM) proposed by Kupershtokh et al. [6]. They claimed that with the use of the EDM and a proper EOS the stability of the model is improved and many of the aforementioned deficiencies could be alleviated to some extent [7, 8], but the problem with the surface tension continued to exist.

To overcome this obstacle, Sun et al. [9] suggested an extra term reflecting the surface tension influence in the LB equation. However, they did not provide ample results to indicate the limitations and strengths of their model. Among all these models, the EDM method [10] seems to be more promising for further development due to its higher stability. Recently, Hu et al. [7] incorporated a constant parameter which is proportional to the surface tension. It is easier to be used, but the surface tension parameter is still restricted and does not follow any particular rule to be adjusted at different temperatures. Furthermore, in all these approaches, the surface tension can only be adjusted indirectly and implicitly.

In this paper, the EDM in pseudo-potential model is modified to improve its applicability for multiphase flow simulations with different surface tensions. The proposed modification is implemented by introducing a surface tension parameter, $k'$, into the pseudo-potential function using a non-dimensional real EOS. The proposed model is successfully applied for the simulation of a flat interface and the Laplace test. It is shown that the introduction of this new parameter has no adverse effects on the accuracy of the calculated densities of the two phases. By adjusting this parameter the surface tension could be specified in a wider range up to an order of magnitude larger. However, by increasing the surface tension the spurious velocities might increase.

## 2  Pseudo-potential Model

In the Lattice Boltzmann method, an equation including the collision and propagation steps with the Bhatnagar-Groos-Krook (BGK) [11] operator and an external force term is given by

$$f_i(x + e_i\delta t, t + \delta t) - f_i(x, t) = (1/\tau)[f_i(x, t) - f_i^{eq}(x, t)] + \Delta F_i(x, t) \qquad (1)$$

in which, f is the particle distribution function at a specific location and time. The $\tau$ represents the relaxation time, $\Delta F$ is the bulk force, $f_i^{eq}$ indicates the equilibrium distribution function given by [12]

$$f_i^{eq}(x, t) = \omega_i \rho(x, y)[1 + \frac{e_i.u}{c_s^2} + \frac{(e_i.u)^2}{c_s^4} + \frac{u^2}{2c_s^2}] \qquad (2)$$

In Eq. (2), $C_s$ is the lattice sound velocity, $\omega_i$ are the weighting factors, and $e_i$ are the discrete velocities. Moreover, $\rho$ and u indicate the macroscopic density and velocity. Most constant parameters are related to the lattice structure. For example, in a D2Q9 lattice (Fig. 1), $C_s = C/\sqrt{3}$ in which $C = \delta x/\delta t$. Therefore, with choosing $\delta x = \delta t = 1$, the C value becomes unity. The $\omega_i$ and $e_i$ for a D2Q9 lattice are given by

$$e_i = \begin{cases} 0 & \alpha = 0 \\ cos\left[\frac{(\alpha-1)\pi}{2}\right].sin\left[\frac{(\alpha-1)\pi}{2}\right] & \alpha = 1, 2, 3, 4 \\ \sqrt{2}cos\left[\frac{(\alpha-5)\pi}{2} + \frac{\pi}{4}\right].sin\left[\frac{(\alpha-5)\pi}{2} + \frac{\pi}{4}\right] & \alpha = 5, 6, 7, 8 \end{cases} \qquad (3)$$

**Fig. 1** The schematic figure of a two dimensional lattice with nine velocities

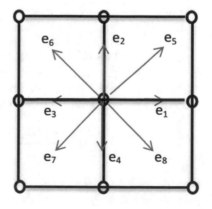

$$\omega_i = \begin{cases} 4/9 & i = 0 \\ 1/9 & i = 1, 2, 3, 4 \\ 1/36 & i = 5, 6, 7, 8 \end{cases} \tag{4}$$

In this method, the macroscopic density and momentum are obtained by

$$\rho = \sum_i f_i \tag{5}$$

$$\rho u = \sum_i e_i \, f_i \tag{6}$$

and the viscosity is related to the relaxation time by $v = (\tau - 0.5)/3$. In the EDM, the bulk force is considered as (7) [6]

$$\Delta F_i(x, t) = f_i^{eq}\left(\rho, u + (F_i(x, t)\delta t)/\rho\right) - f_i^{eq}(\rho, u) \tag{7}$$

The force term in Eq. (7) is the inter-particle interaction force written as [3]

$$F_i(x, t) = \left((1 - 2A)\psi(x) \sum_i \left(\omega_i \psi(x, x')e_i\right) + A \sum_i \left(\omega_i \psi^2(x, x')e_i\right)\right)/\alpha h, \tag{8}$$

where A is a constant parameter that improves the accuracy of the model. The $\alpha$ for the D2Q9 lattice is equal to 1.5. This force term is an approximation of two other force terms, local approximation and mean-value approximation. In addition, $\psi(x)$ is the pseudo-potential function. To adjust the surface tension as an independent parameter, an extra coefficient, $k'$, is introduced in this study, which is shown in the following equation.

$$\psi = \sqrt{(k' \, \bar{p} - \bar{\rho} c_s^2)}. \tag{9}$$

If $k'$ is set to 1 the original model, suggested by Kupershtokh et al. [6], is obtained. In the following sections, the influences of this parameter on the model applicability, accuracy and stability are further investigated. Similarly, Kupershtokh et al. [6] proposed a non-dimensional EOS to be used in the pseudo-potential function.

$$\bar{p} = k\left(\frac{c\bar{\rho}R\bar{T}(1 + b\,\bar{\rho} + (b\,\bar{\rho})^2 - (b\,\bar{\rho})^3)}{(1 - b\,\bar{\rho})^3} - a\bar{\rho}^2\right), \tag{10}$$

where $\bar{T} = T/T_{cr}$, $\bar{p} = p/p_{cr}$ and $\bar{\rho} = \rho/\rho_{cr}$ are non-dimensional temperature, pressure and density, respectively and $T_{cr}$, $p_{cr}$ and $\rho_{cr}$ are the corresponding critical values. Since water is one of the most abundant fluids in nature and is used frequently in the literature as the working fluid, it is more convenient to compare our results with those reported by others. Hence, water is chosen for present simulations. The EOS constant parameters, $a$, $b$ and $c$ are set to $a = 3.852462257$, $b = 0.130443884$, $and$ $c = 2.785855166$ [6]. The details of non-dimensionalisation form of the Carnahan-Starling [13] are provided in reference [6]. Furthermore, the corresponding critical values for water are $p_{cr} = 0.004416$, $\rho_{cr} = 0.1341$, and $T_{cr} = 0.09433$ in the lattice unit. For instance, equivalent water critical temperature in physical unit is 647.15 degree Kelvin. It is worth mentioning that in the present model other fluids could also be used instead of water, provided that the EOS can predict their properties. The proposed EOS also includes an extra term, $k$, which is related to the critical parameters of the given EOS as follows:

$k = p_{cr} \, \Delta t^2 / \rho_{cr} \, h^2$, where $\Delta t$ and $h$ are the lattice time and space units, respectively. For most fluids $k \approx 0.01$ [6]. Based on water critical values, the exact value would be $k = 0.03293$.

# 3 Results

## 3.1 The Laplace Test

The Laplace test is a standard benchmark to validate multiphase models. In this test a blob of liquid is located inside its saturated vapour. After the simulation is done, a circular droplet (in two dimensional simulations) of fluid is formed for which the following relation holds:

$$\sigma = R(P_{in} - P_{out}), \tag{11}$$

where $P_{in}$ and $P_{out}$ are the pressure inside and outside of the droplet, respectively, $R$ is the droplet radius and $\sigma$ is the surface tension.

In the pseudo-potential model, in spite of surface tension importance in numerous phenomena such as bubbles or droplets merging [14], it could not be specified a priori, rather, it can only be calculated after the simulation is done. This fact limits the applicability of the multiphase model. The proposed coefficient in this study ($k'$), removes this limitation and provides the user with an adjustable parameter to explicitly manipulate the value of the surface tension.

To perform the Laplace test, a $200 \times 200$ lattice is used and the computational domain is a square box with periodic boundary conditions. Fluids are at rest at the beginning of the simulation. The Carnahan-Starling EOS is used with a constant reduced temperature of 0.5.

To determine the influence of the $k'$ coefficient on the surface tension, a series of simulations is done with a range of $k'$ from 0.1 to 4. Figure 2 shows the results. The horizontal and vertical axes represent $1/R$ and $p^* = \Delta p / p_{cr}$, respectively. As it is shown in Fig. 2, $p^*$ varies linearly versus $1/R$ for each $k'$ as expected (Eq. 11)

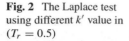

**Fig. 2** The Laplace test using different $k'$ value in $(T_r = 0.5)$

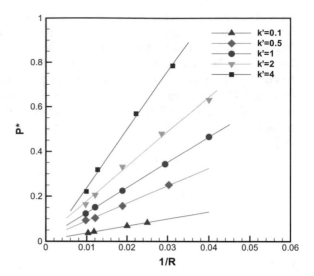

and the slope of each line can be interpreted as the surface tension for the assumed temperature.

It is evident that by employing the $k'$ coefficient, different values for the surface tension can be obtained, which is a desired capability for realistic applications of the multiphase model. Theoretical manipulation of the proposed model shows that the resultant surface tension should be directly proportional to the employed $k'$ value. However, numerical results show that finer lattices are required to capture this behaviour.

## 3.2 Effects on the Interface Thickness

The employment of the proposed coefficient, $k'$, shows some effects on the interface thickness. To investigate these effects, a droplet with a radius of 50 lattice units is placed at the center of the computational domain.

Three $k'$ values are used in the simulations. The variation of the calculated density along the centerline of the computational domain is shown in Fig. 3. As it can be found from this figure, the parameter $k$ does not noticeably alter the densities of the two phases.

However, the density variations are different right at the interface. It is shown that the thickness of the interface is adapted to the employed $k'$ value. Figure 3 shows when a smaller $k'$ value is used, the interface thickness increases.

**Fig. 3** Density profile for three $k' = 0.5, 1, 2$

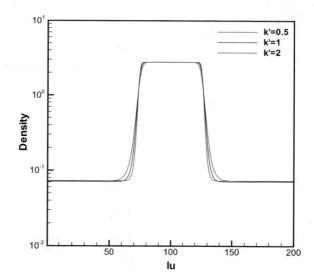

## 3.3 Effects on Phase Pressures

Basically, surface tension parameter impacts on density distribution in the interface between two phases. As the density distribution changes, the corresponding pressure alters; and consequently, a different surface tension can be obtained. Therefore, the resultant surface tension is directly proportional to the employed $k'$ value, and it is expected that the computed pressure difference across the interface is also multiplied by $k'$. To numerically investigate this behaviour, a two phase flow with a flat interface is simulated. It should be noted that in this simulation, a layer of liquid is placed between two layers of its saturated vapour. A reduced temperature of 0.7 is used. Figure 4 shows the variation of the pressure distribution across the flat interface. As shown in Fig. 4, the pressure within both phases remains equally constant which is consistence with the Maxwell Construction [8]. Moreover, the value of the pressure for $k' = 0.5$ is approximately reduced by half compared to that of $k' = 1$. A nonphysical pressure overshoot is also observed within the gas layers adjacent to the interface, which increases as the $k'$ value increases.

## 3.4 Spurious Velocity

The term "spurious velocity" refers to a nonphysical velocity field which exists in almost all LBM multiphase models due to the force term added to the equilibrium velocity. Figure 5 demonstrates the maximum spurious velocity magnitude in a static droplet simulation at $T_r = 0.7$. From Fig. 5 it is evident that with the increase of the surface tension coefficient, the maximum spurious velocity within the computational

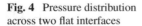

**Fig. 4** Pressure distribution across two flat interfaces

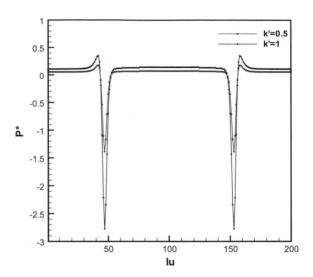

domain also increases. Physically, this observation can be explained by noting the fact that a higher force gradient at the interface occurs when the surface tension is larger. In fact, in all multiphase LBM models, with an increase in surface tension or density ratio the induced spurious velocity increases no matter what approach is utilized [15]. Consequently, a higher spurious velocity is produced as an outcome of a greater surface tension at interface. It is worth mentioning that a value of 0.01 for the surface tension is high enough for most simulations in comparison with that of used in other multiphase models. For most cases, a smaller value (in the order of 0.001) would be required [15]. In spite of favorable influences of surface tension parameter when $k'$ is smaller than unity in terms of reducing the spurious velocity, for $k'$ larger than 4 the magnitude of spurious velocity is high, so using other methods like the Multirange pseudo-potential approach [5, 16] seems to be necessary.

## 4   Conclusion

The proposed surface tension coefficient is applicable to the pseudo-potential model for adjusting the surface tension as an independent, initial parameter. The Laplace test illustrates that a wide range of surface tension could be achieved by employing this new coefficient. Using fine meshes could improve the accuracy of the computed surface tension to obtain precise surface tension values consistent with that of predicted by theory. Moreover, pressure and density profiles indicate that there the use of this new coefficient does not deteriorate the accuracy of the numerical results except within the region at the interface. Due to the undesired effect of the surface tension coefficient on the spurious velocity field, especially when large values are

**Fig. 5** Maximum spurious velocity magnitude for different $k'$

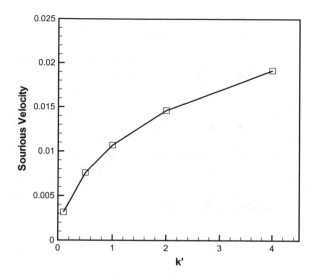

used, the use of extra techniques might be necessary to reduce the magnitude of the nonphysical spurious velocities.

# References

1. Succi, S.: The Lattice Boltzmann Equation: For Fluid Dynamics and Beyond. Oxford University Press, Oxford (2001)
2. Huang, H., Sukop, M., Lu, X.: Multiphase Lattice Boltzmann Methods: Theory and Application. Wiley, New York (2015)
3. Shan, X., Chen, H.: Lattice Boltzmann model for simulating flows with multiple phases and components. Phys. Rev. E **47**(3), 1815 (1993)
4. Yuan, P., Schaefer, L.: Equations of state in a lattice Boltzmann model. Phys. Fluids **18**(4), 042101 (2006)
5. Sbragaglia, M., Benzi, R., Biferale, L., Succi, S., Sugiyama, K., Toschi, F.: Generalized lattice Boltzmann method with multirange pseudopotential. Phys. Rev. E **75**(2), 026702 (2007)
6. Kupershtokh, A., Medvedev, D., Karpov, D.: On equations of state in a lattice Boltzmann method. Comput. Math. Appl. **58**(5), 965–974 (2009)
7. Hu, A., Li, L., Chen, S., Liao, Q., Zeng, J.: On equations of state in pseudo-potential multiphase lattice Boltzmann model with large density ratio. Int. J. Heat Mass Transf. **67**, 159–163 (2013)
8. Gong, S., Cheng, P.: Numerical investigation of droplet motion and coalescence by an improved lattice Boltzmann model for phase transitions and multiphase flows. Comput. Fluids **53**, 93–104 (2012)
9. Sun, K., Wang, T., Jia, M., Xiao, G.: Evaluation of force implementation in pseudopotential-based multiphase lattice Boltzmann models. Phys. A Stat. Mech. Appl. **391**(15), 3895–3907 (2012)
10. Zheng, L., Zhai, Q., Zheng, S.: Analysis of force treatment in the pseudopotential lattice Boltzmann equation method. Phys. Rev. E **95**(4), 043301 (2017)

11. Bhatnagar, P.L., Gross, E.P., Krook, M.: A model for collision processes in gases. I. Small amplitude processes in charged and neutral one-component systems. Phys. Rev. **94**(1–12), 511–525 (1954)
12. McNamara, G.R., Zanetti, G.: Use of the Boltzmann equation to simulate lattice-gas automata. Phys. Rev. Lett. **61**(20), 2332 (1988)
13. Carnahan, N.F., Starling, K.E.: Equation of state for nonattracting rigid spheres. J. Chem. Phys. **51**(2), 635–636 (1969)
14. Nie, D., Lv, Y., Zhang, X., Qiu, L.: Research on gas bubble merging through the lattice Boltzmann method. J. Comput. Methods Sci. Eng. **16**(1), 99–109 (2016)
15. Ye, F., Di, Q., Wang, W., Chen, F., Chen, H., Hua, S.: Comparative study of two lattice Boltzmann multiphase models for simulating wetting phenomena: implementing static contact angles based on the geometric formulation. Appl. Math. Mech. **39**(4), 513–528 (2018)
16. Qin, F., Mazloomi Moqaddam, A., Kang, Q., Derome, D., Carmeliet, J.: Entropic multiple-relaxation-time multirange pseudopotential lattice Boltzmann model for two-phase flow. Phys. Fluids **30**(3), 032104 (2018)

# Magnetohydrodynamic Flow in a Rectangular Duct

Canan Bozkaya

**Abstract** The magnetohydrodynamic (MHD) flow of an incompressible, viscous and electrically conducting fluid in a rectangular duct with insulated and perfectly conducting walls is investigated numerically in the presence of hydrodynamic slip. The flow is fully developed and driven by a constant pressure gradient in the axial direction under the effect of an externally applied uniform and inclined magnetic field. A direct boundary element method (BEM) using a fundamental solution which enables to treat the governing MHD flow equations in their original coupled form is employed and the validity of the code is also ascertained. The numerical simulations are carried out for several values of slip length, Hartmann number and the inclination angle of the external magnetic field. It is well-observed from the equivelocity and induced current lines that the velocity increases through the duct and the Hartmann layers weaken while the side layers become thicker with an increase in slip length especially at low values of Hartmann number irrespective of the conductivity of the walls.

**Keywords** MHD · Duct flow · BEM

## 1 Introduction

The magnetohydrodynamic flow investigating the motion of electrically conducting fluid in the presence of a magnetic field, has enormous engineering applications in MHD pumps, generators, magnetic flow meters, plasma confinement for the fusion reactors, propulsion and flight control for rockets and hypersonic aerodynamic vehicles. Thus, the classic MHD flow considering the effect of induced magnetic field in rectangular ducts with no-slip conditions has been intensively studied for various wall conductivities [2–4, 7, 12]. However, there have been very few works on the solution of MHD flow with slip condition although a slip boundary condition must be

C. Bozkaya (✉)

Department of Mathematics, Middle East Technical University, 06800 Ankara, Turkey

e-mail: bcanan@metu.edu.tr

© Springer Nature Switzerland AG 2018

D. M. Kilgour et al. (eds.), *Recent Advances in Mathematical and Statistical Methods*, Springer Proceedings in Mathematics & Statistics 259, https://doi.org/10.1007/978-3-319-99719-3_16

171

employed in some applications, such as microfluid and nanofluid devices, in which the slip behavior is typical when the surface to volume ratio is large and the viscous effect on the boundary is negligible [16]. In these works, besides a closed form of analytical solutions derived to the flow of incompressible fluids subject to Navier's slip on the boundary [9], a special case of MHD flow in rectangular ducts under the influence of an horizontal external magnetic field when the vertical walls are conducting with slip on horizontal walls [11] and when all walls are insulated with slip on vertical walls [16] are solved analytically by using a series expansion. As mentioned in [16], the proposed analytical technique can not be employed under more general boundary conditions, e.g. slip on all walls, and a numerical or asymptotic approach is required.

On the other hand, MHD flow subject to slip velocity conditions has been considered mainly over infinite surfaces and channels [1, 6, 10, 14, 15], and rarely in rectangular ducts [13, 17]. They have conducted a parametric study to analyze the effects of slip condition and the magnetic field on the flow field. In these studies the magnetic Reynolds number is taken so small that the induced magnetic field is neglected, however, the present work focuses on the effect of slip conditions on both the induced magnetic field and the velocity.

In the present study, we investigate the influence of the hydrodynamic slip on the numerical solution of the MHD duct flow with general boundary conditions involving both the insulated and/or perfectly conducting walls and the mixed type slip boundary condition constructed as a linear combination of the slip velocity and the tangential stress. An effective numerical technique is utilized for the solution of MHD slip flow. That is, the governing partial differential equations coupled in velocity and induced magnetic field are discretized in their original coupled form by a direct approach of boundary element method using the fundamental solution derived in [4]. The resulting system of discretized BEM equations rearranged according to the given boundary conditions, which involves the unknown values of velocity and induced magnetic field only on the boundary of the duct, is small in size and can be solved at one stroke with no iteration. Thus, the BEM results are obtained with considerably less computational effort which is one of the basic advantage of the boundary element method. This technique has already been used in the works [4, 5, 18] for the solution of MHD flow problems in rectangular ducts with no-slip velocity conditions. However, the insertion of the slip velocity condition, which is the basis of the present work, needs a special treatment that leads to modifications in the resulting BEM system obtained in the previous works [4, 5, 18]. Thus, it can be counted as a contribution of the present study in terms of the application of the numerical method. In addition, the effect of the direction of the magnetic field is further investigated by considering an external magnetic field which makes a positive angle with the vertical axis.

## 2 Mathematical Model

The steady, laminar flow of a viscous, incompressible electrically conducting fluid is investigated in a rectangular duct subject to a constant and uniform inclined magnetic field. The flow is driven by a constant pressure gradient in a sufficiently long pipe in the $z$-direction and becomes two-dimensional for a fully developed flow in the rectangular cross-section of the pipe. The equations governing the MHD duct flow are derived by the interaction of Navier-Stokes equations of fluid dynamics and the Maxwell's equations of electromagnetism through Ohm's law. Thus, the non-dimensional form of the MHD flow equations are given as [8]

$$\nabla^2 V + M_x \frac{\partial B}{\partial x} + M_y \frac{\partial B}{\partial y} = -1$$
$$\text{in } \Omega \qquad (1)$$
$$\nabla^2 B + M_x \frac{\partial V}{\partial x} + M_y \frac{\partial V}{\partial y} = 0$$

which are coupled in velocity $V(x, y)$ and the induced magnetic field $B(x, y)$ in $z$-direction through the rectangular duct $\Omega = \{(x, y) : -a \le x \le a, -b \le y \le b\}$. The externally applied uniform magnetic field of intensity $B_0$ is $\mathbf{M} = (M_x, M_y)$ with the components $M_x = M \sin \gamma$ and $M_y = M \cos \gamma$, where the norm of $\mathbf{M}$ is the Hartmann number $M(= B_0 L_0 \sqrt{\sigma} / \sqrt{\mu}$, $L_0$: characteristic length, $\sigma$: electrical conductivity, $\mu$: viscosity coefficient); and $\gamma$ is the angle between the magnetic field and the positive $y$-axis (see Fig. 1). The walls of the cavity are considered to be either insulated ($B = 0$) or perfectly conducting ($\partial B / \partial n = 0$) in the presence of slip. The boundary condition for the velocity through the slipping walls is given by ($V + \alpha \partial V / \partial n = 0$), where $\alpha$ is the dimensionless slip length (see [16]).

The corresponding homogeneous equations to Eq. 1 are obtained by using the particular solution $\mathbf{u_p} = [V_p \ B_p]^T$ where $V_p = 0$ and $B_p = -x/M_x$ (or $B_p = -y/M_y$ when the magnetic field is applied vertically i.e. $\gamma = 0$). Thus, by taking $\mathbf{u} = \mathbf{u_h} + \mathbf{u_p}$ the homogeneous solution $\mathbf{u_h} = [V_h \ B_h]^T$ satisfies

**Fig. 1** The rectangular cross-section of the pipe

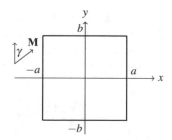

$$\nabla^2 V_h + M_x \frac{\partial B_h}{\partial x} + M_y \frac{\partial B_h}{\partial y} = 0$$

$$\text{in } \Omega \qquad (2)$$

$$\nabla^2 B_h + M_x \frac{\partial V_h}{\partial x} + M_y \frac{\partial V_h}{\partial y} = 0$$

with the corresponding boundary conditions:

On insulated walls: $\quad B_h = \dfrac{x}{M_x} \text{ (or } B_h = \dfrac{y}{M_y}\text{)}, \qquad V_h + \alpha \dfrac{\partial V_h}{\partial n} = 0,$

$$\qquad (3)$$

On conducting walls: $\dfrac{\partial B_h}{\partial n} = \dfrac{n_x}{M_x} \text{ (or } \dfrac{\partial B_h}{\partial n} = \dfrac{n_y}{M_y}\text{)}, \quad V_h + \alpha \dfrac{\partial V_h}{\partial n} = 0$

where $\mathbf{n} = (n_x, n_y)$ is the outward unit normal on the duct walls and $\alpha = 0$ correspondences to the no-slip condition (i.e. $V_h = 0$). To keep the notation simple in the equations obtained through the application of the boundary element method, the homogeneous solution $\mathbf{u_h} = [V_h \ B_h]^T$ will be taken as $\mathbf{u} = [V \ B]^T$.

## 3 Application of the Numerical Method

A direct boundary element method is used for the discretization of the homogeneous MHD flow equations. BEM is a boundary only nature technique which transforms the differential equations into equivalent boundary integral equations by inherent use of the fundamental solution of the governing equations. Thus, Eq. (2) is weighted with the fundamental solution ($\mathbf{W} = [\mathbf{w_1} \ \mathbf{w_2}]$, where $\mathbf{w_1} = [V_1^* \ B_1^*]^{\mathbf{T}}$ and $\mathbf{w_2} = [V_2^* \ B_2^*]^{\mathbf{T}}$) of the coupled MHD equations via Galerkin principle to obtain the boundary integral equations for the velocity and induced magnetic field. The components of the fundamental solution derived in [4] are

$$V_1^* = B_2^* = \frac{1}{2\pi} K_0(\frac{Mr}{2}) \cosh(\frac{\mathbf{M.r}}{2}), \quad V_2^* = B_1^* = \frac{1}{2\pi} K_0(\frac{Mr}{2}) \sinh(\frac{\mathbf{M.r}}{2})$$

where $K_0$ is the modified Bessel function of the second kind of order zero, $r$ is the distance from the source point to the field point and is also the magnitude of vector $\mathbf{r} = (r_x, r_y)$. Then, the discretization of the boundary $\Gamma$ with $N$ constant boundary elements $\Gamma_j, j = 1, \ldots, N$, leads to the following matrix boundary integral equation

$$-c_A \begin{Bmatrix} V(A) \\ B(A) \end{Bmatrix} + \begin{bmatrix} H & G \\ G & H \end{bmatrix} \begin{Bmatrix} V \\ B \end{Bmatrix} + \begin{bmatrix} \bar{H} & \bar{G} \\ \bar{G} & \bar{H} \end{bmatrix} \begin{Bmatrix} \partial V/\partial n \\ \partial B/\partial n \end{Bmatrix} = \begin{Bmatrix} 0 \\ 0 \end{Bmatrix} \qquad (4)$$

where $c_A$ is either $1/2$ or $1$ when the fixed point $A$ is on the boundary or inside, respectively, and the entries of $H, G, \bar{H}$ and $\bar{G}$ are as given in [4]. However, Eq. (4) is rearranged according to the given boundary conditions taking into account the slip. Once the obtained new system is solved, the unknown values for homogeneous velocity, induced magnetic field and their normal derivatives are obtained on the boundary, however, one can easily obtain the values of $V$ and $B$ inside the computational domain $\Omega$ by taking $c_A = 1$ in Eq. (4). The solution to the inhomogeneous equation (1) is further calculated by adding the particular solution to the obtained homogeneous solution.

## 4   Results and Discussions

The MHD flow subject to an external inclined magnetic field is considered in a rectangular duct with various types of wall conditions involving insulated or conducting walls which exhibit slip. The computational domain is determined by taking the lengths of the rectangle $a = b = 1$ and boundary is discretized by a maximum number of $N = 160$ constant boundary elements when $M = 100$. The flow characteristics under the influence of the slip are examined for the values of Hartmann number $M = 10, 100$ and the inclination angle $\gamma = 0, \pi/4, \pi/3, \pi/2$. The effect of the slip on the velocity field is measured by the slip ratio $s$ which is defined by the ratio of the slip length $\alpha$ to the thickness of the boundary layer $\delta$, i.e. $s = \alpha/\delta$. In MHD duct flows, the walls perpendicular to the applied magnetic field are called Hartmann walls while the parallel ones are called side walls. It is well-known that with no-slip velocity conditions the MHD flow exhibits boundary layers whose thickness scales as $\delta_{Ha} = 1/M$ along the Hartmann walls and $\delta_{side} = 1/\sqrt{M}$ along the side walls. Hence, the slip ratio becomes, $s = \alpha M$ and $s = \alpha\sqrt{M}$ for the Hartmann and side walls, respectively. Slip ratio is an important parameter which determines the relative contribution of the magnetic field effect and the slip itself. In the strong slip $s > 1$, the flow is fully controlled by the slip phenomenon. However, if $s < 1$, the effect of magnetic field is dominant. When the slip ratio is unity, both MHD and slip effects are important.

### 4.1   Problem 1: MHD Flow in an Insulated Duct with Slip on the Vertical Walls

MHD flow in an insulated duct of which the vertical walls exhibit slip is studied in the presence of an inclined magnetic field. First, the case when the magnetic field is applied horizontally, that is $\gamma = \pi/2$, is considered to compare the present results with the analytical results reported by Smolentsev [16]. The effect of the slip length $\alpha$ on the velocity distribution $V/V_m$ ($V_m$ is the mean bulk velocity of the flow) is visualized in Fig. 2 and the obtained results are in very well agreement with the ones given in the work of Smolentsev (see Fig. 7 in [16]). It is observed that the velocity at the core of the cavity increases with an increase in slip length.

**Fig. 2** Effect of slip length
on velocity profile $V/V_m$ at
$M = 100, \gamma = \pi/2$

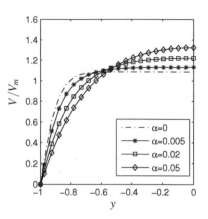

Figures 3 and 4 show the equivelocity and the induced current lines, respectively, for the slip ratio $s = \alpha M = 0, 0.4, 4$ at $M = 10, 100$. The velocity decreases and becomes stagnant at the center of the duct, and as a result the equivelocity lines are concentrated towards the walls forming boundary layers with an increase in Hartmann number. The velocity increases and the thickness of the side layers becomes thicker as $s$ increases; and hence the core of the uniform velocity becomes vertically thinner compared to no-slip ($\alpha = 0$) case. However, the increase rate in velocity is less at high $M = 100$ compared to $M = 10$ since the slip effect on the core velocity is suppressed by the strong magnetic field at high $M$. The thickness of the Hartmann layer is not significantly affected when $s < 1$, however, it diminishes for small $M = 10$ when $s > 1$ since flow is fully controlled with the slip phenomenon. On the other hand, the slip ratio has no significant effect on the profiles of current lines especially at $M = 10$. However, at $M = 100$ the side layers weaken when $s > 1$ and the core of current lines shrinks vertically. An increase in slip length results in a slight decrease in the magnitude of current lines when $M = 10$ whereas at $M = 100$ the magnitude is same at each $\alpha$. Moreover, the magnitude of current lines decreases as $M$ advances, which is the well-known flattening tendency in MHD flow.

The effects of the inclination angle $\gamma = 0, \pi/4, \pi/3$ and slip length $\alpha = 0, 0.01, 0.3$ on the velocity distribution at $M = 100$ are shown in Fig. 5. Equivelocity lines extend in the direction of the applied magnetic field where the flow becomes stagnant. As $\alpha$ advances velocity increases and the core of the uniform velocity becomes smaller compared the no-slip case whereas it enlarges as $\gamma$ increases form $\pi/4$ to $\pi/3$. The boundary layers are concentrated near the corners in the direction of the applied magnetic field when $\gamma = \pi/4, \pi/3$. The magnetic field is applied vertically when $\gamma = 0$, so that the horizontal walls become Hartmann walls while the vertical walls are side walls. Thus, the slip is on the side walls. The side layers weaken and finally vanishes following the formation of a flow circulation as $\alpha$ increases due to the strong slip effect opposite to the case when $\gamma = \pi/2$. On the other hand, the thickness of Hartmann layers remains almost the same for each $\alpha$ at $M = 100$ while it slightly diminishes in the case of horizontally applied magnetic field $\gamma = \pi/2$.

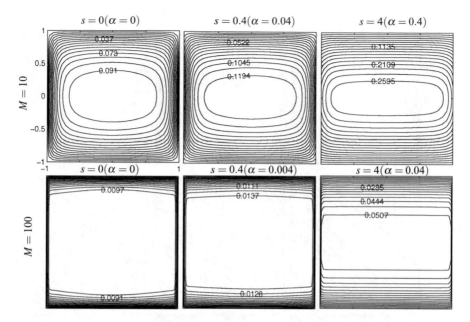

**Fig. 3** Effect of slip ratio $s$ on equivelocity lines at $M = 10, 100, \gamma = \pi/2$

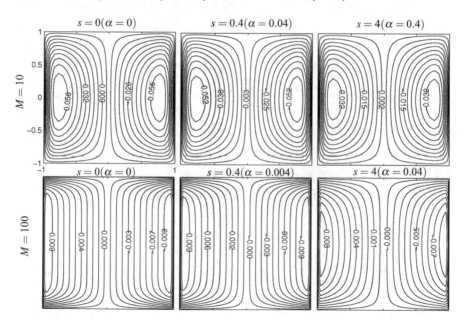

**Fig. 4** Effect of slip ratio $s$ on current lines at $M = 10, 100, \gamma = \pi/2$

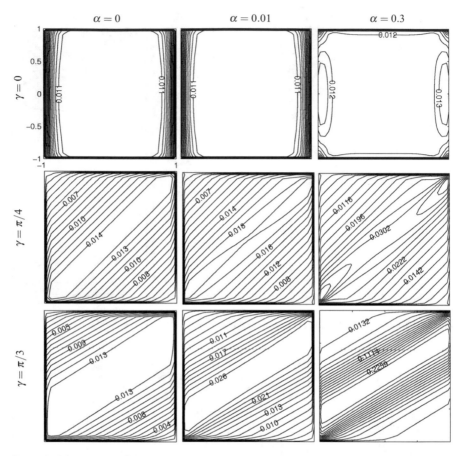

**Fig. 5** Effects of the inclination angle $\gamma$ and slip length $\alpha$ on equivelocity lines at $M = 100$

## 4.2 Problem 2: MHD Flow in Duct with Perfectly Conducting Walls and Slip on Vertical Walls

MHD flow in a duct all of which walls are perfectly conducting is considered under the influence of an horizontally applied magnetic field. That is, the boundary conditions for the induced magnetic field are $\partial B / \partial n = 0$ on all walls, and the vertical Hartmann walls exhibit slip as in Problem 1. The effect of the slip ratio $s = \alpha M$ on the velocity and induced magnetic field is displayed, respectively, in Figs. 6 and 7 when $M = 10, 100$ and $\gamma = \pi/2$. Similar to the insulated duct case, an increase in $\alpha$ leads to the enhancement of the velocity in the core of the duct and the side layers get thicker while Hartmann layers diminish at $M = 10$. However, when compared to insulated duct case the profile of equivelocity lines alters significantly at $M = 100$, that is, two circulations are formed along the side walls. As slip gets stronger the

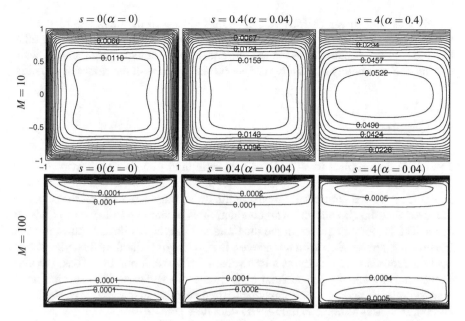

**Fig. 6** Effect of slip ratio $s$ on equivelocity lines at $M = 10, 100, \gamma = \pi/2$

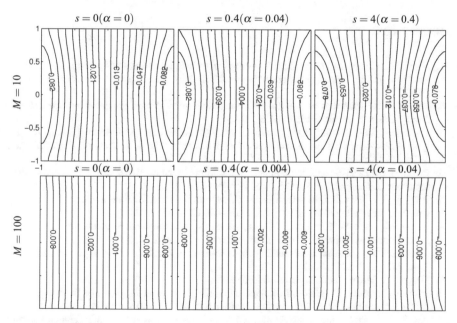

**Fig. 7** Effect of slip ratio $s$ on current lines at $M = 10, 100, \gamma = \pi/2$

circulations start to vanish following a slight increase in the thickness of the side layers. Moreover, the thin Hartmann layers almost vanish when $s > 1$. On the other hand, due to the conducting walls the current lines become perpendicular to walls and distribute smoothly especially at $M = 100$ irrespective of the values of slip ratio.

# 5 Conclusion

The MHD flow subject to an inclined magnetic field in a duct with insulated and conducting walls which exhibit slip on vertical walls (i.e. on Hartmann walls when $\gamma = \pi/2$) is solved numerically by using the direct boundary element method. It is observed that the slip and the wall conductivities essentially influence the flow in ducts. The velocity increases in the duct and the side layers become thicker while Hartmann layers weaken with an increase in slip length for both insulated and conducting duct walls especially at a low value of Hartmann number. Thus, the core of the uniform velocity gets smaller compared to no-slip case. On the other hand, both the velocity and the induced magnetic field decrease in magnitude as Hartmann number increases as in the classic MHD duct flow with no-slip.

# References

1. Ahmad, S., Chishtie, F., Mahmood, A.: Analytical technique for magnetohydrodynamic (MHD) fluid flow of a periodically accelerated plate with slippage. Eur. J. Mech. B Fluids 65, 192–198 (2017)
2. Barrett, K.E.: Duct flow with a transverse magnetic field at high Hartmann numbers. Int. J. Numer. Meth. Eng. 50(8), 1893–1906 (2001)
3. Bourantas, G.C., Skouras, E.D., Loukopoulos, V.C.: An accurate, stable and efficient domain-type meshless method for the solution of MHD flow problems. J. Comput. Phys. 228(21), 8135–8160 (2009)
4. Bozkaya, C., Tezer-Sezgin, M.: Fundamental solution for coupled magnetohydrodynamic flow equations. J. Comput. Appl. Math. 203, 125–144 (2007)
5. Bozkaya, C., Tezer-Sezgin, M.: A direct BEM solution to MHD flow in electrodynamically coupled rectangular channels. Comput. Fluids 66, 177–182 (2012)
6. Buren, M., Jian, Y., Chang, L., Liu, Q., Zhao, G.: AC magnetohydrodynamic slip flow in microchannel with sinusoidal roughness. Microsyst. Technol. 23, 3347–3359 (2017)
7. Carabineanu, A., Lungu, E.: Pseudospectral method for MHD pipe flow. Int. J. Numer. Meth. Eng. 68(2), 173–191 (2006)
8. Dragoş, L.: Magnetofluid Dynamics. Abacus Press, London (1975)
9. Hron, J., Le Roux, C., Málek, J., Rajagopal, K.R.: Flows of incompressible fluids subject to Navier's slip on the boundary. Comput. Math. Appl. 56, 2128–2143 (2008)
10. Ijaz, S., Saleem, N., Munawar, S.: Slip effect on the magnetohydrodynamics channel flow in the presence of the across mass transfer phenomenon. J. Appl. Mech. Tech. Phy. 58, 54–62 (2017)
11. Ligere, E., Dzenite, I., Matvejevs, A.: The Proceedings of 10th PAMIR International Conference-Fundamental and Applied MHD, Cagliari, Italy, 20–24 June 2016

12. Loukopoulos, V.C., Bourantas, G.C., Skouras, E.D., Nikiforidis, G.C.: Localized meshless point collocation method for time-dependent magnetohydrodynamics flow through pipes under a variety of wall conductivity conditions. Comput. Mech. **47**(2), 137–159 (2011)
13. Ortiz-Pérez, A.S., García-Ángel, V., Acuña-Ramírez, A., Vargas-Osuna, L.E., Pérez-Barrera, J., Cuevas, S.: Magnetohydrodynamic flow with slippage in an annular duct for microfluidic applications. Microfluid. Nanofluid. **21**, 138 (2017)
14. Reddy, P.B.A., Suneeth, S., Reddy, N.B.: Numerical study of magnetohydrodynamics (MHD) boundary layer slip flow of a Maxwell nanofluid over an exponentially stretching surface with convective boundary condition. Propul. Power Res. **6**(4), 259–268 (2017)
15. Seth, G.S., Mishra, M.K.: Analysis of transient flow of MHD nanofluid past a non-linear stretching sheet considering Navier's slip boundary condition. Adv. Powder Technol. **28**, 375–384 (2017)
16. Smolentsev, S.: MHD duct flows under hydrodynamic slip condition. Theor. Comput. Fluid Dyn. **23**, 557–570 (2009)
17. Srinivasacharya, D., Himabindu, K.: Analysis of entropy generation due to micropolar fluid flow in a rectangular duct subjected to slip and convective boundary conditions. J. Heat Trans. **139**, 072003-1-9 (2017)
18. Tezer-Sezgin, M., Bozkaya, C.: Boundary element method solution of magnetohydrodynamic flow in a rectangular duct with conducting walls parallel to applied magnetic field. Comput. Mech. **41**, 769–775 (2008)

# The Effects of Thermal Radiation on a Reactive Hydromagnetic Internal Heat Generating Fluid Flow Through Parallel Porous Plates

Anthony R. Hassan, Jacob A. Gbadeyan and Sulyman O. Salawu

**Abstract** This study analyses the influence of thermal radiation on an electrically conducting, incompressible and steady flow of a reactive hydromagnetic fluid with heat source within two parallel porous plates; under the reaction of different chemical kinetics. The dimensionless nonlinear governing equations are determined using the modified Adomian decomposition Method (mADM). The velocity and the temperature profiles are investigated for different physical parameters, especially the porous medium and thermal radiation parameters.

**Keywords** Thermal radiation · Reactive fluid · Porous plates
Internal heat generation · Modified Adomian decomposition method (mADM)

## 1 Introduction

In view of quantity in applications of fluid mechanics in industries, engineering and technology; the interest in the study has tremendously increased during the last few years with different physical properties. This development has been strongly influenced by its numerous applications to engineering, environment and biological sciences which can be modeled or approximated as stated in [1]; as a matter of fact, many deep perceptive studies have been done on reactive hydromagnetic fluid flow,

A. R. Hassan (✉)
Department of Mathematical Sciences, University of South Africa,
Pretoria 0003, South Africa
e-mail: anthonyhassan72@yahoo.co.uk

A. R. Hassan
Department of Mathematics, Tai Solarin University of Education, Ijagun, Nigeria

J. A. Gbadeyan · S. O. Salawu
Department of Mathematics, University of Ilorin, Ilorin, Nigeria
e-mail: j.agbadeyan@yahoo.com

S. O. Salawu
e-mail: salawukunle@gmail.com

© Springer Nature Switzerland AG 2018
D. M. Kilgour et al. (eds.), *Recent Advances in Mathematical
and Statistical Methods*, Springer Proceedings in Mathematics & Statistics 259,
https://doi.org/10.1007/978-3-319-99719-3_17

few of those studies are mentioned in [2–4]. In their study, [5] observed that due to the diversity of fluids in nature, surveys through investigative studies explained that a lot of models have been proposed to describe fluid behavior in different circumstances and physical properties such as fluid flowing through porous media [1, 6]. Also, fluid flowing with the impact of an internal heat source or sink was investigated in [3, 4, 7]. In addition to that, fluid flowing under the influence of thermal radiation were investigated in [1, 8, 9]. Other physical properties like the impact of the magnetic field intensity were studied in [2–4, 10, 11] and it also plays another important role in fluid behaviour.

Meanwhile, compound effects of physical properties may determine fluid behaviour. These effects have been examined by various researchers in stating the effects that range from magnetic influence, heat transfer, heat source/sink, viscosity and thermal radiation effects to mention few. Comprehensive survey for some of these effects are discussed extensively in [1, 2] and references therein. Additionally, [10] extended [2] by respectively investigating the thermal stability and entropy generation analysis of a reactive fluid flow through a channel under various chemical kinetics and further extended the investigation in [3, 4] by respectively analysing the effect of internal heat generation on the entropy generation in a reactive hydromagnetic fluid flow only under Arrhenius kinetics and for various chemical kinetics.

In order to have clear and more understanding on the fluid behaviour, there exists a need to investigate the thermal radiative effects on the fluid flow through parallel porous plates earlier examined in [2–4, 10] because of its importance in engineering, industries and physics applications which are investigated as stated in [12]. This study in [12] revealed the importance of radiation heat transfer in space technology and the role it plays to control polymer processing in industries where the quality of the final product depends on the heat controlling factors to some extent.

Hence, in this present study, the studies in [2–4, 10] are further extended to investigate the impact of thermal radiation on an internal heat generating reactive hydromagnetic fluid flow within parallel porous plates under different chemical kinetics. The dimensionless governing equations of the fluid flow are obtained using the mADM. The momentum and energy distributions are investigated for different physical parameters especially with respect to the impact of thermal radiation.

## 2  Mathematical Formulation

The steady flow of an incompressible reactive hydromagnetic fluid flow through parallel porous plates is investigated, with the given width as (a) and length (L) under constant wall temperature together with the impact of transversely applied magnetic field $(B_0)$ and thermal radiation $(q_r)$. The horizontal parallel porous walls are at a distance of $2a$ located at $y = -a$ and $y = a$ as shown in Fig. 1. Following [2, 10], the differential equations governing the fluid flow in non-dimensionless forms is given as:

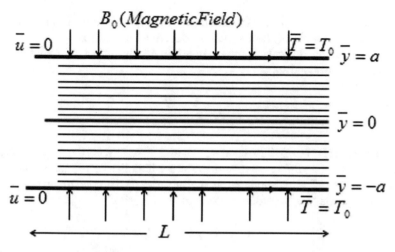

**Fig. 1** Geometry of the problem

$$-\frac{d\overline{p}}{d\overline{x}} + \mu\frac{d^2\overline{u}}{d^2\overline{y}} - \sigma_0 B_0^2\overline{u} - \frac{\mu}{K}\overline{u} = 0 \tag{1}$$

$$k\frac{d^2\overline{T}}{d^2\overline{y}} + \mu\left(\frac{d\overline{u}}{d\overline{y}}\right)^2 + QC_0A\left(\frac{k\overline{T}}{v\ell}\right)^m e^{-\frac{E}{R\overline{T}}} + \sigma_0 B_0^2\overline{u}^2$$

$$+ \frac{\mu}{K}\overline{u}^2 + Q_0\left(\overline{T} - T_0\right) - \frac{dq_r}{d\overline{y}} = 0 \tag{2}$$

with the symmetric conditions along the channel centreline given as

$$\frac{d\overline{u}}{d\overline{y}} = \frac{d\overline{T}}{d\overline{u}} = 0 \quad \text{on} \quad \overline{y} = 0 \quad \text{and} \quad \overline{u} = \overline{T} = 0 \quad \text{on} \quad \overline{y} = a \tag{3}$$

Note that the bar on any of the variables signify the dimensionless version of the variable. Here $p$ represents pressure, $\mu$ is fluid viscosity, $u$ is the fluid velocity, $T$ is the fluid temperature, $\sigma_0$ represents electrical conductivity and $K$ is Darcy's permeability constant. Also, $Q$ is the heat of the reaction term, $k$ is the thermal conductivity coefficient, $C_0$ is the reactant species initial concentration, $v$ denotes vibration frequency, $E$ is the activation energy and $\ell$ is Planck's number. Meanwhile, $A$ and $R$ respectively stand for the constants of reaction rate and universal gas. Also, $Q_0$ is the dimensional heat generation coefficient, $q_r$ is the radiative heat flux and $T_0$ is the wall temperature. The numerical exponents $m \in \{-2, 0, 0.5\}$ respectively represent the rate of chemical reaction for sensitized, Arrhenius and bimolecular kinetics.

Notably, the last term in (1) and fifth in (2) are formulated from Darcy's law of porosity modified by Brinkman [13, 14]. The sixth term in (2) is the effect of internal heat source as in [4, 7, 15] and the last term in (2) is with respect to the impact of thermal radiation within the flow system as described in [1, 16].

According to the Rosseland approximation for the effect of radiation $q_r$ as described in [1, 16] is given as:

$$q_r = -\frac{4\sigma}{3k^*}\frac{\mathrm{d}\overline{T}^4}{\mathrm{d}\overline{y}} \tag{4}$$

such that $\sigma$ is the Stefan-Boltzmann constant and $k^*$ represents the mean absorption coefficient where the difference in temperature within the flow system is described in such a way that $T^4$ is expanded using Taylor series on the free-stream temperature $(T_\infty)$ and neglecting higher orders as done in [1, 16], yield:

$$T^4 \equiv 4T_\infty^3 T - 3T_\infty^4 \tag{5}$$

such that

$$\frac{\mathrm{d}q_r}{\mathrm{d}\overline{y}} = -\frac{16\sigma T_\infty^3}{3k^*}\frac{\mathrm{d}^2\overline{T}}{\mathrm{d}\overline{y}^2}. \tag{6}$$

Therefore (2) becomes

$$k\frac{\mathrm{d}^2\overline{T}}{\mathrm{d}^2\overline{y}} + \mu\left(\frac{\mathrm{d}\overline{u}}{\mathrm{d}\overline{x}}\right)^2 + QC_0A\left(\frac{k\overline{T}}{v\ell}\right)^m e^{-\frac{E}{R\overline{T}}} + \sigma_0 B_0^2\overline{u}^2 + \frac{\mu}{K}\overline{u}^2$$

$$+ Q_0\left(\overline{T} - T_0\right) + \frac{16\sigma T_\infty^3}{3k^*}\frac{\mathrm{d}^2\overline{T}}{\mathrm{d}\overline{y}^2} = 0. \tag{7}$$

We thereby introduce non-dimensional variables and parameters as follows:

$$y = \frac{\overline{y}}{a}, \quad x = \frac{\overline{x}}{a}, \quad u = \frac{\overline{u}}{U}, \quad T = \frac{E\left(\overline{T} - T_0\right)}{RT_0^2}, \quad Br = \frac{E\mu U^2}{kRT_0^2},$$

$$\delta = \frac{RT_0}{E}, \quad \gamma = \frac{\mu U^2}{QAa^2C_0}\left(\frac{v\ell}{kT_0}\right)^m e^{\frac{E}{RT_0}}, \quad H^2 = \frac{\sigma_0 B_0^2 a^2}{\mu},$$

$$G = -\frac{\mathrm{d}p}{\mathrm{d}x}, \quad p = \frac{a\overline{p}}{\mu U}, \quad \alpha = \frac{a^2}{K}, \quad \lambda = \frac{QEAa^2C_0}{KRT_0^2}\left(\frac{kT_0}{v\ell}\right)^m e^{-\frac{E}{RT_0}},$$

$$R_d = \frac{16\sigma T_\infty^3}{3kk^*} \quad \text{and} \quad \beta = \frac{Q_0RT_0^2}{QAEC_0}\left(\frac{v\ell}{kT_0}\right)^m e^{\frac{E}{RT_0}} \tag{8}$$

such that, $G$ represents the pressure gradient, $a$ stands for the channel half width, $U$ is the mean velocity. $H$ and $Br$ are respectively Hartmann and Brinkman numbers. In addition to that, $\gamma$, $\lambda$, $R_d$, $\alpha$, $\delta$, and $\beta$ respectively represent parameters for viscous heating, Frank–Kamenettski, conduction-radiation, porous permeability, activation energy and the heat source.

With the introduction of (8) in (1), (3) and (7), we obtain equations governing the fluid flow under the influence of thermal radiation in dimensionless form as:

$$\frac{d^2u}{dy^2} - \left(H^2 + \alpha\right)u + G = 0 \tag{9}$$

$$\frac{d^2T}{dy^2} + \frac{\lambda}{1 + R_d}\left[(1 + \delta T)^m\, e^{\frac{T}{1+\delta T}} + \gamma\left(\left(\frac{du}{dy}\right)^2 + \left(H^2 + \alpha\right)u^2\right) + \beta T\right] = 0 \tag{10}$$

together with the boundary conditions

$$\frac{du}{dy} = \frac{dT}{dy} = 0 \quad \text{on} \quad y = 0 \quad \text{and} \quad u = T = 0 \quad \text{on} \quad y = \pm 1. \tag{11}$$

## 3  Modified Adomian Decomposition Method (mADM)

The momentum and energy profiles (9)–(10) with the boundary conditions (11) that govern the flow system with the effect of thermal radiation are solved using mADM as in [3, 4, 10, 17]. The momentum equation (9) has a general exact solution obtained as:

$$u(y) = \frac{e^{-y\sqrt{\alpha+H^2}}\left(-e^{\sqrt{\alpha+H^2}} + e^{y\sqrt{\alpha+H^2}} + e^{(y+2)\sqrt{\alpha+H^2}} - e^{(2y+1)\sqrt{\alpha+H^2}}\right)G}{\left(e^{2\sqrt{\alpha+H^2}} + 1\right)\left(\alpha + H^2\right)} \tag{12}$$

To solve the energy equation (10) with the boundary condition (11), Eq. (12) shall be used to solve Eq. (10) as follows:

$$\frac{d^2T}{dy^2} = -\frac{\lambda}{1 + R_d}\left[(1 + \delta T)^m\, e^{\frac{T}{1+\delta T}} + \gamma\left(\left(\frac{du}{dy}\right)^2 + \left(H^2 + \alpha\right)u^2\right) + \beta T\right] \tag{13}$$

We now solve Eq. (13) with the numerical exponent ($m$), for different chemical kinetics by integrating equation (13) twice together with boundary conditions (11), we obtain:

$$T(y) = a_0 - \frac{\lambda}{1 + R_d}\int_0^y \int_0^y \left[(1 + \delta T)^m\, e^{\frac{T}{1+\delta T}}\right.$$
$$\left. + \gamma\left(\left(\frac{du}{dy}\right)^2 + \left(H^2 + \alpha\right)u^2\right) + \beta T\right] dy\, dy \tag{14}$$

where $a_0 = T(0)$. This will be determined with the other boundary condition in (11). The mADM requires the introduction of a series solution such that:

$$T(y) = \sum_{n=0}^{\infty} T_n(y) \tag{15}$$

where the components $T_0, T_1, T_2, \ldots, T_k$ are to be determined. Thus, substitute (15) into (14) gives

$$T(y) = a_0 - \frac{\lambda}{1 + R_d} \int_0^y \int_0^y \left[ \left( 1 + \delta \left( \sum_{n=0}^{\infty} T_n(y) \right) \right)^m e^{\frac{\left( \sum_{n=0}^{\infty} T_n(y) \right)}{1 + \delta \left( \sum_{n=0}^{\infty} T_n(y) \right)}} \right.$$

$$\left. + \gamma \left( \left( \frac{du}{dy} \right)^2 + (H^2 + \alpha) u^2 \right) + \beta \left( \sum_{n=0}^{\infty} T_n(y) \right) \right] dy \, dy \tag{16}$$

However, the following series can be used to represent the non–linear term in (16) to determine the components $T_0, T_1, T_2, \ldots, T_k$.

$$\sum_{n=0}^{\infty} A_n(y) = \left( 1 + \delta \left( \sum_{n=0}^{\infty} T_n(y) \right) \right)^m e^{\frac{\left( \sum_{n=0}^{\infty} T_n(y) \right)}{1 + \delta \left( \sum_{n=0}^{\infty} T_n(y) \right)}} \tag{17}$$

The expression in (17) is binomially expanded in such a way that the following are obtained:

$$A_0 = e^{\frac{T_0(y)}{\delta T_0(y) + 1}} \left( \delta T_0(y) + 1 \right)^m,$$

$$A_1 = T_1(y) e^{\frac{T_0(y)}{\delta T_0(y) + 1}} \left( \delta T_0(y) + 1 \right)^{m-2} \left( \delta m + \delta^2 m T_0(y) + 1 \right),$$

$$A_2 = \frac{1}{2} e^{\frac{T_0(y)}{\delta T_0(y) + 1}} \left( \delta T_0(y) + 1 \right)^{m-4} \left( 2T_2(y) \left( \delta T_0(y) + 1 \right)^2 \left( \delta m + \delta^2 m T_0(y) + 1 \right) \right.$$

$$\left. + T_1(y)^2 \left( \delta(m-1)(\delta m + 2) + \delta^2(m-1) T_0(y) \left( 2\delta m + \delta^2 m T_0(y) + 2 \right) + 1 \right) \right), \tag{18}$$

Here, the components $A_0, A_1, A_2, \ldots$, are referred to as Adomian polynomials. Then, (16) reduces to

$$T(y) = a_0 - \frac{\lambda}{1 + R_d} \int_0^y \int_0^y \left[ \sum_{n=0}^{\infty} A_n(y) + \gamma \left( \left( \frac{du}{dy} \right)^2 + (H^2 + \alpha) u^2 \right) \right.$$

$$\left. + \beta \left( \sum_{n=0}^{\infty} T_n(y) \right) \right] dy \, dy \tag{19}$$

Taking the zeroth component of (19), we obtain the following:

$$T_0(y) = 0 \tag{20}$$

$$T_1(y) = a_0 - \frac{\lambda}{1 + R_d} \int_0^y \int_0^y \left[ A_0(y) + \gamma \left( \left( \frac{du}{dy} \right)^2 + \left( H^2 + \alpha \right) u^2 \right) \right.$$
$$\left. + \beta \left( T_0(y) \right) \right] dy \, dy \tag{21}$$

$$T_{n+1}(y) = -\frac{\lambda}{1 + R_d} \int_0^y \int_0^y \left[ A_n(y) + \beta T_n(y) \right] dy \, dy \qquad n \geq 1 \tag{22}$$

Finally, the solution of the energy equation is approximately given as:

$$T(y) = \sum_{n=0}^{k} T_n(y) \tag{23}$$

With the use of Mathematica software package, Eqs. (20)–(22) are solved to obtain the approximate solution in (23) together with (12) which are then in presenting the numerical results in tables and graphs in Sect. 5.

## 4  Discussion of Results

The respective solutions of velocity and temperature distributions in (12) and (23) are used to obtain figures to show the impact of thermal radiation and other physical properties on a reactive hydromagnetic heat generating fluid flow within parallel porous plates under different chemical kinetics. The rapid convergence for the series solution of temperature profile in (23) is shown in Table 1. This shows the efficiency of the mADM used for the given values.

Also, Table 2 displays the numerical results of the temperature distribution of [2] where perturbation method was used and the present result where mADM is used. Notably, our results shall be equivalent to [2] when $\beta$, $\alpha$, $R_d$ and the numerical

**Table 1** Rapid convergence for the series solution

| $H = G = \lambda = 1, \gamma = \delta = \beta = 0.1, \alpha = y = 0.5, m = 0$ | | |
|---|---|---|
| $n$ | $T_n$ | $\sum_{n=0}^{k} T_n(y)$ |
| 0 | 0 | 0 |
| 1 | 0.448552 | $4.48552 \times 10^{-1}$ |
| 2 | −0.475575 | $4.001 \times 10^{-1}$ |
| 3 | −0.008249 | $3.927 \times 10^{-1}$ |
| 4 | −0.0004900387 | $3.922 \times 10^{-1}$ |
| 5 | 0.000060615 | $3.922 \times 10^{-1}$ |
| 6 | −0.000130686 | $3.922 \times 10^{-1}$ |

**Table 2** Numerical results for the temperature distribution

| $H = G = \delta = \gamma = 1, \lambda = 0.5, m = 0$ | | | |
|---|---|---|---|
| −1.0 | 0 | $-1.59595 \times 10^{-15}$ | $1.596 \times 10^{-15}$ |
| −0.75 | 0.1556934861 | 0.1554686717 | $2.2481 \times 10^{-4}$ |
| −0.50 | 0.2660663845 | 0.2657578071 | $3.0858 \times 10^{-4}$ |
| −0.25 | 0.3323243479 | 0.3319573254 | $3.6702 \times 10^{-4}$ |
| 0 | 0.3544502181 | 0.3540586156 | $3.9160 \times 10^{-4}$ |
| 0.25 | 0.3323243479 | 0.3319573254 | $3.6702 \times 10^{-4}$ |
| 0.50 | 0.2660663845 | 0.2657578071 | $3.0858 \times 10^{-4}$ |
| 0.75 | 0.1556934861 | 0.1554686717 | $2.2481 \times 10^{-4}$ |
| 1.0 | 0 | $-1.596 \times 10^{-15}$ | $1.596 \times 10^{-15}$ |

**Fig. 2** Effect of $\alpha$ on $u(y)$

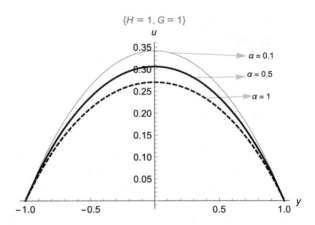

exponent ($m$) are all zero. The results showed that the approximate solution is with average difference of order $10^{-4}$.

The velocity profile for variations in the porous permeability parameter ($\alpha$) and magnetic field parameter ($H$) are shown in Figs. 2 and 3. It is observed that the maximum velocity occurred at the least values of the porous permeability parameter ($\alpha$) in Fig. 2 and magnetic field parameter ($H$) in Fig. 3. The retardation is caused due to the electromagnetic force and the resistance encountered within the flow system.

The temperature profile for variations in the numerical exponent ($m$) representing each chemical kinetics, is displayed in Fig. 4. The observation is that the fluid temperature increases with respect to the increasing values of $m$ from −2 to 0.5. This is normal as the temperature measures the average amount of kinetic energy present in the fluid particles and the more the particles vibrates, the greater the temperature of the fluid. In this sense, energy is transfer from the centreline causing the average kinetic energy of the fluid to increase and hereby causing the temperature to rise as the chemical kinetics exponent $m$ increases as shown in Fig. 4. Moreover, the temperature profile for variations in conduction–radiation parameter ($R_d$) under Arrhenius chemical kinetics ($m = 0$) is displayed in Fig. 5. It is clearly noticed that

**Fig. 3** Effect of $H$ on $u(y)$

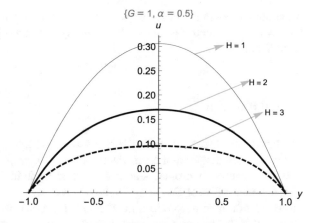

**Fig. 4** Different chemical kinetics for $T(y)$

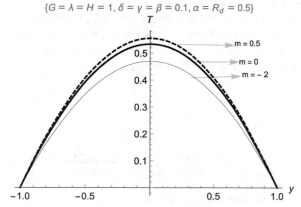

**Fig. 5** Effect of $R_d$ on $T(y)$ when $m = 0$

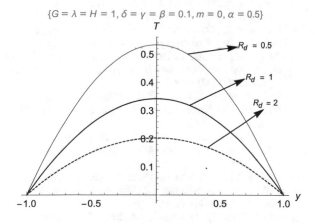

maximum temperature occurred with the least value which is due to the transfer of energy from the centreline to the plate walls symmetrically until thermal equilibrium is maintained.

## 5 Conclusion

The present study extends extensively the work in [2, 4, 10] to investigate the significance of thermal radiation on an electrically conducting, incompressible and steady flow of a reactive hydromagnetic heat generating fluid flow within parallel porous plates; under different chemical kinetics. The energy equation is obtained using the modified Adomian decomposition method (mADM). However, the present results showed that the maximum velocity occurred at the least values of the porous permeability parameter ($\alpha$) and magnetic field parameter ($H$). Also, temperature increases with respect to increasing values of chemical kinetics exponents, $m$ from $-2$ to $0.5$ while a reduction in temperature is noticed with variations in conduction-radiation parameter under Arrhenius kinetics.

## References

1. Rashad, A.M.: Effects of radiation and variable viscosity on unsteady MHD flow of a rotating fluid from stretching surface in porous medium. J. Egypt. Math. Soc. **22**(1), 134–142 (2014)
2. Makinde, O.D., Beg, O.A.: On inherent irreversibility in a reactive hydromagnetic channel flow. J. Therm. Sci. **19**(1), 72–79 (2010)
3. Hassan, A.R., Gbadeyan, J.A.: A reactive hydromagnetic internal heat generating fluid flow through a channel. Int. J. Heat Technol. **33**(3), 43–50 (2015)
4. Hassan, A.R., Maritz, R.: The analysis of a reactive hydromagnetic internal heat generating Poiseuille fluid flow through a channel. SpringerPlus **5**(1), 1–14 (2016)
5. Akhtar, W., Fetecau, C., Tigou, V., Fetecau, C.: Flow of Maxwell fluid between two sides wall induced by a constantly accelerating plates. Int. J. Z. Angew. Maths Phys. (2008). https://doi.org/10.1007/s00033008-7129-8
6. Mukhopadhyay, S., Layek, G.C.: Effects of thermal radiation and variable fluid viscosity on free convective flow and heat transfer past a porous stretching surface. Int. J. Heat Mass Transf. **51**(9), 2167–2178 (2008)
7. Jha, B.K., Ajibade, A.O.: Free convective flow of heat generating/absorbing fluid between vertical porous plates with periodic heat input. Int. Commun. Heat Mass Transf. **36**(6), 624–631 (2009)
8. Uwanta, I.J., Hamza, M.M.: Unsteady/Steady hydromagnetic flow of reactive viscous fluid in a vertical channel with thermal diffusion and temperature dependent properties. J. Appl. Fluid Mech. **9**(1), 169–176 (2016)
9. Hayat, T., Shafiq, A., Alsaedi, A.: Effect of Joule heating and thermal radiation in flow of third grade fluid over radiative surface. Plos one **9**(1), 1–12 (2014)
10. Hassan, A.R., Gbadeyan, J.A.: Entropy generation analysis of a reactive hydromagnetic fluid flow through a channel. Univ. Politech. Buchar. Sci. Bull. Ser. A **77**(2), 285–296 (2015)
11. Saha, S., Chakrabarti, S.: Impact of magnetic strength on magnetic fluid flow through a channel. Int. J. Eng. Res. Technol. (IJERT) **7**(2), 1–8 (2013)

12. Mukhopadhyay, S.: Effects of radiation and variable fluid viscosity on flow and heat transfer along a symmetric wedge. J. Appl. Fluid Mech. 2(2), 29–34 (2009)
13. Chauhan, D.S., Rastogi, P.: Heat transfer and entropy generation in MHD flow through a porous medium past a stretching sheet. Int. J. Energy Tech. 3, 1–13 (2011)
14. Bejan, A., Dincer, I., Lorente, S., Miguel, A., Reis, H.: Porous and Complex Flow Structures in Modern Technologies. Springer Science & Business Media, New York (2013)
15. El-Amin, M.F.: Combined effect of internal heat generation and magnetic field on free convection and mass transfer flow in a micro polar fluid with constant suction. J. Magn. Magn. Mater. 270, 130–135 (2004)
16. Isa, S.M., Ali, A.: Thermal radiation effect on hydromagnetic flow of dusty fluid over a stretching vertical surface. Jurnal Teknologi 77(5), 1–12 (2014)
17. Wazwaz, A.M., El-Sayed, S.M.: A new modification of the Adomian decomposition method for linear and nonlinear operators. Appl. Math. Comput. 122, 393–405 (2001)

# Exponential Stability of Discrete Impulsive Switched Singular Systems with Time Delay

Humeyra Kiyak, Mohamad S. Alwan and Xinzhi Liu

**Abstract** This paper addresses the exponential stability problem for discrete impulsive switched singular systems with time delay where the impulsive effects occur as a result of switching among the subsystems. Some sufficient conditions on the exponential stability of the system are established. The stability conditions are investigated by using the multiple Lyapunov functions along with the average dwell time switching signal and by resorting the Halanay lemma. Finally, numerical examples with simulations are provided.

**Keywords** Discrete singular systems · Impulsive systems · Switched systems
Time delay · Exponential stability · Average dwell time

## 1 Introduction

Singular systems are also referred to as descriptor systems or differential algebraic systems whose behaviours are described by differential equations (or difference equations) and algebraic equations. Readers may refer to [1, 2].

Time delay inevitably exists in various engineering systems and is the main source for causing instability and poor performance of dynamical systems. As a special class of time delay systems, singular time delay systems have attracted much attention from the mathematics and control community (see [3–5]).

In addition, physical systems can be characterized by the fact that they exhibit switching from one operating mode to another at a certain moment of time. Such systems are modeled as switched systems consisting of multi-dynamical subsystems

H. Kiyak · M. S. Alwan (✉) · X. Liu
University of Waterloo, Waterloo, Canada
e-mail: malwan@uwaterloo.ca

H. Kiyak
e-mail: hkiyak@uwaterloo.ca

X. Liu
e-mail: xinzhi.liu@uwaterloo.ca

© Springer Nature Switzerland AG 2018
D. M. Kilgour et al. (eds.), *Recent Advances in Mathematical and Statistical Methods*, Springer Proceedings in Mathematics & Statistics 259,
https://doi.org/10.1007/978-3-319-99719-3_18

and a switching signal to manage switching between subsystems. When subsystems of a switched system are singular systems, the switched system becomes a class of switched singular systems (SSS).

Impulsive systems are dynamical systems subject to sudden jumps or changes (often called impulses) in the system states at specific time moments. The presence of these impulses in the systems of differential equations results in different circumstances. For instance, they may destabilize some stable system (i.e., considered as a perturbation), they may stabilize some other unstable systems (i.e., play as a stabilizing role for the system and the system, in this case, might be called "impulsive control system"), or they may violate some fundamental features of the system, such as existence of a global unique solution, and vice versa. On the other hand, impulses may arise as a result of mode (or subsystem) switching. For these reasons, the study of impulsive control systems have become very important. The coexistence of "mode switching" and "impulsive effects" in one system leads to *impulsive switched systems*. In this paper, we consider impulsive switched singular systems (ISSS); that is, the system modes are considered to be singular systems. Readers may refer to [6–9] for further study of the system.

Stability analysis of linear discrete impulse-free SSS has been investigated in [10–12]. Particularly, in [10] the stability result was established for systems switch among all stable modes, where the matrices of the system modes are required to satisfy the matrix commutative property. The latter condition, in fact, is very restrictive from practical, theoretical perspectives. In [11], a time delay was considered in the system states where the method of Lyapunov functional was used to study the stability property. In this work, we consider time-delayed ISSS consisting of stable and unstable modes subject to nonlinear perturbing terms. To investigate the stability property, we apply the Halanay lemma to obtain the decay rates of the stable modes, and, as for the unstable ones, we have developed a new result that enables us to calculate the growth rates. Also, we use the methodology of multiple Lyapunov functions along with the average dwell-time (ADT) switching signal. The ADT has the role of switching among the system modes and it has been proven to be more practical and efficient in analyzing the stability property.

The rest of the paper is organized as follows: In Sect. 2, the problem formulation and some preliminaries are introduced. In Sect. 3, we state and prove the main theorems. Numerical examples are presented in Sect. 4 to clarify the proposed approach. Finally, a conclusion is given in Sect. 5.

## 2 Problem Formulation and Preliminaries

Let $\mathbb{R}^N$ be the $N$-dimensional real space, $\mathbb{R}^{N \times N}$ denote the set of all $N \times N$ square matrices, $\mathbb{C}$ the complex numbers, $\mathbb{Z}^+$ the positive integers, $\mathbb{N}$ the natural numbers, and for some positive integer $d$, let $\mathbb{N}_{-d} = \{-d, -d+1, \ldots, -1, 0\}$. Let $C = \{\phi : \mathbb{N}_{-d} \to \mathbb{R}^N\}$. Let $\| \cdot \|$ be the Euclidean norm. The Euclidean norm of $x \in \mathbb{R}^N$ is $\|x\| = \sqrt{x^T x}$. For any $\phi \in C$, we define $\|\phi\|_d = \max_{\theta \in \mathbb{N}_{-d}}\{\|\phi(\theta)\|\}$. Consider the impulsive switching singular discrete system with time delay:

$$E_{\sigma(n)} x(n+1) = A_{\sigma(n)} x(n) + f_{\sigma(n)}(n, x(n-d)), \qquad n_{k-1}^+ < n \le n_k$$
$$\Delta x(n) = B_k x(n), \qquad\qquad\qquad n = n_k, \quad k \in \mathbb{N} \qquad (1)$$
$$x_{n_0^+} = \phi,$$

where $x \in \mathbb{R}^N$, $n_0 \in \mathbb{Z}^+$, $f_{\sigma(n)}(n, x(n-d)) : \mathbb{Z}^+ \times \mathbb{R}^N \to \mathbb{R}^N$, $\phi \in C$ and $x_{n_0} \in C$ is defined by $x_{n_0}(s) = x(n_0 + s)$ for any $s \in \mathbb{N}_{-d}$ with $d \in \mathbb{N}$ representing the delay in system (1). $A_{\sigma(n)}, B_k, E_{\sigma(n)} \in \mathbb{R}^{N \times N}$ are system coefficient matrices where $E_{\sigma(n)}$ being singular with $\text{rank}(E_{\sigma(n)}) = r < N$, $A_{\sigma(n)}$ being invertible, and $B_k$ being constant matrices. $\sigma(n) : \mathbb{N} \to \mathscr{S}$ is a switching rule taking values $\sigma(n) = i$ in a finite compact set $\mathscr{S} = \{1, 2, \ldots, M\}$ for some $M \in \mathbb{N}$. $\{n_k\}_{k=0}^\infty$ are the impulsive times that form an increasing sequence satisfying $n_{k-1} < n_k$ and $\lim_{k \to \infty} n_k = \infty$. $\Delta x(n_k) = x(n_k^+) - x(n_k)$ where $x(n_k^+)$ is the value of $x$ at $n_k$ with impulse, and $x(n_k)$ is the value of $x$ at $n_k$ without impulse. We assume $f_{\sigma(n)}(n, 0) \equiv 0$ and for all $(n, x), (n, x^*) \in \mathbb{Z}^+ \times \mathbb{R}^N$

$$\| f_{\sigma(n)}(n, x) - f_{\sigma(n)}(n, x^*) \| \le \| F_{\sigma(n)}(x - x^*) \| \qquad (2)$$

where $F_{\sigma(n)}$ are constant matrices with appropriate dimension.

**Assumption 1** Suppose that the matrix pairs $(E_i, A_i)$ for any $i \in \mathscr{S}$ are regular.

**Definition 1** The solution of system (1) is said to be exponentially stable if for any initial condition $x_{n_0^+}(s) = \phi(s)$ for $s \in \mathbb{N}_{-d}$ there exist constants $0 < \varepsilon < 1$ and $M \ge 1$ such that $\| x(n; n_0, \phi) \| \le M \| E\phi \|_d \varepsilon^{n-n_0}$ for any $n \ge n_0$.

**Definition 2** ([1, 6]) Matrix pair $(E_i, A_i)$ for any $i \in \mathscr{S}$ is *regular* if there exists a constant scalar $\gamma \in \mathbb{C}$ such that $\det(\gamma E_i - A_i) \ne 0$. The matrix pair $(E_i, A_i)$ is said to be *impulse free* if $\deg(\det(\gamma E_i - A_i)) = \text{rank}(E_i)$.

**Definition 3** ([1, 6]) System (1) is admissible if it is stable and impulse-free.

**Lemma 1** ([1, 6]) *If for any $i \in \mathscr{S}$ the matrix pairs $(E_i, A_i)$ in system (1) are regular and impulse free, then there exist nonsingular matrices $\tilde{Q}_i, \tilde{P}_i$ such that $\tilde{Q}_i = \begin{bmatrix} \tilde{Q}_i^1 \\ \tilde{Q}_i^2 \end{bmatrix}$ and $\tilde{P}_i = \begin{bmatrix} \tilde{P}_i^1 & \tilde{P}_i^2 \end{bmatrix}$ where $\tilde{Q}_i^1 \in \mathbb{R}^{r \times N}$, $\tilde{Q}_i^2 \in \mathbb{R}^{(N-r) \times N}$, $\tilde{P}_i^1 \in \mathbb{R}^{N \times r}$, $\tilde{P}_i^2 \in \mathbb{R}^{N \times (N-r)}$ and the following standard decomposition holds: $\tilde{Q}_i E_i \tilde{P}_i = \text{diag}(I_r, 0)$, $\tilde{Q}_i A_i \tilde{P}_i = \text{diag}(A_{1_i}, I_{N-r})$, $\tilde{Q}_i f_i(n, x_n) = \begin{bmatrix} \tilde{Q}_i^1 f_i(n, x_n) \\ \tilde{Q}_i^2 f_i(n, x_n) \end{bmatrix}$, and $\tilde{P}_i^{-1} x(n) = \begin{bmatrix} x_1(n) \\ x_2(n) \end{bmatrix}$, where $r = \text{rank}(E_i)$, $A_{1_i} \in \mathbb{R}^{r \times r}$, $x_1 \in \mathbb{R}^r$, and $x_2 \in \mathbb{R}^{N-r}$.*

**Lemma 2** (Discrete Halanay) ([13]) *Let $d > 0$ be a natural number, and $\{x_n\}_{n \ge -d}$ be a sequence of real numbers satisfying the inequality $\Delta x_n \le -a x_n + b \max\{x_n, x_{n-1}, \ldots, x_{n-d}\}$, $n \ge 0$, where $\Delta x_n = x_{n+1} - x_n$. If $0 < b < a \le 1$, then there exists a constant $\lambda_0 \in (0, 1)$ such that $x_n \le \max\{0, x_0, x_{-1}, \ldots, x_{-d}\} \lambda_0^n$, $n \ge 0$. Moreover,*

$\lambda_0$ can be chosen as the smallest root in the interval $(0, 1)$ of the equation $\lambda^{d+1} + (a - 1)\lambda^d - b = 0$.

Since we consider unstable modes in this paper, we have developed the following lemma which enables us to evaluate the growth rate of the unstable modes.

**Lemma 3** *Let $d > 0$ be a natural number, and $\{x_n\}_{n \geq -d}$ be a sequence of positive real numbers satisfying the inequality $\triangle x(n) \leq ax(n) + b \max_{s \in \mathbb{N}_{-d}}\{x(n + s)\}, n \geq n_0$, where $\triangle x(n) = x(n + 1) - x(n)$. Assume that $0 < a$ and $0 < b$, then there exists a constant $\lambda_0 \geq 1$ such that $x(n) \leq \max_{s \in \mathbb{N}_{-d}}\{x(n_0 + s)\}\lambda_0^{n-n_0}$, where $\lambda_0 = a + b + 1$.*

*Proof* Consider

$$\triangle y(n) = ay(n) + b \max_{s \in \mathbb{N}_{-d}}\{y(n + s)\}, \quad n \geq n_0 \tag{3}$$

with the initial condition $y(n) = x(n)$, for all $n \in \{n_0 - d, \ldots, n_0 - 1, n_0\}$. Since $a > 0$ and $b > 0$ in difference equation (3), $y(n)$ is increasing. Thus, $\max_{s \in \mathbb{N}_{-d}}\{y(n + s)\} = y(n)$ for all $n \geq n_0$. As a result, equation (3) becomes $\triangle y(n) = (a + b)y(n)$, where $\triangle y(n) = y(n + 1) - y(n)$. Thus, the solution of this delay difference equation is $y(n) = (a + b + 1)^{n-n_0} \max_{s \in \mathbb{N}_{-d}}\{y(n_0 + s)\}, \quad n \geq n_0$. Claim that $x(n) \leq y(n)$ for all $n \geq n_0$. If this were not true, there would exist $n^*$ such that $x(n^* + 1) > y(n^* + 1)$ and $x(n) \leq y(n)$ for all $n_0 \leq n \leq n^*$. Thus, $\triangle y(n^*) < \triangle x(n^*) \leq ay(n^*) + b \max_{s \in \mathbb{N}_{-d}}\{y(n^* + s)\}$. That is, $\triangle y(n^*) < ay(n^*) + b \max_{s \in \mathbb{N}_{-d}}\{y(n^* + s)\}$ which contradicts with equation (3). That means the claim $x(n) \leq y(n)$ for all $n \geq n_0$ is correct. In other words, we obtain that $x(n) \leq (a + b + 1)^{n-n_0} \max_{s \in \mathbb{N}_{-d}}\{y(n_0 + s)\}, \quad n \geq n_0$. By using the initial condition, we conclude the solution of delay difference equation as $x(n) \leq (a + b + 1)^{n-n_0} \max_{s \in \mathbb{N}_{-d}}\{x(n_0 + s)\}$ for all $n \geq n_0$.

## 3 Main Results

**Theorem 1** *For any $i \in \mathscr{S}$, assume that each subsystem of (1) is admissible. Then, the trivial solution of (1) is exponentially stable if the following assumptions hold:*

(i)   *For any $i, j \in \mathscr{S}$ there exists $\gamma_k > 1$ ($k \in \mathbb{N}$) such that*

$$(I + B_k)^T E_j^T X_j E_j (I + B_k) \leq \gamma_k E_i^T X_i E_i, \tag{4}$$

   *where $X_i > 0$ satisfying the Lyapunov equation $A_i^T X_i A_i - E_i^T X_i E_i = -Y_i$, for any $Y_i > 0$.*

(ii)   *For any $n_0$, the switching law satisfies ADT which is $N(n_0, n) \leq N_0 + \frac{n-n_0}{T_a}$ where $N(n_0, n)$ denotes the number of switchings in $(n_0, n)$, $T_a$ is the average dwell time and $N_0$ is the chatter bound.*

*Proof* Let $x(n) = x(n; n_0, \phi)$ be the solution of the system (1). For $n \in (n_{k-1}, n_k]$, define $V_i(x(n)) = x^T(n)E_i^T X_i E_i x(n)$, $i = \sigma(n)$ as a Lyapunov function candidate for the $i$th subsystem. Thus, the variation of $V_i$ relative to system (1) is

$$\Delta V_i(x(n)) = -x^T(n)Y_i x(n) + 2f_i^T(n, x(n-d))X_i A_i x(n)$$
$$+ f_i^T(n, x(n-d))X_i f_i(n, x(n-d))$$

where $-Y_i = A_i^T X_i A_i - E_i^T X_i E_i$ for any $Y_i > 0$ since each subsystem of (1) is stable. Using Lipschitz condition (2), we obtain that

$$2f_i^T(n, x(n-d))X_i A_i x(n) \leq \frac{1}{\varepsilon_i}\|F_i x(n-d)\|^2 + \varepsilon_i\|A_i x(n)\|^2 \lambda_{max}(X_i^2), \text{ and}$$
$$f_i^T(n, x(n-d))X_i f_i(n, x(n-d)) \leq \lambda_{max}(X_i)\|F_i x(n-d)\|^2.$$

Thus, we obtain

$$\Delta V_i(x(n)) \leq \left[-\lambda_{min}(Y_i) + \varepsilon_i\|A_i\|^2 \lambda_{max}(X_i^2)\right]\|x(n)\|^2$$
$$+ \left[\frac{1}{\varepsilon_i} + \lambda_{max}(X_i)\right]\|G_i\|^2\|E_i x_n\|_d^2 \leq -\alpha_i V_i(x(n)) + \beta_i \max_{s \in \mathbb{N}_{-d}} V_i(x(n+s))$$

$$(5)$$

where $\alpha_i = \frac{\lambda_{min}(Y_i) - \varepsilon_i\|A_i\|^2 \lambda_{max}(X_i^2)}{\lambda_{max}(E_i^T X_i E_i)} > 0$, $\beta_i = \frac{[1+\varepsilon_i\lambda_{max}(X_i)]\|G_i\|^2}{\varepsilon_i\lambda_{min}(X_i)} > 0$, and $F_i = G_i E_i$ such that $Ex(n+s) \neq 0$ for $s \in \mathbb{N}_{-d}$. By Lemma 2 we obtain the solution of (5) for $n \in (n_{k-1}^+, n_k]$ as

$$V_i(x(n)) \leq \max_{\theta \in \mathbb{N}_{-d}}\{V_i(x(n_{k-1}^+ + \theta))\}\lambda_{0_i}^{(n-n_{k-1})} \qquad (6)$$

where $\lambda_{0_i}$ is the smallest root in the interval $(0, 1)$ of the equation $\lambda^{d+1} + (\alpha_i - 1)\lambda^d - \beta_i = 0$. On the other hand, for $n = n_k$, $k = 1, 2, \ldots$, suppose $\sigma(n_k) = j$, it follows from (1) and (4) that

$$V_j(x(n_k^+)) = x^T(n_k)(I + B_k)^T E_j^T X_j E_j(I + B_k)x(n_k) \leq \gamma_k V_i(x(n_k)). \quad (7)$$

Using (6) and (7) successively on each subinterval leads to the following general result for $n \in (n_{k-1}^+, n_k]$:

$$V_{i_k}(x(n)) \leq \gamma_1\gamma_2\ldots\gamma_{k-1}\max_{\theta \in \mathbb{N}_{-d}}\{V_{i_1}(x(n_0^+ + \theta))\}\lambda_{0_{i_1}}^{(n_1-d-n_0)}\lambda_{0_{i_2}}^{(n_2-d-n_1)}\ldots\lambda_{0_{i_k}}^{(n-n_{k-1})}.$$

Let $\lambda = \max\{\lambda_{0_{i_j}}, i \in \mathbb{N}, j = 1, 2, \ldots, k\}$, so the last inequality becomes

$$V_{i_k}(x(n)) \leq \gamma_1\lambda_{0_{i_1}}^{-d}\gamma_2\lambda_{0_{i_2}}^{-d}\ldots\gamma_{k-1}\lambda_{0_{i_{k-1}}}^{-d}\max_{\theta \in \mathbb{N}_{-d}}\{V_{i_1}(x(n_0^+ + \theta))\}\lambda^{(n-n_0)}. \qquad (8)$$

Let $\gamma = \max\{\gamma_i,\ i = 1, 2, \ldots, k-1\}$ and $\tilde{\lambda} = \min\{\lambda_{0_{i_j}},\ i \in \mathbb{N},\ j = 1, 2, \ldots, k-1\}$, so by (8) we obtain

$$V_{i_k}(x(n)) \le \lambda^{(n-n_0)\left[\frac{(k-1)\ln\mu}{(n-n_0)\ln\lambda}+1\right]} \max_{\theta\in\mathbb{N}_{-d}}\{V_{i_1}(x(n_0^+ + \theta))\} \text{ where } \mu = \gamma\tilde{\lambda}^{-d}. \quad (9)$$

For simplicity, if we choose $N_0 = 0$ in assumption (ii), then we obtain $\frac{N(n_0,n)}{n-n_0} \le \frac{1}{T_a}$ where $N(n_0, n) = k - 1$. Thus, using this we can write down inequality (9) as

$$V_{i_k}(x(n)) \le \lambda^{\rho(n-n_0)} \max_{\theta\in\mathbb{N}_{-d}}\{V_{i_1}(x(n_0^+ + \theta))\} \text{ where } \rho = \frac{\ln\mu}{T_a\ln\lambda} + 1 > 0. \quad (10)$$

Let

$$\tilde{P}_i^{-1}x(n) = \begin{bmatrix} x_1(n) \\ x_2(n) \end{bmatrix}, \text{ and } \tilde{Q}_i^{-T}X_i\tilde{Q}_i^{-1} = \begin{bmatrix} X_{1i} & X_{2i} \\ X_{2i}^T & X_{3i} \end{bmatrix} \quad (11)$$

where $x_1(n)$ and $x_2(n)$ are called slow and fast sub-state of system (1), respectively. Then, it follows from the standard decomposition form system (1) is equivalent to

$$x_1(n+1) = A_{1_i}x_1(n) + \tilde{Q}_i^1 f_i(n, x(n-d)) \quad (12)$$

$$0 = x_2(n) + \tilde{Q}_i^2 f_i(n, x(n-d)) \quad (13)$$

where $i = 1, 2, \ldots, M$, $x_1 \in \mathbb{R}^r$, $x_2 \in \mathbb{R}^{N-r}$, $\tilde{Q}_i = \begin{bmatrix} \tilde{Q}_i^1 & \tilde{Q}_i^2 \end{bmatrix}^T$, $\tilde{Q}_i^1 \in \mathbb{R}^{r\times N}$, $\tilde{Q}_i^2 \in \mathbb{R}^{(N-r)\times N}$, $\tilde{P}_i = \begin{bmatrix} \tilde{P}_i^1 & \tilde{P}_i^2 \end{bmatrix}$, $\tilde{P}_i^1 \in \mathbb{R}^{N\times r}$, and $\tilde{P}_i^2 \in \mathbb{R}^{N\times(N-r)}$.
Using the relationship (11), the Lyapunov function can be rewritten as

$$V_i(x(n)) = x_1^T(n)X_{1i}x_1(n) > 0, \quad \forall x_1(n) \ne 0. \quad (14)$$

Then, one can obtain from (10) by using (14) that

$$\|x_1(n)\| \le \sqrt{\frac{\lambda_{\max}(X_{i_1})}{\lambda_{\min}(X_{1i_k})}} \max_{\theta\in\mathbb{N}_{-d}}\{\|E_i x(n_0^+ + \theta)\|\}\lambda^{\rho(n-n_0)/2}, \quad n \ge n_0$$

which shows $x_1$ is exponentially stable. We need to show that $x_2$ is also exponentially stable. It follows from the Lipschitz condition (2) and (13) that

$$\|x_2(n)\| \le \frac{\|\tilde{Q}_i^2\|\|F_i\tilde{P}_i^1\|}{1 - \|\tilde{Q}_i^2\|\|F_i\tilde{P}_i^2\|}\sqrt{\frac{\lambda_{\max}(X_{i_1})}{\lambda_{\min}(X_{1i_k})}} \max_{\theta\in\mathbb{N}_{-d}}\{\|E_i x(n_0^+ + \theta)\|\}\lambda^{\rho(n-d-n_0)/2}$$

where $1 > \|\tilde{Q}_i^2\|\|F_i\tilde{P}_i^2\|$. Thus, the entire system is exponentially stable.

**Theorem 2** *For any $i \in \mathcal{S} = \mathcal{S}_{\mathcal{U}} \cup \mathcal{S}_{\mathcal{S}}$, where $\mathcal{S}_{\mathcal{U}}$ and $\mathcal{S}_{\mathcal{S}}$ represent the index sets of unstable and stable subsystems, respectively, assume that each subsystem* *of (1) is impulse free. Then, the trivial solution of (1) is exponentially stable if the following assumptions hold:*

*(A1)  For any $i, j \in \mathscr{S}$ there exists $\gamma_k > 1$ $(k \in \mathbb{N})$ such that*

$$(I + B_k)^T E_j^T X_j E_j (I + B_k) \leq \gamma_k E_i^T X_i E_i, \tag{15}$$

*where $X_i$ is positive definite matrix satisfying the Lyapunov equation $A_i^T X_i A_i - E_i^T X_i E_i = -Y_i$ for any $Y_i > 0$.*

*(A2)  Let $\lambda_+ = \max\{\lambda_{0_{ij}}^* : j = 1, 2, \ldots, l\}$, $\lambda_- = \max\{\lambda_{0_{ip}} : p = l+1, l+2, \ldots, k\}$ where $\lambda_{0_{ij}}^* = \alpha_i^* + \beta_i^* + 1$ with $\alpha_i^*, \beta_i^*$ are positive numbers defined later in the proof, and $\lambda_{0_{ip}}$ is the smallest root in the interval $(0, 1)$ of the equation $\lambda^{d+1} + (\alpha_i - 1)\lambda^d - \beta_i = 0$ with $\alpha_i, \beta_i$ are positive numbers defined later in the proof as well. Let also $T^+(n_0, n)$ be the total activation time of unstable modes, $T^-(n_0, n)$ be the total activation time of stable modes, and for any $n_0$, assume that the switching law guarantees that $\dfrac{T^-(n_0, n)}{T^+(n_0, n)} > \dfrac{\ln \lambda_+ - \ln \lambda_*}{\ln \lambda_* - \ln \lambda_-}$ where $0 < \lambda_- < \lambda_* < 1$. Furthermore, for any $n_0$, the switching law satisfies the ADT condition.*

*Proof* Let $x(n) = x(n; n_0, \phi)$ be the solution of the system (1). Similar to the proof of Theorem 1, the variation of Lyapunov function candidate for ith subsystem $V_i$ relative to system (1) is obtained as

$$\triangle V_i(x(n)) = x^T(n)\left[A_i^T X_i A_i - E_i^T X_i E_i\right]x(n) + 2f_i^T(n, x(n-d))X_i A_i x(n)$$
$$+ f_i^T(n, x(n-d))X_i f_i(n, x(n-d)) \tag{16}$$

In the proof of Theorem 1, we already obtain the variation of $V_i$ for $i \in \mathscr{S}_S$ as

$$\triangle V_i(x(n)) \leq -\alpha_i V_i(x(n)) + \beta_i \max_{s \in \mathbb{N}_{-d}} V_i(x(n+s)) \tag{17}$$

where $\alpha_i = \dfrac{\lambda_{min}(Y_i) - \varepsilon_i \|A_i\|^2 \lambda_{max}(X_i^2)}{\lambda_{max}(E_i^T X_i E_i)} > 0$, $\beta_i = \dfrac{[1 + \varepsilon_i \lambda_{max}(X_i)]\|G_i\|^2}{\varepsilon_i \lambda_{min}(X_i)} > 0$ and $F_i = G_i E_i$ such that $Ex(n+s) \neq 0$ for $s \in \mathbb{N}_{-d}$, and the solution of (17) for $n \in (n_{k-1}^+, n_k]$ as

$$V_i(x(n)) \leq \max_{s \in \mathbb{N}_{-d}} \{V_i(x(n_{k-1}^+ + s))\}\lambda_{0_i}^{(n-n_{k-1})}, \tag{18}$$

where $\lambda_{0_i}$ is the smallest root in the interval $(0, 1)$ of the equation $\lambda^{d+1} + (\alpha_i - 1)\lambda^d - \beta_i = 0$.

Let $\delta_i$ $(i \in \mathscr{S}_u)$ be a positive constant such that all eigenvalues of the matrix pairs $(E_i + \delta_i E_i, A_i)$ are located in the unit circle. Then, for each $Y_i > 0$ there exists $X_i > 0$ satisfying $A_i^T X_i A_i - (E_i + \delta_i E_i)^T X_i(E_i + \delta_i E_i) = -Y_i$. Plugging this equation into (16) we obtain

$$\Delta V_i(x(n)) \leq x^T(n)\left[-Y_i + \delta_i^2 E_i^T X_i E_i + 2\delta_i E_i^T X_i E_i\right]x(n)$$
$$+ 2f_i^T(n, x(n-d))X_i A_i x(n) + f_i^T(n, x(n-d))X_i f_i(n, x(n-d)). \tag{19}$$

Following the similar steps in stable subsystems case, for any $\varepsilon_i > 0$ and $\zeta_i > 0$, inequality (19) becomes

$$\Delta V_i(x(n)) \leq \alpha_i^* V_i(x(n)) + \beta_i^* \max_{s\in\mathbb{N}_{-d}} V_i(x(n+s)) \tag{20}$$

where $\alpha_i^* = \frac{-\lambda_{\min}(Y_i) + \varepsilon_i\|A_i\|^2\lambda_{\max}(X_i^2) + (\delta_i^2 + 2\delta_i)\lambda_{\max}(X_i)\|E_i\|^2}{\|E_i\|^2\lambda_{\min}(X_i)}$ and $\beta_i^* = \frac{[1 + \varepsilon_i\lambda_{\max}(X_i)]\|G_i\|^2}{\varepsilon_i\lambda_{\min}(X_i)}$. By Lemma 3 the solution of (20) is obtained for $n \in (n_{k-1}^+, n_k]$ as

$$V_i(x(n)) \leq \max_{s\in\mathbb{N}_{-d}}\{V_i(x(n_{k-1}^+ + s))\}\lambda_{0_i}^{*(n-n_{k-1})}, \quad \text{where } \lambda_{0_i}^* = \alpha_i^* + \beta_i^* + 1. \tag{21}$$

On the other hand, we have

$$V_j(x(n_k^+)) \leq \gamma_k V_i(x(n_k)). \tag{22}$$

Using (18) and (22) successively on each subinterval leads to the following general result for $n \in (n_{k-1}^+, n_k]$, $V_{i_k}(x(n)) \leq \gamma_1\gamma_2\ldots\gamma_{k-1}\max_{\theta\in\mathbb{N}_{-d}}\{V_{i_1}(x(n_0^+ + \theta))\}$
$\lambda_{0_{i_1}}^{(n_1-d-n_0)}\lambda_{0_{i_2}}^{(n_2-d-n_1)}\ldots\lambda_{0_{i_k}}^{(n-n_{k-1})}$.
Now, using (21) and (22) successively on each subinterval we obtain the general result for $n \in (n_{k-1}^+, n_k]$, $V_{i_k}(x(n)) \leq \gamma_1\gamma_2\ldots\gamma_{k-1}\max_{s\in\mathbb{N}_{-d}}\{V_{i_1}(x(n_0^+ + s))\}\lambda_{0_{i_1}}^{*(n_1-n_0)}$
$\lambda_{0_{i_2}}^{*(n_2-n_1)}\ldots\lambda_{0_{i_k}}^{*(n-n_{k-1})}$.
To obtain a general estimate, let us run $l$ unstable modes and switch $l$ times from an unstable mode, and run $m - l$ stable modes and switch $m - l - 1$ times from a stable mode. Then, for $n \in (n_{k-1}, n_k]$, $V_{m_k}(n) \leq \prod_{j=1}^{l}\gamma_j\lambda_{0_{m_j}}^{*(n_j-n_{j-1})} \times \prod_{p=l+1}^{m-1}\gamma_p\lambda_{0_{m_p}}^{-d}\lambda_{0_{m_p}}^{(n_p-n_{p-1})}$
$\times \max_{s\in\mathbb{N}_{-d}}\{V_{m_1}(x(n_0^+ + s))\}\lambda_{0_{m_k}}^{(n-n_{m-1})}$. Let $\lambda_+ = \max\{\lambda_{0_{i_j}}^* : j = 1, 2, \ldots, l\}$, $\lambda_- = \max\{\lambda_{0_{i_p}} : p = l + 1, l + 2, \ldots, k\}$ and denote by $T^+(n_0, n)$ and $T^-(n_0, n)$ the total activation time of unstable and stable modes, respectively. Then, for $n \in (n_{k-1}, n_k]$, we have $V_{m_k}(n) \leq \prod_{j=1}^{l}\gamma_j\lambda_+^{T^+} \times \prod_{p=l+1}^{m-1}\gamma_p\lambda_{0_{m_p}}^{-d}\lambda_-^{T^-} \times \max_{s\in\mathbb{N}_{-d}}\{V_{m_1}(x(n_0^+ + s))\}$. Choose $\lambda_*$ such that $0 < \lambda_- < \lambda_* < 1$, and assume that the switching law satisfies (A2), then we obtain

$$V_{m_k}(n) \le \lambda_*^{(n-n_0)\left[\frac{(m-1)\ln \mu}{(n-n_0)\ln \lambda_*}+1\right]} \max_{\theta \in \mathbb{N}_{-d}} \{V_{m_1}(x(n_0^+ + \theta))\} \qquad (23)$$

where $\mu = \gamma \tilde{\lambda}^{-d}$, $\gamma = \max\{\gamma_p, \ p = 1, 2, \ldots, m-1\}$, and $\tilde{\lambda} = \min\{\lambda_{0_{m_p}}, \ m \in \mathbb{N}, \ p = 1, 2, \ldots, m-1\}$. By following the same ADT concept as in Theorem 1, we can write down inequality (9) as

$$V_{m_k}(x(n)) \le \lambda_*^{\rho(n-n_0)} \max_{\theta \in \mathbb{N}_{-d}} \{V_{m_1}(x(n_0^+ + \theta))\} \text{ where } \rho = \frac{\ln \mu}{T_a \ln \lambda_*} + 1 > 0. \quad (24)$$

By using decomposition of the system (1), we can similarly obtain following inequalities which show the sub-states $x_1$ and $x_2$ are exponentially stable

$$\|x_1(n)\| \le \sqrt{\frac{\lambda_{\max}(X_{m_1})}{\lambda_{\min}(X_{1m_k})}} \max_{\theta \in \mathbb{N}_{-d}} \{\|E_m x(n_0^+ + \theta)\|\} \lambda_*^{\rho(n-n_0)/2},$$

$$\|x_2(n)\| \le \frac{\|Q_m^2\| \|F_m \tilde{P}_m^1\|}{1 - \|Q_m^2\| \|F_m \tilde{P}_m^2\|} \sqrt{\frac{\lambda_{\max}(X_{m_1})}{\lambda_{\min}(X_{1m_k})}} \max_{\theta \in \mathbb{N}_{-d}} \{\|E_m x(n_0^+ + \theta)\|\} \lambda_*^{\rho(n-d-n_0)/2}.$$

## 4 Numerical Examples

*Example 1* Consider the discrete ISSSD given by (1) where $x = \begin{bmatrix} x_1(n) \ x_2(n) \ x_3(n) \end{bmatrix}^T$,

$\sigma(n) \in \mathscr{S} = \{1, 2\}, E_1 = E_2 = \begin{bmatrix} 1 & 0 & 0 \\ 0 & 1 & 0 \\ 0 & 0 & 0 \end{bmatrix}, B_k = 1.005I, A_1 = \begin{bmatrix} -1.1 & 0.2 & 0.1 \\ -0.3 & -2.3 & 0 \\ -0.5 & 1 & 1 \end{bmatrix},$

$f_1(n, x(n-1)) = \begin{bmatrix} \frac{1}{10} \tanh(x_1(n-1)) & \frac{1}{10} \tanh(x_2(n-1)) \end{bmatrix}^T,$     $A_2 =$

$\begin{bmatrix} 1 & -0.1 & 0 \\ 0.2 & 0.6 & 0 \\ 0.05 & 0.01 & -1 \end{bmatrix}$  $f_2(n, x(n-1)) = \begin{bmatrix} \frac{1}{15} \tanh(x_1(n-1)) & \frac{1}{15} \tanh(x_2(n-1)) \end{bmatrix}^T.$

The initial function is given by $\phi(n) = [5 - n \ \ 4 + n \ \ 2 + n]^T$. The Lipschitz condition (2) is satisfied with $F_1 = \frac{1}{10}I$ in stable subsystem 1 and $F_2 = \frac{1}{15}I$ in unstable

subsystem 2. $X_1 = \begin{bmatrix} 14.2547 & -2.7361 & 0 \\ -2.7361 & 2.2984 & 0 \\ 0 & 0 & 1 \end{bmatrix} > 0$ satisfies $A_1^T X_1 A_1 - E_1^T X_1 E_1 =$

$-Y_1 \quad$ for $\quad Y_1 = \begin{bmatrix} -1.6445 & 6.0722 & 1.9859 \\ 6.0722 & -13.9475 & -1.9144 \\ 1.9859 & -1.9144 & -1.1425 \end{bmatrix}.$ $\quad$ Similarly, $\quad X_2 =$

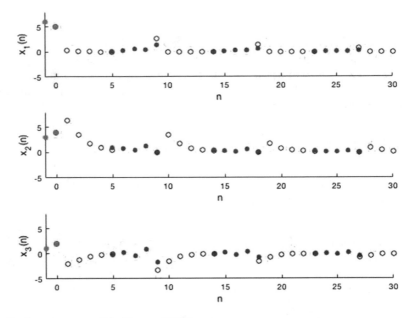

**Fig. 1** State responses of the discrete ISSSD

$$\begin{bmatrix} 1.0503 & -0.0932 & 0 \\ -0.0932 & 1.1942 & 0 \\ 0 & 0 & 1 \end{bmatrix} > 0 \quad \text{satisfying} \quad (A_2 - E_2)^T X_2 (A_2 - E_2) - E_2^T X_2 E_2 =$$

$-Y_2$ for any $Y_2 = \begin{bmatrix} -0.013 & -0.0779 & 0.05 \\ -0.0779 & 0.7425 & 0.01 \\ 0.05 & 0.01 & -1 \end{bmatrix}$. Thus, we compute that $\alpha_1 = 0.8666$,

$\beta_1 = 0.3485$, $\alpha_1^* = 2.0886$ and $\beta_1^* = 0.9995$. By Lemmas 2 and 3, we computed $\lambda_{0_1} = 0.6608$ and $\lambda_{0_1}^* = 4.0881$. Also, $\gamma_k = 4.0200$ so that the inequality $(I + B_k)^T E^T X_j E (I + B_k) \le \gamma_k E^T X_i E$ is satisfied. Thus, the system is exponentially stable under ADT switching with $T_a > 4.3592$ seconds. The simulation is shown in Fig. 1.

## 5 Conclusion

We discussed discrete ISSSD in two mode cases; in the first case, the switching occurs between all stable modes, while in the second case, the system consists of stable and unstable modes. The focus is on establishing the problems of stability of these systems by designing switching laws to organize the switching among either all stable or a mix of stable and unstable subsystems. In the stability analysis, we considered ADT approach together with the technique of multiple Lyapunov functions.

# References

1. Duan, G.: Analysis and Design of Descriptor Linear Systems. Springer, New York (2010)
2. Dai, L.: Singular Control Systems. Springer, Berlin (1989)
3. Halanay, A.: Differential Equations: Stability, Oscillations, Time Lags. Academic Press Inc., New York (1966)
4. Driver, R.D.: Ordinary and Delay Differential Equations. Springer, New York (1977)
5. Li, X., Cao, J.: An impulsive delay inequality involving unbounded time-varying delay and applications. IEEE Trans. Autom. Control **62**(7), 3618–3625 (2017)
6. Feng, G., Cao, J.: Stability analysis of impulsive switched singular systems. IET Control Theory Appl. **9**(6), 863–870 (2015)
7. Alwan, M.S., Kiyak, H., Liu, X.: Stability properties of switched singular systems subject to impulsive effects. In: Mathematical and Computational Approaches in Advancing Modern Science and Engineering. Springer International Publishing, pp. 355–365 (2016)
8. Yin, Y.J.: Stability of switched linear singular systems with impulsive effects. Elsevier Sci. **33**(4), 446–448 (2007)
9. Liu, Y.: The impulsive property of switched singular systems and its stability. In: Proceeding of the 7th World Congress on Intelligent Control and Automation, Changqing, China, pp. 6369–6372 (2008)
10. Zhai, G., Xu, X., Imae, J., Kobayashi, T.: Qualitative analysis of switched discrete-time descriptor systems. Int. J. Control Autom. Syst. **7**(4), 512–519 (2009)
11. Zhang, L., Zhao, J., Qi, X., Li, F.: Exponential stability for discrete-time singular switched time-delay systems with average dwell time. In: Proceedings of the 30th Chinese Control Conference, July 2011, pp. 1789–1794
12. Chen, Y., Fei, S., Zhang, K.: Stability analysis for discrete-time switched linear singular systems: average dwell time approach. IMA J. Math. Control Inf. **30**, 239–249 (2013)
13. Liz, E.: Stability of non-autonomous difference equations: simple ideas leading to useful results. J. Differ. Equ. Appl. **17**, 203–220 (2011)

# Experimental Investigation of ABB Effect on Unbalanced Rotor Vibration

**Michael Makram, Mohamed K. Khalil, Ahmed F. Nemnem and Guirguis Samer**

**Abstract** Rotor vibration due to unbalance causes a lot of problems during operation. Passive balancing devices represent one of the simplest ways to reduce rotor vibration. A $(2 + n)$ degrees of freedom mathematical model is derived with respect to a Cartesian co-ordinate system for the unbalanced rotor with the automatic ball balancer. The model equations are expressed as state equations then solved numerically. Experimental rig is developed with a data acquisition system to enable measuring the rotor vibration amplitudes. A four balls automatic ball balancer (ABB) is designed, manufactured, and attached to the rotor. The numerical solutions of rotor vibration with and without the balancer are obtained and compared to the measured data to validate the mathematical model. The applied effect of the automatic ball balancer on vibration amplitudes is presented at different speed ranges.

**Keywords** Rotor vibrations · Online balancing · Passive balancing
Automatic ball balancer · Dynamic balancer

## 1 Introduction

Rotors are commonly used in several systems including vehicle wheels, electrical motors, machine tools, turbo machinery, helicopter blades, and so on. Vibrations affects all these systems. Vibrations have many causes, but mass imbalance is still one of the primary sources of vibrations, which occurs when the principal inertia axis

M. Makram (✉) · M. K. Khalil · A. F. Nemnem · G. Samer
Military Technical College, Cairo, Egypt
e-mail: Michael@mtc.edu.eg

M. K. Khalil
e-mail: M_khalil@mtc.edu.eg

A. F. Nemnem
e-mail: Farid_nemnem@mtc.edu.eg

G. Samer
e-mail: Samer_guirguis_2000@yahoo.com

© Springer Nature Switzerland AG 2018
D. M. Kilgour et al. (eds.), *Recent Advances in Mathematical and Statistical Methods*, Springer Proceedings in Mathematics & Statistics 259,
https://doi.org/10.1007/978-3-319-99719-3_19

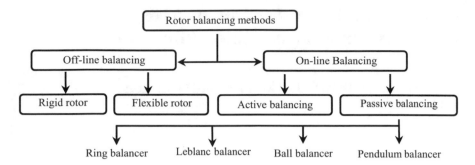

**Fig. 1** Balancing methods classification

of the rotor does not coincide with its rotational axis. An imbalance can arise through imperfections in the manufacturing process or resulting from wear, missing balance weights or damage. A heavy spot in a rotating component will cause vibration when the unbalanced weight rotates around the rotor axis, creating a centrifugal force. As rotor speed changes, the effects of imbalance may become higher. In some cases, imbalances can be factors in poor performance, high noise levels, reduced bearing life, and reduced human comfort.

Balancing techniques can be classified to two common balancing methods as shown in Fig. 1, one method is off-line balancing in which the rotating machine stops, and masses are redistributed. Where the second method is on-line balancing in which the mass distribution rearrangement occurs during rotation. On-line balancing method is more effective especially if balancing of machine components is usually needed to be done, or in case of difficult machine assembly and disassembly. There are two types of automatic balancers, active and passive. Active devices utilize computers and sensors which continuously read the vibrations, then apply control laws to counteract these vibrations. But its complexity, expensive cost and high weight reduce its usage in some applications. Where the passive balancers depend on the automatic balancing phenomenon of the free balancing masses without any interference. Simplicity, reliability, and relatively low cost of passive balancing systems make them a very attractive solution, and thus they have been significant subjects for past research.

Passive balancing techniques especially pendulum and ball automatic balancers have received a great deal of attention. Pendulum balancers tend to be costlier to construct than ball balancers, and the weight of the pendulums must be supported in special ways, which leads to additional mechanical complexity. The ball balancer is still more popular than the pendulum balancer and successfully applied to different fields. A traditional ball-type balancer is composed of several balls moving only in tangential direction along a fixed circular orbit. The ball balancer which was first designed in a detailed experimental study by Thearle [1] in 1932.

Thearle [2] also compared several different types of automatic dynamic balancers, such as a ring, pendulum and ball balancers and concluded that ball balancers were a superior system. Balancer applications include optical disc drives [3, 4], and rotary machinery. In 1998, Rajalingham [5] examining a vertical rotor with an ABB. A band of instability that decreased in size as the operating speed increased was showed. However, the unstable operation appeared at speeds below the critical speed of the rotor, the balancer was seen to improve rotor performance.

## 2  Mathematical Model

The rotor shaft system is considered as a 2 degree of freedom system taking in to consideration Jeffcott model assumptions. The model, as shown in Fig. 2, consists of: a vertical simply-supported massless flexible shaft, and a disk mounted at the mid span of the shaft rotating in a horizontal plane with a radial mass imbalance causing a shift between its geometry center and its center of gravity. The disk model has two-degrees of freedom, x and y, which are mutually orthogonal linear displacements in the same horizontal plane. The model is symmetric, having the same spring stiffness $k_x$, $k_y$ and damping coefficient ($c_x$, $c_y$) in both directions, and ideal friction bearing is assumed.

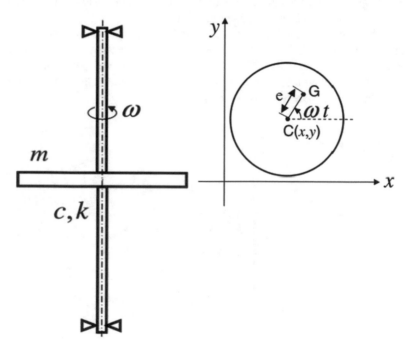

**Fig. 2**  Jeffcott model

The differential equations of motion:

$$m\ddot{x} + c\dot{x} + kx = -me\omega^2\cos(\omega t)$$
$$m\ddot{y} + c\dot{y} + ky = -me\omega^2\sin(\omega t) \tag{1}$$
$$C = C_x = C_y, k = k_x = k_y \tag{2}$$

The analytical solution of the radially unbalanced system is:

$$A(t) = \frac{\omega^2 e}{\sqrt{\left(\frac{k}{\omega} - \omega^2\right)^2 + \left(\frac{c\omega}{m}\right)^2}} \tag{3}$$

Each ball in the ABB reaches its own angular coordinate ($\theta$), and this coordinate is independent on the linear coordinates of the rotor. So that the rotor and the ABB can be modeled by a (2 + n) DOF system, where (n) is the number of balancing balls. An eccentric rotating disc is studied with an ABB consisting of several balls free to move in a race filled partially with a viscous fluid, and positioned at (a) fixed distance from the center of rotation of the disc. This set-up is shown schematically in Fig. 3. Point (G) represents the center of mass of the disc (without the balancing balls) and is located a distance (e) from the center of rotation (C).

The equations of motion of the proposed model are derived, where the assumption that all motion is confined to the two-dimensional plane. Also, it is assumed that no interactions between the balls. This assumption is valid provided the balls are in an equilibrium state. Note that neglecting impacts between the balls makes this study similar to that of an ABB with double ball races [9].

**Fig. 3** Schematic drawing of an ABB

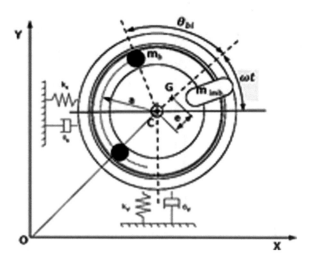

$$m\ddot{x} + c\dot{x} + kx = -me\omega^2\cos(\omega t)$$
$$- \sum_{n=1}^{i} m_{bn} a \left[ \theta_{bn} \sin(\omega t + \theta_{bn} + (\omega + \theta_{bn})^2 \cos(\omega t + \theta_{bn})) \right] \quad (4)$$

$$m\ddot{y} + c\dot{y} + ky = -me\omega^2\sin(\omega t)$$
$$- \sum_{n=1}^{i} m_{bn} a \left[ \ddot{\theta}_{bn} \cos(\omega t + \theta_{bn} + (\omega + \dot{\theta}_{bn})^2 \sin(\omega t + \theta_{bn})) \right] \quad (5)$$

$$m_{bn} a^2 \ddot{\theta}_{bn} + c_{bn} a^2 \dot{\theta}_{bn} = -m_{bn} a \left[ \ddot{x} \sin(\omega t + \theta) - \ddot{y} \cos(\omega t + \theta_{bn}) \right] \quad (6)$$

Equations (4) and (5) describe the horizontal and vertical displacements in the same plane. Equation (6) is the moment equation of ball about the center, and for more than one ball ABB this equation is repeated for each ball.

## 3 Numerical Solution

The state equations can be conveniently used in solving the model equations, and these equations are solved numerically using MATLAB software (ode-45). Let us rewrite the model equations in the form of state equations. To do this, it is necessary to denote new symbols as shown:
Let:

$$x_1 = x \qquad x_2 = y \qquad x_{2+i} = \theta_{bi} \ldots\ldots\ldots\ldots x_{2+n} = \theta_{bn}$$
$$x_{3+n} = \dot{x} \qquad x_{4+n} = \dot{y} \qquad x_{4+n+i} = \dot{\theta}_{bi} \ldots\ldots\ldots\ldots x_{4+2n} = \dot{\theta}_{bn} \quad (7)$$

The equations of motion can be expressed as the state equations which are $(2n + 4)$ first order differential equations. The state equations may be written in a matrix vector equation.

$$x = \dot{A}(x)x + B \quad (8)$$

$$x = \left[ x_1 x_2 x_{2+i} \ldots\ldots\ldots\ldots x_{2+n} x_{3+n} \ldots\ldots\ldots\ldots x_4 \right]$$
$$\dot{x}_{2n} = \left[ \dot{x}_1 \dot{x}_2 \dot{x}_{2+i} \ldots\ldots\ldots\ldots \dot{x}_{2+n} \dot{x}_{3+n} \ldots\ldots\ldots\ldots \dot{x}_{4+2n} \right]$$

$$A(x) = \begin{bmatrix} I & 0 \\ 0 & M \end{bmatrix} \quad (9)$$

where
I is (2 + n) (2 + n) identity matrix,
M is (2 + n) (2 + n) matrix determined from the above equations,
B is (4 + 2n) (4 + 2n) matrix determined from the model equations.

## 4 Experimental Investigation

### 4.1 Experimental Rig

Rotor Kit Tm620 is used after some modification to suit the aim of experiment as shown in Fig. 4. The rotor consists of an elastic 6 mm thick shaft of high-strength steel. One steel disc is clamped at mid span of the shaft. To prevent impermissibly high oscillation amplitudes which may lead to the rotor being destroyed, the mass discs are provided with safety bearings. The bearing gap is large enough that no contact takes place between the disc lug and the safety bearing during measuring rotor amplitudes. Angularly movable self-aligning ball bearing is used. The driven motor has sufficient power to be able to run through critical speeds quickly. The speed measurement takes place via an inductive sensor on the motor shaft. The speed is displayed digitally in the switchbox.

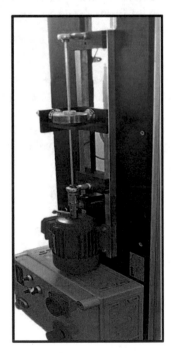

**Fig. 4** Rotor Kit

The rotor kit is modified to be used in investigating the effect of the ABB on unbalanced vertical rotor vibration, so that two main adaptations were needed, the first is to support the kit in vertical position in a safe way taking in to consideration the measurement accuracy. The totor kit is vertically supported on a test rig using four screw bolts with rubber spacers for vibration damping not to transfer the resulted vibration to the rig. And the second was a fixation of two orthogonal displacement sensors to enable the measurement of vibration amplitudes. A manufactured part is added to the kit to enable the clamping of two orthogonal displacement sensors as shown in Fig. 5, so that the vibration amplitude value can be measured.

A four balls ABB is designed and manufactured according to the rotor parameters. It is attached fine to the rotor with avoiding any relative rotation. ABB design enable the usage of balls of different diameters and masses. Also, the required imbalance mass can be clamped by two bolts as shown in Fig. 6.

A data acquisition system is built up to enable a simple way in vibration measurement; the system consists of: two inductive non-contact displacement sensors are connected to the sensor supply module TM 151 then to a module in the cDAQ-1988 then to PC via USB port. A simple program is resolved using LabVIEW software as shown in Fig. 7. By deducing sensor transfer function from calibration curves, the voltage signal transferred to the measured values in mm. By measuring the vibration maximum amplitude at several speeds, it is being able to draw the resonance diagram for the rotor which shows a relation between angular speed (in rpm) and vibration amplitudes (in meters).

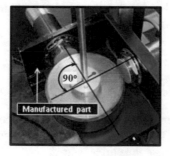

**Fig. 5** Sensors clamping

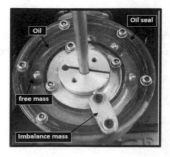

**Fig. 6** Manufactured ABB

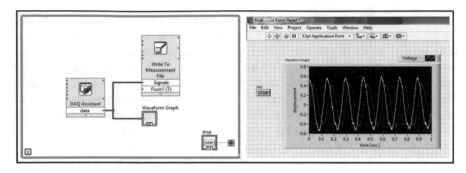

**Fig. 7** Measuring resolved software

## 5 Critical Speed Calculation

The critical speeds are calculated first to be passed quickly on rotor operating. As known that the critical speed is accompanied by high dynamic load and great vibration which make it too difficult to be determined practically. So, it is very important to determine the value of the critical speeds. Two methods are used to calculate the critical speeds of proposed model, the first is the transfer matrix method which is analytical method, where the other is computational method using ANSYS package. The calculated first critical speed ($\omega_{cr}$) equals to 85 rad/s which corresponds to 811 rpm. So, that the all measurements can be taken at fixed speeds away from the critical speed, some are below the critical speed and the others are above the critical speed.

### 5.1 Model Validation

All measurements are taken at fixed speeds away from the calculated critical speed. These speeds are shown in Table 1. The first three speeds are below the critical speed, and the other speeds are above the critical speed.

#### 5.1.1 Rotor Without ABB

The rotor without ABB includes the unbalanced rotor itself with the main body of the balancer, without balls and oil inside the balancer track as shown in Fig. 8a. This to

**Table 1** Angular speeds of practical measuring

| $0.25\omega_{cr}$ | $0.5\omega_{cr}$ | $0.75\omega_{cr}$ | $1.5\omega_{cr}$ | $2\omega_{cr}$ | $2.5\omega_{cr}$ | $3\omega_{cr}$ | $3.5\omega_{cr}$ |
|---|---|---|---|---|---|---|---|
| 202 rpm | 404 rpm | 606 rpm | 1217 rpm | 1623 rpm | 2029 rpm | 2435 rpm | 2840 rpm |

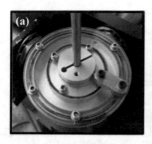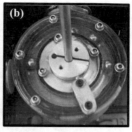

**Fig. 8** **a** Rotor without ABB **b** Rotor with four balls ABB

**Table 2** Experimental model parameters

| Parameter | Value | Parameter | Value |
|---|---|---|---|
| Rotor mass [$m$] | 1 kg | Imbalance radial distance [$a$] | 3 cm |
| Rotor thickness [$t$] | 2.5 cm | Balancing ball mass [$m_b$] | 3 gm |
| Rotor inner radius [$r_i$] | 3 mm | Shaft length [$l$] | 45 cm |
| Rotor outer radius [$r_o$] | 4 cm | Shaft diameter | 6 mm |
| Imbalance mass [$m_{im}$] | 10.14 gm | | |

avoid adding any residual imbalance may be resulted during balancer manufacture, the model and balancer parameters are shown in Table 2.

The vibration amplitudes are measured and recorded for the unbalanced rotor model without ABB. Then these readings are compared to the rotor response curve obtained from the proposed mathematical model. This comparison is shown in Fig. 9. The numerical solution is represented by a continuous curve, where the green points represent the experimental reading and the error bars for each point represent the uncertainty range with 99.8% level of confidence.

With zooming the curve at the speeds above the critical speed, it is observed that all the numerical results of the proposed model lie in the measured experimental ranges.

### 5.1.2 Rotor with Four Balls ABB

After adding four balls each of mass three grams and little amount of low viscous fluid as shown in Fig. 8b. This fluid has two effective functions, the first is reducing the friction between balancing balls and balancer walls, where the second is damping motions of the balancing ball. Vibration amplitudes are measured and recorded for the unbalanced rotor model with the four balls ABB. Then these readings are compared to the rotor response curve obtained from the proposed mathematical model (at $c = 0.4$, and $c_b = 0.00002$).

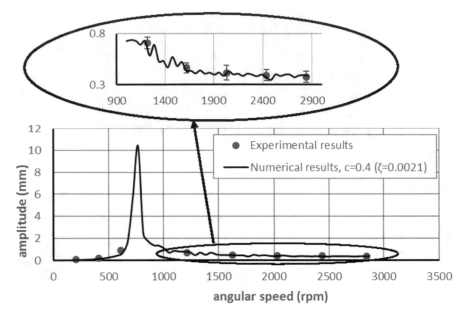

**Fig. 9** Rotor response curve without ABB

Figure 10 shows a comparison between the numerical solution represented by a continuous curve, and the experimental reading represented by the thick points with error bar for each reading which denotes the uncertainty range with 99.8% level of confidence. With zooming the curve at the speeds away the critical speed. It is observed that all the numerical results of the proposed model lie in the measured experimental ranges except the point indicated with a circle in Fig. 10, as the safety bearing prevent the rotor from exceeding this vibration value.

## 6    Effect of ABB

From the above figures, the experimental results for vibration amplitudes of the unbalanced rotor model without ABB and the rotor with a four balls ABB can be presented.

Figure 11 compares the results to show the experimental effect of the ABB. The range of speed out of reading represents the range of the critical speed. Figure 11 shows clearly the effect of a four ball ABB on the vibration of unbalanced rotor. ABB decreases vibration amplitude at angular speeds above the critical speed. Where this role is opposed at speeds below the critical speeds. This experimental reflection agrees greatly with the numerical solutions, and both accept the theory.

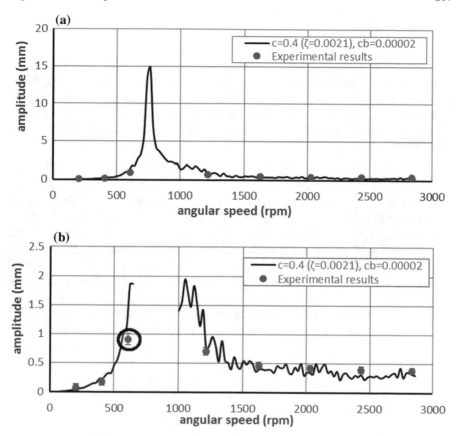

**Fig. 10** Rotor with a four balls ABB validation curves. **a** Resonance diagram. **b** Zooming at speeds away from critical speeds

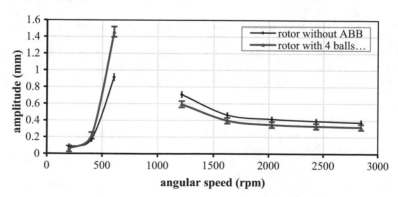

**Fig. 11** ABB effect on rotor vibrations

# 7   Conclusion

The aim of this paper is to investigate experimentally the role of ABB on rotor vibrations. First A mathematical model is proposed and solved numerically using MATLAB. For experimental investigation, an experimental rig was created and setup to assess the suitability of ABB at improving the vibration characteristics of the rotor. The intended measuring system can sense the effect of the attached ABB in rotor vibration characteristics.

(1) A proposed model is validated to be used in rotor shaft systems with ABB simulation. This model can be used in ABB design and best chosen of its parameters.
(2) Experimental investigation with accurate intended measuring system is done to the ABB effect on unbalanced vertical rotor. The practical effect of ABB is presented by the difference between the experimental measurements of rotor vibration with and without the balancer. The ABB effectively reduced the vibrations above the critical speed. While it increases vibrations below the critical speed. This result is approved practically and agreed greatly with the numerical solutions.
(3) More studies should take place in the future work on the mechanisms that can be combined with the ABB to improve its performance and cancel its effect on low speeds.

# References

1. Thearle, E.L.: A new type of dynamic-balancing machine. Trans. ASME (Appl. Mech.) pp. 131–141 (1932)
2. Thearle, E.L.: Automatic dynamic balancers (part 2- ring, pendulum, ball balancers). Machine Des. **22**, 103–106 (1950)
3. Kim, W., et al. Three-dimensional modeling and dynamic analysis of an automatic ball balancer in an optical disk drive. J. Sound Vib. (2005)
4. Huang, W.Y., Chao, C.P.: The application of ball-type balancers for radial vibration reduction of high-speed optic disk drives. J. Sound Vib. **250**, 415–430 (2002)
5. Rajalingham, C., et al.: Automatic balancing of flexible vertical rotors using a guided ball. Int. J. Mechanical Sci. (1998)
6. Yang, Q., et al.: Study on the influence of friction in an automatic ball balancing system. J. Sound vib. (ELSEVIER) (2005)
7. Royzman, V., Drach, I.: Improving theory for automatic balancing of rotating rotors with liquid self-balancers. MECHANIKA (2005)
8. Kim, T., Na, S.: New automatic ball balancer design to reduce transient-response in rotor system. Mechanical Syst. Signal Process. pp. 265–275 (2013)
9. Hwang, C.H., Chung, J.: Dynamic analysis of an automatic ball balancer with double races. Jsme Int. J. pp. 265–272 (1999)
10. Evaluation of measurement data — Guide to the expression of uncertainty in measurement. JCGM (2008)

# Optimization of a Flanged DAWT Using a CFD Actuator Disc Method

**Mohammad Hassan Ranjbar, Seyyed Abolfazl Nasrazadani and Kobra Gharali**

**Abstract** For improving the efficiency of horizontal axis wind turbines, shrouded or ducted wind turbines have become state of the art research topics. Getting energy from a wind turbine more than the Betz limit is a great motivation for researchers. Recent Computational Fluid Dynamics (CFD) simulations and experimental techniques show the effects of dominant factors such as the length of the duct, the angle of the diffuser, the height of the flange. In the current study, a ducted wind turbine is simulated numerically combined with an Actuator Disc (AD) method. The first step is to find the maximum velocity in the duct by improving the angles of the flange to finalize the geometry of the duct. Then, the power of the bare wind turbine and the Diffuser Augmented Wind Turbine (DAWT) are compared numerically while an AD method is used for modeling the rotor of the horizontal axis wind turbine. For the numerical simulation, the $K - \omega$ turbulent model is applied. For the 2D axisymmetric geometry, more than 0.5 million cells are used. The results show that the axial velocity can be enhanced more than 60%. The CFD analysis proves that the angle of the flange dominates the efficiency of the DAWTs and DAWT plays a key role in the enhancement of the power extraction of horizontal axis wind turbines. With a DAWT more power from a low wind speed can be extracted.

**Keywords** Wind turbine · Actuator disc · Betz limit · DAWT · CFD

M. H. Ranjbar · S. A. Nasrazadani · K. Gharali (✉)
Faculty of Engineering, College of Mechanical Engineering,
University of Tehran, Tehran, Iran
e-mail: kgharali@ut.ac.ir

M. H. Ranjbar
e-mail: mhranjbar@ut.ac.ir

S. A. Nasrazadani
e-mail: a.nasrazadani@ut.ac.ir

© Springer Nature Switzerland AG 2018
D. M. Kilgour et al. (eds.), *Recent Advances in Mathematical and Statistical Methods*, Springer Proceedings in Mathematics & Statistics 259,
https://doi.org/10.1007/978-3-319-99719-3_20

219

# 1 Introduction

A well-known and fundamental concept in wind turbines is that the wind power is proportional to the cube of wind speed. To enhance the power extraction, one of the main focuses is to increase the velocity near the wind turbine by using nozzles, diffusers, ducts, and flanges. Hjort and Larsen [3] studied the coefficient of performance a ducted wind turbine with the numerical and computational approaches. Also, Hjort and Larsen [4] focused on Hansen Diffuser Augmented Wind Turbine (Hansen DAWT) using Actuator Disc (AD) theory. Moeller and Visser [8] combined the AD and computational methods. Govindharajan [12] observed that the low-pressure region is more pronounced bumped configuration with brim by CFD method and found a significant increase in mass flow rate available for the wind turbine. Kale and Sapali [5] indicated that the inclined flange DAWT produce approximately 2.23 times more power than that of the bare wind turbine for the tested velocity range. Many specifications of the DAWT were studied by them such as the length of the duct, the angle of the diffuser, the height of the flange. It was showed by Ohya et al. that a wind turbine equipped with a flanged diffuser shroud can augment the power by a factor of about 4–5 compared to a standard (bare) wind turbine [9, 10]. The angle of a flange was investigated by El-Zahaby et al. and Kale et al. [1, 6]. El-Zahaby et al. study [1] indicated an optimum flange angle of 15° (between the vertical axis and the flange) with an enhanced entrance air velocity; also, the generated power was increased about 5% due to optimum flange angle. Kale et al. [6] examined different geometries of a diffuser. They found that the diffuser with an inclined flange shows 40.3% increase, the diffuser with a vertical flange shows 34.28% increase and the diffuser without a flange shows 18.57% increase in the velocity along the central axis of the rotor. They excluded the effects of the inlet geometry. Lipian Michal et al. [7] compared two direct and actuator-based models for analyzing the DAWT. The actuator model showed a good correlation with the experiment method in terms of wind turbine power prediction. Ghenai et al. [2] modeled shrouded horizontal axis wind turbine using the RANS method. They calculated induction factor and the power coefficient ($C_p$) from the computed velocity profiles. Also, the shrouded turbine power increased by a four folds compared to the unshrouded turbine power. Sorribes-Palmer et al. [13] used a one dimensional analytical model. The model predicted the DAWT performance coefficients and to compare with the Betz limit. In the present study, first, a DAWT is simulated without inlet and the results are compared with available experimental data [10]. Then, the DAWT is simulated to find the optimal angle of the flange with the presence of the inlet. Finally, the maximum available power based on the AD theory and the CFD method are calculated. The effects of the inlet and the optimum flange geometry are discussed in details.

# 2 Theory

Werle and Presz [15] provided the equations of the power in the ducted wind turbine based on the Actuator Disc (*AD*) theory. The equations were based on the momentum, pressure losses and the kinetic energy. By assuming an inviscid incompressible flow, any axial pressure changes due to the energy extraction by a wind turbine expanded or contracted the flow streamlines which results in rising the velocity component normal to the shroud. Because of this, the *Kutta–Joukowski* theorem which used for the calculation of the force of any two-dimensional bodies required an axial induced force ($F_s$) on the shroud [15]. On the other hand, $F_s$ comes from the interaction between the induced velocity component normal to the shroud axis and the ring-vortex vector associated with the aerodynamic circulation. Axial force coefficient, $C_s$, was defined as:

$$C_s \equiv \frac{F_s}{A_p(p_{p2} - p_{p1})}. \tag{1}$$

By setting $\frac{\partial P}{\partial V_0}$ to zero, the maximum power was

$$P_{max} = -\frac{16}{27}(1 + C_s)(\frac{1}{2}\rho A_p V_a^3) \tag{2}$$

which gives,

$$C_{Pmax} = -\frac{16}{27}(1 + C_s). \tag{3}$$

If $C_s = 0$, Eq. (3) recovers the classical *Betz* limit of $\frac{16}{27}$. For the DAWT the extracted power passes the *Betz* limit [15]. The results of these formulations will be used in the CFD post-processing.

## 3 Case Study

The aim of the present work is to analyze numerically the aerodynamic behaviors of a DAWT operating at different flange angles with a constant wind speed of 5 m/s. For the validation purpose, the geometry and all assumptions agree with those of the experimental study of Ohya et al. [10]. The geometrical details [10] are summarized in Table 1.

**Table 1** Main geometrical features of the experimental geometry, see Fig. 1 [10]

| Parameter | Value (cm) | Explanations |
| --- | --- | --- |
| $D_1$ | 20 | The throat diameter |
| $D_2$ | 24 | The major diameter |
| $h$ | 10 | The height of the flange |
| $L$ | 30 | The length of the diffuser |

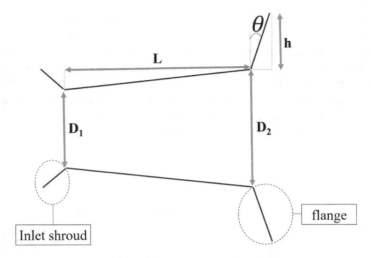

**Fig. 1** Schematic of a wind turbine equipped with a flanged diffuser shroud, adapted from [10]

## 4  Numerical Approach

### 4.1  *Computational Grid, Solver and Validation*

Different mesh sizes, from $1.2 \times 10^5$ to $0.5 \times 10^7$ cells, were examined considering the *y-plus*, $y^+$, and the convergence criteria. With $2.8 \times 10^5$ elements, $y^+$ is less than 2.6. The mentioned pattern of mesh selection is used for all simulations. The growth rate of boundary cells is 1.15. The width and height of the computational domain are set about 30 and 20 times the rotor radius, respectively. The inlet and outlet boundary conditions are the velocity inlet and the pressure outlet. The symmetry boundary condition is used for the upper wall. The bottom boundary is defined as the axis. The final mesh and the boundary conditions are shown in Fig. 2.

The partial differential equations are solved based on the SIMPLE (Semi-Implicit Method) algorithm introduced by Patanker [11]. The second order upwind spatial discretization is used. The flow is assumed to be 2D axisymmetric, steady, turbulent,

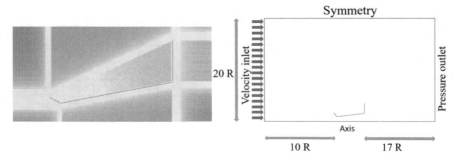

**Fig. 2**  The final mesh of the 2D DAWT (left) and the boundary conditions of the domain (right)

incompressible. In this part, considering experimental setup [10], the geometry consists of the flange and the diffuser (Fig. 3). Both $K - \varepsilon$ and $K - \omega$ SST turbulence models were used. The results have a good agreement with those of the experimental data but the $K - \omega$ SST turbulence model shows a better agreement; so, the $K - \omega$ SST turbulence model is used. The maximum relative error of the velocity ratio is %5. Figure 4 shows the velocity ratio in the central axis of the DAWT versus the length ratio ($\frac{X}{L}$). The maximum value of the velocity ratio using the $K - \omega$ SST turbulence model is 1.532.

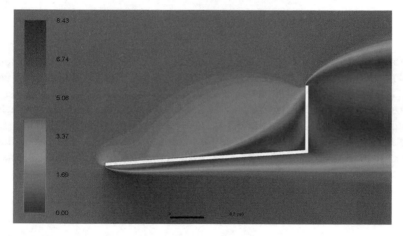

**Fig. 3** Velocity contours (m/s) for the validation with no inlet

**Fig. 4** Maximum velocity in the central axis of the DAWT; +-+-+: experimental data [10]; the rest: the current simulations

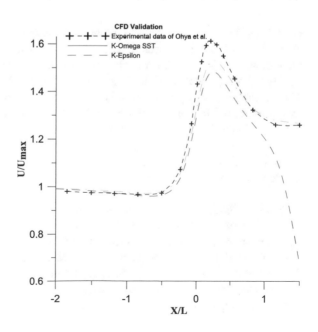

## 4.2   Angle of Flange

To optimize the angle of the flange, the DAWT consists of an inlet, a diffuser and a flange. All simulations run with the $K - \omega$ SST turbulence model, the SIMPLE algorithm and the second order upwind spatial discretization. The domain is axisymmetric. The angle of the flange, $\theta$, is varied from $0°$ to $15°$ by the step of $2.5°$. The wind speed is 5 m/s in all cases.

## 4.3   Maximum Power of DAWT

According to Eq. (3), the maximum power of a DAWT is more than that of a bare turbine. In this section, the axial force coefficient, $C_s$, and the power coefficient, $C_{Pmax}$, will be obtained. The numerical setup is the same as previous sections. The ADs are used for generating wake velocity deficits. The concept can be applied to both experimental and numerical techniques. The flow field behind the wind turbine rotor is simulated to mimic the energy extraction from a wind turbine without modeling a specific rotor [14]. The AD is modeled by a porous jump. In the post-processing, the magnitude of the velocity and the pressure drop in the vicinity of the AD were used to calculate $C_s$ and $C_{Pmax}$.

## 5   Results and Discussion

First the AD was simulated without a duct in the free stream which gave the power coefficient of 0.592 as expected. Then, the DAWT is simulated for the maximum ideal power extraction. The velocity contours of the DAWT with AD are illustrated in Fig. 5. Various angles of the flange from $0°$ to $15°$ by the step of $2.5°$ are tried. The maximum velocity ratios in the central axis direction of the DAWT versus the length ratio are illustrated in Fig. 6 for the all angles. Also, the maximum velocity ratio magnitude for each angle of the flange is shown in Fig. 7.

Considering the optimum angle of the flange, the AD is modeled using the porous jump method. The results of $C_s$ and $C_{Pmax}$ (Eq. (3)) based on the AD theory with the duct and without the duct are reported in Table 2. The streamlines are shown in Fig. 8.

In Fig. 7, initially the velocity ratio increases up to $5°$ then it falls down until $15°$. For the vertical flange ($\theta = 0$), the maximum velocity ratio is 1.604 and the optimum (maximum) velocity ratio is 1.615 in $5°$. The minimum velocity ratio is 1.596 in $15°$. For the first geometry of the DAWT without any inlet or nozzle (Fig. 3), the maximum velocity ratio is 1.532. By adding inlet or nozzle, the velocity ratio can increase up to 4.7% with the vertical flange and to 5.4% with the optimum angle of the flange ($\theta = 5$). Figures 3, 5 and 8 illustrate that by adding an inlet or a

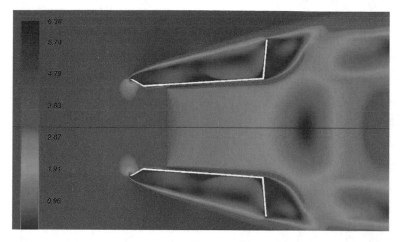

**Fig. 5** The velocity contours with an AD

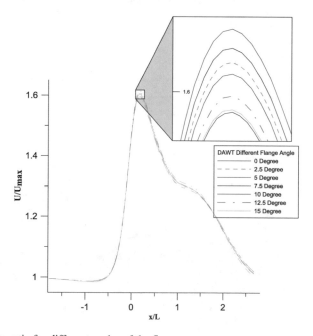

**Fig. 6** Velocity ratio for different angles of the flange

small nozzle to the DAWT, a new vortex is generated which can change the pressure differences. Adding the nozzle influences the stream lines; also, the angle of the nozzle can change the DAWT efficiency by changing the strength of the vortex. The streamlines are expanded in the downwind of the DAWT (Fig. 8). That means, the velocity magnitude decreases in the large area and a low pressure region is generated in comparison with the bare wind turbine. This results in more power extraction. Based on the AD theory, the maximum power coefficients are 0.59 and 1.44 for the

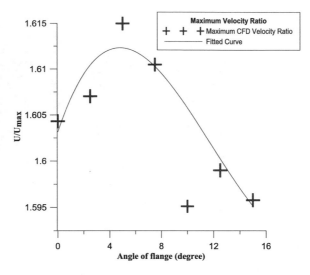

**Fig. 7** Velocity ratio versus angle of the flange

**Table 2** Results of the $C_s$ and $C_{Pmax}$

| Parameters | DAWT | Bare |
|------------|------|------|
| $C_s$ | 1.43 | 0 |
| $C_{Pmax}$ | 1.44 | 0.59 |

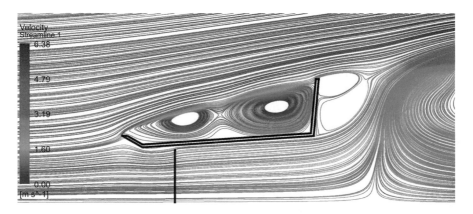

**Fig. 8** Streamlines for the DAWT, obtained with the AD method

bare wind turbine and the DAWT, respectively. That means for the mentioned DAWT geometry, it is not possible to increase the coefficient of the power more than 1.44. Results of the AD simulation show that the combination of the inlet, diffuser and the flange can increase the maximum power coefficient 2.44 times. The axial velocity can be enhanced more than 60% in the flange type of a DAWT.

# 6 Conclusion

Using a DAWT enhances the power extraction from a small scale wind turbine especially in the *low wind speed* since a common wind turbine cannot work properly under low wind speed. The CFD analysis proved that the angle of the flange can dominate the efficiency of the DAWT. An optimized combination of a inlet, a diffuser and a flange plays a key role in the enhancement of the power extraction of a horizontal axis wind turbine. The DAWT was modeled based on the AD theory. Comparing the experimental data with the numerical results (the $K - \omega$ SST turbulence model) confirms the reliability of the simulation with the maximum relative error of 5% for the velocity ratio. The optimum angle of the flange was determined 5° with the inlet. The inlet or the small nozzle increased the maximum velocity ratio up to 5.4%. Using the DAWT with the optimum angle of the flange, the maximum available coefficient of performance was increased 2.44 times. Also, the axial velocity can be enhanced more than 60%.

# References

1. El-Zahaby, A.M., Kabeel, A.E., Elsayed, S.S., Obiaa, M.F.: CFD analysis of flow fields for shrouded wind turbines diffuser model with different flange angles. Alexandria Eng. J. **56**(1), 171–179 (2017)
2. Ghenai, C., Salameh, T., Janajreh, I.: Modeling and simulation of shrouded horizontal axis wind turbine using RANS method. Jordan J. Mech. Ind. Eng. **11**(4), 235–243 (2017)
3. Hjort, S., Larsen, H.: A multi-element diffuser augmented wind turbine. Energies **7**(5), 3256–3281 (2014)
4. Hjort, S., Larsen, H.: Rotor design for diffuser augmented wind turbines. Energies **8**(10), 10736–10774 (2015)
5. Kale, S., Sapali, S.N.: Development and field testing of an inclined flanged compact diffuser for a micro wind turbine. In: ASME 2014 International Mechanical Engineering Congress and Exposition, pp. 70–76. American Society of Mechanical Engineers (2014)
6. Kale, S.A., Gunjal, Y.R., Jadhav, S.P., Tanksale, A.N.: CFD analysis for optimization of diffuser for a micro wind turbine. In: 2013 International Conference on Energy Efficient Technologies for Sustainability (ICEETS), pp. 257–260. IEEE (2013)
7. Michał, L., Maciej, K., Jakub, M., Krzysztof, J.: Numerical simulation methodologies for design and development of diffuser-augmented wind turbines-analysis and comparison. Open Eng. **6**(1), 235–240 (2016)
8. Moeller, M., Visser, K.: Experimental and numerical studies of a high solidity, low tip speed ratio DAWT. In Proceedings of the 48th AIAA Aerospace Sciences Meeting and Exhibit, Orlando, FL, USA, pp. 4–7 (2010)
9. Ohya, Y., Karasudani, T.: A shrouded wind turbine generating high output power with wind-lens technology. Energies **3**(4), 634–649 (2010)
10. Ohya, Y., Karasudani, T., Sakurai, A., Abe, K., Inoue, M.: Development of a shrouded wind turbine with a flanged diffuser. J. Wind Eng. Ind. Aerodyn. **96**(5), 524–539 (2008)
11. Patankar, S.V.: Numerical Heat Transfer and Fluid Flow. Taylor & Francis (1980). Technical report, ISBN 978-0-89116-522-4
12. Parammasivam, K.M., Govindharajan, R., Vivek, V., Vishnu Priya, R.: Numerical investigation and design optimization of brimmed diffuser–wind lens around a wind turbine. In: The Eighth

Asia-Pacific Conference on Wind Engineering, pp. 1204–1210. Research Publishing, Singapore (2013)
13. Sorribes-Palmer, F., Sanz-Andres, A., Ayuso, L., Sant, R., Franchini, S.: Mixed CFD-1D wind turbine diffuser design optimization. Renewable Energy **105**, 386–399 (2017)
14. Sturge, D., Sobotta, D., Howell, R., While, J., Lou, A.: A hybrid actuator disc-full rotor CFD methodology for modelling the effects of wind turbine wake interactions on performance. Renewable Energy **80**, 525–537 (2015)
15. Werle, M.J., Presz Jr., W.M.: Ducted wind/water turbines and propellers revisited. J. Propul. Power **24**(5), 1146–1150 (2008)

# Axisymmetric Simulations of Nonlinear Sound Propagation in a Trumpet

Janelle Resch, Andrew Giuliani, Lilia Krivodonova
and John Vanderkooy

**Abstract** An axisymmetric model to simulate the evolution of nonlinear waves through a trumpet is presented. In particular, we simulate the time pressure waveform of a musical note as it travels through the instrument. The flare expansion and curvature of the initial tubing near the mouthpiece shank is carefully modeled. For the mathematical model, we chose the compressible Euler equations and solved them numerically using a GPU implementation of the discontinuous Galerkin method. We compare our numerical results with a full three-dimensional model. We find that axisymmetric simulations exhibit less numerical diffusion while providing better resolution without additional mesh refinement. Moreover, axisymmetric simulations significantly reduce runtime and required memory.

**Keywords** Nonlinear acoustics · Sound wave propagation
Compressible Euler equations · Discontinuous Galerkin method · Axisymmetric
Three-dimensional · Brass instruments · Sound pressure measurements

## 1 Introduction

We present results of axisymmetric simulations of sound propagation in a trumpet and compare them to full three-dimensional simulations. The main advantage of axisymmetric simulations is the reduction in computing time and required memory.

J. Resch (✉) · A. Giuliani · L. Krivodonova
Department of Applied Mathematics, University of Waterloo,
200 University Ave. W., Waterloo, ON N2L 3G1, Canada
e-mail: jresch@uwaterloo.ca

A. Giuliani
e-mail: agiulian@uwaterloo.ca

L. Krivodonova
e-mail: lgk@uwaterloo.ca

J. Vanderkooy
Department of Physics and Astronomy, University of Waterloo,
200 University Ave. W., Waterloo, ON N2L 3G1, Canada
e-mail: jv@uwaterloo.ca

© Springer Nature Switzerland AG 2018
D. M. Kilgour et al. (eds.), *Recent Advances in Mathematical
and Statistical Methods*, Springer Proceedings in Mathematics & Statistics 259,
https://doi.org/10.1007/978-3-319-99719-3_21

Axisymmetric formulations exploit the axial symmetry of the problem, in our case, the trumpet. With this, five equations in the Euler system describing the motion of an inviscid compressible fluid reduce to four equations and the three-dimensional (3D) domain is simplified to a two-dimensional (2D) one. The reduction of one spatial dimension allows us to create finer meshes and improve the solution's resolution. Conversely, the required number of elements is reduced by several orders of magnitude for the same resolution. This might be of importance for graphic processing unit (GPU) computing where memory is limited.

While 3D and axisymmetric equations are the same from an analytical point of view, the simulation results can be different due to the presence of numerical artifacts. For instance, unstructured tetrahedral meshes lack axial symmetry. As a result, the 3D numerical solution will also lack axial symmetry. This is due to numerical diffusion which depends on the size and orientation of the tetrahedra in the mesh. For the flows we are interested in, the differences should be small. A more important numerical artifact is due to imperfect approximation of the physical domain by a computational one. The surface of the computational domain in 3D consists of triangular faces of tetrahedra, i.e., it is not smooth when straight faced tetrahedra discretization is used. It is well known that the accuracy of the simulations will then suffer from spurious entropy production at the vertices and edges of the mesh. The proper way to treat such geometry is to use higher order mesh elements. But this does not always work well for complicated geometries and is difficult to deal with numerically. Axisymmetric simulations do not suffer from this problem, except possibly at the expansion of the flare.

In this paper, we present some findings of comparing 3D and axisymmetric finite element simulations of wave propagation through a simplified trumpet geometry. We take a similar approach to the work presented in [1] and assume nonlinear effects can be examined separately from viscothermal losses. However, instead of only simulating acoustic pulses within musical instruments (e.g., [2–4]) or an approximation of a musical note (e.g., [1]), we present numerical results of generating a realistic musical note recorded in the lab. In particular, comparisons are made on simulations of the $B_3^b$ musical note [5]. For our study, we created a geometric trumpet that attempts to accurately model the flare expansion and initial tubing variations near the mouthpiece shank (instead of assuming the initial bore is of uniform diameter. In order to maintain the axial symmetry, the bends and valves will not be included. As we argued in [5], the bends do not greatly influence the sound production for the $B_3^b$ note.

## 2  Numerical Setup

We write the general conservation law in a domain $\Omega$ as

$$\frac{\partial \mathbf{u}}{\partial t} + \nabla \cdot \mathbf{f}(\mathbf{u}) = \mathbf{0}, \qquad \mathbf{x} \in \Omega, \qquad t > 0, \tag{1a}$$

$$\mathbf{u} = \mathbf{u}^0, \qquad t = 0, \tag{1b}$$

where $\mathbf{f}(\mathbf{u})$ is the flux function and the solution is $\mathbf{u}(\mathbf{x}, t) = (u_1, u_2, ..., u_m)^t$, $(\mathbf{x}, t) \in \Omega \times [0, T]$. The solution $\mathbf{u}(\mathbf{x}, t)$ on each element is approximated by a vector function $\mathbf{U}_j$ whose components are written as a linear combination of the orthogonal basis functions $\{\varphi_j\}$.

We model nonlinear sound wave propagation through a trumpet using the compressible Euler equations in which we describe the flow as an inviscid, isentropic fluid. The equations of motion will be written using the 3D Cartesian coordinate system $(x, y, z)$ as well as the 2D axisymmetric system $(x, r)$ where r is the radial component and x is the horizontal. For the formulations which will be defined below, we write the variables as so: $\rho$ is the gas density; $\rho\mathbf{u} = (\rho u, \rho v, \rho w)$ are the momenta in the x, y and z direction, respectively; p is the internal pressure; and E is the total energy. For the axisymmetric model, the momenta in the axial and radial directions are described by $\rho x$ and $\rho r$, respectively. The specific heat ratio $\gamma \approx 1.4$ for air [6].

## 2.1 Three-Dimensional Formulation

The 3D compressible Euler equations in Cartesian coordinates $(x, y, z)$ are given by

$$\frac{\partial \mathbf{U}}{\partial t} + \frac{\partial \mathbf{F}(\mathbf{U})}{\partial x} + \frac{\partial \mathbf{G}(\mathbf{U})}{\partial y} + \frac{\partial \mathbf{H}(\mathbf{U})}{\partial z} = \mathbf{0}, \tag{2}$$

where $\mathbf{U}$ is the vector of conserved variables and the flux vectors are

$$\mathbf{F}(\mathbf{U}) = \begin{bmatrix} \rho u \\ \rho u^2 + p \\ \rho u v \\ \rho u w \\ u(E + p) \end{bmatrix}, \quad \mathbf{G}(\mathbf{U}) = \begin{bmatrix} \rho v \\ \rho u v \\ \rho v^2 + p \\ \rho v w \\ v(E + p) \end{bmatrix}, \quad \mathbf{H}(\mathbf{U}) = \begin{bmatrix} \rho w \\ \rho u w \\ \rho v w \\ \rho w^2 + p \\ w(E + p) \end{bmatrix}. \tag{3}$$

The equation of state for an ideal gas connects E to the other variables and closes the system

$$E = \frac{p}{\gamma - 1} + \frac{\rho}{2}(u^2 + v^2 + w^2). \tag{4}$$

## 2.2 Axisymmetric Formulation

We can also formulate the problem by exploiting the axial symmetry in which the solution is independent from the angular coordinate $\theta$. To avoid the singularity at

$r = 0$, the surface integral is not computed along the axis of symmetry and $\mathbf{U}$ is multiplied by r. The system (2–4) in $(x, r)$ coordinates is now written as

$$\frac{\partial[r\mathbf{U}]}{\partial t} + \frac{\partial[r\mathbf{F}(\mathbf{U})]}{\partial x} + \frac{\partial[r\mathbf{G}(\mathbf{U})]}{\partial r} = \mathbf{S}(\mathbf{U}), \qquad (5)$$

where the source term is

$$\mathbf{S}(\mathbf{U}) = \begin{bmatrix} 0, & 0, & p, & 0 \end{bmatrix}^{\mathsf{T}}. \qquad (6)$$

## 2.3  Numerical Test Case

We simulated the time pressure waveform of the recorded $B_3^b$ musical note (see [5] for details) shown in the left plot of Fig. 1. This pressure measurement was obtained by mounting a quarter-inch microphone on a $B^b$ Barcelona BTR-200LQ trumpet approximately 4.5 cm from the beginning of the mouthpiece. This area of the trumpet is known as the *mouthpiece shank*. The wave profile (Fig. 1, left) was prescribed as the boundary condition on pressure at the inlet boundary of the computational trumpet for the simulations presented in Sect. 3. We wrote an expression for the pressure by applying Fourier synthesis to one period of the recorded waveform. The series was truncated at the 31st term and is written as

$$p = A_0 + 2 \sum_{i=1}^{30} A_i \cos\left(2\pi f_i t + \phi_i\right), \qquad (7)$$

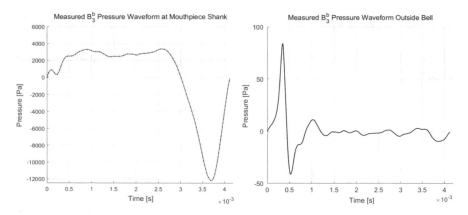

**Fig. 1**  Left: Measured pressure waveform of the $B_3^b$ at the mouthpiece. Right: Measured pressure waveform of the $B_3^b$ outside the bell

where $f_i$ denotes an integer multiple of the fundamental frequency $f_1 \approx 242\,\text{Hz}$; $A_i$ and $\phi_i$ is the amplitude and phase corresponding to each harmonic component, respectively; and $A_0$ is the term corresponding to the direct current.

We locally related pressure and velocity at the mouthpiece boundary using the planar expression derived from linear acoustic theory. This relation between pressure and velocity reproduced the measured mouthpiece pressure waveform accurately. Finally, the density was prescribed assuming the adiabatic relation between pressure and density from compressible flow theory. In summary, the dimensionless boundary conditions at the mouthpiece of the computational trumpet are given by

$$\begin{cases} \hat{p} = \hat{A}_0 + \sum_{i=1}^{N_f} 2\hat{A}_i \cos\left(2\pi \hat{f}_i t + \hat{\phi}_i\right), \\ \hat{\rho} = \gamma \hat{p}^{\frac{1}{\gamma}}, \\ \hat{u} = \frac{\hat{p}-p_o}{\rho_o c}, \\ \hat{v} = 0.0, \\ \hat{w} = 0.0, \\ \hat{E} = \frac{\hat{p}}{\gamma-1} + \frac{\hat{\rho}}{2}(\hat{u}^2 + \hat{v}^2 + \hat{w}^2), \end{cases} \tag{8}$$

where $\hat{A}_i$, $\hat{f}_i$, and $\hat{\phi}_i$ denote the amplitude, frequency and phase shift, respectively, for the harmonics of the measured note [5].

The simulated pressure was sampled 16 cm outside the computational trumpet. This corresponds to the position where another microphone was placed along the central axis of the real instrument. The microphones simultaneously recorded the $B_3^b$ pressure profile so we could examine the evolution of the waveform as it traveled through the instrument. One period of the pressure measurement outside the flare is shown in the right plot of Fig. 1. Comparing the experimental waveform outside the bell with our numerical outputs allowed us to test the validity of our model.

## 2.4 Initial and Boundary Conditions

We modeled a trumpet where the flare opens into an open domain. We assumed that the flow initially was at rest. For all simulations, the flow (8) is introduced into the domain at the left vertical boundary of the bore which corresponds to the mouthpiece boundary. Along the far-field, pass-through boundary conditions were used in which the ghost state was prescribed to be the free flow state, i.e., the initial state. We experimentally determined the size of the computational domain so that reflections at the far-field would not influence the waveform solution. We prescribed reflective boundary conditions (i.e., solid wall boundary conditions) on the inner and outer walls of the computational trumpet. At the ghost state, the normal velocity was taken to be the inner value with a negative sign. The density, pressure and tangential velocity were unchanged from the corresponding values inside the cell (see [7] for more details).

## 2.5  Computational Trumpet Geometries

We now present the computational trumpet that was used for our numerical simulations. The computational geometry describes the physical shape of the 1.48 m
long trumpet where the initial 24 cm of tubing and the flare expansion are carefully measured and approximated. Slight inaccuracies in these regions can produce
exaggerated discrepancies in numerical simulations as we discusssed in [8].

For our trumpet geometry, the tubing between $x \in [0 \text{ cm}, 24 \text{ cm}]$ was reconstructed from measurements taken at eight points. The outline of the inner trumpet tubing
whose cross-section is shown in Fig. 2 was interpolated using these measurements.
This was followed by a cylindrical bore in the region $x \in [24 \text{ cm}, 102 \text{ cm}]$ and then
the flare expansion for $x \in [102 \text{ cm}, 148 \text{ cm}]$. To obtain a realistic flare shape, a pho-
tograph of the trumpet bell was taken. The *grabit* software (Math Works Inc.) was
then used to trace out the trumpet flare by a series of points. We used these points
to interpolate the bell shape by cubic splines. The resulting curve is shown in Fig. 3
and was passed to the mesh generating software GMSH.

We added vertical lines about the axis of symmetry $r = 0$ and at the far-field
boundary $r = 2.5$ m to the curve depicted in Fig. 3. A rotational extrusion about the
x-axis was then carried out on the axisymmetric geometry to obtain the equivalent
3D trumpet geometry. For convenience, the axisymmetric and 3D geometry will be
referred to as $Geo_{axi}$ and $Geo_{3D}$, respectively. We used adaptive element sizes to
accurately resolve the geometric features of the trumpet. The refinement chosen in
GMSH was defined to be the same for both $Geo_{axi}$ and $Geo_{3D}$. We generated a second

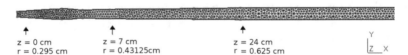

$z = 0$ cm          $z = 7$ cm              $z = 24$ cm
$r = 0.295$ cm      $r = 0.43125$cm         $r = 0.625$ cm

**Fig. 2**  A longitudinal cross-section of the 3D geometric shape of the tubing near the mouthpiece
boundary used to construct the computational trumpet

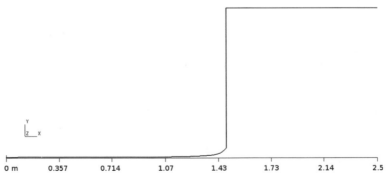

0 m      0.357      0.714      1.07      1.43      1.73      2.14      2.5

**Fig. 3**  The profile used in GMSH to create the computational trumpet meshes and surrounding
area via a rotational extrusion about the x-axis

**Table 1** Number of cells and $L^2$ errors associated with the Geo$_{axi}$ and Geo$_{3D}$ simulations sampled 16 cm outside the trumpet bell

| Name of geometry | Number of cells | Min. inscribed circle | $L^2$ error (%) |
|---|---|---|---|
| Geo$_{axi}$ | 70,595 | 2.198080e−04 | 6.5649 |
| Geo$_{axi-ref}$ | 368,361 | 8.418355e−05 | 6.3915 |
| Geo$_{3D}$ | 1,317,219 | 2.668689e−05 | 5.8741 |

axisymmetric mesh that had over five times as many cells. We will refer to this mesh as Geo$_{axi-ref}$. The minimum inscribed radius or circle and the total number of triangles or tetrahedra for each mesh can be found in Table 1. We ran the additional simulation on Geo$_{axi-ref}$ to determine if the mesh was sufficiently fine along the central axis.

## 3  Simulation Results

The 2D axisymmetric and 3D Cartesian compressible Euler equations were solved on Geo$_{axi}$, Geo$_{axi-ref}$ and Geo$_{3D}$. All three simulated pressure waveforms were sampled outside the trumpet bell and plotted along with the experimental profile in Fig. 4.

We observe that the numerical and experimental waveforms match rather well, especially Geo$_{3D}$. The relative error between the experimental and numerical curves was computed using the $L^2$ norm

$$\text{error}(\%) = \left( \frac{||p_{\text{experimental}} - p_{\text{numerical}}||_2}{||p_{\text{experimental}}||_2} \right) * 100 \% \tag{9}$$

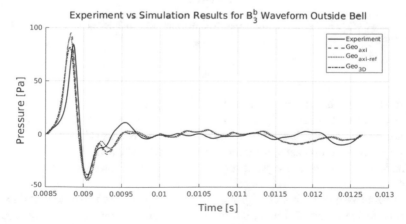

**Fig. 4** Pressure waveform of experimental data with the Geo$_{axi}$, Geo$_{axi-ref}$ and Geo$_{3D}$ simulation results sampled outside of the instrument

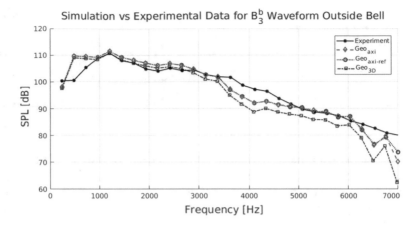

**Fig. 5** Frequency spectra of experimental data and the Geo$_{axi}$, Geo$_{axi-ref}$ and Geo$_{3D}$ simulations

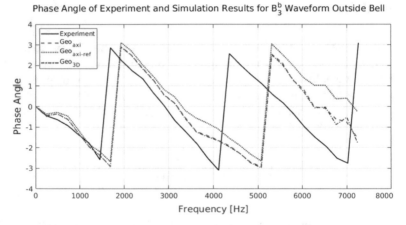

**Fig. 6** Phase angle in frequency domain of experimental data and Geo$_{axi}$, Geo$_{axi-ref}$ and Geo$_{3D}$ simulations

and reported in Table 1. We see that the errors in the simulations are similar, with Geo$_{3D}$ computations being slightly more accurate. In addition, although Geo$_{axi-ref}$ is much finer than Geo$_{axi}$, the difference in relative error is only 0.1734%.

The spectral components of the pressure waveforms shown in Fig. 4 are plotted in Fig. 5. The corresponding phase angles as a function of frequency are plotted in Fig. 6.

We find that the 3D result aligns slightly better with the experimental data for frequencies lower than 2800 Hz; but only by a decibel at most. The axisymmetric simulations better match the experiment for the remaining range. Comparing the Geo$_{axi}$ and Geo$_{axi-ref}$ SPLs only, we see the results are almost identical with the exception of the last harmonic. There are very small variations ($<0.5$ dB) between these numerical solutions, specifically for frequencies in the 4800–6900 Hz range.

As seen in Fig. 6, $Geo_{3D}$ and $Geo_{axi/axi-ref}$ phases are very similar. Furthermore, there is little difference between the $Geo_{axi}$ and $Geo_{axi-ref}$ phase angles. In particular, they are in better agreement with each other than with the experimental data. For all simulated waveforms, the phase angles best match the experiment for harmonics whose frequencies are lower than approximately 1500 Hz. These are the harmonic waves that reflect the most at the trumpet bell [9].

# 4 Conclusion

Computational results presented in Figs. 4, 5 and 6 indicate that the proposed axisymmetric and 3D models produce similar results for the first five frequencies in (7). Variations between the models are observed for the remaining spectra.

The differences between the models may be partly due to the use of straight-side mesh elements. Such elements better approximate the complex geometry of the trumpet in 2D than in 3D for reasons discussed in Sect. 1. Assuming the $Geo_{axi}$ mesh was sufficiently refined, this would explain why the $Geo_{axi}$ and $Geo_{axi-ref}$ results are almost the same. However, true comparison between the models is difficult to make, especially when using nonuniform meshes. Axial symmetry is not guaranteed for 3D meshes and hence, 3D simulations. Furthermore, mesh generation slightly differs in 2D and 3D, particularly for local refinement [7].

Nonetheless, if the computational trumpet is better modeled in 2D, the axisymmetric simulations in principle should have less numerical diffusion. From comparing our results presented in Fig. 5, we see some evidence of this: the harmonic distribution of the $Geo_{3D}$ and $Geo_{axi/axi-ref}$ numerical curves (i.e., the shape of the numerical outputs) is the same, but the distance between the solutions slowly increases as a function of frequency. Since higher frequencies are usually diffused more, and this is what we see in our results, we believe the gap between our results is due to numerical diffusion. This would also be consistent with the similarity seen in the phase shifts in Fig. 6.

Comparing the experimental data to the numerical solutions reveals that the evolution of the higher harmonics is well modeled. However, the second and third harmonics in the numerical curves deviate from the measured SPLs. This discrepancy could be due to neglecting the valves as their geometry is quite complex and would preferentially influence the lower frequencies (since a large portion of the energy is reflected from the bell and hence, confined within the bore). Another possible explanation for the observed variation is the plane wave approximation for velocity that was prescribed for the inlet boundary condition. This simplification was made since accurately measuring velocity in the narrow mouthpiece shank in the lab is technically difficult.

In conclusion, our results demonstrate that axisymmetric simulations can offer better resolution for our problem while greatly reducing runtimes and memory requirements. Runtime for the $Geo_{axi}$ simulation is faster than the corresponding 3D simulation, with equivalent mesh refinement and runtimes of 4165.8 and 39328.7 s, respectively. Runtime for the $Geo_{axi}$ simulation is over nine times shorter than the corresponding 3D simulation, with equivalent mesh refinement.

**Acknowledgements** This research was supported in part by the Alexander Graham Bell PGS-D grant 365873. We also acknowledge and thank the support of NVIDIA Corporation with the donation of the Titan X Pascal GPU used for this research.

# References

1. Msallam, R., Dequidt, S., Caussé, R., Tassart, S.: Physical model of the trombone including nonlinear effects. Application to the sound synthesis of loud tones. Acta Acustica United Acustica **86**(4), 725–736 (2000)
2. Erickson, R.R., Zinn, B.T.: Modeling of finite amplitude acoustic waves in closed cavities using the Galerkin method. J. Acoust. Soc. Am. **113**(4), 1863–1870 (2003)
3. Richter, A., Stiller, J., Grundmann, R.: Stablized discontinous Galerkin method for flow-sound interaction. J. Comput. Acoust. **15**, 123–143 (2007)
4. Wolkov, A.V., Petrovskaya, N.B.: Higher order discontinuous Galerkin method for acoustic pulse problem. Comput. Phys. Commun. **181**(7), 1186–1194 (2010)
5. Resch, J., Krivodonova, L., Vanderkooy, J.: A two-dimensional study of finite amplitude sound waves in a trumpet using the discontinuous Galerkin method. J. Comput. Acoust. **22**(3), 27 (2014)
6. Warburton, T., Hesthaven, J.S.: Nodal Discontinuous Galerkin Methods: Algorithms, Analysis, and Applications. Springer, New York (2008)
7. Flaherty, J.E., Krivodonova, L., Remacle, J.F., Shephard, M.S.: Some aspects of discontinuous Galerkin methods for hyperbolic conservation laws. J. Finite Elem. Anal. Des. **38**(10), 889–908 (2002)
8. Resch, J., Krivodonova, L., Vanderkooy, J.: A comparison between two and three-dimensional simulations of finite amplitude sound waves in a trumpet. In: Mathematical and Computational Approaches in Advancing Modern Science and Engineering, pp. 481–492. Springer International Publishing (2016)
9. Fletcher, N.H., Rossing, T.D.: The Physics of Musical Instruments. Springer Science & Business Media, New York (2012)

# Turbulent Diffusion of Inertial Particle Pairs Such as in Pollen and Sandstorms

Syed M. Usama and Nadeem A. Malik

**Abstract** We explore the concept of local and non-local diffusion processes [Malik N. A., PLoS ONE 12(12): e0189917 (2017)] in application to the diffusion of inertial particle pairs in the limit of Stoke's drag. Inertial particles are arguably more important than fluid particles because most real world applications are related to inertial particle motion, from hail and pollen to sandstorms. The inertial pair diffusion regimes depend upon the local Stokes' number $St(l)$, where $l$ is the pair separation distance. For $St(l) \ll 1$, the inertia dominates and we observe ballistic motion for inertial pair separation. For $St(l) \gg 1$, the turbulent energy dominates the diffusion process which asymptotes to the fluid non-local pair regime for very large inertial ranges. A numerical model, Kinematic Simulations, is used to generate inertia particle trajectories and we observe the predicted inertial pair diffusion regimes in the limit of large inertial subranges.

**Keywords** Turbulence · Diffusion · Pair diffusion · Inertial particles
Stokes drag · Kinematic Simulation · Modeling and simulation

## 1 Introduction

The transport of particles in turbulent flows is ubiquitous in industrial applications and in natural phenomena such as in atmospheric dust storms, the dispersion of pollens, and in suspensions of droplets, bubbles, and finite-size particles convected by turbulent flows [1–5].

Understanding the transport processes governing inertial particle motion and their statistical properties is therefore of paramount importance in many areas of science and engineering. This is especially true in todays' world where climate, pollution, and bio-diversity are major concerns for the future of the planet. In all of these areas, the motion of inertial particles plays important roles. The movement of water laden

S. M. Usama · N. A. Malik (✉)
Department of Mathematics and Statistics, King Fahd University
of Petroleum and Minerals, Dhahran 31261, Saudi Arabia
e-mail: nadeem_malik@cantab.net

© Springer Nature Switzerland AG 2018
D. M. Kilgour et al. (eds.), *Recent Advances in Mathematical and Statistical Methods*, Springer Proceedings in Mathematics & Statistics 259,
https://doi.org/10.1007/978-3-319-99719-3_22

239

clouds, hail, snow, and other forms of percipitation are central to the ecological cycle and climate modeling. Pollution from soot, and plastics, and the like in the atmosphere and oceans are mostly in the form of small particles, sometimes chemically reacting. Pollens and seeds, also inertial particles carried by the wind and ocean currents, are essential for life.

Fluid particles follow streamlines, but inertial particles deviate from streamlines which makes theoretical and numerical modeling of inertial particle transport especially difficult. Fluid particle motion is easy to compute if the flow field is known, but the transport equations that describe the motion of individual inertial particles (particles with weight, friction, size, and density) is not fully developed yet, although simplified descriptions in specific contexts have been proposed, in particular by Maxey and Riley [6]. Furthermore, the suspended particles have finite size, and density different from that of the carrier fluid. As a consequence, interactions between the particle and the underlying flow structures plays an important role; it is well known, for instance, that heavy particles are expelled out of vortical structures, while light particles tend to concentrate in their cores, leading to preferential concentration and the formation of strong inhomogeneities in the particle spatial distribution [7].

## 2  Turbulent Pair Diffusion

The relative motion of groups of particles is important to understand phenomena such as dust storms, and pollen dispersion, and the like. This can usually be related to the relative motion of two particles, or pair diffusion. In 1926 Richardson [8] proposed a theory of pair diffusion of fluid particles based upon the idea of a scale dependent pair diffusivity, $K_f(l)$, where $l$ is the distance between two particles, and on the locality hypothesis in which only energy in the turbulent scales which are of a similar size to the pair separation itself is effective in further increasing the pair separation. This yields the 4/3-scaling for the diffusion coefficient, $K_f(l) \sim l^{4/3}$. Obukhov [9] showed that this is equivalent to $\sigma_l^2 = \langle l^2 \rangle \sim t^3$ known as the $t^3-$ regime. $\langle \cdot \rangle$ is the ensemble average. In the ensuing discussions, we follow the usual convention of replacing the scaling on $l$ with its rms value, i.e. $l \sim \sigma_l$.

However, recent studies in turbulent particle pair diffusion [10–13] has suggested that both local and non-local processes govern pair diffusion in high Reynolds number turbulence. For Kolomogrov energy spectrum, $E(k) \sim k^{-5/3}$, $k_1 < k \leq k_\eta$, in the limit of very large inertial subrange, $R_k = k_\eta/k_1 \to \infty$, the theory predicts the scalings, $K_f(l) \sim \sigma_l^\gamma$ where $\gamma > 4/3$; in [10] simulations yielded $K_f(l) \sim \sigma_l^{1.53}$.

## 2.1  Inertial Particles

A natural extension of this new non-local theory is to inertial particles. Diffusion of inertial particle pairs has received less attention than pair diffusion of fluid particles in the past, although a few recent works have appeared such as the DNS of Bec et al. [14] in the limit of Stoke's drag, and Kelken et al. [15] who consider inertial particle pair diffusion in the presence of gravity. Bragg et al. [16, 17] consider the form of the diffusion coefficient in forward and backward time dispersion. Other recent works include [18–21].

In [17], the diffusion coefficient for inertial particles is derived using PDF phase-space theories, and it involves two contributions, one of which is the second order inertial particle-pair relative velocity structure function, which dominates the behavior of the diffusion coefficient for $St \geq O(1)$ in the dissipation range. This structure function is known to have a power law behavior in the dissipation range, where the exponent is related to the correlation dimension for the inertial particle spatial distribution.

Here, our interest is the inertial subrange scalings for the inertial pair diffusion coefficient. We want to examine the extension of the local-non-local concept which was first developed for fluid pair diffusion in the inertial subrange in [10, 12] to inertial particles. As such, we will not be considering dissipation range scaling.

A complete theory of inertia particle transport is unknown, but the theory of Maxey and Riley [6] has gained widespread acceptance. However, even this theory contains up to seven terms, dealing with added mass, density differences, and gravity and memory effects.

Like Bec et al. and others, we consider the simplest case where we neglect all terms except the Stoke's drag term. We investigate numerically turbulent pair diffusion of inertial particles in high Reynolds number turbulence in the limit of large inertial subrange, $R_k \to \infty$, and in the Stokes drag limit. The particle trajectory is then obtained by integrating,

$$\frac{d\mathbf{x}}{dt} = \mathbf{v}(t) \tag{1}$$

$$\frac{d\mathbf{v}}{dt} = -\frac{1}{\tau_p} \left( \mathbf{v}(t) - \mathbf{u}(\mathbf{x}, t) \right) \tag{2}$$

where $\mathbf{u}(\mathbf{x}, t)$ is the fluid velocity at $(\mathbf{x}, t)$, and $\mathbf{v}(t)$ is the particle velocity at the same location and time, and $\tau_p$ is the particle relaxation time which accounts for the particle inertia.

The global Stokes number is,

$$St = \frac{\tau_p}{t_\eta} \tag{3}$$

where $t_\eta \sim \varepsilon^{-1/3} \eta^{2/3}$ is the Kolmogorov time scale of the turbulence. A local Stoke's number depending on the local separation can also be defined,

$$St = \frac{\tau_p}{t_l} \tag{4}$$

where $t_l \sim \varepsilon^{-1/3} l^{2/3}$ is the turbulence time scale at lengths scale $\sim 1/l$. $\varepsilon$ is the rate of energy dissipation per unit mass, and $\eta$ is the Kolmogorov length scale.

Equations (1) and (2) are particle transport equation for inertial particles in a fluid flow – they are not field equations like that for diffusion of a scalar in fluid flow. It is an assumption that turbulent particle transport can be described by a diffusion equation with a scale dependent diffusion coefficient. Similar concerns have been expressed about the correctness of a diffusion equation for turbulent fluid pair diffusion; however, it is accepted that in the limit of point source release, then fluid particle pair diffusion can be described by a diffusion equation.

We extend this idea to inertial particle pair diffusion. We consider an effective point source release of inertial particles and assume that inertial pair diffusion can also be described by a diffusion equation with a scale dependent diffusion coefficient. In the limit to Stoke's drag, the diffusion coefficient will then be a function of two variables, $K_p = K_p(l, St)$.

For small separations, the particle inertia is expected to dominate over the small scale turbulent energy, thus we should observe ballistic motion, and the inertia pair diffusivity should be linear in the separation,

$$K_p(l, St) \sim \sigma_l^1, \qquad \sigma_l \ll \sigma_l^* \tag{5}$$

where $\sigma_l^*$ is the scale where the inertia and turbulent energies are balanced, which is expected to occur when the timescales are equal, i.e. when $St(\sigma_l^*) = 1$, so that $t_{\sigma_l^*} = \tau_p$, [14].

At very large times, the turbulent energy is expected to be dominant, and we expect the inertia pair diffusion to asymptote towards the fluid pair diffusion provided that the inertial subrange is big enough for the pair separation to still remain within the subrange. Thus,

$$K_p(l, St) \rightarrow K_f(l) \sim \sigma_l^{1.53}, \qquad \sigma_l \gg \sigma_l^*. \tag{6}$$

As the Stokes' number increases, we expect the ballistic regime to penetrate further in to the inertial subrange before transition.

## 3 Numerical Simulations

The Lagrangian diffusion model Kinematic Simulations (KS) was used to obtain the statistics of particle pair diffusion. In KS one specifies the second order Eulerian structure function through the power spectrum, [10, 22, 23]. In principle, you can specify any form of spectra, like $E(k) \sim k^{-p}$, $k_1 \leq k \leq k_\eta$ for any $p$; although here we examine Kolmogorov turbulence with $p = 5/3$. KS can generate inertial subranges sufficiently large to test pair diffusion scaling laws over extended inertial subranges.

KS generates turbulent-like non-Markovian particle trajectories by releasing particles in flow fields which are prescribed as sums of energy-weighted random Fourier modes. By construction, the velocity fields are incompressible and the energy is distributed among the different modes by a prescribed Eulerian energy spectrum, $E(k)$. The essential idea behind KS is that the flow structures in it - eddying, straining, and streaming zones - are similar to those observed in turbulent flows, although not precisely the same, which is sufficient to generate turbulent-like particle trajectories.

KS has been used to examine single particle diffusion [24, 25], and pair diffusion [23, 26–29]. KS has also been used in studies of turbulent diffusion of inertial particles [30, 31]. Meneguz and Reeks [30] found that the statistics of the inertial particle segregation in KS generated flow fields for statistically homogeneous isotropic flow fields are similar to those generated by DNS.

KS pair diffusion statistics have been found to produce close agreement with DNS at low Reynolds numbers, incuding the flatness factor of pair separation [28].

However, in the past KS has been criticised for producing pair diffusion scalings that are not consistent with Richardson's 4/3-scaling law [29, 32, 33]. It has been speculated by these authors that this is because KS does not possess the correct dynamical sweeping of the small inertial scales by the large convective scales, leading to larger than expected power law scalings for the diffusion coefficient. However, these concerns have recently been addressed in [10] where a detailed mathematical analysis has shown that such errors are in fact very small, and therefore it is the hypothesis of locality that is in error not KS, an issue that was never addressed by the cited authors.

## 3.1   The KS Velocity Fields and Energy Spectra

An individual Eulerian turbulent flow field realization in KS is generated as a truncated Fourier series,

$$
\mathbf{u}(\mathbf{x}, t) = \sum_{n=1}^{N_k} \left( (\mathbf{A}_n \times \hat{\mathbf{k}}_n) \cos(\mathbf{k}_n \cdot \mathbf{x} + \omega_n t) + (\mathbf{B}_n \times \hat{\mathbf{k}}_n) \sin(\mathbf{k}_n \cdot \mathbf{x} + \omega_n t) \right) \quad (7)
$$

where $N_k$ is the number of representative wavenumbers, typically hundreds for very long spectral ranges, $R_k \gg 1$. $\hat{\mathbf{k}}_n$ is a random unit vector; $\mathbf{k}_n = k_n \hat{\mathbf{k}}_n$ and $k_n = |\mathbf{k}_n|$. The coefficients $\mathbf{A}_n$ and $\mathbf{B}_n$ are chosen such that their orientations are randomly distributed in space and uncorrelated with any other Fourier coefficient or wavenumber, and their amplitudes are determined by $\langle \mathbf{A}_n^2 \rangle = \langle \mathbf{B}_n^2 \rangle \propto E(k_n)dk_n$, where $E(k)$ is the energy spectrum in some wavenumber range $k_1 \leq k \leq k_\eta$. The angled brackets $\langle \cdot \rangle$ denotes the ensemble average over space and over many random flow fields. The associated frequencies are proportional to the eddy-turnover frequencies, $\omega_n = \lambda \sqrt{k_n^3 E(k_n)}$. There is some freedom in the choice of $\lambda$, so long as $0 \leq \lambda < 1$. The construction in Eq. (7) ensures that the Fourier coefficients are normal to their wavevector which automatically ensures incompressibility of each flow realization, $\nabla \cdot u = 0$. The flow field ensemble generated in this manner is statistically homogeneous, isotropic, and stationary.

The energy spectrum $E(k)$ can be chosen freely within a finite range of scales, even a piecewise continuous spectrum, or an isolated single mode are possible. To incorporate the effect of large scale sweeping of the inertial scales by the energy containing scales, the simulations are carried out in the sweeping frame of reference by setting $E(k) = 0$ in the largest scales, for $k < k_1$ [10]. We choose the energy spectrum in the inertial subrange,

$$E(k) = C_k \varepsilon^{2/3} k^{-5/3}, \qquad k_1 \leq k \leq k_\eta \tag{8}$$

where $C_k$ is a constant. The largest represented scale of turbulence is $2\pi/k_1$ and smallest is the Kolmogorov micro-scale $\eta = 2\pi/k_\eta$. A particle trajectory, $\mathbf{x}(t)$, is obtained by solving Eqs. (1) and (2) in time. Pairs of trajectories are harvested from a large ensemble of flow realizations and pair statistics are then obtained from it for analysis.

## 4  Results

We ran KS with the spectrum of $E(k) \sim k^{-5/3}$, for an ensmeble of about 30,000 inertial particle pairs, and the results are presented below for several inertial subranges and for different Stoke's numbers.

Figure 1 shows the pair diffusion coefficient, $K_p/\eta v_\eta$, against the rms separation, $\sigma_l/\eta$. The inertial subrange size is $R_k = 10^1$. Cases for Stokes number of, $St = 0.1, 0.5, 1, 5$ are shown. The $St = 0.1$ case is close to fluid particles, while the $St = 5$ case is far from it. A line of slope 1 is shown for comparison with ballistic motion, and a line of slope $4/3$ is shown for comparison with the Richardson's locality

**Fig. 1** Log-log of the inertial pair diffusion coefficient $K_p/\eta v_\eta$ against the rms pair separation $\sigma_l/\eta$ from KS simulations with energy spectrum $E(k) \sim k^{-5/3}$ and inertial subrange of size $R_k = 10^1$, and for different Stokes numbers $St = 0.1, 0.5, 1.0$, and 5.0

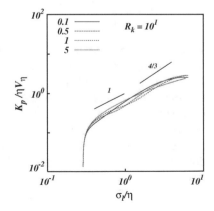

hypothesis. The inertial subrange is short and we observe an approximate inertial subrange scaling only for the smallest Stoke's number; for larger Stoke's number and the ballistic regime penetrates through almost the entire inertial subrange.

Figures 2, 3, and 4 are similar except for the inertial subrange sizes of, $R_k = 10^2$, $10^3$ and $R_k = 10^4$ repectively.

**Fig. 2** Log-log of the inertial pair diffusion coefficient $K_p/\eta v_\eta$ against the rms pair separation $\sigma_l/\eta$ from KS simulations with energy spectrum $E(k) \sim k^{-5/3}$ and inertial subrange of size $R_k = 10^2$, and for different Stokes numbers $St = 0.1, 0.5, 1.0$, and $5.0$

**Fig. 3** Log-log of the inertial pair diffusion coefficient $K_p/\eta v_\eta$ against the rms pair separation $\sigma_l/\eta$ from KS simulations with energy spectrum $E(k) \sim k^{-5/3}$ and inertial subrange of size $R_k = 10^3$, and for different Stokes numbers $St = 0.1, 0.5, 1.0$, and $5.0$

**Fig. 4** Log-log of the inertial pair diffusion coefficient $K_p/\eta v_\eta$ against the rms pair separation $\sigma_l/\eta$ from KS simulations with energy spectrum $E(k) \sim k^{-5/3}$ and inertial subrange of size $R_k = 10^4$, and for different Stokes numbers $St = 0.1, 0.5, 1.0$, and $5.0$

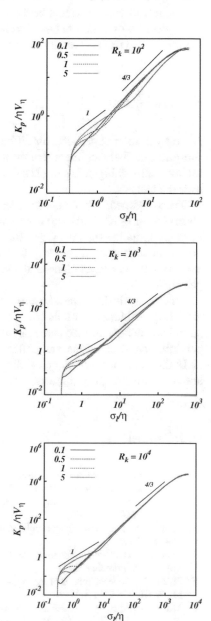

The results show initial ballistic regimes, Eq. (5) that penetrate further in to the inertial subrange as Stoke's number increases. The long time fluid pair diffusion, Eq. (6) is less clear – it will require bigger subrange to fully confirm – nevertheless the diffusion coefficient appears to be asymptoting in the correct manner towards the fluid non-local regime $K_p \to K_f \sim \sigma_L^{1.53}$ as $R_k \to \infty$, [10, 12].

The results also show that between the two asymptotic cases, there exists a transition over an extended range of scales which is so long that it qualifies as a third regime in own right – the transition regime.

## 5  Discussion

A theory of inertial particle pair diffusion has been developed in which we predict a short time ballistic regime where the inertia is dominant, and a long time asymptotic regime approaching fluid particle pair diffusion where the turbulent energy dominates over the inertia.

These regimes for Kolmogorov energy spectrum, $E(k) \sim k^{-5/3}$, have been broadly observed using KS, although it will take larger inertial subranges to fully confirm. For very large inertial subranges, the long time regime approches the fluid particle non-local scaling predicted in [10, 12], which vindicates our inital assumption of extending the concept of local and non-local diffusional processes to inertial particle pair diffusion.

This study is important because of its possible application to the theory and modeling of inertial particle transport and to the spreading of groups of inertial particles. Such phenomena are ubiguitous in nature such as in, the spread of clouds, percipitation, dust storms, and pollen dispersion, and much more.

In the future we will complete the paramteric study for larger inertial subranges, and for more generalised inverse power law energy spectra.

## References

1. Calzavarini, E., Kerscher, M., Lohse, D., Toschi, F.: Dimensionality and morphology of particle and bubble clusters in turbulent flow. J. Fluid Mech. **607**, 1324 (2008)
2. Falkovich, G., Pumir, A.: Sling effect in collision of water droplet in turbulent clouds. J. Atm. Sci. **64**, 44974505 (2007)
3. Shaw, R.A.: Particle-turbulence interactions in atmospheric clouds. Ann. Rev. Fluid Mech. **35**, 183227 (2003)
4. Sofiev, M.: Airborne pollen transport. In: Sofiev, M., Bergmann, K.C. (eds.) Allergenic Pollen. Springer, Dordrecht (2013)
5. Toschi, F., Bodenschatz, E.: Lagrangian properties of particles in turbulence. Ann. Rev. Fluid Mech. **41**, 375404 (2009)
6. Maxey, M.R., Riley, J.R.: Equation of motion for a small rigid sophere in a non-uniform flow. Phys. Fluids **26**, 883 (1983). https://doi.org/10.1063/1.864230

7. Qureshi, N.M., Bourgoin, M., Baudet, C., Cartellier, A., Gagne, Y.: Turbulent transport of material particles: an experimental study of finite size effects. Phys. Rev. Lett. **99**, 184502 (2007)
8. Richardson, L.F.: Atmospheric diffusion shown on a distance-neighbour graph. Proc. Roy. Soc. Lond. A **100**, 709–737 (1926)
9. Obukhov, A.: Spectral energy distribution in a turbulent flow. Izv. Akad. Xauk. SSSR. Ser. Geogr. i Geojz **5**, 453–466 (1941). (Translation : Ministry of Supply. p. 21 1097)
10. Malik, N.A.: Residual sweeping errors in turbulent pair diffusion in a Lagrangian diffusion model. PLoS ONE **12**(12), e0189917 (2017). https://doi.org/10.1371/journal.pone.0189917
11. Malik N.A.: Ninety years in the hunt for turbulent pair diffusion laws. IMA Conference on Turbulence, Waves and Mixing. 6–8 July, Cambridge (2016)
12. Malik, N.A.: Turbulent Particle Pair Diffusion: a theory based on local and non-local diffusional processes. Accepted on August 14 for publication in PLoS ONE, to appear soon (2018)
13. Malik, N.A.: Turbulent particle pair diffusion: numerical simulations. submitted to Plos One (2018)
14. Bec, J., Biferale, L., Lanotte, A., Scagliarini, A., Toschi, F.: J. Fluid Mech. **645**, 497 (2010)
15. Chang, K., Benedict, J.M., Shaw, R.A.: Turbulent pair dispersion in the presence of gravity. New J. Phys. **17**(3), 033010 (2015)
16. Bragg, A.D., Ireland, P.J., Collins, L.R.: Forward and backward in time dispersion of fluid and inertial particles in isotropic turbulence. Phys. Fluids **28**(1) (2016)
17. Bragg, A.D.: Analysis of the forward and backward in time pair-separation probability density functions for inertial particles in isotropic turbulence. J. Fluid Mech. **830**, 63–92 (2017)
18. Bec, J., Biferale, L., Cencini, M., Lanotte, A.S., Toschi, F.: Intermittency in the velocity distribution of heavy particles in turbulence. J. Fluid Mech. **646**, 527536 (2010)
19. Gustavsson, K., Mehlig, B.: Distribution of relative velocities in turbulent aerosols. Phys. Rev. E **84**, 045304 (2011)
20. Gustavsson, K., Vajedi, S., Mehlig, B.: Clustering of particles falling in a turbulent flow. Phys. Rev. Lett. **112**, 214501 (2014)
21. Bragg, A.D., Collins, L.R.: New insights from comparing statistical theories for inertial particles in turbulence: II. relative velocities of particles. New J. Phys. **16**, 055014 (2014)
22. Kraichnan, R.H.: Diffusion by a random velocity field. Phys. Fluids **13**, 22–31 (1970)
23. Fung, J.C.H., Hunt, J.C.R., Malik, N.A., Perkins, R.J.: Kinematic simulation of homogeneous turbulence by unsteady random Fourier modes. J. Fluid Mech. **236**, 281 (1992)
24. Turfus, C., Hunt, J.C.R.: A stochastic analysis of the displacements of fluid element in inhomogeneous turbulence using Kraichnan's method of random modes. In: Comte-Bellot, G., Mathieu, J. (eds.) Advances in Turbulence, pp. 191–203. Springer, Berlin (1987)
25. Murray, S., Lightstone, M.F., Tullis, S.: Single-particle Lagrangian and structure statistics in kinematically simulated particle-laden turbulent flows. Phys. Fuids **28**, 033302 (2016)
26. Malik N.A. :Structural diffusion in 2D and 3D random flows. In: S. Gavrilakis et al. (eds.) Adv. in Turbulence vol. VI, pp. 619–620 (1996)
27. Fung, J.C.H., Vassilicos, J.C.: Two-particle dispersion in turbulent-like flows. Phys. Rev. E **57**, 1677 (1998)
28. Malik, N.A., Vassilicos, J.C.: A Lagrangian model for turbulent dispersion with turbulent-like flow structure: comparison with direct numerical simulation for two-particle statistics. Phys. Fluids **11**, 1572–1580 (1999)
29. Nicolleau, F.C.G.A., Nowakowski, A.F.: Presence of a Richardson's regime in kinematic simulations. Phys. Rev. E **83**, 056317 (2011)
30. Meneguz, E., Reeks, M.W.: Statistical properties of particle segregation in homogeneous isotropic turbulence. J. Fluid Mech. **686**, 338–351 (2011)
31. Farhan, M., Nicolleau, F.C.G.A., Nowakowski, A.F.: Effect of gravity on clustering patterns and inertial particle attractors in kinematic simulations. Phys. Rev. E **91**, 043021 (2001)
32. Thomson, D.J., Devenish, B.J.: Particle pair separation in kinematic simulations. J. Fluid Mech. **526**, 277–302 (2005)
33. Eyink, G.L., Benveniste, D.: Suppression of particle dispersion by sweeping effects in synthetic turbulence. Phys. Rev. E **87**, 023011 (2013)

# Coupled Axial, In Plane and Out of Plane Bending Vibrations of Cable Harnessed Space Structures

**Karthik Yerrapragada and Armaghan Salehian**

**Abstract** A distributed parameter model is presented to study the effect of a cable harness on the vibration characteristics of space structures. A cable is attached at an offset distance along the beam. Positioning the cable at an offset position induces coupling between various coordinates of motion such as the in plane bending, out of plane bending and the axial modes. The system is modeled using energy methods and the governing coupled partial differential equations of the cable harnessed beam are developed using the Extended Hamilton's principle. The natural frequencies obtained from the coupled and decoupled partial differential equations are compared to the natural frequencies obtained from the Finite Element Analysis formulation.

**Keywords** Cabled beam · Coupled vibrations · Straight cable harness

## 1 Introduction

Cables account for about 10–30% of the total weight of modern day spacecraft [1]. Many researchers in the recent past reported that these cables play a significant role on the dynamic behaviour of the whole structure. To obtain a deeper physical insight into the problem, Refs. [1, 2] model both the host structures and cables as beams. Goodding et al. [3] attached the cable to the beam with the help of tie-down structures and determined the dynamic response of the cabled-beam using the Finite Element Analysis (FEA).

The goal of current work is to develop a distributed parameter model as they are computationally less expensive and can be used for feedback control applications. Choi et al. [4] and Spak et al. [5] developed distributed parameter models to study the out-of-plane bending vibrations of cable harnessed beams. Continuum model

K. Yerrapragada (✉) · A. Salehian
University of Waterloo, Waterloo, ON N2L 3G1, Canada
e-mail: kyerrapr@uwaterloo.ca

A. Salehian
e-mail: salehian@uwaterloo.ca

© Springer Nature Switzerland AG 2018
D. M. Kilgour et al. (eds.), *Recent Advances in Mathematical and Statistical Methods*, Springer Proceedings in Mathematics & Statistics 259, https://doi.org/10.1007/978-3-319-99719-3_23

developed by Martin et al. [6, 7] assume the host structure behaves as a Euler-Bernoulli beam and the authors include the effect of pre-tension and Young's modulus of the cable. The bending stiffness of the cable is assumed negligible by Martin et al. [6–8]. The analytical models of Refs. [4–8] neglect the effect of coupling between various coordinates of motion.

This research builds on the continuum model developed by Martin et al. [6–8]. In the current work, the cable is attached at an offset distance along the beam and we seek to investigate the effect of coupling in the structure between various vibration degrees of freedom such as the in-plane bending, out-of-plane bending and the axial modes using Euler Bernoulli (EB) theory. The continuum model is developed using linearized displacement field and higher degree strain tensor. Hamilton's principle [9] is used to develop the coupled partial differential equations of the cable-harnessed beam. Complex exponential method developed by Salehian et al. [10–16] is used to find the natural frequencies of the cabled structure from the coupled partial differential equations. Finally, the natural frequencies obtained from the decoupled analytical model and coupled analytical model are compared to the Finite Element Analysis (FEA) results.

## 2 Mathematical Modeling

Figure 1 shows the schematic of cable harnessed structure along with the coordinate axes. The cable is positioned, at an offset distance along the y-axis. To develop the continuum model of the cable-harnessed structure, the following assumptions [7] apply:

1. The cable stays in contact with the beam at all times while the structure vibrates.
2. The strain and kinetic energies of the cable at the centroid of the cross-section are equal to the strain and kinetic energies at other points of its cross-section.

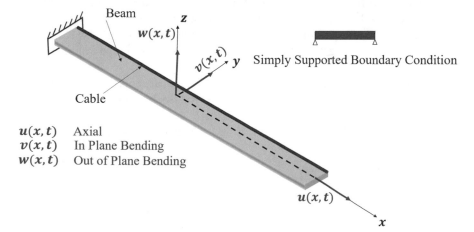

**Fig. 1** Representation of the cable harness beam along with the coordinate axes

3. The cable is assumed to be pre-tensioned and it is also assumed that the tension in the cable induces pre-compression in the beam.

The procedure to develop the continuum model for the cable-harnessed beam is outlined in the next few steps. The linearized three-dimensional displacement field using Euler-Bernoulli (EB) beam theory is given by Stoykov et al. [17] and shown in Eq. (1)

$$
\begin{aligned}
X\,(x, y, z, t) &= u\,(x, t) - y\frac{\partial v(x,t)}{\partial x} - z\frac{\partial w(x,t)}{\partial x} \\
Y\,(x, y, z, t) &= v\,(x, t) \\
Z\,(x, y, z, t) &= w\,(x, t)
\end{aligned}
\tag{1}
$$

where $u\,(x, t)$, $v\,(x, t)$, $w\,(x, t)$ are the motions in the axial, in-plane bending and out-of-plane bending respectively. The expressions for Green-Lagrange strain tensor are as [17] (Eq. 2). A beam is a structure whose length is significantly larger than the width and thickness, the direct strains in the $y$ and $z$ directions can be neglected [18].

$$
\varepsilon_{xx} = \frac{\partial X}{\partial x} + \frac{1}{2}\left(\frac{\partial X}{\partial x}\right)^2 + \frac{1}{2}\left(\frac{\partial Y}{\partial x}\right)^2 + \frac{1}{2}\left(\frac{\partial Z}{\partial x}\right)^2
\tag{2}
$$

where $\varepsilon_{xx}$ is the direct strain in the $x$ direction.

$$
U = \frac{1}{2}[\iiint_V E_c(\varepsilon_{xx})_c{}^2]dV + \frac{1}{2}[\iiint_V E_b(\varepsilon_{xx})_b{}^2]dV
\tag{3}
$$

The strain induced in the cable and beam as result of pre-tension $T$ in the cable and pre-compression in the beam are $(\varepsilon_{xx})_c = T/E_cA_c + \varepsilon_{xx}$ and $(\varepsilon_{xx})_b = -T/E_bA_b + \varepsilon_{xx}$ respectively. The negative sign in $(\varepsilon_{xx})_b$ is because of pre-compression induced in the beam due to tension in the cable. $E_b$ is the Young's Modulus of the beam. $E_c$ is the Young's Modulus of the cable. $T$ is the pre-tension in the cable. $A_b$ is the area of the cross-section of the beam and $A_c$ is the area of cross-section of the cable. where $I_{zz}$ and $I_{yy}$ are the area moment of inertia of the beam about z-axis and y-axis respectively. $\rho_b$ is the density of the beam. $\rho_c$ is the density of the cable. $y_c$ and $z_c$ are the position coordinates of the cable. The strain and kinetic energy expressions for a cable harnessed Euler-Bernoulli are as follows.

$$
U = \frac{1}{2}\int_0^l [b_1(u')^2 + b_2(v'')^2 + b_3(w'')^2 + 2b_4(v'')(w'') + 2b_5(u')(v'')
$$
$$
+ 2b_6(u')(w'')]dx
\tag{4}
$$

$$
T = \frac{1}{2}\int_0^l [k_1(\dot{u})^2 + k_2(\dot{v})^2 + k_3(\dot{w})^2]dx
\tag{5}
$$

The constants of the above strain and kinetic energy expressions are as follows:

$$b_1 = E_b A_b + E_c A_c$$
$$b_2 = E_b I_{zz} + E_c A_c y_c^2 + T y_c^2 - \frac{T I_{zz}}{A_b}$$
$$b_3 = E_b I_{yy} + E_c A_c z_c^2 + T z_c^2 - \frac{T I_{yy}}{A_b}$$
$$b_4 = E_c A_c y_c z_c + T y_c z_c$$
$$b_5 = (E_c A_c + T)(-y_c)$$
$$b_6 = (E_c A_c + T)(-z_c)$$
$$k_1 = \rho_b A_b + \rho_c A_c$$
$$k_2 = \rho_b A_b + \rho_c A_c$$
$$k_3 = \rho_b A_b + \rho_c A_c \tag{6}$$

where superscript dash $()'$ denotes partial derivative with respect to spatial coordinate $x(\frac{\partial}{\partial x})$ and superscript dot $()$ denotes partial derivative with respect to time $t(\frac{\partial}{\partial t})$.

It is assumed there are no external loads acting on the system. Therefore, the Lagrangian of the system is $L = T - U$. As per Hamilton's principle, $\delta \int_{t_1}^{t_2} L \, dt = 0$ gives the governing partial differential equations of the system.

$$- k_1 \ddot{u} + b_1 u'' + b_5 v''' + b_6 w''' = 0 \tag{7}$$

$$- k_2 \ddot{v} - b_2 v'''' - b_5 u''' - b_4 w'''' = 0 \tag{8}$$

$$-k_3 \ddot{w} - b_3 w'''' - b_6 u''' - b_4 v'''' = 0 \tag{9}$$

The boundary conditions for a simply-supported end are as follows.

$$u = v = w = 0|_{x=0 \ or \ l}$$
$$b_2 v'' + b_4 w'' + b_5 u' = 0|_{x=0 \ or \ l}$$
$$b_3 w'' + b_4 v'' + b_6 u' = 0|_{x=0 \ or \ l} \tag{10}$$

The general solution to the coupled PDEs is assumed as follows.

$$\begin{Bmatrix} u \\ v \\ w \end{Bmatrix} = \begin{Bmatrix} U \\ V \\ W \end{Bmatrix} e^{\alpha x} e^{i\omega t} \tag{11}$$

The temporal solution of the PDEs is assumed to be harmonic (represented by the complex exponential $e^{i\omega t}$) and the spatial solution is assumed to be of the form $e^{\alpha x}$. Where $\omega$ is the frequency and $\alpha$ is the mode shape parameter. Substituting Eq. (11) in Eqs. (7)–(9), we obtain three simultaneous algebraic equations which are converted into matrix form as follows.

$$[A]_{3 \times 3} \begin{Bmatrix} U \\ V \\ W \end{Bmatrix}_{3 \times 1} = \{0\}_{3 \times 1} \tag{12}$$

where $[A]$ is given by:
$$\begin{bmatrix} b_1 \alpha^2 + k_1 \omega^2 & b_6 \alpha^3 & b_5 \alpha^3 \\ b_5 \alpha^3 & -b_2 \alpha^4 + k_2 \omega^2 & -b_4 \alpha^4 \\ b_6 \alpha^3 & -b_4 \alpha^4 & -b_3 \alpha^4 + k_3 \omega^2 \end{bmatrix}.$$

For non-trivial solution, the determinant $|A(\alpha, \omega)| = 0$, we then get a polynomial in terms of mode shape parameter $\alpha$ and frequency $\omega$. Solving the above polynomial, we get ten roots for $\alpha$ in terms of $\omega$.

We know from Eq. (12) that

$$a_{31} U + a_{32} V + a_{33} W = 0 \tag{13}$$

where $a_{3i}$ for $i \rightarrow 1$ to 3 represent the elements of the third row of matrix $[A]$. For the linear dependency between $U$, $V$ and $W$ to be satisfied, the spatial solutions for different coordinates of motion should be as follows.

$$U_n = \left| (-1)^{3+1} M_{31} \right|$$
$$V_n = \left| (-1)^{3+2} M_{32} \right|$$
$$W_n = \left| (-1)^{3+3} M_{33} \right| \tag{14}$$

where $M_{3i}$ for $i \rightarrow 1$ to 3 represent the minors of the elements $a_{3i}$ for $i \rightarrow 1$ to 3 of matrix $[A]$. The general solution of the coupled PDEs is expanded as follows.

$$\begin{Bmatrix} u(x, t) \\ v(x, t) \\ w(x, t) \end{Bmatrix} = \sum_{n=1}^{10} d_n \begin{Bmatrix} U_n(\alpha = \alpha_n) \\ V_n(\alpha = \alpha_n) \\ W_n(\alpha = \alpha_n) \end{Bmatrix} e^{\alpha_n x} e^{i\omega t} \tag{15}$$

where $d_n$ is a solution constant for $n \rightarrow 1$ to 10. At each end of the beam, we need five boundary conditions. The boundary conditions for a simply-supported end is given by Eq. (10). After applying the boundary conditions, we would end up with ten simultaneous algebraic equations and after casting them into matrix form, we obtain

$$[L(\omega)]_{10 \times 10} \left\{ \vec{d} \right\}_{10 \times 1} = \{0\}_{10 \times 1} \tag{16}$$

where $\vec{d} = \{d_1, d_2, d_3, d_4, d_5, d_6, d_7, d_8, d_9, d_{10}\}^T$.

For non-trivial solution, the determinant of the matrix $[L(\omega)]_{10 \times 10}$ should be set to zero. The determinant results in a transcendental equation in terms of $\omega$, the roots of which give the natural frequency.

# 3 Results and Discussions

In this section, for the cable-harnessed beam shown in Fig. 1, the natural frequencies of the coupled analytical model, decoupled analytical model and the finite element analysis are presented and compared against each other.

The cross-section of the beam is assumed to be rectangular and the cross-section of the cable is assumed to be circular. The structure is assumed to be simply-supported at both the ends. The parameters used in the numerical simulations are presented in Table 1. Where $l$ is the length of the beam. $b$ is the width of the beam. $h$ is the thickness of the beam. $r_c$ is the radius of the cable. As depicted in Fig. 1, the cable is positioned at an offset distance of $y_c = \frac{b}{2} - r$. First, using the parameters shown in Table 1, the natural frequencies corresponding to the out-of-plane, the in-plane bending and the axial modes are calculated by solving the decoupled partial differential equations and are presented in the first column of Table 2.

The notations in the Table 2 OP, IP and A stand for out of plane bending, in-plane bending and the axial degrees of freedom respectively. The natural frequencies obtained from coupled set of partial differential equations are presented in the third column of Table 2. The results obtained from the finite element analysis are presented in column 4 of Table 2. The frequencies obtained from the coupled and decoupled analytical are compared to those of finite element analysis and the resulting error percentages are presented in the last two columns of Table 2. The mode shapes corresponding to all the natural frequencies are shown in Fig. 2. For the first two modes, the out-of-plane bending is dominant and for the third mode, the in-plane bending is dominant. The mode shape for higher frequency where the axial mode is dominant

**Table 1** Numerical parameters of the cable and the beam

| Beam parameters | Cable parameters |
|---|---|
| $l = 0.25$ m; $b = 0.01$ m; $h = 0.0015$ m; | $T = 25$ N; $r_c = 0.7$ mm; |
| $E_b = 68.9 \times 10^9$ N/m$^2$; $\rho_b = 2700$ kg/m$^3$ | $E_c = 150 \times 10^9$ N/m$^2$; |
| | $\rho_c = 1400$ kg/m$^3$; |
| | $z_c = \frac{h}{2} + r_c$; $y_c = \frac{b}{2} - r_c$ |

**Table 2** Natural frequencies, simply supported boundary condition

| Decoupled nat. Frequency (Hz) | Mode no | Coupled nat. Frequency (Hz) | FEA nat. Frequency (Hz) | Error % decoupled and FEA | Error % coupled and FEA |
|---|---|---|---|---|---|
| 100.29 OP1 | 1 | 86.3575 | 86.32 | 13.9296 | 0.0434 |
| 401.18 OP2 | 2 | 334.243 | 334.03 | 16.7381 | 0.0637 |
| 436.76 IP1 | 3 | 436.562 | 434.98 | 0.4075 | 0.3624 |
| 10889.0 A1 | Higher | 10797.1 | 10783.9 | 0.9652 | 0.1223 |

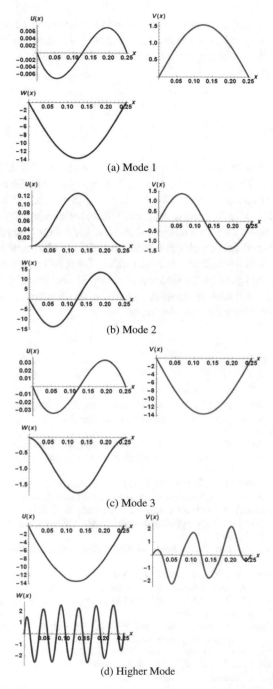

(a) Mode 1

(b) Mode 2

(c) Mode 3

(d) Higher Mode

**Fig. 2** Coupled vibration mode shapes for a simply supported boundary condition

is also shown in Fig. 2.The frequencies obtained from the coupled partial differential equations are lower than that of the decoupled model. The natural frequencies of the coupled model match very well with that of finite element analysis when compared to the decoupled model.

# 4 Conclusion

A distributed parameter model was presented to study the vibrations of a cable-harnessed structure. The mathematical model took into account the effect of coupling between various coordinates of motion such as the in-plane, out-of-plane bending and the axial modes. The coupled set of partial differential equations were solved for the natural frequencies using the analytical method for a simply supported boundary condition. The natural frequencies obtained from the coupled model and decoupled model were compared to the finite element model. The results demonstrate that when the cable is positioned at an offset distance, the coupling between various coordinates of motion is significant and the coupled distributed parameter model predicted the natural frequencies better than the decoupled model.

# References

1. Coombs, D.M., Goodding, J.C., Babuska, V., Ardelean, E.V., Robertson, L.M., Lane, S.A.: Dynamic modeling and experimental validation of a cable-loaded panel. J. Spacecraft Rockets **48**, 958–973 (2011)
2. Goodding, J.C., Ardelean, E.V., Babuška, V., Robertson III, L.M., Lane, S.A.: Experimental techniques and structural parameter estimation studies of spacecraft cables. J. Spacecraft Rockets **48**, 942–957 (2011)
3. Goodding, J.C., Babuška, V., Griffith, D.T., Ingram, B.R., Robertson, L.: Study of free-free beam structural dynamics perturbations due to mounted cable harnesses. In: Proceedings of the 48th aiaa/asme/asch/ahs/asc sdm conference, honolulu, hi (2007)
4. Choi, J., Inman, D.J.: Spectrally formulated modeling of a cable-harnessed structure. J. Sound Vib. **333**, 3286–3304 (2014)
5. Spak, K., Agnes, G., Inman, D.: Parameters for modeling stranded cables as structural beams. Exp. Mech. **54**, 1613–1626 (2014)
6. Martin, B., Salehian, A.: Dynamic modelling of cable-harnessed beam structures with periodic wrapping patterns: a homogenization approach. Int. J. Modell. Simul. **33**, 185–202 (2013)
7. Martin, B., Salehian, A.: Mass and stiffness effects of harnessing cables on structural dynamics: continuum modeling. AIAA J. (2016)
8. Martin, B., Salehian, A.: Homogenization modeling of periodically wrapped string-harnessed beam structures: experimental validation. AIAA J. (2016)
9. Rao, S.S.: Vibration of Continuous Systems. Wiley (2007)
10. Salehian, A., Cliff, E.M., Inman, D.J.: Continuum modeling of an innovative space-based radar antenna truss. J. Aerospace Eng. **19**, 227–240 (2006)
11. Salehian, A., Inman, D.J.: Dynamic analysis of a lattice structure by homogenization: experimental validation. J. Sound Vib. **316**, 180–197 (2008)
12. Salehian, A., Seigler, T.M., Inman, D.J.: Dynamic effects of a radar panel mounted on a truss satellite. AIAA J. **45** (2007)

13. Salehian, A., Inman, D.: Micropolar continuous modeling and frequency response validation of a lattice structure. J. Vib. Acoust. **132**, 011010 (2010)
14. Salehian, A., Inman, D.J., Cliff, E.M.: Natural frequency validation of a homogenized model of a truss. In: Proceedings of the xxiv-international modal analysis conference (2006)
15. Salehian, A., Chen, Y.: On strain-rate dependence of kinetic energy in homogenization approach: theory and experiment. AIAA J. **50**, 2029–2033 (2012)
16. Salehian, A., Inman, D.J.: Thermally induced oscillations of an inflatable space structure with a repeated element pattern. Int. J. Acoust. Vib. **16**, 3 (2011)
17. Stoykov, S., Ribeiro, P.: Nonlinear forced vibrations and static deformations of 3d beams with rectangular cross section: the influence of warping, shear deformation and longitudinal displacements. Int. J. Mechanical Sci. **52**, 1505–1521 (2010)
18. Stoykov, S., Ribeiro, P.: Vibration analysis of rotating 3d beams by the pversion finite element method. Finite Elem. Anal. Des. **65**, 76–88 (2013)

# Part IV
# Mathematical Modelling and Computation in Physical and Chemical Sciences

# A Comparison of the Magnus Expansion and Other Solvers for the Chemical Master Equation with Variable Rates

**Khanh Dinh and Roger Sidje**

**Abstract** Many traditional approaches for solving the chemical master equation (CME) cannot be used in their basic form when reaction rates change over time, for instance due to cell volume or temperature. One technique is to use the Magnus expansion to represent the solution to the CME as the action of a matrix exponential, for which Krylov-based approximation methods can be applied. In this paper, we compare two variants of the Magnus scheme with some popular ordinary differential equations (ODE) solvers, such as Adams-Bashforth, Runge-Kutta and Backward-differentiation formula (BDF). Our numerical tests show that the Magnus variants are remarkably efficient at computing the transient probability distributions of a transcriptional regulatory system where propensities vary over time due to cell volume increase.

**Keywords** Chemical master equation · Magnus expansion · Matrix exponential

## 1 Introduction

Consider a chemical reaction system consisting of $N$ molecular species $S_1, \ldots, S_N$ that interact through $M$ reactions. The *reaction rates* $c_k(t)$ are time-dependent scale factors for how likely the reaction $k$ occurs at time $t$. The *state vector* of the system is defined as

$$x(t) = (x_1, \ldots, x_N)^T,$$

K. Dinh (✉) · R. Sidje
Department of Mathematics, University of Alabama, Tuscaloosa, USA
e-mail: kdinh@crimson.ua.edu

R. Sidje
e-mail: roger.b.sidje@ua.edu

© Springer Nature Switzerland AG 2018
D. M. Kilgour et al. (eds.), *Recent Advances in Mathematical and Statistical Methods*, Springer Proceedings in Mathematics & Statistics 259,
https://doi.org/10.1007/978-3-319-99719-3_24

where $x_l$ is the count for species $S_l$ at time $t$. The *propensity function* $\alpha_k(x(t), t)$ of reaction $R_k$ at the current state $x(t)$ and current time $t$ is defined so that the probability of such a reaction occurring during the infinitesimal time interval $[t, t + dt)$ is equal to $\alpha_k(x(t), t)dt$. If the reaction occurs, the state vector is updated as $x(t) := x(t) + v_k$, where the *stoichiometric vector* $v_k$ stores the changes in species counts.

The chemical master equation (CME) [1] seeks $P(x, t) = \text{Prob}\{x(t) = x\}$, the probability that the system is in state $x$ at time $t$:

$$\frac{dP(x, t)}{dt} = \sum_{k=1}^{M} \alpha_k(x - v_k, t) P(x - v_k, t) - \sum_{k=1}^{M} \alpha_k(x, t) P(x, t). \quad (1)$$

Let $X = \{x_1, \ldots, x_n\}$ be the ordered set of $n$ possible states, where $x_i = (x_{1i}, \ldots, x_{Ni})^T$. We can rewrite (1) as a system of ordinary differential equations (ODEs) governing the change in $p(t) = (P(x_1, t), \ldots, P(x_n, t))^T$ from the known initial distribution $p_0$:

$$\begin{cases} \dot{p}(t) = A(t) \cdot p(t), \\ p(0) = p_0, \end{cases} \quad (2)$$

where the transition rate matrix $A(t) = [a_{ij}(t)] \in \mathbb{R}^{n \times n}$ is defined as

$$a_{ij} = \begin{cases} -\sum_{k=1}^{M} \alpha_k(x_j, t), & \text{if } i = j, \\ \alpha_k(x_j, t), & \text{if } x_i = x_j + v_k, \\ 0, & \text{otherwise.} \end{cases}$$

Note that $A$ changes over time due to the time-dependency of the reaction rates $c_k$.

The state space $X$ can be infinite in theory, but is kept finite in practice, although $n$ can be very large. In this case, we can apply the finite state projection (FSP) [2], which reduces the state space to only the probable states during the time period of interest. The vectors $p(t)$, $p_0$ and matrix $A(t)$ in (2) are then truncated to only values of this reduced finite state space. It is important to note that the CME is traditionally solved indirectly by drawing a large number of trajectories from Monte Carlo methods, such as the stochastic simulation algorithm (SSA) [3] or first reaction method (FRM) [4], and then computing the frequency at the desired time point. Their resulting error is statistical, in contrast to the analytical bound on the error when the CME is solved directly by employing the FSP. We only consider solving the CME directly in this study, and the results are compared against the frequencies from a large number of FRM trajectories.

We will discuss different approaches for solving the ODE system (2) in the next sections. For convenience, we will denote the ODE problem as

$$\dot{p}(t) = f(t, p(t)) \equiv A(t) \cdot p(t).$$

## 2 ODE Solvers

### 2.1 Adams

Adams methods form a family of linear multi-step methods, among which are explicit Adams-Bashforth and implicit Adams-Moulton. We use the **ADAMS-PECE** scheme by Shampine and Gordon [5], which implements the implicit Adams-Moulton according to

$$t_{k+1} = t_k + h_k,$$
$$p_{k+1} = p_k + h_k \left( \beta_r^{AM} f_{k+1} + \beta_{r-1}^{AM} f_k + \cdots + \beta_0^{AM} f_{k-r+1} \right),$$
$$f_{k+1} = f(t_{k+1}, p_{k+1}),$$

where $\{\beta_i^{AM}\}_{i=0}^r$ are given analytically. The unknown $p_{k+1} \approx p(t_{k+1})$ is involved in both sides of the formula, leading to a nonlinear problem that is solved with a fixed-point scheme starting from the solution of the explicit Adams-Bashforth.

### 2.2 Runge-Kutta

Runge-Kutta methods form a class of multistage, one-step iteration ODE solvers. The explicit Runge-Kutta of order $r$ proceeds with

$$t_{k+1} = t_k + h_k,$$
$$y_i = p_k + h_k \sum_{j=1}^{i-1} m_{ij}^{RK} f(t_k + h_k c_j^{RK}, y_j); \quad i = 1, \ldots, r,$$
$$p_{k+1} = p_k + h_k \sum_{j=1}^{r} b_j^{RK} f\left(t_k + h_k c_j^{RK}, y_j\right),$$

in which the coefficients $\left\{m_{ij}^{RK}\right\}_{i,j=1}^s$, $\{b_i^{RK}\}_{i=1}^s$ and $\{c_i^{RK}\}_{i=1}^s$ are defined by the Butcher-tableau.

In this comparison, we use the solver **RK78** from the RKSUITE by Brankin et al. [6], which is a reputed Runge-Kutta method that controls the error and stepsize by using embedded Runge-Kutta formulae with orders 7 and 8.

### 2.3 Backward-Differentiation Formula

Backward-differentiation formula (BDF) methods are linear multi-step and follow the formula of order $r$:

$$t_{k+1} = t_k + h_k,$$
$$p_{k+1} = h_k \beta_r^{BDF} f(t_{k+1}, p_{k+1}) + \alpha_{r-1}^{BDF} f_k + \cdots + \alpha_0^{BDF} f_{k-r+1},$$
$$f_{k+1} = f(t_{k+1}, p_{k+1}),$$

where the coefficients $\{\alpha_i^{BDF}\}_{i=0}^{r-1}$ and $\beta_r^{BDF}$ are given analytically. The formula forms a nonlinear problem, because $p_{k+1}$ appears on both sides.

We use the VODPK/BDF implementation [7] which has different options for solving the nonlinear problem:

1. **BDF-FI**: directly by functional iteration.
2. **BDF-GM-LU**: Newton root finding scheme; each linear system during the scheme is solved by SPIGMR (Scaled Preconditioned Incomplete GMRES), preconditioned by the LU decomposition.
3. **BDF-GM-LU0**: Newton root finding scheme; SPIGMR preconditioned by the incomplete LU decomposition, which discards elements not in the sparsity pattern of $A$.
4. **BDF-LU**: each linear system during the Newton scheme is solved directly by LU decomposition.
5. **BDF-LU0**: the linear system is solved directly by incomplete LU decomposition.

## 3   The Magnus-Based Methods

### 3.1   *Magnus Expansion*

The Magnus expansion [8] seeks to express the solution to (2) in the form of

$$p(t) = \exp(\boldsymbol{\Omega}(t)) \cdot p_0, \tag{3}$$

where $\boldsymbol{\Omega}(t)$ is an infinite series consisting of integrals and matrix commutators of $A(t)$.

Originally a theoretical method in physics, there has been increasing interest to transform the Magnus expansion into a numerical solver for initial value problems (IVPs) in the form of (2). One such approach [9, 10], denoted **MAGNUS** in our comparative tests, truncates the Magnus series after 4 terms and approximates the integrals by the Gauss-Legendre quadrature, resulting in a fourth-order numerical scheme with constant stepsize $h$:

$$t_{k+1} = t_k + h,$$
$$A_1 = A\left(t_k + \left(\tfrac{1}{2} - \tfrac{\sqrt{3}}{6}\right)h\right), \quad A_2 = A\left(t_k + \left(\tfrac{1}{2} + \tfrac{\sqrt{3}}{6}\right)h\right),$$
$$\sigma = \tfrac{h}{2}(A_1 + A_2) + \tfrac{h\sqrt{3}}{12}(A_2 A_1 - A_1 A_2),$$
$$p_{k+1} = \exp(\sigma) \cdot p_k,$$

We approximate $p_{k+1}$ by the matrix-free Krylov technique of EXPOKIT that only uses the action of $\sigma$ on vectors. See [11] for more details, and also [12] for a comparison with traditional ODE solvers in the context where $A$ is time-independent, i.e. constant, in (2).

## 3.2 Magnus with an Adaptive SSA-based State Space

During the integration time of any ODE solver for (2), most of the values in $p(t)$ will be extremely small and therefore computing the full distribution can be expensive without gaining much accuracy. For CME problems with time-independent rates, the FSP-SSA method [13] reduces the state space $X$ at each step to only states with potentially large probabilities during the small interval $[t_k, t_k + h]$. This is done by running SSA trajectories [3] from states in the current state space, and updating the state space to contain all states that the SSA trajectories travel through. The 'holes' in the state space are then patched by the $r$-step reachability [2], which seeks all states that can be connected to the state space with $r$ reactions or less, and expands the state space to include those. We incorporate this adaptive SSA-based state space expansion scheme into the **MAGNUS-SSA** method:

$$t_{k+1} = t_k + h,$$

$X$ is reduced to states with probability $> 10^{-16}$,

$X$ is expanded by SSA over $[t_k, t_k + h]$ and $r$-step reachability with $r = 5$,

$$A_1 = A\left(t_k + \left(\frac{1}{2} - \frac{\sqrt{3}}{6}\right)h\right), \quad A_2 = A\left(t_k + \left(\frac{1}{2} + \frac{\sqrt{3}}{6}\right)h\right),$$

$$\sigma = \frac{h}{2}(A_1 + A_2) + \frac{h\sqrt{3}}{12}(A_2 A_1 - A_1 A_2),$$

$$p_{k+1} = \exp(\sigma) \cdot p_k.$$

Note that the SSA only serves here as a method for expanding the state space over the small time-stepping interval, and accounts for less than 5% of the computational runtime in the numerical tests. Computing $p_{k+1}$ via EXPOKIT is the most time-consuming part of the algorithm. In this initial implementation, the stepsize $h$ is constant. We developed this method further in another work [14] to control the error and allow for adaptive stepsizes that can be either rejected or accepted.

## 4 Numerical Comparisons

### 4.1 The Alabama Supercomputer

All numerical tests reported here utilized resources of the Alabama Supercomputer, which houses two supercomputers called SGI UV and DMC. The user can request a job to be executed on either of them, or can simply let the operating system select the more suitable system depending on the workload and availability. All codes were written in FORTRAN 77 and were run on the large queue of the SGI UV with 1 processor core (Xeon E5-4640 CPU operating at 2.4 GHz), 360 hr time limit and 120 GB memory limit.

## 4.2   The Transcriptional Regulatory Problem

The biological problem for comparing the ODE solvers depicts a transcriptional regulatory system [15]. The problem consists of six species:

$$M : \text{protein (monomer)},$$
$$D : \text{transcription factor (dimer)},$$
$$DNA : \text{DNA template, free of dimers},$$
$$DNA.D : \text{DNA template, bound at one binding site},$$
$$DNA.2D : \text{DNA template, bound at both binding sites},$$
$$RNA : \text{mRNA produced by transcription},$$

which can interact through ten reactions:

$$
\begin{aligned}
RNA &\xrightarrow{c_1} RNA + M; & M &\xrightarrow{c_2} \emptyset; \\
DNA.D &\xrightarrow{c_3} RNA + DNA.D; & RNA &\xrightarrow{c_4} \emptyset; \\
DNA + D &\xrightarrow{c_5} DNA.D; & DNA.D &\xrightarrow{c_6} DNA + D; \\
DNA.D + D &\xrightarrow{c_7} DNA.2D; & DNA.2D &\xrightarrow{c_8} DNA.D + D; \\
M + M &\xrightarrow{c_9} D; & D &\xrightarrow{c_{10}} M + M.
\end{aligned}
$$

The reaction rates are:

$$
\begin{aligned}
c_1 &= 0.043s^{-1}; & c_2 &= 0.0007s^{-1}; \\
c_3 &= 0.078s^{-1}; & c_4 &= 0.0039s^{-1}; \\
c_5 &= \frac{0.012 \cdot 10^9}{A \cdot V(t)} s^{-1}; & c_6 &= 0.4791s^{-1}; \\
c_7 &= \frac{0.00012 \cdot 10^9}{A \cdot V(t)} s^{-1}; & c_8 &= 0.8765 \cdot 10^{-11} s^{-1}; \\
c_9 &= \frac{0.05 \cdot 10^9}{A \cdot V(t)} s^{-1}; & c_{10} &= 0.5s^{-1},
\end{aligned}
$$

where $A$ is the Avogado's constant, and $V(t)$ is the cell volume at time $t$, which increases from the initial value $V(0) = 10^{-15}$ in accordance to

$$V(t) = V(0)e^{\ln(2)t/\tau}$$

during the entire cell cycle time period $\tau = 35$ minutes until the cell divides.

We wish to follow the distributions of the count of each species from the initial state where the cell has two dimers and the DNA is unbound:

$$
\begin{aligned}
\text{M} &= 0; & \text{D} &= 2; \\
\text{DNA} &= 1; & \text{DNA.D} &= 0; \\
\text{DNA.2D} &= 0; & \text{RNA} &= 0.
\end{aligned}
$$

The distributions from solving (2) by the ODE solvers are compared with the frequency from 100,000 FRM trajectories. The fixed FSP state space for the ODE solvers is found by finding the maximum and minimum of each species count during these trajectories, except for **MAGNUS-SSA**, which does not require a priori fixed FSP bounds and changes the state space adaptively instead. In practice, these bounds can be defined based on the knowledge of the biological problem or the experimental data, and may not require stochastic simulations.

As noted before, both **MAGNUS** and **MAGNUS-SSA** schemes were implemented here with constant stepsize, taken as $h = 1$ s in the reported numerical experiments. We also compared the actual execution times of the methods with that of the 100,000 trajectories of the FRM method (which obviously becomes more time-consuming as more trajectories are sampled, and is used here instead of the standard SSA because the reaction rates are time-dependent), and we observed that the FRM runtime was comparable to the Magnus-based methods.

## 4.3 Numerical Results

We performed two numerical tests. The first test has small end time point and therefore results in a small state space, whereas the second one has longer end time point with a much larger state space and poses a large stiff problem for the ODE solvers. The error tolerance for all ODE solvers is $tol = 10^{-5}$.

### 4.3.1 Numerical Test 1

We seek the probability distribution at $t_f = 30s$. The FRM trajectories suggest the FSP bounds:

$$
\begin{aligned}
0 &\leq \text{M} \leq 8; & 0 &\leq \text{D} \leq 3; \\
0 &\leq \text{DNA} \leq 1; & 0 &\leq \text{DNA.D} \leq 1; \\
0 &\leq \text{DNA.2D} \leq 1; & 0 &\leq \text{RNA} \leq 4.
\end{aligned}
$$

$X$ has $n = 1440$ states and $A$ has $nz = 8233$ nonzero elements.

The probability distributions at $t_f$ from all ODE solvers are displayed in Fig. 1. Their results agree with each other and fit the frequency from FRM.

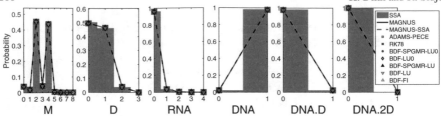

**Fig. 1** Probability distributions at $t_f = 30s$ from the ODE solvers in test 1

### 4.3.2 Numerical Test 2

We now attempt to find the probability distribution at $t_f = 10$ m. Because of the larger time range, the FSP bounds suggested by the FRM trajectories are more extensive:

$$0 \le \quad M \quad \le 46; 0 \le \quad D \quad \le 59;$$
$$0 \le \quad DNA \quad \le 1; 0 \le DNA.D \le 1;$$
$$0 \le DNA.2D \le 1; 0 \le \quad RNA \quad \le 12,$$

resulting in $n = 293280$ states in $X$ and $nz = 2091993$ nonzero elements in $A$. The results from the ODE solvers are listed in Table 1.

Among the ODE solvers, ADAMS-PECE and RK78 did not finish, detecting that the problem was stiff. BDF-LU and BDF-FI also did not finish and reported that they are not appropriate solvers for the problem. BDF-SPGMR-LU failed before reaching $t_f$ because there was not sufficient storage, even though the work array was extended to the maximum size allowed on the Alabama Supercomputer.

The probability distributions from MAGNUS, MAGNUS-SSA and BDF-SPGMR-LU0, BDF-LU0 are compared in Fig. 2. While BDF-SPGMR-LU0 and BDF-LU0 produce wrong results, the distributions from MAGNUS and MAGNUS-SSA agree with the FRM frequencies. The Magnus-based methods are therefore the only reliable ODE solvers for this biological problem.

**Table 1** Reports from the ODE solvers in test 2

| ODE solver | Results |
| --- | --- |
| MAGNUS | Distributions at $t_f$ are in agreement with FRM frequencies |
| MAGNUS-SSA | Distributions at $t_f$ are in agreement with FRM frequencies |
| ADAMS-PECE | Fails before reaching $t_f$ (stiff problem detected - flag 5) |
| RK78 | Fails before reaching $t_f$ (stiff problem detected - flag 4) |
| BDF-SPGMR-LU0 | Distributions at $t_f$ do not fit the FRM frequencies |
| BDF-LU0 | Distributions at $t_f$ do not fit the FRM frequencies |
| BDF-SPGMR-LU | Reports that there is insufficient storage |
| BDF-LU | Reports that it is a wrong solver for this problem |
| BDF-FI | Reports that it is a wrong solver for this problem |

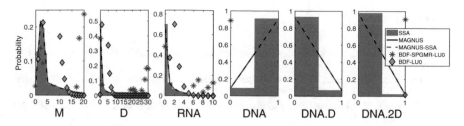

**Fig. 2** Probability distributions at $t_f = 10$ m from the ODE solvers in test 2

## 5 Conclusion

The ODE solvers in this comparison have been tested in [12] across problems in the form of (2) where $A$ is time-independent, in which case the solution is $p(t) = \exp(tA) \cdot p_0$. The authors showed that EXPOKIT [11] and BDF-LU0 [7] are the most efficient among the ODE solvers. We have considered solvers for the CME with time-dependent rates, with EXPOKIT embedded in the Magnus schemes. To our knowledge, such numerical comparisons of Magnus-based methods against other ODE solvers for large biological problems are just starting to appear in the literature.

That Adams, Runge-Kutta and BDF-FI solvers fail for $t_f = 10$ m is to be expected. The reaction rates in the transcriptional regulatory problem differ greatly in magnitude, suggesting that the ODE system is stiff. These ODE solvers behave like explicit methods and therefore are not suitable choices.

Among the remaining four BDF implementations, those relying on the complete LU decomposition are too expensive for this large problem. The incomplete LU0 decomposition, on the other hand, loses important information along the integration and therefore their solutions are unreliable.

The Magnus-based methods were the only solvers to successfully predict the probability distributions at $t_f = 10$ m, suggesting that they can be a powerful tool for solving stiff CME problems with time-dependent rates. Especially, the MAGNUS-SSA possesses the powerful advantage of flexibly changing the state space to follow the probability mass. It therefore does not demand the FSP bounds from the user, which are problem-dependent and require knowledge about the biological problem, and does not follow the entire probability distribution, which is expensive without offering meaningful accuracy. Disadvantages in current Magnus implementations, however, include the lack of an adaptive time-step scheme and the fact that the constant stepsize $h$ for the Magnus methods has to be chosen efficiently. We pursued adaptive time-stepping strategies in [14], which also contains more numerical comparisons.

# References

1. Gillespie, D.: A rigorous derivation of the chemical master equation. Phys. A **188**(1–3), 404–425 (1992)
2. Munsky, B., Khammash, M.: The finite state projection algorithm for the solution of the chemical master equation. J. Chem. Phys. **124**(4), 044104 (2006)
3. Gillespie, D.: Exact stochastic simulation of coupled chemical reactions. J. Phys. Chem. **81**(25), 2340–2361 (1977)
4. Purtan, R., Udrea, A.: A modified stochastic simulation algorithm for time-dependent intensity rates. In: 19th International Conference on Control Systems and Computer Science (2013)
5. Shampine, L.F., Gordon, M.K.: Computer solution of ordinary differential equations: the initial value problem. W.H. Freeman and Co. (1975)
6. Brankin, R.W., Gladwell, I., Shampine, L.F.: RKSUITE: a suite of Runge-Kutta codes for the initial value problem for ODEs, Softreport 91–1. Math. Dept., Southern Methodist University, Dallas, TX, USA, Technical report (1991)
7. Brown, P.N., Byrne, G.D., Hindmarsh, A.C.: VODE: a variable-coefficient ODE solver. SIAM J. Sci. Comput. **10**(5), 1038–1051 (1989)
8. Magnus, W.: On the exponential solution of differential equations for a linear operator. Comm. Pure Appl. Math. **7**(4), 649–673 (1954)
9. Iserles, A., Nørsett, S.P., Rasmussen, A.F.: Time symmetry and high-order Magnus methods. Appl. Numer. Math. **39**(3–4), 379–401 (2001)
10. MacNamara, S., Burrage, K.: Stochastic modeling of naive T cell homeostasis for competing clonotypes via the master equation. Multiscale Model. Simul. **8**(4), 1325–1347 (2010)
11. Sidje, R.B.: EXPOKIT: a software package for computing matrix exponentials. ACM Trans. Math. Softw. (TOMS) **24**(1), 130–156 (1998)
12. Sidje, R.B., Stewart, W.J.: A numerical study of large sparse matrix exponentials arising in Markov chains. Comput. Stat. Data Anal. **29**(3), 345–368 (1999)
13. Sidje, R.B., Vo, H.D.: Solving the chemical master equation by a fast adaptive finite state projection based on the stochastic simulation algorithm. Math. Biosci. **269**, 10–16 (2015)
14. Dinh, K.N., Sidje R.B.: An adaptive Magnus expansion method for solving the Chemical Master Equation with time-dependent propensities. J. Coupled Syst. Multiscale Dyn. https://doi.org/10.1166/jcsmd.2017.1124.
15. Goutsias, J.: Quasiequilibrium approximation of fast reaction kinetics in stochastic biochemical systems. J. Chem. Phys. **122**(18), 184102 (2005)

# Temperature Effect on Sound Scattering by Fine Bubbles in Viscoelastic Liquid

S. Levitsky

**Abstract** Effect of liquid temperature on nonlinear sound scattering by small gas bubbles in a polymeric solution is studied. The analysis is based on the model accounting for liquid rheology manifestation in a close vicinity of the liquid-gas interface where the main velocity gradients at the bubble pulsations are developed. The normalized scattering cross-section of a bubble at the basic frequency and nonlinear cross-section at the frequency of second harmonics are calculated and studied numerically for macromolecular liquids with different polymer concentrations in a temperature range far from the liquid boiling temperature. The temperature dependence of the rheological parameters is accounted for on the basis of Spriggs approximation for relaxation times distribution and the time-temperature superposition principle. The results indicate that the main effect of the temperature is localized in the vicinity of the bubbles resonance frequency and reveals itself in the scattering enhancement with temperature. Temperature dependence of the resonant frequency and the impact of polymer concentration are discussed as well.

**Keywords** Gas bubble · Sound scattering · Viscoelastic liquid
Temperature effect · Second harmonics

## 1 Introduction

The presence of fine bubbles is a characteristic feature of polymeric solutions and melts because self-evacuation of free gas in such systems is complicated by usually high viscosity [1]. Final properties of polymeric products are sensitive to small gas inclusions; therefore, diagnostics of microbubbles is an important part of different technological processes [2]. One of the potentially efficient diagnostic methods is based on the acoustic technique, using registration of sound waves scattered by bubbles [3, 4]. Theoretical background of such technique for polymeric fluids with an

S. Levitsky (✉)
Shamoon College of Engineering, Beer-Sheva, Israel
e-mail: levits@sce.ac.il

© Springer Nature Switzerland AG 2018
D. M. Kilgour et al. (eds.), *Recent Advances in Mathematical and Statistical Methods*, Springer Proceedings in Mathematics & Statistics 259,
https://doi.org/10.1007/978-3-319-99719-3_25

emphasis on the liquid rheology impact on bubble dynamics and sound propagation in non-Newtonian two-phase systems was developed in a number of studies starting from the paper [5]. Basic publications in the field until 1995 were summarized in [6]; more recent results were reported in [7–9], etc. Nonlinear scattering of sound by gas bubbles with an account for liquid viscoelasticity was described in [10] in quadratic approximation; the important contribution [11] should be noted also. The existing results relate to isothermal conditions, so the question of the liquid temperature influence on sound scattering by bubbles is still open. The current analysis is focused on this question; it is supposed that in the studied temperature range the interface mass transfer can be neglected.

## 2   Thermorheological Description of Liquid

It is supposed hereafter, similar to [3, 10] that rheological, thermal and acoustic losses at bubble pulsations in the acoustic field can be accounted for as additive factors. Rheological behavior of polymeric liquid, surrounding the bubble, is described by generalized linear Maxwell model [12]:

$$\tau_{ij} = 2 \int_{-\infty}^{t} \int_{0}^{\infty} F(\theta) e^{-(t-t_1)/\theta} s_{ij}(t_1) d\theta dt_1 + 2\eta_s s_{ij}, \tag{1}$$

$$s_{ij} = e_{ij} - \frac{1}{3}(\nabla \cdot \mathbf{v})I, \quad e_{ij} = \frac{1}{2}(\frac{\partial v_i}{\partial x_j} + \frac{\partial v_j}{\partial x_i}).$$

Here $F(\theta)$ describes the spectrum distribution of relaxation times $\theta$; $\tau_{ij}$, $s_{ij}$ - deviators of stress and rate-of-strain tensors, respectively; $\eta_s$ - low-molecular solvent viscosity; $\mathbf{v}$ - liquid velocity. Rheological Eq. (1) doesn't account for relaxation features at bulk deformations of liquid in the sound wave. It is shown in [6] that the input of liquid volume viscoelasticity in bubble dynamics is small in a wide range of conditions, as compared with other sources of dispersion and dissipation.

Dynamic behavior of viscoelastic liquid at periodic deformations with a frequency $\omega$ of the sound wave is described by complex dynamic module [12]. To write it in a non-dimensionless form, suppose that the pressure in the incident wave is described by the relation $p = p_0 + p_a$, where $p_0$ and $p_a$ are the equilibrium pressure and its disturbance, proportional to $e^{i\omega t}$. Introducing dimensionless variables with characteristic time defined as $t_0 = a_0\sqrt{\rho/p_0}$, where $a_0$, $\rho$ are equilibrium bubble radius and liquid density, we come, in the case of a discrete spectrum, to the following relation for the non-dimensional complex dynamic module $G^*$:

$$(i\Omega)^{-1} G^* = \bar{\eta}' - i\bar{\eta}'' = \frac{\bar{\eta}_p - \bar{\eta}_s}{z(\alpha)} \sum_{k=1}^{\infty} \frac{k^\alpha - i\Omega\bar{\theta}_1}{k^{2\alpha} + (\Omega\bar{\theta}_1)^2}, \tag{2}$$

$$\bar{\theta} = \theta/t_0, \quad \Omega = \omega t_0, \quad \bar{\eta}_{p,s} = \eta_{p,s}/(p_0 t_0),$$

where $\eta_p$ is Newtonian (low-frequency) viscosity of the polymeric solution, which can be estimated from the Martin relation $\eta_p = (1 + \beta \exp(k_M\beta))\eta_s$, and $\bar{\eta}'$, $\bar{\eta}''$ are frequency-dependent components of dynamic viscosity. Here $k_M$ is the Martin constant, $\phi$ - polymer concentration, $\beta = \phi[\eta]$- reduced polymer concentration, $R_G$ - the universal gas constant, $T$ - the absolute temperature and $[\eta]$ - characteristic viscosity of solution calculated below from the Mark-Houwink relation $[\eta] = KM^b$, where $M$ is the polymer molecular mass and $K, b$ are constants for a given polymer-solvent pair at a given temperature over a certain range of molecular mass variation. The parameter $b$ (Mark-Houwink exponent) lies in the range 0.5–0.6 for solutions of flexible chains polymers in thermodynamically bad solvents and in the range 0.7–0.8 for good solvents [1]. For the former ones the constant $K \approx 10^{-2}$ (if the intrinsic viscosity $[\eta]$ is measured in cm$^3$/g), while for the latter $K \approx 10^{-3}$. The Spriggs law $\theta_k = \theta_1/k^\alpha$ is used below [12]; in this case $z(\alpha)$ is the Riemann zeta function of the spectral distribution parameter $\alpha$. The main relaxation time in the spectrum $\theta_1$ can be estimated from the Rouse formula:

$$\theta_1 = 0.608 \frac{(\eta_p - \eta_s)M}{\phi R_G T}. \tag{3}$$

The temperature dependence of viscosity is described by the activation theory:

$$\eta_p = \eta_{p0} \exp[E_p(R_G T_0)^{-1}(T_0/T - 1)], \tag{4}$$
$$\eta_s = \eta_{s0} \exp[E_s(R_G T_0)^{-1}(T_0/T - 1)].$$

where $E_p$, $E_s$ are activation energies of the solution and the solvent, respectively; $\eta_{p0} = \eta_p(T_0)$, $\eta_{s0} = \eta_s(T_0)$ and $T_0$ is the reference temperature. The $E_s$ value is usually about 10–20 kJ/mol. For low-concentrated solutions of polymers with moderate molecular masses, the difference between these two activation energies, $\Delta E = E_p - E_s$, does not exceed usually 10 kJ/mol [1]. Temperature dependence of the relaxation characteristics of polymeric liquids is described by the time-temperature superposition (TTS) principle [12], which states that with a change in temperature the spectrum of relaxation times shifts as a whole in a self-similar manner along the $T$ axis, according to the value of the temperature-shift factor $a_T$:

$$a_T = \frac{\rho(T_0)T_0(\eta_p(T) - \eta_s(T))}{\rho(T)T(\eta_p(T_0) - \eta_s(T_0))}. \tag{5}$$

With $\Omega a_T$ for an argument, it becomes possible to use the temperature-invariant description of the complex dynamic module $G^*$ dependency from frequency.

## 3   Second Harmonics Generation by Bubble in Temperature-Dependent Polymeric Solution

As it is well known, a spherical bubble in liquid is a monopole scatterer with prominent nonlinearity. It is supposed that thermodynamic behavior of gas within the bubble follows the polytropic law with exponent $\gamma$, dissipation and nonlinearity at sound propagation in a quiescent liquid have an only minor impact [13]. Then the equation of bubble dynamics with an account for liquid rheology and the relation for pressure in the wave scattered by a bubble can be defined in the form [10]:

$$\rho(a\ddot{a} + 3/2\dot{a}^2) = \Delta p_g - p_a + 2\sigma a_0^{-1}(1 - a_0 a^{-1}) \tag{6}$$
$$-4\int_{-\infty}^{t}\int_{0}^{\infty} F(\theta)\exp(-\frac{t - t'}{\theta})\dot{a}(t')a^{-1}(t')d\theta\, dt' - 4\eta_s\dot{a}a^{-1},$$

$$p_s(r, t) = \rho\left(\frac{a^2(t_r)\ddot{a}(t_r) + 2a(t_r)\dot{a}^2(t_r)}{r} - \frac{a^4(t_r)\dot{a}^2(t_r)}{2r^4}\right), \tag{7}$$
$$\Delta p_g = p_g - p_{g0}, \quad p_{g0} = p_0 + 2\sigma a_0^{-1}.$$

Here $\sigma$ - surface tension coefficient, index $g$ refers to gas, $r$ is the radial coordinate with the origin in the bubble center, and retarded time $t_r = t - r/c_0$ is introduced to account for finite sound speed $c_0$ in liquid. Further analysis is based on the volume approach [3], according to which the disturbance of the bubble's volume $\Delta V = (4\pi/3)(a^3 - a_0^3)$ is introduced instead of the radius $a$. Equations (6) and (7), are written in the far-field approximation [3], keeping all terms up to $\Delta V^2$, and using non-dimensional variables $v = \Delta V(4/3\pi a_0^3)^{-1}$, $\tau = t/t_0$, $\bar{r} = r/R_0$, $\bar{p}_s = p_s/p_0$, $\tau_r = t_r/t_0$. The solution of the resulting system of equations is searched in the form $v = v_1 + v_2$, $\bar{p}_s = \bar{p}_1 + \bar{p}_2$, $\{v_1, \bar{p}_1\} = \frac{1}{2}\{V_1, P_1\}e^{i\Omega\tau} + c.c.$, $\{v_2, \bar{p}_2\} = \{V_{20}, 0\} + \frac{1}{2}\{V_2, P_2\}e^{2i\Omega\tau} + c.c.$, $\bar{p}_a = \frac{1}{2}P_a e^{i\Omega\tau} + c.c.$, $V_1 \sim P_a$, $V_2 \sim P_a^2$. The calculations follow the procedure described in detail in [3, 14] and yield the following relations for the pressure amplitudes of the basic and second harmonics and the normalized scattering cross-sections $\sigma_1$, $\sigma_2$ of the bubble for the basic and second harmonics:

$$|P_1| = \Omega^2 |V_1|(3\bar{r})^{-1}, \quad |V_1| = 3P_a((\Omega^2 - \beta_1)^2 + \Omega^2\mu_1^2)^{-1/2}, \tag{8}$$
$$|P_2| = \Omega^2 \left|\Omega^2 - \bar{\omega}_0^2(\gamma + 1)\right| |V_1|^2 \{3\bar{r}[(4\Omega^2 - \beta_2)^2 + 4\Omega^2\mu_2^2]^{1/2}\}^{-1},$$
$$\beta_1 = \bar{\omega}_{0\sigma}^2 + 4\Omega\bar{\eta}_{\Omega}'', \quad \bar{\omega}_{0\sigma}^2 = \bar{\omega}_0^2 - 2\bar{\sigma}, \quad \bar{\omega}_0^2 = 3\gamma(1 + 2\bar{\sigma}), \quad \mu_1 = 4(\bar{\eta}_s + \bar{\eta}_{\Omega}')$$
$$+ \Omega^2/\bar{c}_0 + Re\{H(\Omega)\}, \quad H(\Omega) = 3(p_{g0}/p_0)\Gamma Pe(i\Omega Pe - 3(1 - \Gamma)z)^{-1},$$
$$z = (i\Omega Pe)^{1/2}cth\left((i\Omega Pe)^{1/2} - 1\right), \quad \bar{c}_0 = c_0 t_0 R_0^{-1}, \quad Pe = a_g^{-1}R_0(p_0/\rho)^{1/2},$$
$$\beta_2 = \bar{\omega}_{0\sigma}^2 + 8\Omega\bar{\eta}_{2\Omega}'', \quad \mu_2 = 4(\bar{\eta}_s + \bar{\eta}_{2\Omega}') + 4\Omega^2/\bar{c}_0 + Re\{H(2\Omega)\},$$
$$a_g = \chi_g(\rho_{g0}c_{gp})^{-1}, \quad \sigma_1 = 4\bar{r}^2(|P_1|/P_a)^2, \quad \sigma_2 = 4\bar{r}^2(|P_2|/P_a)^2.$$

Here $\Gamma$ is the ratio of gas specific heats, $\rho_{g0}$ - equilibrium gas density, $\chi_g$ - heat conductivity of gas, $c_{gp}$ - specific heat capacity of gas at a constant pressure, $\bar{\eta}'_\Omega$, $\bar{\eta}''_\Omega$ and $\bar{\eta}'_{2\Omega}$, $\bar{\eta}''_{2\Omega}$ are dimensionless components of dynamic viscosity of the polymeric liquid at frequencies $\Omega$ and $2\Omega$, respectively, $\mu_{1,2}$ is the total loss constant of a gas bubble in a compressible polymeric liquid at frequencies $\Omega$ and $2\Omega$, respectively [6]. Note that rheological parameters in Eq. (8) are supposed to be temperature-dependent, according to the relations (3)–(5).

# 4 Results and Discussion

Nonlinear scattering of sound by gas bubble was studied numerically. The values of the system parameters in the relations (8), chosen for simulations, are collected below. Note that physical properties of polymeric liquids are extremely diverse and their complex estimation represents a separate problem, sketched in Sect. 2 and discussed in more detail in [1, 6]. The data, used in simulations, were calculated in accordance with this discussion, and can be approximately related to the solution of high molecular polystyrene ($M \sim 10^6$) in Aroclor:

$$p_0 = 10^5\,\text{Pa}, \quad \eta_s = 0.1\,\text{Pa} \cdot \text{s}, \quad \rho = 10^3\,\text{kg/m}^3, \quad c_f = 1500\,\text{m/s}, \quad k_M = 0.4, \quad (9)$$
$$E_s = 12\,\text{kJ/mol}, \quad E_p = 16\,\text{kJ/mol}, \quad A = 500, \quad \bar{\sigma} = 0.03, \quad T_0 = 293\,\text{K}, \quad \alpha = 2$$

The studied temperature range is equal approximately 60 K. The chosen value of the Spriggs distribution parameter $\alpha$ corresponds to Rouse distribution.

Results of simulations are presented in the Figs. 1, 2, 3 and 4. For all plots $a_0 = 5 \cdot 10^{-4}$ m, the studied non-dimensional frequency range for the chosen parameter values corresponds approximately to dimensional frequency $1.5 < f < 11\,\text{kHz}$, $f = \omega/2\pi$.

As it follows from the Fig. 1, scattering cross-section of the bubble at the incident wave frequency undergoes drastic changes with polymer concentration – the bubble ability to scatter sound becomes less in more concentrated solution. This result relates both to linear and second harmonics and is explained by the rheological dissipation increase with $\beta$. The temperature effect is localized mainly in the linear resonance region; the temperature rise yields the scattering enhancement. The data indicate that despite the absolute value of the scattering cross section for second harmonics is less than for the basic one, the relative impact of liquid temperature on nonlinear sound scattering is more pronounced. This conclusion follows also from the plots on the Fig. 2, where the projection of the 3D plot $\sigma = \sigma(\Omega, T)$ on the $\sigma - \Omega$ plane is presented. The figure illustrates the range of changes in the scattering cross-section with temperature; it can be seen that for second harmonics this range is larger. Both basic and second resonance frequencies decrease slightly with temperature.

The plots in Fig. 3 aim to illustrate the manifestation of liquid viscoelasticity at nonlinear sound scattering by a bubble. We can conclude that the relative amplitude of second harmonics (with respect to the basic one) in polymeric liquid exceeds

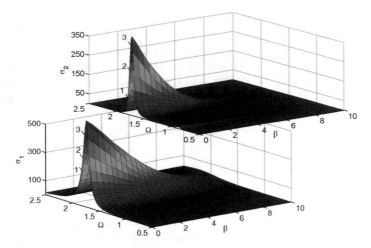

**Fig. 1** Temperature effect on the scattering cross-section for basic and second harmonics. 1 - $T = 1$; 2 - $T = 1.08$; 3 - $T = 1.2$

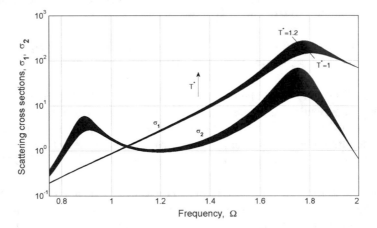

**Fig. 2** Temperature effect on the scattering cross sections for basic and second harmonics (projection of the 3D plot $\sigma = \sigma(\Omega, T)$ on the $\sigma - \Omega$ plane). For both plots $\beta = 3.6$

essentially that one for a similar pure viscous liquid, which is explained by dynamic viscosity reduction with frequency. Temperature rise yields an increase in the relative amplitude of the scattered signal at any frequency, but especially near the frequency of linear resonance.

The amplitude of the signal scattered at the frequency of second harmonics is always less than at the basic frequency, besides a narrow region near the second resonance. Note that for pure viscous liquid the temperature rise in this region may change monotonic dependence of the relative pressure amplitude from frequency to the resonance-like one. As a result, the amplitude of the second harmonics may

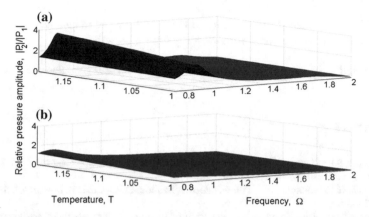

**Fig. 3** Temperature and rheology effect on the relative pressure amplitude of the basic and second harmonics. For both plots $\beta = 3.6$; **a** – viscoelastic liquid, **b** – pure viscous liquid with $\eta = \eta_p$

**Fig. 4** Normalized pressure amplitudes of the basic and second harmonics versus polymer concentration at sub-resonance frequencies. $T^* = 1.1$, dashed lines correspond to pure viscous liquid with $\eta = \eta_p$

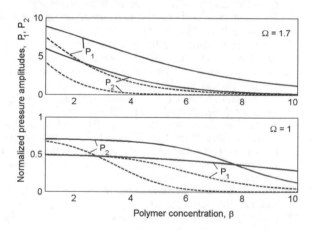

exceed the amplitude of the basic one and to reverse the relation between $|P_1|$ and $|P_2|$. The data in Fig. 4 describes the dependence of normalized amplitudes of the basic and second harmonics from polymer concentration at sub-resonance frequencies and a fixed temperature. Increase in $\beta$ value yields a decrease in the scattered wave intensity; however, for viscoelastic liquid, this effect is less than in pure viscous one with an equivalent viscosity. Interesting to note that at the frequency $\Omega = 1$, which is close to the second resonance, the amplitude of the second harmonics is more sensitive to polymer concentration than that one of the basic harmonics. It is explained by the fact that dependence of $|P_1|$ on polymer concentration, the same as on temperature, is localized mainly in the first resonance range which is sufficiently far from $\Omega = 1$.

It can be summarized that the study has revealed an essential impact of liquid temperature on nonlinear sound scattering by bubbles in the polymeric liquid. The main effect is localized in the vicinity of basic and second resonances and consists in the scattering enhancement with the temperature growth.

**Acknowledgements** The study was supported by the Shamoon College of Engineering (SCE).

# References

1. Levitsky, S.P.: Shulman, Z.P. In: Wypych, G. (eds.) Handbook of Solvents, vol. 1 pp. 367–399. ChemTec Publishing, Toronto (2014)
2. Astarita, G., Maffettone, P.L.: Polymer devolatilization: State of the art. Macromol. Symp. **68**, 1–12 (1993)
3. Zabolotskaya, E.A., Soluyan, S.I.: Emission of harmonic and combination frequency waves by air bubbles. Sov. Phys. Acoust. **18**, 396–398 (1972)
4. Leighton, T.G., Ramble, D.G., Phelps, A.D., Morfey, C.L., Harris, P.P.: Acoustic detection of gas bubbles in a pipe. Acta Acust. **84**, 801–814 (1998)
5. Yang, W.J., Yeh, H.C.: Approximate method for the determining of bubble dynamics in non-Newtonian fluids. Phys. Fluids. **8**, 758–760 (1965)
6. Levitsky, S.P., Shulman, Z.P.: Bubbles in Polymeric Liquids. Dynamics, Heat and Mass Transfer. Technomics Publish. Co., Lancaster (1995)
7. Allen, J.S., Roy, R.A.: Dynamics of gas bubbles in viscoelastic fluids. I. Linear viscoelasticity. J. Acoust. Soc. Am. **107**, 3167–3178 (2000)
8. Warnez, M.T., Johnsen, E.: Numerical modeling of bubble dynamics in viscoelastic media with relaxation. Phys. Fluids. **27**, 063103.1–063103.28 (2015)
9. Zhang, Y., Li, S.: Mass transfer during radial oscillations of gas bubbles in viscoelastic mediums under acoustic excitation. Int. J. Heat Mass. Transfer. **69**, 106–116 (2014)
10. Levitsky, S.: On nonlinear scattering of sound by small bubble in polymeric liquid. In: Rudenko, O., Sapozhnikov, O. (eds.) Nonlinear Acoustics at the Beginning of the 21st Century, vol. 2, pp. 927–930. MSU, Moscow (2002)
11. Khismatullin, D.B.: Resonance frequency of microbubbles: effect of viscosity. J. Acoust. Soc. Am. **116**, 1463–1473 (2004)
12. Bird R.B., Armstrong R.C., Hassager O.: Dynamics of Polymeric Liquids. Fluid Mechanics, vol. 1. Wiley, NY (1987)
13. Nakoryakov, V.E., Pokusaev, B.G., Shreiber, I.R.: Wave Propagation in Gas-Liquid Media. CRC Press, NY (1993)
14. Sutin, A.M., Yoon, S.W., Kim, E.J., Didenkulova, I.N.: Nonlinear acoustic method for bubble density measurements in water. J. Acoust. Soc. Am. **103**, 2377–2384 (1998)

# A Fourth-Order Compact Numerical Scheme for Three-Dimensional Acoustic Wave Equation with Variable Velocity

**Wenyuan Liao and Ou Wei**

**Abstract** In this paper we proposed an accurate and efficient numerical algorithm for solving the acoustic wave equation in three-dimensional heterogeneous media. Numerical solution of the wave equation has been used in various science and engineering applications, such as the seismic full waveform inversion (FWI) problem. FWI is a computationally intensive procedure, in which the acoustic wave equation is numerically solved (forward modelling) repeatedly during the iterative process. Therefore, efficiency and accuracy of the numerical method for solving the acoustic wave equation is critical in the success of seismic full waveform inversion. The new method is obtained by combining the Padé approximation and a novel algebraic manipulation with the Alternative Directional Implicit (ADI) method. Numerical experiments have shown that the new method is accurate, efficient and stable.

**Keywords** Alternative Direction Implicit · Compact finite difference
Acoustic wave equation

## 1 Introduction

Finite difference (FD) method has been widely used in various science and engineering applications since the analytical solution is not available in general. In particular, the high-order FD methods have attracted the interests of many researchers working on seismic modelling (see [1–4] and references therein) due to the high-order accuracy and effectiveness in suppressing numerical dispersion.

W. Liao (✉)
Department of Mathematics and Statistics, University of Calgary,
Calgary, AB T2N 1N4, Canada
e-mail: wliao@ucalgary.ca

O. Wei
Department of Computer Science, Nanjing University of Aeronautics
and Astronautics, Nanjing, China
e-mail: owei@nuaa.edu.cn

© Springer Nature Switzerland AG 2018                                         279
D. M. Kilgour et al. (eds.), *Recent Advances in Mathematical
and Statistical Methods*, Springer Proceedings in Mathematics & Statistics 259,
https://doi.org/10.1007/978-3-319-99719-3_26

Recently, a great deal of efforts have been devoted to develop high-order FD schemes for the acoustic equations, and many accurate and efficient methods have been reported. Levander [5] addressed the cost-effectiveness of solving real problems using high-order spatial derivatives to allow a more coarse spatial sample rate. In [3], the authors used a plane wave theory and the Taylor series expansion to develop a low dispersion time-space domain FD scheme with error $O(\tau^2 + h^{2M})$ for 1-D, 2-D and 3-D acoustic wave equations, where $\tau$ and $h$ represent the time step and spatial grid size, respectively. It was then shown that, along certain fixed directions the error can be improved to $O(\tau^{2M} + h^{2M})$. In [2], Cohen and Poly extended the works of Dablain [6], Shubin and Bell [7] and Bayliss et al. [8] and developed a fourth-order accurate explicit scheme with error of $O(\tau^4 + h^4)$ to solve the heterogeneous acoustic wave equation. Moreover, it has been reported that highly accurate numerical methods are very effective in suppressing the annoying numerical dispersion [9, 10]. High-order FD method is of particular importance for large-scale 3D acoustic wave equation, as it requires less grid points [11].

These methods are accurate but are non-compact, which give rise to two issues: efficiency and difficulty in boundary condition treatment. To resolve these issues, a variety of compact higher-order FD schemes to approximate the spatial derivatives have been developed for hyperbolic, parabolic and elliptical partial differential equations. In [12], the authors developed a family of fourth-order three-point combined difference schemes to approximate the first- and second-order spatial derivatives. For more recent compact higher-order difference methods, the readers are referred to [13].

For three-dimensional problems, an implicit scheme results in a block tri-diagonal system, which is required to be solved at each time step. Direct solution of such large block linear system is very inefficient, therefore, some operator splitting techniques are used to convert the three-dimensional problem into a sequence of one-dimensional problems. One widely used method is the ADI method, which was originally introduced by Peaceman and Rachford [14]. Combined with Padé approximation, some efficient and high-order compact finite difference methods have been developed to solve the acoustic wave equations in 2D and 3D with constant velocity [15, 16]. However when the velocity is a spatially varying function, it is difficult to apply this technique because the algebraic manipulation is not applicable here. Nevertheless, some research work on accurate and low-dispersion numerical simulation of acoustic wavefields in heterogeneous media have been reported [10, 17], although these methods are either non-compact or focus on special case only, such as layered media.

Recently a new fourth-order compact ADI FD scheme was reported in [18] for solving the 2D case. Here we extend this method and the Padé approximation based high-order compact FD scheme in [15] to the 3D acoustic wave equation with non-constant velocity. The new method is compact and efficient, with fourth-order accuracy in both time and space.

The rest of the paper is organized as follows. We first give a brief introduction of the acoustic wave equation and some standard second-order central FD schemes, compact higher-order FD schemes for spatial derivatives and some other related high-order method in Sect. 2, then derive the new compact fourth-order ADI FD scheme in Sect. 3, which is followed by two numerical examples in Sect. 4. Finally, the conclusions are discussed in Sect. 5.

## 2  Acoustic Wave Equation and Existing Algorithms

Consider the 3D acoustic wave equation

$$u_{tt} = v^2(x, y, z)(u_{xx} + u_{yy} + u_{zz}) + s(x, y, z, t), \quad (x, y, z, t) \in \Omega \times [0, T], \tag{1}$$

$$u(x, y, z, 0) = f_1(x, y, z), \quad (x, y, z) \in \Omega, \tag{2}$$

$$u_t(x, y, z, 0) = f_2(x, y, z), \quad (x, y, z) \in \Omega \tag{3}$$

$$u(x, y, z, t) = g(x, y, z, t), \quad (x, y, z, t) \in \partial\Omega \times [0, T], \tag{4}$$

where $u(x, y, z, t)$ represents the acoustic pressure at the location $(x, y, z)$ and time $t$, $v(x, y, z)$ represents the wave velocity. Here $f_1$, $f_2$ and $g$ are sufficiently smooth functions that specify the initial and boundary conditions of the acoustic wave equation. $\Omega \subset R^3$ is a finite computational domain and $s(x, y, z, t)$ is the source function. We denote $c(x, y, z) = v^2(x, y, z)$ for the sake of simple notation.

First assume that $\Omega$ is a 3D rectangular box : $[x_0, x_1] \times [y_0, y_1] \times [z_0, z_1]$, which is discretized into an $N_x \times N_y \times N_z$ grid with spatial grid sizes $h_x$, $h_y$ and $h_z$, where $N_x$, $N_y$ and $N_z$ are numbers of grid points in $x-$, $y-$ and $z-$ directions, respectively. Therefore, the grid sizes are given by

$$h_x = \frac{x_1 - x_0}{N_x - 1}, \quad h_y = \frac{y_1 - y_0}{N_y - 1}, \quad h_z = \frac{z_1 - z_0}{N_z - 1}.$$

Let $\tau$ be the time stepsize, $u_{i,j,k}^n$ denotes the numerical solution at the grid point $(x_i, y_j, z_k)$ and time level $n\tau$. The standard second-order central FD schemes are given by

$$u_{tt}(x_i, y_j, z_k, t_n) \approx \delta_t^2 u_{i,j,k}^n / \tau^2 = (u_{i,j,k}^{n-1} - 2u_{i,j,k}^n + u_{i,j,k}^{n+1})/\tau^2, \tag{5}$$

$$u_{xx}(x_i, y_j, z_k, t_n) \approx \delta_x^2 u_{i,j,k}^n / h_x^2 = (u_{i-1,j,k}^n - 2u_{i,j,k}^n + u_{i+1,j,k}^n)/h_x^2, \tag{6}$$

$$u_{yy}(x_i, y_j, z_k, t_n) \approx \delta_y^2 u_{i,j,k}^n / h_y^2 = (u_{i,j-1,k}^n - 2u_{i,j,k}^n + u_{i,j+1,k}^n)/h_y^2, \tag{7}$$

$$u_{zz}(x_i, y_j, z_k, t_n) \approx \delta_z^2 u_{i,j,k}^n / h_z^2 = (u_{i,j,k-1}^n - 2u_{i,j,k}^n + u_{i,j,k+1}^n)/h_z^2. \tag{8}$$

To improve the method to fourth-order accurate in space, we can approximate these derivatives with high-order accuracy. The conventional high-order FD method was derived by approximating the spatial derivatives using more than three points in one direction, which results in larger stencil. The conventional high-order FD method is accurate in space but suffers severe numerical dispersion. Another issue is that it requires more points near the boundary.

To improve the accuracy in time, a class of time-domain high-order FD methods have been derived by Liu and Sen [3]. The idea of the time-domain high-order FD method is to determine coefficients using time-space domain dispersion. As a result, the coefficient will be a function of $\frac{v\tau}{h}$.

To develop high-order compact ADI FD scheme, we apply Padé approximation to the second-order central FD operators defined in Eqs. (5)–(8). Let $\lambda_x = \tau^2/h_x^2$, $\lambda_y = \tau^2/h_y^2$, $\lambda_z = \tau^2/h_z^2$. Substituting the fourth-order Padé approximations into Eq. (1) gives

$$
\frac{\delta_t^2}{(1 + \frac{1}{12}\delta_t^2)} u_{i,j,k}^n = \left[ \frac{\lambda_x c_{i,j,k} \, \delta_x^2}{(1 + \frac{1}{12}\delta_x^2)} + \frac{\lambda_y c_{i,j,k} \, \delta_y^2}{(1 + \frac{1}{12}\delta_y^2)} + \frac{\lambda_z c_{i,j,k} \, \delta_z^2}{(1 + \frac{1}{12}\delta_z^2)} \right] u_{i,j,k}^n + \tau^2 s_{i,j,k}^n.
$$

(9)

Truncation error analysis shows that the algorithm is fourth-order accurate in time and space with the truncation error $O(\tau^4 + h_x^4 + h_y^4 + h_z^4)$, provided the solution $u(x, y, z, t)$ and $c(x, y, z)$ satisfy certain smooth conditions. As shown in [18], the difficulty to develop high-order compact scheme for wave equation with variable velocity is that the operator $(1 + \delta_t^2/12)(1 + \delta_x^2/12)(1 + \delta_y^2/12)(1 + \delta_z^2/12)$ cannot be multiplied to both sides of Eq. (9) to cancel the operators $(1 + \delta_t^2/12)^{-1}$, $(1 + \delta_x^2/12)^{-1}$, $(1 + \delta_y^2/12)^{-1}$ and $(1 + \delta_z^2/12)^{-1}$.

## 3    Derivation of the Compact High-Order ADI Method

Now we extend the novel algebraic manipulation introduced in [18] to the 3D acoustic wave equation with heterogeneous velocity. The obtained method is fourth-order accurate in time and space and compact, which allows efficient ADI implementation. Multiplying $(1 + \frac{\delta_t^2}{12})$ to Eq. (9) yields

$$
\delta_t^2 u_{i,j,k}^n = c_{i,j,k} \left[ \lambda_x \left(1 + \frac{\delta_t^2}{12}\right) \frac{\delta_x^2}{(1 + \delta_x^2/12)} + \lambda_y \left(1 + \frac{\delta_t^2}{12}\right) \frac{\delta_y^2}{(1 + \delta_y^2/12)} + \right.
$$
$$
\left. \lambda_z \left(1 + \frac{\delta_t^2}{12}\right) \frac{\delta_z^2}{(1 + \delta_z^2/12)} \right] u_{i,j,k}^n + \tau^2 \left(1 + \delta_t^2/12\right) s_{i,j,k}^n.
$$

(10)

Collecting the term $\delta_t^2 u_{i,j,k}^n$, we have

$$\left[1 - \frac{\lambda_x c_{i,j,k}}{12} \frac{\delta_x^2}{(1 + \frac{1}{12}\delta_x^2)} - \frac{\lambda_y c_{i,j,k}}{12} \frac{\delta_y^2}{(1 + \frac{1}{12}\delta_y^2)} - \frac{\lambda_y c_{i,j,k}}{12} \frac{\delta_z^2}{(1 + \frac{1}{12}\delta_z^2)}\right] \delta_t^2 u_{i,j,k}^n =$$

$$c_{i,j,k} \left[\frac{\lambda_x \delta_x^2}{(1 + \delta_x^2/12)} + \frac{\lambda_y \delta_y^2}{(1 + \delta_y^2/12)} + \frac{\lambda_z \delta_z^2}{(1 + \delta_z^2/12)}\right] u_{i,j,k}^n + \tau^2 \left(1 + \frac{\delta_t^2}{12}\right) s_{i,j,k}^n.$$

$$(11)$$

Factoring the left-hand side of Eq. (11) yields

$$\left[1 - \frac{c_{i,j,k}}{12} \frac{\lambda_x \delta_x^2}{1 + \frac{1}{12}\delta_x^2}\right] \cdot \left[1 - \frac{c_{i,j,k}}{12} \frac{\lambda_y \delta_y^2}{1 + \frac{1}{12}\delta_y^2}\right] \cdot \left[1 - \frac{c_{i,j,k}}{12} \frac{\lambda_z \delta_z^2}{1 + \frac{1}{12}\delta_z^2}\right] \delta_t^2 u_{i,j,k}^n =$$

$$c_{i,j,k} \left[\frac{\lambda_x \delta_x^2}{1 + \frac{1}{12}\delta_x^2} + \frac{\lambda_y \delta_y^2}{1 + \frac{1}{12}\delta_y^2} + \frac{\lambda_z \delta_z^2}{1 + \frac{1}{12}\delta_z^2}\right] u_{i,j,k}^n + \tau^2 \left(1 + \frac{\delta_t^2}{12}\right) s_{i,j,k}^n + ERR,$$

$$(12)$$

where the factorization error is given by

$$ERR = \frac{\lambda_x}{144} c_{i,j,k} \frac{\delta_x^2}{(1 + \delta_x^2/12)} \lambda_y c_{i,j,k} \frac{\delta_y^2}{(1 + \delta_y^2/12)} \delta_t^2 u_{i,j,k}^n +$$

$$\frac{\lambda_y}{144} \frac{c_{i,j,k}}{1 + \delta_y^2/12} \frac{\delta_y^2}{1 + \delta_y^2/12} \lambda_z \frac{c_{i,j,k}}{1 + \delta_z^2/12} \frac{\delta_z^2}{1 + \delta_z^2/12} \delta_t^2 u_{i,j,k}^n + \frac{\lambda_x}{144} \frac{c_{i,j,k}}{1 + \delta_x^2/12} \frac{\delta_x^2}{1 + \delta_x^2/12} \lambda_z \frac{c_{i,j,k}}{1 + \delta_z^2/12} \frac{\delta_z^2}{1 + \delta_z^2/12} \delta_t^2 u_{i,j,k}^n$$

$$- \frac{\lambda_x}{1728} \frac{c_{i,j,k}}{(1 + \delta_x^2/12)} \frac{\delta_x^2}{(1 + \delta_y^2/12)} \lambda_y \frac{c_{i,j,k}}{(1 + \delta_y^2/12)} \frac{\delta_y^2}{(1 + \delta_z^2/12)} \lambda_z \frac{c_{i,j,k}}{(1 + \delta_z^2/12)} \frac{\delta_z^2}{(1 + \delta_z^2/12)} \delta_t^2 u_{i,j,k}^n.$$

$$(13)$$

Using Taylor series, it is easy to verify that $ERR = O(\tau^6)$, provided that $c(x, y, z)$ and $u(x, y, z, t)$ satisfy certain smooth conditions.

Ignoring ERR leads to the following compact fourth-order FD method

$$\left[1 - \frac{\lambda_x c_{i,j,k}}{12} \frac{\delta_x^2}{1 + \delta_x^2/12}\right] \cdot \left[1 - \frac{\lambda_y c_{i,j,k}}{12} \frac{\delta_y^2}{1 + \delta_y^2/12}\right] \cdot \left[1 - \frac{\lambda_z c_{i,j,k}}{12} \frac{\delta_z^2}{1 + \delta_z^2/12}\right] \delta_t^2 u_{i,j,k}^n$$

$$= c_{i,j,k} \left[\frac{\lambda_x \delta_x^2}{1 + \delta_x^2/12} + \frac{\lambda_y \delta_y^2}{1 + \delta_y^2/12} + \frac{\lambda_z \delta_z^2}{1 + \delta_z^2/12}\right] u_{i,j,k}^n + \tau^2 \left(1 + \delta_t^2/12\right) s_{i,j,k}^n.$$

$$(14)$$

Using ADI method, Eq. (14) can be efficiently solved in three steps

$$\left(1 - \frac{\lambda_x c_{i,j,k}}{12} \frac{\delta_x^2}{1 + \delta_x^2/12}\right) u_{i,j,k}^{**} = \left[\frac{c_{i,j,k} \lambda_x \delta_x^2}{1 + \delta_x^2/12} + \frac{c_{i,j,k} \lambda_y \delta_y^2}{1 + \delta_y^2/12} + \frac{c_{i,j,k} \lambda_z \delta_z^2}{1 + \delta_z^2/12}\right] u_{i,j,k}^n$$

$$+ \tau^2 \left(1 + \delta_t^2/12\right) s_{i,j,k}^n, \quad 2 \le j \le N_y - 1, \ 2 \le k \le N_z - 1, \tag{15}$$

$$\left(1 - \frac{\lambda_y c_{i,j,k}}{12} \frac{\delta_y^2}{1 + \delta_y^2/12}\right) u_{i,j,k}^* = u_{i,j,k}^{**}, \quad 2 \le i \le N_x - 1, \ 2 \le k \le N_z - 1, \tag{16}$$

$$\left(1 - \frac{\lambda_z c_{i,j,k}}{12} \frac{\delta_z^2}{1 + \delta_z^2/12}\right) \delta_t^2 u_{i,j,k}^n = u_{i,j,k}^*, \quad 2 \le i \le N_x - 1, \ 2 \le j \le N_y - 1. \tag{17}$$

However all three equations are difficult to implement due to the fractional operators $\left(1 + \delta_x^2/12\right)^{-1}$, $\left(1 + \delta_y^2/12\right)^{-1}$ and $\left(1 + \delta_z^2/12\right)^{-1}$. To implement Eq. (15), we divide by $c_{i,j,k}$ then multiply $\left(1 + \delta_x^2/12\right)$ to both sides,

$$\left[\left(1 + \frac{\delta_x^2}{12}\right) \frac{1}{c_{i,j,k}} - \frac{\lambda_x}{12} \delta_x^2\right] u_{i,j,k}^{**} = \tau^2 \left(1 + \frac{\delta_x^2}{12}\right) \left(1 + \frac{\delta_t^2}{12}\right) \frac{s_{i,j,k}^n}{c_{i,j,k}}$$

$$+ \left[\lambda_x \delta_x^2 + \lambda_y \left(1 + \delta_x^2/12\right) \frac{\delta_y^2}{1 + \delta_y^2/12} + \lambda_z \left(1 + \delta_x^2/12\right) \frac{\delta_z^2}{1 + \delta_z^2/12}\right] u_{i,j,k}^n. \tag{18}$$

Substituting $\frac{\delta_y^2}{1+\delta_y^2/12} u_{i,j,k}^n$ with $\delta_y^2(1 - \delta_y^2/12) u_{i,j,k}^n$, $\frac{\delta_z^2}{1+\delta_z^2/12} u_{i,j,k}^n$ with $\delta_z^2(1 - \delta_z^2/12) u_{i,j,k}^n$, respectively, we obtain

$$\left[\left(1 + \frac{\delta_x^2}{12}\right) \frac{1}{c_{i,j,k}} - \lambda_x \frac{\delta_x^2}{12}\right] u_{i,j,k}^{**} = \tau^2 \left(1 + \frac{\delta_x^2}{12}\right) \left(1 + \frac{\delta_t^2}{12}\right) \frac{s_{i,j,k}^n}{c_{i,j,k}} +$$

$$\left[\lambda_x \delta_x^2 + \lambda_y \left(1 + \frac{\delta_x^2}{12}\right) \delta_y^2 \left(1 - \frac{\delta_y^2}{12}\right) + \lambda_z \left(1 + \frac{\delta_x^2}{12}\right) \delta_z^2 \left(1 - \frac{\delta_z^2}{12}\right)\right] u_{i,j,k}^n. \tag{19}$$

Note the difference between Eqs. (18) and (19) is $O(h_y^6 + h_z^6)$ [18], thus the method is fourth-order in space. Similarly, Eqs. (16) and (17) can be transformed into

$$\left[\left(1 + \delta_y^2/12\right)\left(1/c_{i,j,k}\right) - \lambda_y \, \delta_y^2/12\right] u_{i,j,k}^* = \left(1 + \delta_y^2/12\right)\left(u_{i,j,k}^{**}/c_{i,j,k}\right) \tag{20}$$

and

$$\left[\left(1 + \delta_z^2/12\right)\left(1/c_{i,j,k}\right) - \lambda_z \, \delta_z^2/12\right] \delta_t^2 u_{i,j,k}^n = \left(1 + \delta_z^2/12\right)\left(u_{i,j,k}^*/c_{i,j,k}\right). \tag{21}$$

Note that Eq. (21) is a three-level FD scheme since $\delta_t^2 u_{i,j,k}^n = u_{i,j,k}^{n+1} - 2u_{i,j,k}^n + u_{i,j,k}^{n-1}$.

All three linear systems given in Eqs. (19)–(21) can be efficiently solved using Thomas algorithm. Here some one-sided fourth-order approximations are needed for boundary condition approximations in these equation systems. For example, in Eq. (21), the following fourth-order one-sided approximations will be used to approximate $u^*_{i,j,1}$ and $u^*_{i,j,N_z}$, respectively:

$$u^*_{i,j,1} = 4u^*_{i,j,2} - 6u^*_{i,j,3} + 4u^*_{i,j,4}4 - u^*_{i,j,5},$$
$$u^*_{i,j,N_y} = 4u^*_{i,j,N_z-1} - 6u^*_{i,j,N_z-2} + 4u^*_{i,j,N_z-3} - u^*_{i,j,N_z-4},$$

for $i = 2, 3, \cdots, N_x - 1$, $j = 2, 3, \cdots, N_y - 1$.

The boundary conditions needed by Eq. (20) can be obtained by setting $j = 1$ and $j = N_y$ in Eq. (21), respectively.

$$\left(1 + \frac{\delta_z^2}{12}\right)\frac{u^*_{i,1,k}}{c_{i,1,k}} = \left[\left(1 + \frac{\delta_z^2}{12}\right)\frac{1}{c_{i,1,k}} - \frac{\lambda_z}{12}\delta_z^2\right]\delta_t^2 u^n_{i,1,k}, \tag{22}$$

$$\left(1 + \frac{\delta_z^2}{12}\right)\frac{u^*_{i,N_y,k}}{c_{i,N_y,k}} = \left[\left(1 + \frac{\delta_z^2}{12}\right)\frac{1}{c_{i,N_y,k}} - \frac{\lambda_z}{12}\delta_z^2\right]\delta_t^2 u^n_{i,N_y,k}. \tag{23}$$

Solving the two tri-diagonal linear systems we can get the boundary conditions for Eq. (20). Similarly, the boundary conditions needed by Eq. (19) can be obtained by letting $i = 1$ and $i = N_x$, respectively.

Equation (21) is a three-level FD scheme, which requires two initial conditions. However only the first initial condition is explicitly specified. To approximate the second initial condition with fourth-order accuracy, we expand $u(x_i, y_j, z_k, t)$ by Taylor series at $t = 0$ to obtain the following fourth-order approximation

$$u^1_{i,j,k} = u^0_{i,j,k} + \tau\frac{\partial u}{\partial t}\Big|^0_{i,j,k} + \frac{\tau^2}{2}\frac{\partial^2 u}{\partial t^2}\Big|^0_{i,j,k} + \frac{\tau^3}{6}\frac{\partial^3 u}{\partial t^3}\Big|^0_{i,j,k} + \frac{\tau^4}{24}\frac{\partial^4 u}{\partial t^4}\Big|^0_{i,j,k} + O(\tau^5), \tag{24}$$

where the high-order derivatives are derived using the method in [18].

## 4 Numerical Examples

In this section two numerical examples are solved by the new method to demonstrate the efficiency and accuracy. The exact solution of the first example is available, so the numerical error can be calculated to validate the order of convergence. In the second example, a problem with the Ricker's wavelet source is solved to demonstrate the effectiveness of the new method.

*Example 1* In this example we solve Eq. (1) on the rectangular domain $[0, \pi] \times [0, \pi] \times [0, \pi]$, and $t \in [0, 1]$, with the coefficient $c(x, y, z) = 1 + \sin^2(x) + \sin^2(y) + \sin^2(z)$. The analytical solution is $u(x, y, z, t) = e^{-t}\cos(x)\cos(y)\cos(z)$. The

**Table 1** Maximal errors for Example 1 with $\tau = 0.0025$ at $T = 1$

| $h$ | $\pi/16$ | $\pi/20$ | $\pi/25$ | $\pi/32$ | $\pi/40$ |
|---|---|---|---|---|---|
| $E_M(h)$ | 5.2701e−05 | 2.5026e−05 | 1.1060e−05 | 4.3147e−06 | 1.8719e-06 |
| Conver. Order | – | 3.3374 | 3.6593 | 3.8132 | 3.7422 |

**Table 2** Maximal errors for Example 1 with various $h$ and $\tau$

| $(h, \tau)$ | $(\pi/16, 1/20)$ | $(\pi/32, 1/40)$ | $(\pi/64, 1/80)$ | $(\pi/128, 1/160)$ |
|---|---|---|---|---|
| $E_M(h, \tau)$ | 5.1391e−05 | 4.2849e−06 | 3.9569e−07 | 2.9088e−08 |
| $\frac{E_M(h, \Delta t)}{E_M(h/2, \Delta t/2)}$ | – | 11.9935 | 10.8289 | 13.6032 |
| Conver. Order | – | 3.5842 | 3.4368 | 3.7659 |

initial condition, boundary condition and source function are chosen accordingly to satisfy the equation. To simplify the discussion, uniform grid size $h$ is used in $x$, $y$ and $z$ directions. To validate the fourth-order convergence in space, we fixed $\tau = 0.0025$ so the temporal truncation error is negligible. The maximal errors obtained by using different $h$ are included in Table 1, which clearly show that the new method is fourth-order accurate in space. We notice that the convergence order is slightly lower than fourth-order, due to the round-off errors.

To show that the method is fourth-order accurate in time, $h$ and $\tau$ are simultaneously reduced by the same factor to ensure that the CFL condition is satisfied. We mention that using very small $h$ to verify the order in time will violate the stability condition. Instead we verify the order of convergence in time using contradiction. Suppose the numerical scheme is $p$th-order accurate in time and fourth-order in space, with $p < 4$, halving $h$ and $\tau$ several times, the truncation error in time will become the dominating error, thus the total error will be reduced by a factor of $2^p < 16$ when $h$ and $\tau$ been halved. In the following numerical test cases, we start from $h = \pi/16$, $\tau = 1/20$ (the parameters are chosen to satisfy the stability condition) and each time we halve both $h$ and $\tau$. The result in Table 2 clearly indicates that the total error is reduced by a factor 16 (roughly) when $h$ and $\tau$ are halved, which confirmed that the convergence order in time is fourth-order. It is worthy to point out that, the new method is an implicit scheme, the computational cost in each time step is higher than that of the explicit method, however the overall computational efficiency has been greatly improved due to the high-order convergence.

*Example 2* In this example we solved the wave equation with a point source located inside a $[0, \ 600\,\text{m}] \times [0, \ 600\,\text{m}] \times [0, \ 600\,\text{m}]$ domain. The velocity model is $v(x, y, z) = 800 + 400(x/x_{max})^2 + 100(y/y_{max})^2 + 800(z/z_{max})^2$. Therefore, the Max and Min wave speeds are 2100 m/s and 800 m/s, respectively. The Ricker's source $s(x, y, z, t) = \delta(x - x_0, y - y_0, z - z_0)\left[1 - 2\pi^2 f_p^2(t - d_r)^2\right]e^{-\pi^2 f_p^2(t-d_r)^2}$ is used to generate the wave, where $f_p = 10\,\text{Hz}$ is the peak frequency, $d_r = 0.5/f_p$ is the temporal delay to ensure zero initial conditions. $(x_0, y_0, z_0)$ is the centre of the

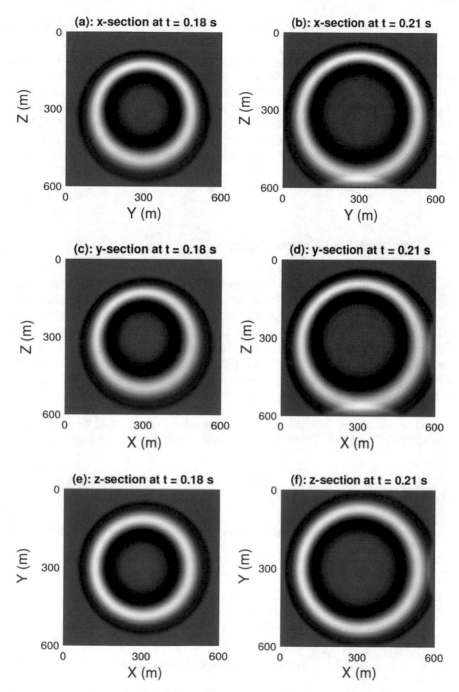

**Fig. 1** Wavefields of x-, y- and z- sections at $t = 0.18,\ 0.21$ s

domain. For all numerical simulations, the uniform grid $h = 5m$ and $\tau = 0.001s$ are used to ensure stability.

We plot the wavefields snapshots for x-, y- and z- sections at $t = 0.18$ s and $t = 0.21$ s in Fig. 1. We first observed that there is no visible numerical dispersions, which indicated that the numerical algorithm is accurate and effective in suppressing numerical dispersion. Secondly, we observed that the wave fronts accurately match the velocity model. For example, as shown in Fig. 1a–b, it clearly shows the wavefront moves faster in z-direction, since the wave speed is higher in z-direction than in y-direction. Moreover, the wave speed increase with $y$ and $z$ increase, so the wavefronts hit the right and bottom boundary earlier. Similar phenomena about the y-, z- sections of the wavefields can be observed in Fig. 1c–f.

## 5 Conclusion and Future Work

A compact fourth-order ADI FD scheme has been developed to solve the three-dimensional acoustic wave equation in heterogeneous media. The new method overcomes the difficulty that were encountered by the existing compact higher-order ADI methods. The fourth-order convergence is validated by a numerical example for which the exact solution is available. Numerical example also demonstrated that the new method is robust, accurate and efficient for numerical seismic modelling on complex geological models. In the future we plan to take more realistic boundary conditions, such as the absorbing boundary condition, into consideration.

**Acknowledgements** The work of the first author is supported by the Natural Sciences & Engineering Research Council of Canada (NSERC) individual Discovery Grant program.

## References

1. Chen, J.B.: High-order time discretizations in seismic modelling. Geophysics **72**(2007), 115–122 (2007)
2. Cohen, G., Joly, P.: Construction and analysis of fourth-order finite difference schemes for the acoustic wave equation in non-homogeneous media. SIAM J. Numer. Anal. **4**(1996), 1266–1302 (1996)
3. Liu, Y., Sen, M.K.: An implicit staggered-grid finite-difference method for seismic modelling. Geophys. J. Int. **179**(2009), 459–474 (2009)
4. Takeuchi, N., Geller, R.J.: Optimally accurate second order time-domain finite difference scheme for computing synthetic seismograms in 2-D and 3-D media. Phys. Earth Planet. Int. **119**(2000), 99–131 (2000)
5. Levander, A.R.: Fourth-order finite-difference P-SV seismograms. Geophysics **53**(11), 1425–1436 (1988)
6. Dablain, M.A.: The application of high order differencing for the scalar wave equation. Geophysics **51**(1), 54–66 (1986)
7. Shubin, G.R., Bell, J.B.: A modified equation approach to constructing fourth-order methods for acoustic wave propagation. SIAM J. Sci. Statis. Comput. **8**(2), 135–151 (1987)

8. Bayliss, A., Jordan, K.E., Lemesurier, B., Turkel, E.: A fourth-order accurate finite difference scheme for the computation of elastic waves. Bull. Seismol. Soc. Amer. **76**(4), 1115–1132 (1986)
9. Finkelstein, B., Kastner, R.: Finite difference time domain dispersion reduction schemes. J. Comput. Phys. **221**(2007), 422–438 (2007)
10. Yang, D.H., Tong, P., Deng, X.Y.: A central difference method with low numerical dispersion for solving the scalar wave equation. Geophysical Prospecting **60**(5), 885–905 (2012)
11. Etgen, J.T., OBrien, M.J.: Computational methods for large-scale 3D acoustic finite-difference modeling: a tutorial. Geophysics **72**(5), SM223–SM230 (2007)
12. Chu, P., Fan, C.: A three-point combined compact difference scheme. J. Comput. Phy. **140**(1998), 370–399 (1998)
13. Shukla, R., Zhong, X.: Derivation of high-order compact finite difference schemes for non-uniform grid using polynomial interpolation. J. Comput. Phy. **204**(2), 404–429 (2005)
14. Peaceman, G.W., Rachford, H.H.: The numerical solution of parabolic and elliptic differential equations. J. Soc. Ind. Appl. Math. **3**(1), 28–41 (1955)
15. Das, S., Liao, W., Gupta, A.: An efficient fourth-order low dispersive finite difference scheme for a 2-D acoustic wave equation. J. Comput. Appl. Mathe. **258**(2014), 151–167 (2014)
16. Liao, W.: On the dispersion, stability and accuracy of a compact higher-order finite difference scheme for 3D acoustic wave equation. J. Comput. Appl. Math. **270**(2014), 571–583 (2014)
17. Zhang, W., Jiang, J.: A new family of fourth-order locally one-dimensional schemes for the three-dimensional wave equation. J. Comput. Appl. Math. **311**(2017), 130–147 (2017)
18. Liao, W., et al.: Efficient and accurate numerical simulation of acoustic wave propagation in a 2D heterogeneous media. Appl. Math. Comput. **321**, 385–400 (2018)

# On Global Properties of Gowdy Spacetimes in Scalar-Tensor Theory

**Makoto Narita**

**Abstract** Recent results show that standard singularity theorem that holds when an energy condition is applied in general relativity also holds when that energy condition is applied to the Bakry-Emery-Ricci tensor which naturally arises in the scalar-tensor theory of gravity. The theory is one of the generalized theories of gravitation and is a low energy effective superstring theory. Thus it is important to investigate global behavior of solutions to the gravitational field equations in the theory. We study the global properties of the Gowdy metrics generated by Cauchy data on $T^3$ in the Brans-Dicke theory which is one of the scalar-tensor theory of gravity. We show that the past boundaries of the maximal Cauchy developments of Gowdy initial data sets are asymptotically velocity-terms dominated singularities. The Kretschmann scalar blows up on the boundary. Thus the maximal Cauchy development cannot extend beyond the boundary and our result shows that the validity of the strong cosmic censorship conjecture.

**Keywords** General relativity · Spacetime singularity
Strong cosmic censorship conjecture · BKL conjecture

## 1 Singularity Theorems and Two Conjectures

General theory of relativity is a gravitational theory. The fundamental equations are the *Einstein equations*, which say relation between spacetime curvature and distribution of matter fields:

$$R_{\mu\nu} = \kappa \left( T_{\mu\nu} - \frac{1}{2} T g_{\mu\nu} \right), \tag{1}$$

$$\nabla_\mu T^{\mu\nu} = 0, \tag{2}$$

M. Narita (✉)
National Institute of Technology, Okinawa College, Nago, Japan
e-mail: narita@okinawa-ct.ac.jp

© Springer Nature Switzerland AG 2018
D. M. Kilgour et al. (eds.), *Recent Advances in Mathematical and Statistical Methods*, Springer Proceedings in Mathematics & Statistics 259, https://doi.org/10.1007/978-3-319-99719-3_27

where $g_{\mu\nu}$ is a $(3 + 1)$-dimensional metric tensor of spacetime with Lorentzian signature, $R_{\mu\nu}$ is the Ricci tensor and $T_{\mu\nu}$ is the energy-momentum tensor. The Einstein equations consists of six (four constraints and two evolution equations) 2nd-order $(3 + 1)$-dimensional nonlinear PDEs. In this theory, important theorems were proved concerning **spacetime singularity**.

**Theorem 1** (Penrose [1]) *Suppose the following conditions hold: (1) a Cauchy surface $\Sigma$ is noncompact, (2) the null convergence condition (for any future-directed null vector field $N$, $R_{\mu\nu}N^\mu N^\nu \geq 0$), (3) $\Sigma$ contains a closed trapped surface. Then the corresponding maximal future development $D^+(\Sigma)$ is incomplete.*

Here, given a Lorentzian manifold, if $\Sigma$ is a spacelike surface, then $D^+(\Sigma)$ is the future of $\Sigma$ which means that, for any point $p$ in spacetime, every inextensible, past-directed, non-spacelike curve through $p$ intersects $\Sigma$. Similarly $D^-(\Sigma)$ is the past of $\Sigma$. If $D(\Sigma) := D^+(\Sigma) \cup \Sigma \cup D^-(\Sigma)$ is the entire spacetime, then $\Sigma$ is a Cauchy surface. Closed trapped surfaces mean that compact spacelike two-surfaces in spacetime such that outgoing null rays perpendicular to the surfaces are not expanding.

**Theorem 2** (Hawking-Penrose [2]) *Suppose the following conditions hold: (1) a Cauchy surface $\Sigma$ is compact, (2) the timelike convergence condition (for any future-directed timelike vector field $T$, $R_{\mu\nu}T^\mu T^\nu \geq 0$), (3) the generic condition. Then the corresponding maximal Cauchy development $D(\Sigma)$ is incomplete.*

Here, the generic condition means $\xi_{[\alpha}R_{\rho]\mu\nu[\sigma}\xi_{\beta]}\xi^\mu\xi^\nu \neq 0$ at some point of each causal geodesic with tangent vector $\xi$.

*Remark 1* The *convergence conditions* mean the positivity of Ricci curvature, which is the positivity of energy density via Einstein equations. The *generic condition* means physically that there exists tidal force.

These theorems say physically reasonable spacetimes have spacetime singularities (incomplete geodesics) in general. However, the theorems do not say us **nature of singularity**, i.e. asymptotic behavior of spacetimes. In addition, **predictability** is breakdown if singularity can be seen. For these problems, two conjecture were proposed as follows.

**Conjecture 1** (Belinskii-Khalatnikov-Lifshitz (BKL) conjecture) *Solutions to the Einstein(-matter) equations should be Kasner-like ones near spacetime singularity.*

In other word, spacetimes would become homogeneous and the Einstein equations would consist of ODEs in time near spacetime singularity. In this case, the curvature of spacetimes should be blow up.

**Conjecture 2** (Strong cosmic censorship (SCC) conjecture) *Generic Cauchy data sets have maximal Cauchy developments which are locally inextendible as Lorentzian manifolds.*

This conjecture was proposed by Penrose and its mathematical formulation was given by Moncrief and Klainerman [3–5]. Roughly speaking, this conjecture says that spacetime singularity cannot be seen by any observer. The most magnificent results of the SCC are the nonlinear stability of the Minkowski space [3, 6, 7] and inextendibility of $T^3$-Gowdy spacetimes [8]. To prove these conjectures, we need to show

- *global existence theorems* of solutions to the Einstein(-matter) equations in suitable coordinates,
- existence of Kasner-like solutions near spacetime singularity *in generic*,
- and *inextendibility* of spacetimes.

## 2 Singularity Theorems in Scalar-Tensor Theories

Recently, singularity theorems for Bakry-Emery-Ricci (BER) tensor

$$R_{\mu\nu}^{\mathrm{BER}} := R_{\mu\nu} + \nabla_\mu \nabla_\nu f,$$

which is the Ricci tensor with another term given by the Hessian of a weight function $f$, have been proved [9]. The BER tensor naturally arises in scalar-tensor (ST) gravitational theories in the conformal gauge (e.g. Jordan-Brans-Dicke (JBD) theory in the Jordan frame) [10, 11].[1] Now we have a question: "Can the SCC and BKL conjectures be solved in the ST theories, which are generalization of the general theory of relativity?" The purpose of the present paper is to answer the above question.

To solve global problems for the (generalized) Einstein equations, some assumptions will be needed, because the equations are very complicated nonlinear PDEs and then we have less mathematical tools to analyze such equations. The ansatz are as follows:

- The JBD theory, which is the simplest ST theory, is considered,
- Existence of two spacelike Killing vectors will be assumed (so called *Gowdy spacetimes*, which are the simplest inhomogeneous ones including dynamical degree of freedom of gravity),
- Topology of spacelike hypersurfaces is three-torus,
- No matter (vacuum) will be assumed.

New results are to show the validity of the SCC and BKL conjectures in the JBD theory which includes the Einstein theory. Methods used here are standard energy estimates, so-called *light cone estimate* [4], and *Fuchsian technique* developed by Kichenassamy-Rendall [16].

---

[1]In the Einstein frame, we have a global existence theorem for the Gowdy symmetric spacetimes with stringy matter [12–15].

## 3 Vacuum Einstein Equations in Gowdy Symmetric Spacetimes

The action for the JBD theory is

$$S = \int d^4x \sqrt{-g} \left[ -\phi R + \omega \frac{\partial_\mu \phi \partial^\mu \phi}{\phi} \right], \tag{3}$$

where $\phi$ is the JBD scalar field and $\omega > 0$ is a constant. Varying the action with respect to the metric and scalar field, we have the Einstein equations and the JBD scalar field equation as follows:

$$R_{\mu\nu} = \frac{\omega}{\phi^2} \partial_\mu \phi \partial_\nu \phi + \frac{1}{\phi} \partial^2_{\mu\nu} \phi, \tag{4}$$

$$\left( \frac{\partial^2}{\partial t^2} - \Delta \right) \phi = 0. \tag{5}$$

Note that if $\phi$ is a constant, the above equations are equal to the vacuum Einstein equations.

The Gowdy metric is given by

$$g = t^{-1/2} e^{\lambda/2} (-dt^2 + d\theta^2) + R[e^P (d\sigma + Q d\delta)^2 + e^{-P} d\delta^2], \tag{6}$$

where $\lambda, R, P$ and $Q$ are functions of $t \in (0, \infty)$ and $\theta \in T^1$. We also assume

$$\phi = e^{\psi(t,\theta)}.$$

From one components of the Einstein equations,

$$\ddot{R} - R'' = 0, \tag{7}$$

one can put $R = t$, which called *areal time coordinate*. Here, dot and prime denote derivative with respect to $t$ and $\theta$, respectively. The constraint equations are

$$\dot{\lambda} = t \left[ \dot{P}^2 + P'^2 + e^{2P} (\dot{Q}^2 + Q'^2) + \left( \omega + \frac{1}{2} \right) \dot{\psi}^2 + \frac{1}{2} \psi'^2 + \ddot{\psi} \right], \tag{8}$$

$$\lambda' = 2t \left[ \dot{P}P' + e^{2P} \dot{Q}Q' + (\omega + 1) \dot{\psi}\psi' + \dot{\psi}' \right]. \tag{9}$$

The evolution equations are

$$\ddot{P} + \frac{\dot{P}}{t} - P'' = e^{2P}(\dot{Q}^2 - Q'^2),\tag{10}$$

$$\ddot{Q} + \frac{\dot{Q}}{t} - Q'' = -2(\dot{P}\dot{Q} - P'Q'),\tag{11}$$

$$\ddot{\psi} + \frac{\dot{\psi}}{t} - \psi'' = \dot{\psi}^2 - \psi'^2.\tag{12}$$

We call this system **JBD-Gowdy system**.

*Remark 2* Thanks to areal time coordinate, the evolution equations decouple with the constraint equations. Then, we can only solve the evolution equations and after that, $\lambda$ can be determined by using the constraint equations.

To analyze the JBD-Gowdy system, a wave map $u : (\mathcal{M}^{2+1}, G) \mapsto (\mathcal{N}^3, h)$ is defined. The system of the evolution equations is equivalent with nonlinear wave equations given by varying the following action:

$$S_{\text{JBDG}} = \int_{S^1} dt d\theta \sqrt{-G}\left(G^{\alpha\beta} h_{AB}\partial_\alpha u^A \partial_\beta u^B\right),\tag{13}$$

where

$$G = -dt^2 + d\theta^2 + t^2 d\Psi^2, \qquad 0 \le \theta, \Psi \le 2\pi,$$

and

$$h = dP^2 + e^{2P}dQ^2 + e^{2\psi}\psi^2.$$

Every functions depend on time $t$ and $\theta$. From the action, the energy-momentum tensor $T_{\alpha\beta}$ for this system is given of the form:

$$T_{\alpha\beta} = h_{AB}\left(\partial_\alpha u^A \partial_\beta u^B - \frac{1}{2}G_{\alpha\beta}\partial_\lambda u^A \partial^\lambda u^B\right).\tag{14}$$

As useful mathematical tools to prove our theorems, the energies are defined as follows:

$$
\begin{aligned}
E(t) &= \int_{S^1} T_{tt} d\theta \\
&= \frac{1}{2} \int_{S^1} \left[ h_{AB} \left( \partial_t u^A \partial_t u^B + \partial_\theta u^A \partial_\theta u^B \right) \right] d\theta \\
&= \int_{S^1} \mathscr{E} d\theta,
\end{aligned}
$$

$$
\begin{aligned}
F(t) &= \int_{S^1} T_{t\theta} d\theta \\
&= \frac{1}{2} \int_{S^1} \left[ h_{AB} \left( \partial_t u^A \partial_\theta u^B + \partial_t u^A \partial_\theta u^B \right) \right] d\theta \\
&= \int_{S^1} \mathscr{F} d\theta,
\end{aligned}
$$

where $\mathscr{E}$ and $\mathscr{F}$ are defined as follows:

$$
\mathscr{E} := \dot{P}^2 + P'^2 + e^{2P} \left( \dot{Q}^2 + Q'^2 \right) + \dot{\psi}^2 + \psi'^2, \tag{15}
$$

and

$$
\mathscr{F} := 2 \left[ \dot{P} P' + e^{2P} \dot{Q} Q' + \dot{\psi} \psi' \right]. \tag{16}
$$

## 4   Global Existence Theorem

The following is the main theorem:

**Theorem 3** *Let* $(M, g)$ *be the maximal Cauchy development of* $C^\infty$ *initial data for the JBD-Gowdy system. Then,* $M$ *can be covered by compact Cauchy surfaces of constant areal time* $t$ *with each value in the range* $(0, \infty)$.

The main part of the proof of Theorem 3 is the following energy estimates:

**Step 1 (Bounds on first derivatives)**

**Lemma 1** (Light cone estimate [4]) $\mathscr{E}$ *is bounded on* $(T_-, T_+) \times S^1$.

*Proof* Define derivaties into the null directions $\partial_\zeta := \partial_t - \partial_\theta$ and $\partial_\xi := \partial_t + \partial_\theta$.

$$
\partial_\zeta (t\mathscr{E} + t\mathscr{F}) = L, \tag{17}
$$

and

$$\partial_\xi (t\mathcal{E} - t\mathcal{F}) = L, \tag{18}$$

where

$$L := \frac{1}{2} \left( -\dot{P}^2 - e^{2P}\dot{Q}^2 - \dot{\psi}^2 + P'^2 + e^{2P}Q'^2 + \psi'^2 \right).$$

Note that $|L| \leq C\mathcal{E}$, where $C$ is a positive constant.

Consider a point $(t, \theta) \in [t_i, T_+) \times S^1$. Integrating the both sides of Eqs. (18) and (18) along null passes, $\partial_\zeta$ and $\partial_\xi$, from points $(t_i, \theta_+)$ and $(t_i, \theta_-)$ to the point $(t, \theta)$, respectively, we have

$$\int \partial_\zeta (t\mathcal{E} + t\mathcal{F}) d\zeta = t\mathcal{E}(t, \theta) + t\mathcal{F}(t, \theta) - t\mathcal{E}(t_i, \theta_+) - t\mathcal{F}(t_i, \theta_+)$$

$$= \int L_+ d\zeta,$$

and

$$\int \partial_\xi (t\mathcal{E} - t\mathcal{F}) d\xi = t\mathcal{E}(t, \theta) - t\mathcal{F}(t, \theta) - t\mathcal{E}(t_i, \theta_-) + t\mathcal{F}(t_i, \theta_-)$$

$$= \int L_- d\xi.$$

Adding these equations and using the inequality $|\mathcal{F}| \leq \mathcal{E}$,

$$t\mathcal{E}(t, \theta) \leq t\mathcal{E}(t_i, \theta_+) + t\mathcal{E}(t_i, \theta_-) + \frac{1}{2} \left[ \int |L_+| d\zeta + \int |L_-| d\xi \right]. \tag{19}$$

Taking supremums over all values of the space coordinate $\theta \in [0, 2\pi]$ on the both sides of the inequality (19), we have

$$\sup_\theta t\mathcal{E}(t, \theta) \leq 2 \sup_\theta t\mathcal{E}(t_i, \theta)$$

$$+ \int_{t_i}^t \frac{1}{s} \left[ C \sup_\theta s\mathcal{E} \right] ds. \tag{20}$$

We now apply Gronwall's lemma to this inequality (20), we have boundedness for $\mathcal{E}$ on $[t_i, T_+) \times S^1$. We can apply the same argument for $t \in (T_-, t_i] \times S^1$, and then we have the conclusion of this lemma. $\qquad$ Q.E.D.

**Step 2 (Bounds on second derivatives)**

If we take time derivatives of the evolution Eqs. (10)–(12) for $P$, $Q$, $\psi$, then we have evolution equations for $P_t := \dot{P}$, $Q_t := \dot{Q}$, $\psi_t := \dot{\psi}$, which we can write in the following form:

$$\ddot{P}_t + \frac{\dot{P}_t}{t} - P''_t = G_1, \tag{21}$$

$$\ddot{Q}_t + \frac{\dot{Q}_t}{t} - Q''_t = G_2, \tag{22}$$

$$\ddot{\psi}_t + \frac{\dot{\psi}_t}{t} - \psi''_t = G_3, \tag{23}$$

where $G_1, G_2, G_3$ consist of terms of the first derivatives below and $\ddot{P}, \ddot{Q}, \ddot{\psi}$. Note that all of the quantities in $G_1, G_2, G_3$ except $\ddot{P}, \ddot{Q}, \ddot{\psi}$ have been shown in the previous step to be controlled. Now we find the following quantities

$$\mathscr{E}_2 := \dot{P}_t^2 + P'^2_t + e^{2P}\left(\dot{Q}_t^2 + Q'^2_t\right) + \dot{\psi}_t^2 + \psi'^2_t, \tag{24}$$

and

$$\mathscr{F}_2 := 2\left[\dot{P}_t P'_t + e^{2P}\dot{Q}_t Q'_t + \dot{\psi}_t \psi'_t\right]. \tag{25}$$

satisfy equations of the form

$$\partial_\zeta (t\mathscr{E}_2 + t\mathscr{F}_2) = L_1, \tag{26}$$

and

$$\partial_\xi (t\mathscr{E}_2 - t\mathscr{F}_2) = L_2, \tag{27}$$

where $L_1, L_2$ involve nothing but controlled quantities, together with terms quadratic in $\dot{P}_t, P'_t, \dot{Q}_t, Q'_t, \dot{\psi}_t, \psi'_t$. Then we repeat the light cone estimate and verify that $\dot{P}_t, P'_t, \dot{Q}_t, Q'_t, \dot{\psi}_t, \psi'_t$ are all bounded. Furthermore, using evolution Eqs. (10)–(12), we get boundedness on $P''$, $Q''$, $\psi''$.

**Step 3 (Bounds on $\lambda$)**

Finally, we have bounds on $\lambda$ by using the constraint Eqs. (8)–(9) because the right hand side in these equations consist of controlled quantities.

Thus, the proof of the Theorem 3 complete.

## 5 Existence Theorem of Kasner-Like Solutions Near Spacetime Singularity

Let us begin with a brief review of the *Fuchsian algorithm*, which is a method to construct exact singular solutions to a PDE system near a singularity ($t = 0$). The algorithm is based on the following idea: near the singularity, decompose the singular formal solutions into a singular part, which depends on a number of arbitrary functions, and a regular part $u$. If the system can be written as a Fuchsian system of the form

$$[D + \mathcal{N}(x)]\, u = t f(t, x, u, \partial_x u), \tag{28}$$

where $D := t \partial_t$ and $f$ is a vector-valued regular function, then the following theorem can be apply:

**Theorem 4** (Kichenassmy-Rendall [16]) *Assume that $\mathcal{N}$ is an analytic matrix near $x = x_0$ such that there is a constant $C$ with $\| \Lambda^{\mathcal{N}} \| \leq C$ for $0 < \Lambda < 1$. In addition, suppose that $f$ is a locally Lipschitz function of $u$ and $\partial_x u$ which preserves analyticity in $x$ and continuity in $t$. Then, the Fuchsian system (28) has a unique solution in a neighborhood of $x = x_0$ and $t = 0$ which is analytic in $x$ and continuous in $t$ and tend to zero as $t \to 0$.*

Thus, the regular part goes to zero and the singular part of the formal solution becomes an exact solution to the original PDE system near the singularity. Now we construct the singular part of the formal solution (Kasner-like solution) by solving asymptotically velocity-terms dominated (AVTD) equations:

$$\ddot{P} + \frac{\dot{P}}{t} = e^{2P} \dot{Q}^2, \tag{29}$$

$$\ddot{Q} + \frac{\dot{Q}}{t} = -2 \dot{P} \dot{Q}, \tag{30}$$

$$\ddot{\psi} + \frac{\dot{\psi}}{t} = \dot{\psi}^2. \tag{31}$$

Now we put the formal solution as follows:

$$P = P_*(\theta) \ln t + P_{**}(\theta) + t^\varepsilon \alpha(t, \theta), \tag{32}$$

$$Q = Q_*(\theta) + t^{2 - 2P_*(\theta)} (Q_{**}(\theta) + \beta(t, \theta)), \tag{33}$$

$$\psi = \psi_*(\theta) + t^\delta (\psi_{**}(\theta) + \gamma(t, \theta)), \tag{34}$$

where $\alpha$, $\beta$, $\gamma$ are regular parts and others are singular part, which are Kasner solutions and $\varepsilon > 0$, $\delta > 0$, $2 - 2P_* > 0$. We can get them by assuming independence of $\theta$ in the JBD-Gowdy system. Put

$$u = (\alpha, D\alpha, t\partial_\theta \alpha, \beta, D\beta, t\partial_\theta \beta, \gamma, D\gamma, t\partial_\theta \gamma),$$

then we have a system consisting of the nine first-order PDEs (Fuchsian system) with $\mathcal{N}$ such that

$$\mathcal{N} = \begin{bmatrix} 0 & -1 & 0 & 0 & 0 & 0 & 0 & 0 & 0 \\ \varepsilon^2 & 2\varepsilon & 0 & 0 & 0 & 0 & 0 & 0 & 0 \\ 0 & 0 & 0 & 0 & 0 & 0 & 0 & 0 & 0 \\ 0 & 0 & 0 & 0 & -1 & 0 & 0 & 0 & 0 \\ 0 & 0 & 0 & 0 & 2P_* & 0 & 0 & 0 & 0 \\ 0 & 0 & 0 & 0 & 0 & 0 & 0 & 0 & 0 \\ 0 & 0 & 0 & 0 & 0 & 0 & 0 & -1 & 0 \\ 0 & 0 & 0 & 0 & 0 & 0 & \delta^2 & 2\delta & 0 \\ 0 & 0 & 0 & 0 & 0 & 0 & 0 & 0 & 0 \end{bmatrix}, \qquad 0 < \varepsilon, 0 < \delta, 0 < P_* < 1.$$

We have the following theorem:

**Theorem 5** *Choose data $\varepsilon > 0$, $\delta > 0$, $0 < P_* < 1$ are satisfied. For any choice of the analytic singular data $P_*(\theta)$, $P_{**}(\theta)$, $Q_*(\theta)$, $Q_{**}(\theta)$, $\psi_*(\theta)$, $\psi_{**}(\theta)$, the BD-Gowdy system has a solution of the form (32)–(34), where $\alpha$, $\beta$ and $\gamma$ tend to zero as $t \to 0$.*

This theorem means that the Kasner-like solution exists near spacetime singularity.

*Remark 3* The Kretschmann scalar $R_{\mu\nu\kappa\lambda}R^{\mu\nu\kappa\lambda}$ goes to infinity as $t \to 0$. Thus, JBD-Gowdy spacetimes are inextendible into the past direction.

*Remark 4* We can generalize this theorem to more generic function space, i.e. analytic to smooth or suitable sovolev space by using theorems in [17–19].

## 6 Summary

We proved the global existence theorem and the existence theorem for Kasner-like solutions to the vacuum Einstein equations with Gowdy symmetric spacetimes in the Jordan-Brans-Dicke theory. These results support the validity of the SCC and BKL conjectures.

# References

1. Penrose, R.: Gravitational collapse and space-time singularities. Phys. Rev. Lett. **14**, 57–59 (1965)
2. Hawking, S.W., Penrose, R.: The singularities of gravitational collapse and cosmology. Proc. Roy. Soc. London Ser. A **314**, 529–548 (1970)
3. Klainerman, S., Nicoló, F.: The Evolution Problem in General Relativity. Progress in Mathematical Physics, vol. 25. Birkhauser Boston, Boston (2003)
4. Moncrief, V.: Global properties of Gowdy spacetimes with $T^3 \times R$ topology. Ann. Phys. **132**, 87–107 (1981)
5. Moncrief, V., Eardley, D.M.: The global existence problem and cosmic censorship in general relativity. Gen. Relativity Gravitation **13**, 887–892 (1981)
6. Christodoulou, D., Klainerman, S.: The Global Nonlinear Stability of the Minkowski Space. Princeton Mathematical Series, vol. 41. Princeton University Press, Princeton (1993)
7. Lindblad, H.: Rodnianski, Igor, The global stability of Minkowski space-time in harmonic gauge. Ann. of Math. 2(171), 1401–1477 (2010)
8. Ringstrom, H.: Strong cosmic censorship in $T^3$-Gowdy spacetimes. Ann. of Math. 2(170), 1181–1240 (2009)
9. Galloway, G.J., Woolgar, E.: Cosmological singularities in Bakry-Emery spacetimes. J. Geom. Phys. **86**, 359–369 (2014)
10. Faraoni, V.: Cosmology in Scalar-Tensor Gravity. Kluwer Academic Publishers (2004)
11. Woolgar, E.: Scalar-tensor gravitation and the Bakry-Emery-Ricci tensor. Classical Quantum Gravity **30**, 085007 (2013)
12. Narita, M.: On the existence of global solutions for $T^3$-Gowdy spacetimes with stringy matter. Classical Quantum Gravity **19**, 6279–6288 (2002)
13. Narita, M.: Global existence problem in $T^3$-Gowdy symmetric IIB superstring cosmology. Classical Quantum Gravity **20**, 4983–4994 (2003)
14. Narita, M.: Global properties of higher-dimensional cosmological spacetimes. Classical Quantum Gravity **21**, 2071–2087 (2004)
15. Narita, M.: On initial conditions and global existence for accelerating cosmologies from string theory. Ann. Henri Poincaré **6**, 821–847 (2005)
16. Kichenassamy, S., Rendall, A.D.: Analytic description of singularities in Gowdy spacetimes. Classical Quantum Gravity **15**, 1339–1355 (1998)
17. Beyer, F., LeFloch, P.G.: Second-order hyperbolic Fuchsian systems and applications. Classical Quantum Gravity **27**, 245012 (2010)
18. Kichenassamy, S.: Fuchsian reduction. Applications to geometry, cosmology, and mathematical physics. Progress in Nonlinear Differential Equations and their Applications, vol. 71. Birkhauser Boston, Inc., Boston (2007)
19. Rendall, A.D.: Fuchsian analysis of singularities in Gowdy spacetimes beyond analyticity. Classical Quantum Gravity **17**, 3305–3316 (2000)

# A Computational Resolution
# of the Inverse Problem of Kinetic
# Capillary Electrophoresis (KCE)

József Vass and Sergey N. Krylov

**Abstract** Determining kinetic rate constants is a highly relevant problem in bio-chemistry, so various methods have been designed to extract them from experimental data. Such methods have two main components: the experimental apparatus and the subsequent analysis, the latter dependent on the mathematical approach taken, which influences the effectiveness of constant determination. A computational inverse problem approach is hereby presented, which does not merely give a single rough approximation of the sought constants, but is inherently capable of determining them from exact signals to arbitrary accuracy. This approach is thus not merely novel, but opens a whole new category of solution approaches in the field, enabled primarily by an efficient direct solver.

**Keywords** Inverse problems · Parameter estimation · Kinetic rate constants
Biochemical interactions · Convection-diffusion equations

# 1 Introduction

## 1.1 Aims and Overview

The direct problem of efficiently generating accurate numerical solutions to the set of partial differential equations of Kinetic Capillary Electrophoresis (KCE) [1] has been resolved earlier via a multimesh algorithm [2], which fully overcomes the typical instability arising from the interaction of the diffusion and convection terms. This potent solution to the direct problem allows the effective resolution of the inverse problem on a reasonable timescale, as we shall hereby discuss and demonstrate. The inversion essentially entails the optimization of a non-linear error objective function, computed between the experimental target signal and the signals generated

J. Vass (✉) · S. N. Krylov
Centre for Research on Biomolecular Interactions,
Department of Chemistry, York University, Toronto, ON M3J 1P3, Canada
e-mail: jvass@yorku.ca

© Springer Nature Switzerland AG 2018
D. M. Kilgour et al. (eds.), *Recent Advances in Mathematical
and Statistical Methods*, Springer Proceedings in Mathematics & Statistics 259,
https://doi.org/10.1007/978-3-319-99719-3_28

numerically at each iteration. Estimating the starting point for the optimization, posed
a challenge in itself [3]. Furthermore, control of the error in the sought parameters is
demonstrated, enabling the resolution of this inverse problem to arbitrary accuracy
for exact target signals.

The KCE system of equations includes kinetic rate constants in the reaction term,
which can be viewed as parameters that the solution functions of this system of
partial differential equations depend on. The aim of the inverse problem is to find
or approximate certain parameters – the rate constants of complex formation and
dissociation – that induce an a priori given exact solution. If such a method can
arbitrarily approximate an exact solution, then it can be applied to experimental data
reliably. Therefore, the goal becomes to minimize an error function between the
given solution and the approximating solutions, which must be generated for each
set of test parameters as the optimization progresses.

The main objective of our research was to develop a robust software [4] that can be
used reliably to analyze experimental data. Our focus was therefore on what works
well, rather than aiming for mathematical rigour. A number of theoretical questions
arose from this computational study, some also mentioned in the concluding remarks
as potential future directions of research. Various other experimental–computational
approaches have been taken in the literature to approximating rate constants, though
not to arbitrary accuracy, which differentiates our method in its novelty. For other
methods see [5–10], and for a survey of KCE-based ones see [3].

## 1.2   The Physical Model

We adopt the physical model and the notations covered in earlier articles [2, 3],
originally introduced in [1, 11, 12].

The concentration vector of reactants $c = (L, \ T, \ C) : \mathbb{R}_+^2 \to \mathbb{R}_+^3$ is a mapping
defined over spacetime points $(t, \ x) \in [0, \ t_{\max}] \times [0, \ x_{\det}]$. It satisfies the equation

$$\partial_t c + v \cdot \partial_x c = D \cdot \partial_x^2 c + R(c)$$

where $v = (v_L, \ v_T, \ v_C) \in \mathbb{R}_+^3$ and $D = (D_L, D_T, D_C) \in \mathbb{R}_+^3$, and $\cdot$ denotes the
Hadamard product. The reaction term takes the form

$$R(c) = (-k_{\mathrm{on}}LT + k_{\mathrm{off}}C, \ -k_{\mathrm{on}}LT + k_{\mathrm{off}}C, \ k_{\mathrm{on}}LT - k_{\mathrm{off}}C) : \mathbb{R}_+^2 \to \mathbb{R}^3$$

where $k = (k_{\mathrm{on}}, \ k_{\mathrm{off}}) \in \mathbb{R}_+^2$. Lastly, define $K_{\mathrm{d}} := k_{\mathrm{off}}/k_{\mathrm{on}}$.

Since as it will become apparent in Sect. 2, the scope of this paper is constrained
by the parameter estimation methods introduced earlier [3], so we only consider
the initial and boundary conditions for the Nonequilibrium Capillary Electrophoresis of Equilibrium Mixtures (NECEEM) [1, 2, 11] for the above partial differential
equations. These initial conditions are given by $\mathrm{IC}(x) = c(0, x) = \bar{c} \cdot \varrho(x/l)$, where
$\bar{c} = (\bar{L}, \ \bar{T}, \ \bar{C}) \in \mathbb{R}_+^3$ (note: $K_{\mathrm{d}} = \bar{L}\bar{T}/\bar{C}$) and $\varrho : \mathbb{R}_+ \to \mathbb{R}_+^3$ is a vector of asymmet-

ric Gaussian density functions, and $l > 0$. The left boundary condition is $c(t, 0) = 0$, while the right one is $\partial_x c(t, x_{\text{det}}) = 0$, for computational purposes.

The signal is defined as the function

$$S[k, \gamma](t) := (L + C)(t, x_{\text{det}}), \quad t \in [0, t_{\text{max}}]$$

parametrized by the above $k$ and the asymmetric Gaussian plug parameters

$$\gamma = (\mu_L, \sigma_L^1, \sigma_L^2, h_L, \mu_T, \sigma_T^1, \sigma_T^2, h_T, \mu_C, \sigma_C^1, \sigma_C^2, h_C)$$

which denote the center, the left and right standard deviations, and the height of the Gaussian initial conditions (dependent on $\bar{c}$).

See our previous articles for further details [1–3], such as the physical meaning of the above constants.

## 2   The Inverse Problem of KCE

### 2.1   Problem Statement

The direct problem of generating a solution to the KCE equations, introduced above, can be inverted to inquire what parameters $(k_*, \gamma_*) \in \mathbb{R}_+^{14}$ induced a given signal $S_* : [0, t_{\text{max}}] \to \mathbb{R}_+$, meaning $S_* = S[k_*, \gamma_*]$ by the earlier notations, which we refer to as the "target signal". Since as we shall see in the next section, the values of $k_*$ and $\gamma_*$ are not independent, we will only need to invert over some of these parameters, denoted by $\omega \in \mathbb{R}_+^{10}$, while updating the definition of the signal mapping $S[\omega]$ to eliminate the redundant parameters.

Define the error function as $E(\omega) := D(S_*, S[\omega])$ $(\omega \in \mathbb{R}_+^{10})$ where $D$ is any metric, typically the Euclidean. This $E$ is the target function to be minimized during inversion, below some required threshold $\varepsilon > 0$. The problem is thus the following.

**Problem 2.1** (KCE Inverse Problem) *Given a threshold $\varepsilon > 0$ and an $S_* : [0, t_{\text{max}}]$ $\to \mathbb{R}_+$ function, induced by unknown KCE parameters $\omega_*$ and defined as $S_* := S[\omega_*]$, find an $\omega$ parameter vector such that $E(\omega) < \varepsilon$.*

This inverse problem may appear at first to be ill-posed, meaning its solution is not necessarily unique, and $E(\omega) = 0$ doesn't trivially imply that $\omega = \omega_*$. The signal mapping $S$ is not only a superposition, but also a slice of a surface, resulting in a significant loss of information relative to the full solution vector $c = (L, T, C)$. However, our computational experiments strongly suggest well-posedness, making it a worthwhile conjecture, equivalent to asserting that the error function possesses a unique minimum.

## 2.2 The Optimization Space

In this section, we clarify how the optimization space over $\omega \in \mathbb{R}_+^{10}$ reduces from the seemingly straightforward variables $(k, \gamma) \in \mathbb{R}_+^{14}$. As mentioned, this reduction is partly necessitated by the interdependencies between the coordinates of the latter vector, which originate in the physicochemical model of KCE [1].

Another reason for the reduction, is that the variation in the $T$-plug parameters in $\gamma$ does not really affect the simulated signal. The standard deviations are not particularly relevant for the effectiveness of the computational inversion. The quantity of the $T$ substance in this chemical reaction can be controlled solely via the height of the $T$-plug, while the plug center may be allowed to vary within 1–2 orders of magnitude. Though the height is in fact dependent on some other parameters, as stated below.

Furthermore, it must be noted that $k_{on}$ typically has little bearing on the NECEEM signal, as reasoned in earlier papers [3, 13], so the optimization process may place a greater emphasis on optimizing in $k_{off}$.

The full vector of parameters

$$(k, \gamma) = (k_{on}, k_{off}, \mu_L, \sigma_L^1, \sigma_L^2, h_L, \mu_T, \sigma_T^1, \sigma_T^2, h_T, \mu_C, \sigma_C^1, \sigma_C^2, h_C)$$

is reduced to the vector of optimization parameters

$$\omega = (k_{off}, \mu_L, \sigma_L^1, \sigma_L^2, h_L, \mu_T, \mu_C, \sigma_C^1, \sigma_C^2, h_C).$$

To make up for the missing coordinates $k_{on}, \sigma_T^1, \sigma_T^2, h_T$, which are still necessary to generate signals $S[\omega]$ for the calculation of the error $E$, some relationships between the coordinates must be observed. Firstly

$$\bar{L} = \sqrt{2\pi}\, \frac{h_L}{l}\, \frac{\sigma_L^1 + \sigma_L^2}{2}$$

and similarly for $\bar{C}$, while $\bar{T} = 1000 T_{ini} - \bar{C}$ where $T_{ini}$ is the initial pre-equilibrium concentration of the $T$-plug. Its height can then be calculated as

$$h_T = \frac{l\bar{T}}{\sqrt{2\pi}} \Big/ \frac{\hat{\sigma}_T^1 + \hat{\sigma}_T^2}{2}$$

where $\hat{\sigma}_T^{1,2}$ are the standard deviation estimates for the asymmetric Gaussian $T$-plug [3]. Using mere estimates does not significantly affect the effectiveness of inversion, as reasoned heuristically above, i.e. the minimization of the error function $E$ below a given threshold. Lastly, $k_{on} = k_{off}\bar{C}/(\bar{L}\bar{T})$ which is simply the relationship mentioned in Sect. 1.2.

Lastly, we remark that the inversion using any optimization algorithm we tested, proved to be significantly more efficient when carried out in logarithmic space, in all independent variables.

## 2.3  Error Control

As stated in the KCE Inverse Problem 2.1, the inversion is formulated as the minimization of the error function $\omega \to E(\omega)$ below some threshold $\varepsilon > 0$, where the signal error is calculated as $E(\omega) = D(S_*, S[\omega])$, typically with the Euclidean metric $D$ and some target signal $S_* = S[\omega_*]$.

It remains unclear, how this minimization can be made practical. For the purpose of scientific applications, our inevitable aim must be to ensure that the error in the $k = (k_{on}, k_{off})$ parameter is minimized below a threshold $\delta > 0$, prescribed a priori. Therefore, the task becomes to determine – or estimate – what $\varepsilon$ threshold above is necessary to ensure this $\delta$.

The matter can be resolved under the rather weak hypothesis that there is a local Lipschitz constant $L$ for some metric $d$, satisfying

$$d(k_*, \ k) \leq d(\omega_*, \ \omega) \leq L \cdot D(S[\omega_*], \ S[\omega]) = L \cdot E(\omega)$$

in a neighborhood of the point $\omega_*$ in the optimization space. Since this point is unknown, computationally we ensure a large enough neighborhood in logarithmic space around our estimate – derived earlier [3] – likely to contain the sought $\omega_*$. Typically, the neighborhood is taken within two orders of magnitude, which proved to be sufficient according to our computational experiments.

The Lipschitz constant $L$ can then be estimated within this neighborhood, by taking random pairs of points $\omega_1$, $\omega_2$ in it, and taking the maximum of the ratios $d(\omega_1, \ \omega_2)/D(S[\omega_1], \ S[\omega_2])$.

Using this estimated $L$, the threshold in the signal error $E(\omega)$ must be taken to be $\delta := \varepsilon/L$, in order to ensure that the error in $k$ falls below the prescribed signal threshold $\varepsilon > 0$.

## 2.4  Implementation

The inverse solver [4] is essentially a non-linear optimization process, which minimizes the error function introduced in Sect. 2.1. At each evaluation of this function, the direct solver must be called to generate a signal $S[\omega]$ for the current iteration of parameters $\omega$. Thus the runtime of the inverse solver is fundamentally implied by that of the direct solver. The stability and efficiency of the direct solver was established in our earlier article [2].

Finding a well-functioning – or perhaps even "ideal" – optimization algorithm, was in itself a challenge, and we have tested several. The **fmincon** MATLAB function with the *interior-point* algorithm proved to be the most robust and efficient. The *bfgs* Hessian approximation option (a dense quasi-Newton approximation [14]) is typically sufficient, but occasionally the *lbfgs* option (a limited-memory, large-scale quasi-Newton approximation [15]) must also be run, in case the *bfgs* option fails to converge below the required signal error threshold within the allocated time. Other tested algorithms include Cuckoo Search [16], Flower Pollination [17], and Harmony Search [18], each of which proved to be less robust than **fmincon**, but are nevertheless available in our package [4].

Each inverter – i.e. error minimization subroutine, with a particular optimization algorithm – was tested for simulated signals induced by known parameters, and then compared to the output parameters in terms of relative error (see Figs. 1 and 3). In practice, the inverters are executed on experimental signals (from unknown parameters), in which case, the accuracy of the result can be gauged via the error control method described in Sect. 2.3, and demonstrated in Sect. 3.


# 3   Performance Analysis

Figure 1 depicts the performance analysis of the primary inverter, running the BFGS and L-BFGS [14, 15] interior point optimization algorithms of MATLAB (**fmincon** with the *interior-point* algorithm, and Hessian approximation methods *bfgs* and *lbfgs*). The target threshold of 0.0001% in the signal error tends to ensure two correct decimal places in $k$ in scientific notation. This threshold is reached by the inverter up to $\log_{10}(k_{on}) \approx 3.45$ on the horizontal axis, but it fails to converge above that value. The ca. 4200 evaluations is the default upper iteration bound that each optimization algorithm is allowed to run, at this $t$-mesh size. The ca. 5000 evaluations at ca. 2.75 results from running the inverter twice, trying both settings (*bfgs* and *lbfgs*).

Figure 2 accompanies Fig. 1, for reference. Apparently for $\log_{10}(k_{on}) > 3.45$ the $C$-peak vanishes, visually elucidating the divergence of the inverter. The necessity of a prominent $C$-peak thus becomes a practical rule of thumb for the reliable inversion of experimental signals.

Figure 3 is a log-log graph (with decreasing horizontal axis), which demonstrates a definite power law relationship on average, with an exponent of ca. 0.7 between the optimization threshold in the signal relative error and the relative error between the original $k_{on}$ value and the one determined by the inverter. The error in $k_{off}$ tends to be close to the same value, or less, so it is not plotted. For lower $k_{on}$ values, the relative error in $k$ apparently stagnates for higher threshold errors in the signal, but does begin to decrease later. The demonstrated power law may be different for other experimental parameter sets.

Interestingly, the **fmincon** optimization subroutine also exhibits a power law relationship between its runtime and the error threshold in the signal, with a negligible exponent of ca. $-0.07$, not considering the outlier. In the outlier $\log_{10}(k_{on}) \approx 2.95$ case, the parameters appear to conspire so that only the *lbfgs* option is able to tackle the inversion (the plotted runtimes include the failed attempts with the *bfgs* option). Nevertheless, the overall linear relationship ensures that the runtime remains predictable for various thresholds.

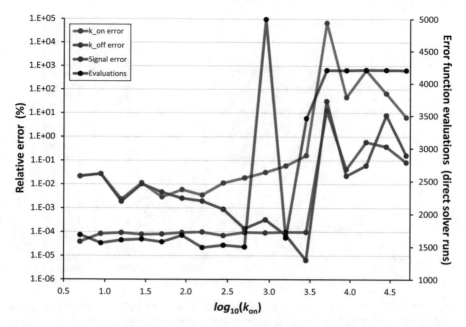

**Fig. 1** Variation of the relative error in $k$ with respect to increasing $\log_{10}(k_{on})$ values, at constant $K_d = 2 \times 10^{-6}\,\mathrm{mol/m^3}$. The $t$-mesh size is 300, and the error threshold is $\varepsilon = 0.0001\%$

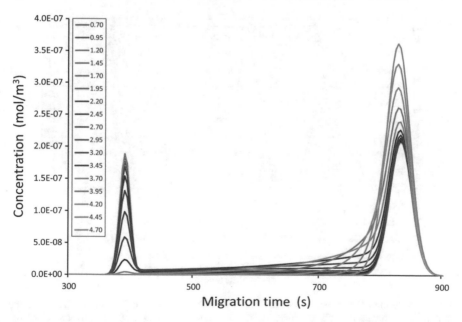

**Fig. 2** Simulated electropherogram signals for increasing $\log_{10}(k_{on})$, at a $t$-mesh size of 300

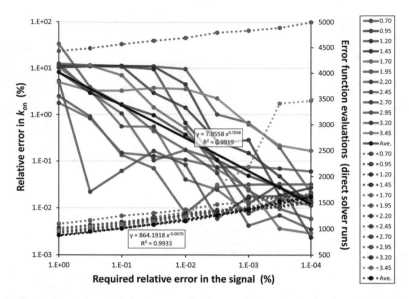

**Fig. 3** Illustration of the correlation between the decrease in the optimization threshold in the signal relative error and the decrease in the $k_{on}$ relative error, for various $\log_{10}(k_{on})$ cases (labeled in the legend). The corresponding runtimes are also plotted. Only the $\log_{10}(k_{on}) \leq 3.45$ cases are plotted, where convergence of the inverter was ensured (see Fig. 1)

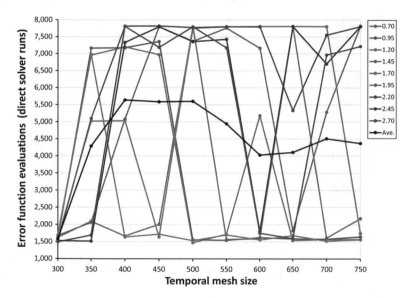

**Fig. 4** Illustration of the variation of runtime with increasing temporal mesh size (to which the spatial is proportional). Only the $\log_{10}(k_{on}) \leq 2.7$ cases are plotted, where convergence of the inverter was ensured within a reasonable timeframe for a temporal mesh size of 300 (see Fig. 1)

Based on Fig. 4, we can conclude that for all the $\log_{10}(k_{on}) \leq 2.7$ test cases, and for all tested mesh sizes, the interior point inverter was successful. The case runtimes, however, did not follow a clear relationship with the increasing mesh size. Taking the average among all cases (in black), however, does exhibit a somewhat clear trend.

## 4 Concluding Remarks

This article aimed to resolve the inverse problem of Kinetic Capillary Electrophoresis, involving a set of partial differential equations, parameterized in the initial and boundary conditions, as well as the equations themselves. The problem was reformulated as the non-linear minimization of a certain error function, each evaluation of which required the generation of a solution with the direct solver.

The main challenge thus became to identify an optimization algorithm capable of carrying out this minimization to arbitrary accuracy, robustly and efficiently, which was accomplished. Furthermore, a local Lipschitz condition was utilized to relate the error in the signal to the error in the sought parameters, in order to control the accuracy in the latter. This is a definite novelty relative to earlier work on this topic.

While this article focused on the design of a computational method and its practical robust implementation, the implied theoretical questions nevertheless project avenues for future research. The most relevant problems being: (1) uniqueness of the global minimizer of the error function; (2) continuous differentiability of the error function. There is strong consistent computational evidence of a unique minimizer, according to our experiments. The second property would imply local Lipschitz continuity (hypothesized in Sect. 2.3), and validate the use of gradient-based optimization algorithms.

**Acknowledgements** This work was supported by the Natural Sciences and Engineering Research Council of Canada (grant: CRDPJ 485321-15).

## References

1. Krylov, S.N.: Kinetic CE: foundation for homogeneous kinetic affinity methods. Electrophoresis **28**(1–2), 69–88 (2007)
2. Vass, J., Krylov, S.N.: A fast stable discretization of the Constant-Convection-Diffusion-Reaction equations of Kinetic Capillary Electrophoresis (KCE). Appl. Numer. Math. **122**, 82–91 (2017)
3. Vass, J., Krylov, S.N.: Estimating kinetic rate constants and plug concentration profiles from simulated KCE electropherogram signals. To be submitted, arXiv:1707.07851 (2017)
4. Vass, J.: KCE Solvers package – direct and inverse solver. GitHub/jzsfvss/KCESolvers (2017)
5. Abdiche, Y., Malashock, D., Pinkerton, A., Pons, J.: Determining kinetics and affinities of protein interactions using a parallel real-time label-free biosensor, the octet. Anal. Biochem. **377**(2), 209–217 (2008)

6.  Al-Soufi, W., Reija, B., Novo, M., Felekyan, S., Kühnemuth, R., Seidel, C.A.: Fluorescence correlation spectroscopy, a tool to investigate supramolecular dynamics: inclusion complexes of pyronines with cyclodextrin. J. Am. Chem. Soc. **127**(24), 8775–8784 (2005)
7.  Hornblower, B., Coombs, A., Whitaker, R.D., Kolomeisky, A., Picone, S.J., Meller, A., Akeson, M.: Single-molecule analysis of DNA-protein complexes using nanopores. Nat. Methods **4**(4), 315–317 (2007)
8.  Li, Y., Augustine, G.J., Weninger, K.: Kinetics of complexin binding to the SNARE complex: correcting single molecule FRET measurements for hidden events. Biophys. J. **93**(6), 2178–2187 (2007)
9.  Rich, R.L., Myszka, D.G.: Higher-throughput, label-free, real-time molecular interaction analysis. Anal. Biochem. **361**(1), 1–6 (2007)
10. Wilson, W.D.: Analyzing biomolecular interactions. Science **295**(5562), 2103–2105 (2002)
11. Berezovski, M., Krylov, S.N.: Nonequilibrium capillary electrophoresis of equilibrium mixtures - a single experiment reveals equilibrium and kinetic parameters of protein-DNA interactions. J. Am. Chem. Soc. **124**(46), 13674–13675 (2002)
12. Petrov, A., Okhonin, V., Berezovski, M., Krylov, S.N.: Kinetic capillary electrophoresis (KCE): a conceptual platform for kinetic homogeneous affinity methods. J. Am. Chem. Soc. **127**(48), 17104–17110 (2005)
13. Okhonin, V., Krylova, S.M., Krylov, S.N.: Nonequilibrium capillary electrophoresis of equilibrium mixtures, mathematical model. Anal. Chem. **76**(5), 1507–1512 (2004)
14. Wikipedia. Broyden–Fletcher–Goldfarb–Shanno algorithm. Link. Accessed 27 June 2017
15. Wikipedia. Limited-memory BFGS. Link. Accessed 27 June 2017
16. Yang, X.-S., Deb, S.: Cuckoo search via Lévy flights. In: 2009 World Congress on Nature & Biologically Inspired Computing (NaBIC), pp. 210–214. IEEE (2009)
17. Yang, X.-S.: Flower pollination algorithm for global optimization. In: International conference on unconventional computing and natural computation, pp. 240–249. Springer (2012)
18. Geem, Z.W., Kim, J.H., Loganathan, G.: A new heuristic optimization algorithm: harmony search. Simulation **76**(2), 60–68 (2001)

# Part V
# Mathematical Modelling in Biological and Environmental Sciences

# A Simulation Study of the Effect of Meso-Scopic Sinusoidal Surface Roughness on Biofilm Growth

**Md. Afsar Ali, Hermann J. Eberl and Rangarajan Sudarsan**

**Abstract** A two-dimensional single species biofilm model is solved under nutrient-rich and nutrient-low conditions to study the effect of mesoscale substratum roughness on biofilm growth activity. Our results indicate that under nutrient-rich conditions, the substratum roughness does not have a pronounced effect on the substrate fluxes and on biofilm growth, leading to formation of biofilms as compact layers. However, under low substrate conditions, substratum roughness has a pronounced effect on both biofilm activity and structure. The overall conclusion is that under low substrate conditions full 2D or 3D simulations are needed to accurately simulate biofilms on irregular surfaces, whereas under nutrient rich conditions, the assumption of flat substrata and 1D models might provide a sufficiently good approximation.

**Keywords** Biofilm structure · Diffusion · Non-orthogonal grid
Surface roughness

## 1 Introduction

Bacterial biofilms are depositions of micro-organisms growing on wetted interfaces, encased in self-secreted slimy glue-like polymeric matrices. They can be found throughout natural and man-made systems wherever environmental conditions are favorable for bacterial growth. For example, in many environmental engineering technologies, biofilms play an important role in degrading pollutants.

Md. A. Ali · H. J. Eberl (✉) · R. Sudarsan
Department of Mathematics and Statistics, University of Guelph,
Guelph, ON N1G 2W1, Canada
e-mail: heberl@uoguelph.ca

Md. A. Ali
e-mail: mali06@uoguelph.ca

R. Sudarsan
e-mail: rsudarsa@uoguelph.ca

© Springer Nature Switzerland AG 2018
D. M. Kilgour et al. (eds.), *Recent Advances in Mathematical
and Statistical Methods*, Springer Proceedings in Mathematics & Statistics 259,
https://doi.org/10.1007/978-3-319-99719-3_29

315

Mathematical modelling has evolved into an effective tool to study biofilm processes and to understand the effect that different reactor operating conditions can have on biofilm performance [1]. In biofilm models, spatio-temporal equations for bacterial growth are coupled with diffusion-reaction equations for nutrients.

The effect of meso-scopic roughness of the surface, on which the biofilm grows (a.k.a substratum), on nutrient diffusivity in the biofilm, as well as on the structure of the biofilm is not well understood. Some experimental studies have been conducted, often with a focus on initial adhesion and early stages growth of biofilms. It was reported that on rough surfaces higher bacterial cell counts are observed than on smooth surfaces [2]. In the food industry, this poses a problem for effective cleaning and sanitizing [3]. It was shown that the adhesion of bacteria to rough surfaces is stronger than to flat surfaces [4, 5]. In [6] it is reported that surface curvature and substrate availability affect biofilm coverage and structure in the early stage of biofilm formation. Based on these observations, to further our understanding, we will systematically address the following two questions in our work:

A. How do mesoscale surface irregularities of the substratum affect the diffusion of substrate into the biofilm, and thus biofilm activity?
B. How do different environmental conditions such as different substrate loadings affect biofilm growth and structure on an irregular substratum?

To answer these questions we use the two-dimensional biofilm model of [7] and simulate biofilm growth in an irregular domain, using a body-fitted grid as introduced in [8]. The traditional biofilm growth model that is used in engineering applications is the one-dimensional Wanner-Gujer model [9], which by construction is able only to describe completely stratified biofilms. Therefore, the answers to the above questions will also shed light on whether one-dimensional mathematical models can be used to adequately model biofilm activity on irregular surfaces.

## 2 Method

### 2.1 Mathematical Model

We make the following modeling assumptions: (i) A single growth limiting substrate diffuses through the aqueous phase into the biofilm and is consumed by bacteria in the biofilm. (ii) Spatial biofilm expansion is due to biomass growth. (iii) The biofilm grows on an impermeable and nonreactive irregular surface.

We use a diffusion-reaction biofilm model that was first proposed in [7]. The dependent variables $u$ and $c$ are the biomass density and substrate concentration. The equations that govern growth and expansion of bacterial biomass, and nutrient distribution in a domain $\Omega \subset \mathbb{R}^2$ for $t > 0$ are

$$u_t = \nabla \cdot (D_u(u)\nabla u) + r_u(u, c) - r_d u, \tag{1}$$

$$c_t = \nabla \cdot (D_c(u)\nabla c) - r_c(u, c). \tag{2}$$

Here, $D_u(u)$ is the diffusion coefficient for biomass, $r_u(u, c)$ is the rate of biomass accumulation, and $r_d$ is the natural decay rate of bacteria. The rate of biomass production $r_u(u, c)$ is described by Monod kinetics as

$$r_u(u, c) = \mu_u \frac{cu}{\kappa + c}, \tag{3}$$

where $\mu_u$ is the maximum specific growth rate and $\kappa$ is the half saturation concentration. Following [7], the density dependent motility function for biomass is

$$D_u(u) = \delta u \left( \frac{u}{u_{max} - u} \right)^4, \tag{4}$$

where $\delta$ is the biomass motility coefficient, and $u_{max}$ is the maximum biomass cell density. In (2), $D_c(u)$ is the diffusion coefficient of the substrate. Diffusion in the biofilm is slower than in the aqueous phase [10]. This is expressed by the convex combination of diffusion coefficient $d_c(0)$ in water and $d_c(1)$ in a fully occupied biofilm

$$D_c(u) = d_c(0) + u/u_{max}(d_c(1) - d_c(0)). \tag{5}$$

The local substrate consumption rate, $r_c(u, c)$ depends on the local concentration of dissolved limiting substrate and is given, in accordance with (3) by

$$r_c(u, c) = \frac{\mu_u u_{max}}{\gamma} \frac{cu}{\kappa + c} = \kappa_s \frac{cu}{\kappa + c} = \frac{u_{max}}{\gamma} r_u(u, c), \tag{6}$$

where $\gamma$ is the yield coefficient of biomass on the substrate, and $\kappa_s$ is the maximum substrate consumption rate.

Equations (1) and (2) are defined in the computational domain $\Omega \subset R^2$. The aqueous phase is $\Omega_1(t) = \{(x, y) \in \Omega : u(t, x, y) = 0\}$. The biofilm phase is $\Omega_2(t) = \{(x, y) \in \Omega : u(t, x, y) > 0\}$. These are separated by the biofilm/water interface, $\Gamma(t) : \Omega_1(t) \cap \bar{\Omega}_2(t)$. Both regions change over time as the biofilm grows. The substratum, on which the biofilm grows, is the bottom surface of the domain.

Equations (1) and (2) are completed by initial and boundary conditions. At time $t = 0$, the substrate is distributed uniformly in the domain and assumed to be at its maximum concentration $C_{bulk}$. To pose initial data for biomass we prescribe the region $\Omega_2(0) \subset\subset \Omega$ and assume that the biomass density there is initially constant with a value $u_0 < u_{max}$, whereas it is nil outside this region. We then have

$$c(0, x, y) = C_{bulk}, \quad (x, y) \in \Omega, \quad u(0, x, y) = \begin{cases} 0, & (x, y) \in \Omega_1(0), \\ u_0, & (x, y) \in \Omega_2(0). \end{cases} \tag{7}$$

We impose homogeneous Neumann boundary conditions for biomass at all boundaries, $\partial_n u = 0$, on $\partial\Omega$, where $n$ is the outward normal direction. For the substrate, we specify the non-homogeneous Dirichlet boundary condition $c = C_{bulk}$ at the top, and homogeneous Neumann boundary conditions at the other boundaries.

The model is non-dimensionalized using the dimensionless variables

$$\bar{x} = \frac{x}{L}, \quad \bar{t} = \mu_u t, \quad \bar{y} = \frac{y}{L}, \quad \bar{c} = \frac{c}{C_{bulk}}, \quad \bar{u} = \frac{u}{u_{max}}. \tag{8}$$

Here, $L$ is the characteristic length scale, $\mu_u$ is the maximum specific growth rate of biomass and $C_{bulk}$ is the substrate bulk concentration. We obtain

$$\bar{u}_{\bar{t}} = \bar{\nabla} \cdot (\bar{D}_u(\bar{u})\bar{\nabla}\bar{u}) + \bar{r}_u(\bar{u}, \bar{c}) - \bar{r}_d u, \tag{9}$$

$$\bar{c}_{\bar{t}} = \bar{\nabla} \cdot (\bar{D}_c(\bar{u})\bar{\nabla}\bar{c}) - \bar{r}_c(\bar{u}, \bar{c}), \tag{10}$$

where

$$\bar{D}_u(\bar{u}) = \frac{D_u(\bar{u})}{L^2\mu_u}, \quad \bar{D}_c(\bar{u}) = \frac{D_c(\bar{u})}{L^2\mu_u}, \bar{\kappa} = \frac{\kappa}{C_{bulk}}, \quad \bar{r}_d = \frac{r_d}{\mu_u}, \quad \bar{\mu}_u = 1, \quad \bar{\kappa}_s = \frac{u_{max}}{\gamma C_{bulk}}.$$

We consider domains with straight lateral and top boundaries and sinusoidal substratum, parameterized by wavelength $\lambda$ and amplitude $A$. The average distance of the substratum to the top of the domain where the substrate is added is in all cases kept the same. For $A = 0$ this describes a rectangular domain which we will use as a reference. A schematic diagram of the domain is depicted in Fig. 1.

The simulation parameters that we use are summarized in Table 1. The ratio of biomass growth rate to substrate transport rate is a crucial dimensionless number to describe biofilm growth and structure [11]. It is given by

**Fig. 1** Schematic of the computational domain with definition of shape parameters wavelength $\lambda$ and amplitude $A$. In all geometries the average height of the domain is the same

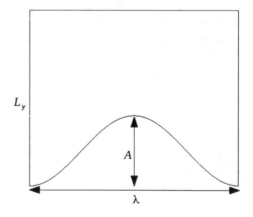

**Table 1** Model parameters

| Parameter | Symbol | Value | Unit | Source |
|---|---|---|---|---|
| Height of system | $L_y$ | 0.0004 | m | Assumed |
| Amplitude of cavity | $A$ | 0.00004, ~ 0.0001 | m | Assumed |
| Wavelength of cavity/length of the domain | $\lambda$ | 0.0002– 0.0006 | m | [11] |
| Monod half saturation constant | $\kappa$ | $3.5 \times 10^{-4}$ | kg m$^{-3}$ | |
| Maximum specific growth rate | $\mu_u$ | $1.52 \times 10^{-5}$ | s$^{-1}$ | [11] |
| Decay rate of bacteria | $r_d$ | $2.3 \times 10^{-6}$ | s$^{-1}$ | [11] |
| Yield coefficient | $\gamma$ | 0.35 | – | [11] |
| Maximum cell density | $u_{max}$ | 70 | kg m$^{-3}$ | [11] |
| Bulk concentration | $C_{bulk}$ | Variable around $4.0 \times 10^{-3}$ | kg m$^{-3}$ | [11] |
| Diffusion coefficient of $c$ in water | $D_c(0)$ | $1.6 \times 10^{-9}$ | m$^2$s$^{-1}$ | [11] |
| Ratio of oxygen diffusion coefficient in biofilm and water : $D_c(1)$ : $D_c(0)$ | $\delta_c$ | 0.9 | – | [11] |
| Biomass motility coefficient | $\delta$ | $8.64 \times 10^{-9}$ | m$^2$s$^{-1}$ | [7] |

$$G = \frac{\text{maximum biomass growth rate}}{\text{maximum substrate transport rate}} = L_y^2 \frac{\mu_u u_{max}}{d_c(0)C_{bulk}}. \qquad (11)$$

Here $L_y$ is a characteristic length scale for diffusive transport. On flat substrata, under low $G$-number regimes homogeneous biofilms are formed, whereas high $G$-numbers lead to irregular biofilm morphologies [7]. We pick for $L_y$ the average system height, i.e., the average of the vertical distance between the top and bottom boundary. This value is kept constant across all simulations. Changes in the $G$-number in our simulations are obtained by changing $C_{bulk}$.

## 2.2 Numerical Method

The biomass Eq. (1) includes two interacting nonlinear diffusion effects, namely a porous medium type degeneracy for $u = 0$ and a super-diffusion singularity for $u = 1$. A semi-implicit numerical method that can handle these two types of degeneracy has been developed in [12] to solve the biofilm model on an orthogonal grid in a rectangular domain. We extended and modified this semi-implicit formulation in [8] for non-orthogonal grids, which allows us to solve the equations on a body-fitted grid in our sinusoidal domain. For our simulations, the transformation is carried out using an elliptic grid generation method [13], as described in [8].

# 3   Results and Discussion

## 3.1   Simulation Setup

In our numerical simulation experiments, we vary the system length $L_x$, whence the dimensionless wave length $\lambda$, and the dimensionless peak-to-peak amplitude of the sinusoidal surface irregularity, $A$. For each of these two parameters, five values are tested, namely $\lambda \in \{0.50, 0.75, 1.0, 1.25, 1.50\}$, corresponding to $L_x \in \{200, 300, 400, 500, 600\,\mu\text{m}\}$, and $A \in \{0, 0.10, 0.15, 0.20, 0.25\}$. $A = 0$ is the reference case of a flat substratum. The average system height $L_y$ is held constant at $400\,\mu\text{m}$ for all simulations. Each simulation is carried out for two different bulk substrate concentrations $C_{bulk} = 52\,\text{g m}^{-3}$ and $C_{bulk} = 5.4\,\text{g m}^{-3}$, corresponding to $G = 2.05$ and $G = 19.7$, respectively. In total, this requires 50 simulations.

The focus of our study is on the effects of substratum irregularity. To avoid effects of irregular inoculation of the substratum overshadowing this, we assume that initially, the entire substratum is covered by a thin film that extends over the first two grid layers, which is $\Omega_2(0)$. To ensure comparability of results between simulations, the initial biomass density in each simulation is constant and determined such that the initial total biomass is the same for all simulations. The simulations are stopped when the size of $\Omega_2(t)$ reaches half of the size of the computational domain.

In order to analyse the results of the numerical simulations, we will present two dimensional visualizations. Furthermore, we report as output quantity the substrate flux into the system, $F_d(t)$, normalised with respect to system length. Since homogeneous Neumann boundary conditions are specified at the bottom and the lateral boundaries, the only contribution to this flux is across the top boundary. Hence,

$$F_d(t) := \frac{1}{\lambda} \int_0^{L_x} D_c(0) \frac{\partial c}{\partial y}(x, L_y, t)\, dx.$$

## 3.2   Effect of Surface Roughness on Biofilm Activity

The substrate flux $F_d(t)$ measures the removal of substrate from the system, i.e., biofilm performance. The characteristic time-scales of substrate diffusion and uptake by the biofilm are orders of magnitude smaller than the characteristic time scales for biofilm growth [7]. Therefore, the substrate flux into the system is a good indicator for biofilm activity.

The substrate flux for the lower $G$-number in Fig. 2 shows that in cases of high substrate availability, surface roughness does not have a pronounced effect on biofilm activity before the stopping criterion is reached. In the case of the higher G-number, cf Fig. 3, the substrate flux is the same for all geometries initially but then starts

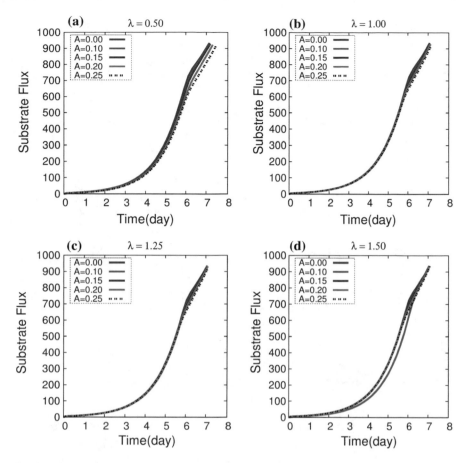

**Fig. 2** Substrate flux into the domain for various wave lengths and amplitudes. The bulk substrate concentration is $C_{bulk} = 52\,\mathrm{g\,m^{-3}}$ (i.e. $G = 2.05$)

diverging at approximately $t = 4$. The flux into the system is larger for geometries with higher amplitude and system wavelength. The substrate flux into the system translates into biomass produced (data not shown).

## 3.3 Effect of Surface Roughness on Biofilm Structure

To investigate the effect of surface roughness on biofilm structure we visualize the simulations in Figs. 4 and 5, where we plot biofilm structure and substrate concentration for different time steps. For all wavelengths similar qualitative results are obtained, but there are quantitative differences. Due to space limitations, not all results can be shown here. We include in detail those for the smallest wavelength,

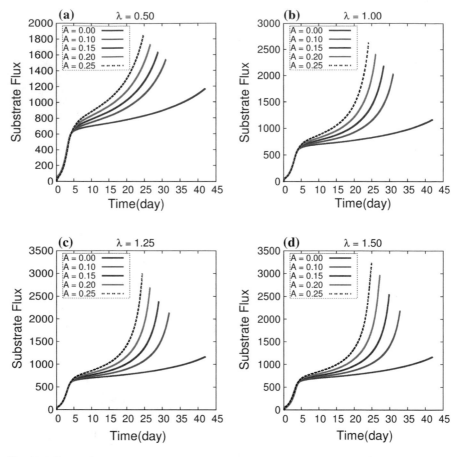

**Fig. 3** Substrate flux into the domain for various wave lengths and amplitudes. The bulk substrate concentration is $C_{bulk} = 5.4\,\mathrm{g\ m^{-3}}$ (i.e. $G = 19.7$)

$\lambda = 0.5$, for which the effects are most pronounced. For $\lambda = 0.75$ and $\lambda = 1.50$, we show the results for amplitude $A = 0.25$ at time $T = 19.45$ for the case $G = 20$ in Fig. 6 as examples.

In the case of the flat surface, the biofilm develops as a homogeneous flat layer. In cases of high substrate availability (low $G$, Fig. 4), a compact biofilm layer covering the substratum develops. In an initial period, the biofilm forms a layer of nearly homogeneous thickness along the substratum. For larger $t$, in the case of small amplitudes, the biofilm overgrows the surface irregularity. For larger wavelengths, biofilm growth remains limited in the deeper regions in the pockets, whereas in the case of smaller wavelength the pockets fill up (simulation data not shown).

In cases of low substrate availability (high $G$, Fig. 5), after an initial period biofilm growth dominates on the hump, closest to the substrate source. Substrate diffusion into the pockets is limited, not allowing biofilm formation. For smaller wavelengths,

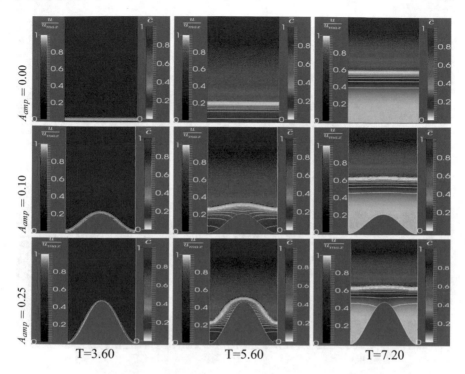

**Fig. 4** Substrate concentration and biofilm structure (shown by biomass density isolines) at various time instances for wavelength $\lambda_1 = 0.50$ and a range of roughness amplitudes. Bulk substrate concentration $C_{bulk} = 52$ g m$^{-3}$ ($G = 2$)

the biofilm colony resembles a mushroom architecture, whereas for larger wavelengths, the local biofilm height is correlated with the distance of the substratum to the substrate source (simulation data not shown).

## 4 Conclusion

Our simulations show that mesoscopic surface irregularity can increase the heterogeneity of biofilm structures. Depending on substrate loading and geometrical parameters of the domain, biofilm growth in pockets can be limited. In many engineering applications, one-dimensional biofilm models are used to simulate biofilm processes and to assess biofilm activity and performance. Our simulation results suggest that such a 1D description might suffice to capture biofilm growth and substrate removal in cases of high substrate availability, particularly, if the surface roughness is mild. On the other hand, if growth conditions are poorer, surface irregularities cannot be neglected, and a full $2D$ simulation is required to describe biofilm activity and structure correctly.

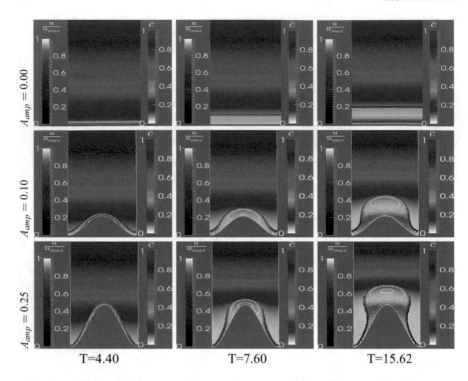

$A_{amp} = 0.00$

$A_{amp} = 0.10$

$A_{amp} = 0.25$

T=4.40                              T=7.60                              T=15.62

**Fig. 5** Substrate concentration and biofilm structure (shown by biomass density isolines) at various time instances for wavelength $\lambda_1 = 0.50$ and a range of roughness amplitudes. Bulk substrate concentration $C_{bulk} = 5.4$ g m$^{-3}$ ($G = 20$)

**Fig. 6** Substrate concentration and biofilm structure (shown by biomass density isolines) for two different wavelengths at amplitude $A = 0.25$ and time $T = 19.45$ with $C_{bulk} = 5.4$ g m$^{-3}$ ($G = 20$)

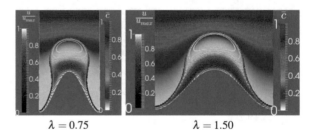

$\lambda = 0.75$                    $\lambda = 1.50$

# References

1. Wanner, O., Eberl, H., Morgenroth, E., Noguera, D., Picioreanu, C., Rittmann, B., van Loosdrecht, M.: Mathematical Modeling of Biofilms. IWA Publishing, London (2006)
2. Percival, S.L., Knapp, J.S., Edyvean, R., Wales, D.S.: Biofilm development on stainless steel in mains water. Wat. Res. **32**(1), 243–253 (1998)
3. Chaturongkasumrit, Y., Takahashi, H., Keeratipibul, S., Kuda, T., Kimura, B.: The effect of polyesterurethane belt surface roughness on Listeria monocytogenes biofilm formation and its cleaning efficiency. Food Control **22**, 1893–1899 (2011)

4. Apilanez, I., Gutierrez, A., Diaz, M.: Effect of surface materials on initial biofilm development. Bioresour. Technol. **66**(3), 225–230 (1998)
5. Characklis, W.G.: Fouling biofilm development: a process analysis. Biotech. Bioeng. **23**, 1923 (1981)
6. Chang, Y.W., Fragkopoulos, A.A., Marquez, M.S., Kim, H.D.: Biofilm formation in geometries with different surface curvature and oxygen availability. New J. Phys. **17**(7), 1367–2630 (2014)
7. Eberl, H.J., Parker, D.F., van Loosdrecht, M.C.M.: A new deterministic spatio-temporal continuum model for biofilm development. J. Theor. Med. **3**, 161–175 (2001)
8. Ali, M.A., Eberl, H.J., Sudarsan, R.: Numerical solution of degenerate, diffusion reaction based biofilm growth model on structured non-orthogonal grids. Commun. Comput. Phys. (in press)
9. Wanner, O., Guejer, W.: Multispecies biofilm model. Biotechnol. Bioeng. **28**, 314–328 (1986)
10. Stewart, P.S.: Diffusion in biofilms. J. Bacteriol. **185**(5), 1485–1491 (2003)
11. Picioreanu, C., Mark, C.M., Loosdrecht, V., Hijnen, J.J.: Mathematical modeling of biofilm structure with a hybrid differential-discrete cellular automation approach. Biotechnol. Bioeng. **58**(1), 101 (1998)
12. Eberl, H.J., Demaret, L.: A finite difference scheme for a degenerated diffusion equation arising in microbial ecology. El. J. Diff. Equs. **15**, 77–95 (2007)
13. Zhang, Y., Jia, Y., Wang, S.S.Y.: An improved nearly-orthogonal structured mesh generation system with smoothness control. J. Comput. Phys. **231**, 5289–5305 (2012)

# Dynamics of a Stage Structured Intraguild Predation Model

Juancho A. Collera and Felicia Maria G. Magpantay

**Abstract** In this paper, we consider a three-species intraguild predation (IGP) model which includes a predator (IG predator) and its prey (IG prey) that share a common resource, and where the IG prey population is partitioned into juvenile and adult stages. The juvenile IG prey are assumed to have little ability for predation and are able to avoid the IG predators by taking refuge. The maturation age of the IG prey population is reflected by a time delay. Conditions for the existence and local stability of all non-negative equilibria are given using the delay as the main parameter. In particular, we show that the positive equilibrium may switch stability at some critical delay value where a Hopf bifurcation occurs. However, this does not lead to destabilization of the system since the stability of the positive equilibrium is passed on to the limit cycle that is created via the Hopf bifurcation. In other words, the introduction of stage structure on the IG prey population enhances the species coexistence through the emergence of limit cycles.

**Keywords** Stage structure · Intraguild predation · Stability switches
Hopf bifurcation · Delay differential equations · Limit cycles

## 1 Introduction

Intraguild predation (IGP), as defined in [9], is killing and eating of potential competitors. An example of IGP is the tri-trophic community module which includes a predator (IG predator) and its prey (IG prey) that share a common resource. Because the IG predator feeds on more than one trophic level, it is a called *omnivorous*. IGP

J. A. Collera (✉)
Department of Mathematics and Computer Science,
University of the Philippines Baguio, Baguio, Philippines
e-mail: jacollera@up.edu.ph

F. M. G. Magpantay
Department of Mathematics and Statistics, Queen's University, Kingston, ON, Canada
e-mail: felicia.magpantay@queensu.ca

© Springer Nature Switzerland AG 2018                                        327
D. M. Kilgour et al. (eds.), *Recent Advances in Mathematical
and Statistical Methods*, Springer Proceedings in Mathematics & Statistics 259,
https://doi.org/10.1007/978-3-319-99719-3_30

is a combination of predation and competition. An IGP model of Lotka-Volterra type considered in [6] showed that IGP could have a destabilizing effect, and a criterion for co-existence of all three species is that the IG prey must be superior than the IG predator in competing for the shared basal resource while the IG predator must gain significantly from its consumption of the IG prey. The following three-species IGP model was examined in [6]:

$$
\begin{aligned}
\dot{x}(t) &= x(t)\left[\, a_0 - a_1 x(t) - a_2 y(t) - a_3 z(t)\right], \\
\dot{y}(t) &= y(t)\left[-b_0 + b_1 x(t) - b_3 z(t)\right], \\
\dot{z}(t) &= z(t)\left[-c_0 + c_1 x(t) + c_2 y(t)\right],
\end{aligned}
\tag{1}
$$

where $x(t)$, $y(t)$, and $z(t)$ denote the densities of the basal resource, the IG prey, and the IG predator, respectively. The parameter $a_0$ represents the basal resource's intrinsic growth rate, while $b_0$ and $c_0$ are, respectively, the death rates of the IG prey and the IG predator. The intraspecific competition or self-regulation coefficient is given by $a_1$; consumption rates are given by $a_2$, $a_3$, and $b_3$; and reproduction rates of the consumer from consumption of the victim are given by $b_1$, $c_1$, and $c_2$. All parameters are assumed to be non-negative, and the initial condition $(x(0), y(0), z(0)) = (x_0, y_0, z_0)$ where $x_0, y_0, z_0 \geq 0$ is used. Discussions on boundedness of solution and permanence of system (1) can be found in [14]. Here, the IG predator depends both on the IG prey and on the basal resource for its sustenance, while the IG prey feeds on the basal resource exclusively [9]. Figure 1a shows a diagram of the interactions between these three species.

IGP models are shown to exhibit rich and interesting dynamics such as multiple stability switches [2, 3], multitype bistability [10], and chaos even if the functional responses are linear [7, 8, 12]. Recent works such as [14] considered a three-species IGP model, like in (1), with stage structure in the IG predator population. In this paper, we study a three-species IGP model of Lotka-Volterra type with stage structure on the IG prey population and use the prey maturation age as the main parameter. Figure 1b shows the diagram of the interactions between species in our stage-structured IGP model. We show that as we vary the maturation age, a stable positive equilibrium may become unstable. However, this does not lead to destabilization of the system since the stability of the positive equilibrium is passed on to the limit cycle that is created by the Hopf bifurcation. That is, all three species still coexist but in a cyclic manner. The introduction of stage structure on the IG prey population enhances the species coexistence.

In the following, we discuss how our model is derived. We use similar assumptions as [13] in incorporating stage structure on the IG prey population. Starting at the equations in (1), we first partition the IG prey population $y(t)$ into immature stage $y_1(t)$ and mature stage $y_2(t)$ where $\tau \geq 0$ is the maturation age with the following assumptions: (i) the immature IG prey have little ability of predation, and (ii) the immature IG prey are able to avoid predation by the IG predators by taking refuge. We obtain the following system

**Fig. 1  a** Three-species IGP
model. **b** IGP model with
stage structured IG prey
population

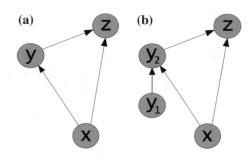

$$\dot{x}(t) = x(t)\left[a_0 - a_1 x(t) - a_2 y_2(t) - a_3 z(t)\right],$$
$$\dot{y}_1(t) = -\mu y_1(t) - b_1 e^{-\mu\tau} x(t-\tau) y_2(t-\tau) + b_1 x(t) y_2(t), \qquad (2)$$
$$\dot{y}_2(t) = -b_0 y_2(t) + b_1 e^{-\mu\tau} x(t-\tau) y_2(t-\tau) - b_3 y_2(t) z(t),$$
$$\dot{z}(t) = z(t)\left[-c_0 + c_1 x(t) + c_2 y_2(t)\right],$$

where $\mu > 0$ is the death rate of immature IG prey, $b_1 e^{-\mu\tau} x(t-\tau) y_2(t-\tau)$ is the number of immature IG prey that was born at time $(t-\tau)$ which still survives at time $t$ and is transferred from the immature stage to the mature stage at time $t$, and $b_1 x(t) y_2(t)$ is number of immature IG prey that are born at time $t$. Note that the equation for the immature IG prey can be separated from the rest of system (2). Renaming $y_2(t)$ to just $y(t)$, we obtain the following system

$$\dot{x}(t) = x(t)\left[a_0 - a_1 x(t) - a_2 y(t) - a_3 z(t)\right],$$
$$\dot{y}(t) = -b_0 y(t) + b_1 e^{-\mu\tau} x(t-\tau) y(t-\tau) - b_3 y(t) z(t), \qquad (3)$$
$$\dot{z}(t) = z(t)\left[-c_0 + c_1 x(t) + c_2 y(t)\right].$$

Observe that when $\tau = 0$, then (3) reduces to (1).

System (3) has five possible non-negative equilibrium solutions: the boundary equilibria $E_0 = (0, 0, 0)$, $E_1 = (K, 0, 0)$, $E_2 = (A, B, 0)$, and $E_3 = (C, 0, D)$ where $K = a_0/a_1$, $A = b_0/b_1 e^{-\mu\tau}$, $B = (a_0 b_1 e^{-\mu\tau} - a_1 b_0)/a_2 b_1 e^{-\mu\tau}$, $C = c_0/c_1$, and $D = (a_0 c_1 - a_1 c_0)/a_3 c_1$, and the positive equilibrium $E_4 = (\frac{P}{S}, \frac{Q}{S}, \frac{R}{S})$ where in $S = a_1 b_3 c_2 - a_2 b_3 c_1 + a_3 b_1 c_2 e^{-\mu\tau}$, $R = (a_0 c_2 - a_2 c_0) b_1 e^{-\mu\tau} - a_1 b_0 c_2 + a_2 b_0 c_1$, $Q = -a_0 b_3 c_1 + a_1 b_3 c_0 - a_3 b_0 c_1 + a_3 b_1 c_0 e^{-\mu\tau}$, and $P = a_0 b_3 c_2 - a_2 b_3 c_0 + a_3 b_0 c_2$.

**Theorem 1**  *For system (3), the equilibrium solutions $E_0$ and $E_1$ always exist, while the boundary equilibria $E_2$ and $E_3$ exist provided $B > 0$ and $D > 0$, respectively. The positive equilibrium $E_4$ exists if the components $P/S$, $Q/S$, and $R/S$ are all positive.*

## 2 Results

We now examine the local stability of the equilibria of system (3). The linearized system around an equilibrium solution $E_* = (x_*, y_*, z_*)$ of system (3) has corresponding characteristic equation given by

$$\det(\lambda I - M_1 - e^{-\lambda \tau} M_2) = 0 \qquad (4)$$

where $[M_1 \mid M_2]$ is given by

$$\begin{bmatrix} a_0 - 2a_1 x_* - a_2 y_* - a_3 z_* & -a_2 x_* & -a_3 x_* & 0 & 0 & 0 \\ 0 & -b_0 - b_3 z_* & -b_3 y_* & b_1 e^{-\mu \tau} y_* & b_1 e^{-\mu \tau} x_* & 0 \\ c_1 z_* & c_2 z_* & -c_0 + c_1 x_* + c_2 y_* & 0 & 0 & 0 \end{bmatrix}.$$

Here the roots $\lambda$ of Eq. (4) depend on $\tau$ and when we want to emphasize this we write $\lambda = \lambda(\tau)$.

At the trivial equilibrium $E_0$, the characteristic Eq. (4) reduces to the polynomial equation $(\lambda - a_0)(\lambda + b_0)(\lambda + c_0) = 0$ with roots $\lambda = a_0 > 0$, $\lambda = -b_0 < 0$, and $\lambda = -c_0 < 0$. Thus, $E_0$ is a saddle and is unstable. At $E_1 = (K, 0, 0)$, Eq. (4) becomes $(\lambda + a_0)(\lambda - a_3 c_1 D / a_1)(\lambda + b_0 - b_1 K e^{-\mu \tau} e^{-\lambda \tau}) = 0$ whose roots include $\lambda = -a_0 < 0$ and $\lambda = a_3 c_1 D / a_1$ which is negative if $D < 0$. Now, notice that if $\lambda$ is a root of $h_1(\lambda, \tau) = 0$ where $h_1(\lambda, \tau) = \lambda + b_0 - b_1 K e^{-\mu \tau} e^{-\lambda \tau}$ with $\mathrm{Re}\, \lambda \geq 0$, then $b_0 \leq |\lambda + b_0| = |b_1 K e^{-\mu \tau} e^{-\lambda \tau}| = b_1 K e^{-\mu \tau} |e^{-\lambda \tau}| \leq b_1 K e^{-\mu \tau}$, or equivalently, $B \geq 0$. That is, if $B < 0$, then the roots of $h_1(\lambda, \tau) = 0$ have negative real parts. Hence, $E_1$ is locally asymptotically stable (LAS) if $B < 0$ and $D < 0$, or equivalently if both $E_2$ and $E_3$ do not exist.

**Theorem 2** *For system (3), the trivial equilibrium $E_0$ is an unstable saddle while the boundary equilibrium $E_1 = (K, 0, 0)$ is LAS whenever $B < 0$ and $D < 0$.*

We now examine the local stability of the remaining boundary equilibria. Suppose $E_2 = (A, B, 0)$ exists, that is, $A > 0$ and $B > 0$. At $E_2$, Eq. (4) becomes $(\lambda - Re^{\mu \tau} / a_2 b_1)(\lambda^2 + (a_1 A + b_0)\lambda + a_1 b_0 A - (\lambda + a_1 A - a_2 B)b_0 e^{-\lambda \tau}) = 0$ whose roots include $\lambda = Re^{\mu \tau} / a_2 b_1$ which is negative if $R < 0$. Now, consider the equation

$$h_2(\lambda, \tau) := \lambda^2 + (a_1 A + b_0)\lambda + a_1 b_0 A - (\lambda + a_1 A - a_2 B)b_0 e^{-\lambda \tau} = 0. \qquad (5)$$

If $\tau = 0$, then (5) reduces to $\lambda^2 + a_1 A \lambda + a_2 b_0 B = 0$ whose roots both have negative real part since both $A$ and $B$ are positive. Consider now the case where $\tau > 0$. First, notice that $\lambda = 0$ is not a root Eq. (5) for any $\tau$ since $B > 0$. Suppose now that $\lambda = i\omega$ with $\omega > 0$ is a root of (5). Then, the imaginary part of the equation $h_2(i\omega, \tau) = 0$ is $(a_1 A + b_0)\omega - b_0 \omega \cos(\omega \tau) + b_0(a_1 A - a_2 B)\sin(\omega \tau) = 0$. Thus,

$$a_1 A\omega + b_0\omega = |b_0\omega \cos(\omega\tau) - b_0(a_1 A - a_2 B) \sin(\omega\tau)|$$
$$\leq b_0\omega |\cos(\omega\tau)| + b_0(a_1 A + a_2 B)| \sin(\omega\tau)|$$
$$\leq b_0\omega + b_0(a_1 A + a_2 B)\omega\tau$$

since $|\cos(\omega\tau)| \leq 1$ and $|\sin(\omega\tau)| \leq |\omega\tau| = \omega\tau$. Hence, $a_1 A \leq b_0(a_1 A + a_2 B)\tau$, or equivalently $\frac{a_1}{a_0 b_1} \leq \tau e^{-\mu\tau}$. That is, if we assume that $\frac{a_1}{a_0 b_1} > \tau e^{-\mu\tau}$, then all roots of (5) have negative real parts. Now suppose that the boundary equilibrium $E_3 = (C, 0, D)$ exists, that is, $C > 0$ and $D > 0$. At $E_3$, the characteristic Eq. (4) reduces to $\left(\lambda^2 + a_1 C\lambda + a_3 c_0 D\right) \left(\lambda + b_0 + b_3 D - b_1 C e^{-\mu\tau} e^{-\lambda\tau}\right) = 0$. Since $C > 0$ and $D > 0$, the roots of $\lambda^2 + a_1 C\lambda + a_3 c_0 D = 0$ both have negative real part. Now, let $\lambda$ be a root of $h_3(\lambda, \tau) := \lambda + b_0 + b_3 D - b_1 C e^{-\mu\tau} e^{-\lambda\tau} = 0$ with Re $\lambda \geq 0$. Then, $(b_0 + b_3 D) \leq |\lambda + b_0 + b_3 D| = |b_1 C e^{-\mu\tau} e^{-\lambda\tau}| = b_1 C e^{-\mu\tau}|e^{-\lambda\tau}| \leq b_1 C e^{-\mu\tau}$. Observe that if $(b_0 + b_3 D) \leq b_1 C e^{-\mu\tau}$, then $Q/a_3 c_1 \geq 0$. Hence, if $Q < 0$, then all roots of $h_3(\lambda, \tau) = 0$ have negative real part. We have the following results.

**Theorem 3** *For system (3), the boundary equilibrium $E_2 = (A, B, 0)$ is LAS if $R < 0$ and $\frac{a_1}{a_0 b_1} > \tau e^{\mu\tau}$, while the boundary equilibrium $E_3 = (C, 0, D)$ is LAS if $Q < 0$.*

We now examine the local stability of the positive equilibrium. Suppose that $E_4 = \left(\frac{P}{S}, \frac{Q}{S}, \frac{R}{S}\right)$ exists. That is, $\frac{P}{S}, \frac{Q}{S}, \frac{R}{S} > 0$. At $E_4$, Eq. (4) reduces to

$$\left[\lambda^3 + a(\tau)\lambda^2 + b(\tau)\lambda + c(\tau)\right] + \left[p(\tau)\lambda^2 + q(\tau)\lambda + r(\tau)\right] e^{-\lambda\tau} = 0 \quad (6)$$

where in $a(\tau) = \left(a_1 P + b_1 e^{-\mu\tau} P\right)/S$, $b(\tau) = \left(a_1 b_1 e^{-\mu\tau} P^2 + a_3 c_1 P R + b_3 c_2 Q R\right]/S^2$, and $c(\tau) = \left[(a_1 b_3 c_2 - a_2 b_3 c_1) P Q R + a_3 b_1 c_1 e^{-\mu\tau} P^2 R\right)/S^3$; $p(\tau) = -b_1 e^{-\mu\tau} P/S$, $q(\tau) = \left[(a_2 Q - a_1 P) b_1 e^{-\mu\tau} P\right]/S^2$, and $r(\tau) = \left[(c_2 Q - c_1 P) a_3 b_1 e^{-\mu\tau} P R\right]/S^3$. These coefficients depend on the time delay $\tau$. For ease of notation, we drop the $\tau$ on these coefficients. We follow the discussions and notations used in [1] in analyzing the roots of characteristic equations with *delay-dependent* coefficients. Note that $(a + p) = a_1 \cdot \frac{P}{S}$, $(b + q) = a_2 b_1 e^{-\mu\tau} \cdot \frac{P}{S} \cdot \frac{Q}{S} + a_3 c_1 \cdot \frac{P}{S} \cdot \frac{R}{S} + b_3 c_2 \cdot \frac{Q}{S} \cdot \frac{R}{S}$, and $(c + r) = \left(a_1 b_3 c_2 - a_2 b_3 c_1 + a_3 b_1 c_2 e^{-\mu\tau}\right) \cdot \frac{P}{S} \cdot \frac{Q}{S} \cdot \frac{R}{S} = S \cdot \frac{P}{S} \cdot \frac{Q}{S} \cdot \frac{R}{S}$. Since the components $\frac{P}{S}, \frac{Q}{S}$, and $\frac{R}{S}$ of $E_4$ are all positive, both $(a + p)$ and $(b + q)$ are positive, while $(c + r)$ is positive (resp. negative) if $S$ is positive (resp. negative). Also, notice that $(a + p)(b + q) - (c + r)$ is given by

$$a_1 \left(a_2 b_1 e^{-\mu\tau} \cdot \frac{Q}{S} + a_3 c_1 \cdot \frac{R}{S}\right) \left(\frac{P}{S}\right)^2 + \left(a_2 b_3 c_1 - a_3 b_1 c_2 e^{-\mu\tau}\right) \cdot \frac{P}{S} \cdot \frac{Q}{S} \cdot \frac{R}{S}.$$

So that if $\left(a_2 b_3 c_1 - a_3 b_1 c_2 e^{-\mu\tau}\right)$ is positive, then $(a + p)(b + q) - (c + r)$ is positive. At $\tau = 0$, characteristic Eq. (6) reduces to $\lambda^3 + \rho\lambda^2 + \sigma\lambda + \varphi = 0$ where the coefficients $\rho = (a + p)|_{\tau=0}$, $\sigma = (b + q)|_{\tau=0}$, and $\varphi = (c + r)|_{\tau=0}$. The Routh-Hurwitz criterion requires $\rho, \sigma, \varphi$, and $(\rho\sigma - \varphi)$ to be all positive so that all roots of this cubic polynomial equation $\lambda^3 + \rho\lambda^2 + \sigma\lambda + \varphi = 0$ have negative real part.

**Theorem 4** *Let $\tau = 0$ in system (3). If $S(0) > 0$ and $(a_2 b_3 c_1 - a_3 b_1 c_2) > 0$, then the positive equilibrium $E_4$ is LAS. If $S(0) < 0$ or if $(\rho\sigma - \varphi) < 0$, then $E_4$ is unstable.*

Consider now the case $\tau > 0$. Since $S \neq 0$, $(c + r) = S \cdot \frac{P}{S}\frac{Q}{S}\frac{R}{S} \neq 0$, and thus $\lambda(\tau) = 0$ is not a root of (6). If $\lambda(\tau) = i\omega(\tau)$, with $\omega(\tau) > 0$, is a root (6), then $\left[-i\omega^3(\tau) - a\omega^2(\tau) + ib\omega(\tau) + c\right] + \left[-p\omega^2(\tau) + iq\omega(\tau) + r\right]e^{-i\omega(\tau)\tau} = 0$. Separating the real and imaginary parts of this equation, we obtain

$$\begin{bmatrix} q\omega(\tau) & -(p\omega^2(\tau) - r) \\ (p\omega^2(\tau) - r) & q\omega(\tau) \end{bmatrix} \begin{bmatrix} \sin(\omega(\tau)\tau) \\ \cos(\omega(\tau)\tau) \end{bmatrix} = \begin{bmatrix} a\omega^2(\tau) - c \\ (\omega^2(\tau) - b)\omega(\tau) \end{bmatrix},$$

which then gives

$$(a\omega^2(\tau) - c)^2 + (\omega^2(\tau) - b)^2\omega^2(\tau) = (p\omega^2(\tau) - r)^2 + q^2\omega^2(\tau). \tag{7}$$

Following [1], we write (7) into the following form

$$F(\omega, \tau) := \omega^6 + \alpha\omega^4 + \beta\omega^2 + \gamma = 0 \tag{8}$$

where $\alpha = a^2 - p^2 - 2b$, $\beta = b^2 - q^2 + 2(pr - ac)$, and $\gamma = c^2 - r^2$. If we let $u = \omega^2$, then (8) can be written as

$$H(u, \tau) := u^3 + \alpha u^2 + \beta u + \gamma = 0. \tag{9}$$

Note that if (9) has a positive root $u_0$, then (8) has a positive root $\omega_0 = \sqrt{u_0}$ and consequently, (6) has a pair of purely imaginary roots $\lambda = \pm i\omega_0$. That is, if (9) has a positive root, then stability switches may occur as $\tau$ is varied. Let $I \subset \mathbf{R}_{+0}$ be the set where $\omega(\tau)$ is a positive root of (8). Define the angle $\theta(\tau) \in [0, 2\pi]$ to be solution to the following

$$\begin{cases} \sin\theta(\tau) = \dfrac{(p\omega^2(\tau) - r)(\omega^2(\tau) - b)\omega(\tau) + q\omega(\tau)(a\omega^2(\tau) - c)}{p^2\omega^4(\tau) + (q^2 - 2pr)\omega^2(\tau) + r^2}, \\[3mm] \cos\theta(\tau) = \dfrac{q\omega^2(\tau)(\omega^2(\tau) - b) - (p\omega^2(\tau) - r)(a\omega^2(\tau) - c)}{p^2\omega^4(\tau) + (q^2 - 2pr)\omega^2(\tau) + r^2}. \end{cases}$$

For $\tau \in I$, that is $\omega(\tau)$ is a positive root of (8), we have $\omega(\tau)\tau = \theta(\tau) + 2n\pi$ for $n \in \mathbf{N}_0$. Hence, we can define the functions $S_n(\tau) = \tau - \tau_n(\tau)$, for $\tau \in I$ and $n \in \mathbf{N}_0$, where $\tau_n(\tau) = (\theta(\tau) + 2n\pi)/\omega(\tau)$. In [1], it was shown that the functions $S_n(\tau)$ are continuous and differentiable.

**Theorem 5** (Beretta and Kuang [1]) *Assume that $\omega(\tau)$ is a positive root of (8) defined for $\tau \in I \subset \mathbf{R}_{+0}$, and at some $\tau^* \in I$, $S_n(\tau^*) = 0$ for some $n \in \mathbf{N}_0$. Then a conjugate pair of simple purely imaginary roots $\lambda_\pm(\tau^*) = \pm i\omega(\tau^*)$ of (6) exists at $\tau = \tau^*$ which crosses the imaginary axis from left to right (resp. from right to left) if $\delta(\tau^*) > 0$ (resp. $\delta(\tau^*) < 0$), where*

$$\delta(\tau^*) = \text{sign} \left\{ \frac{d\text{Re}\lambda}{d\tau} \Big|_{\lambda=i\omega(\tau^*)} \right\} = \text{sign} \left\{ F'_\omega(\omega(\tau^*), \tau^*) \right\} \cdot \text{sign} \left\{ \frac{dS_n(\tau)}{d\tau} \Big|_{\tau=\tau^*} \right\}.$$

From (8) and (9), we get $F'_\omega(\omega(\tau), \tau) = 2\omega(\tau) \cdot H'_u(u(\tau), \tau)|_{u(\tau)=\omega^2(\tau)}$. Since $\omega(\tau) > 0$ for $\tau \in I$, the expression for $\delta(\tau^*)$ in Theorem 5 can be written as

$$\delta(\tau^*) = \text{sign} \left\{ H'_u(u(\tau^*), \tau^*) \right\} \cdot \text{sign} \left\{ \frac{dS_n(\tau)}{d\tau} \Big|_{\tau=\tau^*} \right\}. \tag{10}$$

Also, note that if such $\tau^*$ in Theorem 5 exists and $\delta(\tau^*) \neq 0$, then at $\tau = \tau^*$ system (3) undergoes a Hopf bifurcation at the positive equilibrium $E_4$. See [5, 11] for a statement of the Hopf bifurcation theorem for functional differential equations.

## 3 Numerical Simulations

We use the following parameter values $a_0 = 5.00$, $a_1 = 0.40$, $a_2 = 1.00$, $a_3 = 0.85$, $b_0 = 1.00$, $b_1 = 1.00$, $b_3 = 1.00$, $c_0 = 1.20$, $c_1 = 0.10$, $c_2 = 1.00$, and $\mu = 0.01$. At $\tau = 0$, we get the positive equilibrium $E_4 = (4.0435, 0.7957, 3.0435)$. From Theorem 4, $E_4$ is unstable because $(\rho\sigma - \varphi) < 0$. We want to know if stability switches will occur as $\tau$ is increased from zero. Recall that if the cubic equation $H(u, \tau) = u^3 + \alpha(\tau)u^2 + \beta(\tau)u + \gamma(\tau) = 0$ given in (9) has a simple positive root, then (6) has a pair of simple purely imaginary roots. Figure 2a shows that for values of $\tau$ immediately to the right of zero, the coefficients

$$\alpha(\tau) < 0, \quad \beta(\tau) < 0, \quad \text{and} \quad \gamma(\tau) > 0. \tag{11}$$

If the coefficients of $H(u, \tau)$ satisfy (11), then Eq. (9) has exactly 2 positive simple roots *provided* the relative minimum point $(\bar{u}, H(\bar{u}, \tau))$ of the graph of $H$ satisfies the following condition

$$H(\bar{u}, \tau) < 0. \tag{12}$$

Observe, from Fig. 2a, b that (11) and (12) are satisfied whenever $\tau \in (0, \tau_{end})$ where the value of $\tau_{end}$ is approximately 17.1276.

Consider the set $I = \{ \tau > 0 \mid \alpha(\tau) < 0, \beta(\tau) < 0, \gamma(\tau) > 0, \text{ and } H(\bar{u}, \tau) < 0 \}$. For $\tau \in I$, conditions (11) and (12) are satisfied. Thus, Eq. (9) has 2 positive roots, say $u(\tau) = u_\pm(\tau)$ with $u_+(\tau) > u_-(\tau) > 0$. Consequently, Eq. (8) has 2 positive roots $\omega(\tau) = \omega_\pm(\tau) = \sqrt{u_\pm(\tau)}$. Note that the graph of $H(u(\tau), \tau)$ is decreasing at $u(\tau) = u_-(\tau)$ and is increasing at $u(\tau) = u_+(\tau)$. That is, we have

$$H'_u(u_-(\tau), \tau) < 0 \quad \text{and} \quad H'_u(u_+(\tau), \tau) > 0. \tag{13}$$

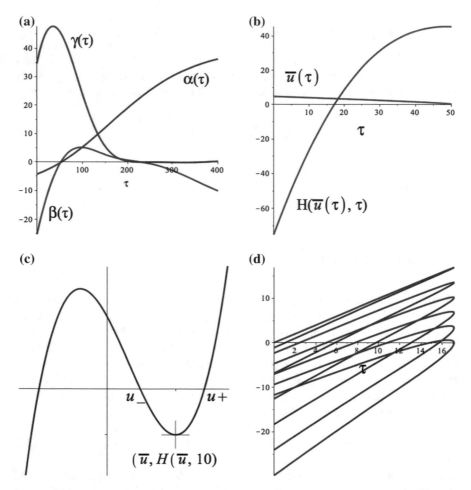

**Fig. 2** **a** Graphs of the coefficients $\alpha(\tau)$, $\beta(\tau)$, and $\gamma(\tau)$ in the cubic polynomial $H(u(\tau), \tau)$. **b** The relative minimum point $(\bar{u}(\tau), H(\bar{u}(\tau), \tau))$ of the graph of $H(u(\tau), \tau)$ has $H(\bar{u}(\tau), \tau) < 0$ for $\tau \in (0, \tau_{end})$, where $\tau_{end} = 17.1276$ approximately. **c** The graph of the cubic polynomial $H(u(\tau), \tau)$ when $\tau = 10$. **d** The graph of the functions $S_n^+(\tau)$ (in blue) and the graph of the functions $S_n^-(\tau)$ (in red) for $n = 0, 1, 2, 3, 4, 5, 6$

Figure 2c shows the graph of the cubic polynomial $H(u, 10)$ whose coefficients satisfy (11) and (12). The positive roots $u_-(10)$ and $u_+(10)$ of $H(u, 10) = 0$ are indicated along with the relative minimum point $(\bar{u}, H(\bar{u}, 10))$. Observe that (11) tells us that the graph of the cubic polynomial intersects the vertical axis at a point above the horizontal axis ($\gamma(\tau) > 0$), and where the graph is decreasing ($\beta(\tau) < 0$) and concave downwards ($\alpha(\tau) < 0$). Meanwhile, (12) assures us that the cubic equation has 2 *simple positive* roots if the relative minimum point is *below* the horizontal axis (i.e. $H(\bar{u}, \tau) < 0$).

In this example, Eq. (6) has 2 conjugate pairs of simple purely imaginary roots $\lambda(\tau_-^*) = \pm i\omega_-(\tau_-^*)$ and $\lambda(\tau_+^*) = \pm i\omega_+(\tau_+^*)$. To find the critical delay values $\tau_\pm^*$ in Theorem 5, where stability switches may occur, we look at the zeros of the functions $S_n^\pm(\tau)$. Figure 2d shows the graph of these functions on the interval $(0, \tau_{end})$ for $n = 0, 1, 2, 3, 4, 5, 6$. In Fig. 3a, we look closer at the graph of the first few $S_n^\pm(\tau)$ and observe that $S_0^+(\tau)$ has no zeros in the interval $(0, \tau_{end})$ while $S_0^-(\tau)$, $S_1^+(\tau)$, $S_2^+(\tau)$, and $S_1^-(\tau)$ has exactly one zero each given approximately by $\tau_0^- = 1.0515$, $\tau_1^+ = 2.4002$, $\tau_2^+ = 4.9575$, and $\tau_1^- = 5.8070$, respectively. To determine the direction of the stability switch at the critical delay value $\tau^*$, we compute $\delta(\tau^*)$ using (10). From Fig. 2d, we see that the functions $S_n^\pm(\tau)$ are all increasing at their respective zeros $\tau = \tau_n^\pm$, so that $\text{sign}\left\{\left.\dfrac{dS_n^\pm(\tau)}{d\tau}\right|_{\tau=\tau_n^\pm}\right\} = +1$. Meanwhile, from (13), we know

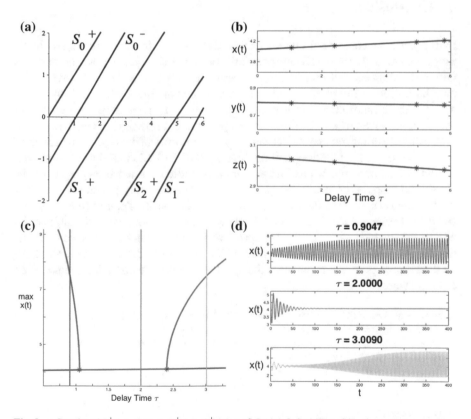

**Fig. 3 a** Graphs of $S_0^+(\tau)$, $S_0^-(\tau)$, $S_1^+(\tau)$, $S_2^+(\tau)$, and $S_1^-(\tau)$. **b** Stability of $E_4$ changes at $\tau = \tau_0^- = 1.0515$ and at $\tau = \tau_1^+ = 2.4002$ marked with black (*) where Hopf bifurcation occurs. Stable parts are in green while unstable parts are in magenta. **c** Stable branches of periodic solutions (shown in green) emanating from the Hopf bifurcations. The vertical axis gives a measure of the maximum value of $x(t)$. **d** Time series of $x(t)$ for different delay values illustrating the existence of a stable periodic solution for $\tau < \tau_0^-$ and $\tau > \tau_1^+$, and the local stability of $E_4$ for $\tau \in (\tau_0^-, \tau_1^+)$

that sign $\left\{ H'_u(u(\tau_n^\pm), \tau_n^\pm) \right\} = \pm 1$. Therefore, we have $\delta(\tau_n^\pm) = \pm 1$. At $\tau = \tau_0^- = 1.0515$, we have a switch from unstable to stable, while at $\tau = \tau_1^+ = 2.4002$ we have a switch from stable to unstable.

Numerical continuation, using DDE-Biftool [4], also confirms these switches on the stability of the positive equilibrium $E_4$ as shown in Fig. 3b. We also mention that at $\tau = \tau_0^-$ and at $\tau = \tau_1^+$, system (3) undergoes a Hopf bifurcation at the positive equilibrium $E_4$. Figure 3c shows the branches of periodic solutions that emerged from these Hopf bifurcation points. In Fig. 3d, we select three different values of the time delay to show that for $\tau < \tau_0^-$ and for $\tau > \tau_1^+$, where $E_4$ is unstable, a stable periodic solution exists, while for $\tau \in (\tau_0^-, \tau_1^+)$, $E_4$ is locally asymptotically stable.

# 4 Conclusion

In this paper, we considered a three-species IGP model with stage structure in the IG prey population, that is, the IG prey population is divided into juvenile and adult stages with maturation age reflected by a delay parameter. We assumed that the juvenile IG prey have little ability of predation and are able to avoid the IG predators by taking refuge. Conditions for the existence and local stability of all non-negative equilibrium solutions are given using the time delay as parameter. In particular, we showed that the positive equilibrium may switch stability at some critical delay value where Hopf bifurcation occurs. Numerical continuation in DDE-Biftool is used to illustrate our results and examine the bifurcating branch of periodic solutions emerging from the Hopf bifurcation. Our results tell us that as we vary the delay parameter, which is the maturation age of the IG prey population, a stable positive equilibrium may lose stability at some critical delay value. However, this does not lead to destabilization of the system since the stability of the positive equilibrium is being passed on to the limit cycle that is created via Hopf bifurcation. The introduction of stage structure on the IG prey population enhances the species coexistence through the emergence of limit cycles.

**Acknowledgements** JAC is grateful to the IMU-CDC for the Abel Visiting Scholars Program grant and to Prof. Felicia Maria G. Magpantay for hosting him at the University of Manitoba in Fall 2016. JAC also acknowledges the support of the University of the Philippines Baguio. FMGM is grateful to NSERC Canada Discovery Grants.

# References

1. Beretta, E., Kuang, Y.: Geometric stability switch criteria in delay differential systems with delay dependent parameters. SIAM J. Math. Anal. **33**, 1144–1165 (2002)
2. Collera, J.A.: Bifurcations in delayed Lotka-Volterra intraguild predation model. Matimyás Matematika **37**, 11–22 (2014)

3. Collera, J.A.: Harvesting in delayed food web model with omnivory. AIP Conf. Proc. **1705**, 020033 (2016)
4. Engelborghs, K., Luzyanina, T., Samaey, G.: DDE-BIFTOOL v. 2.00: A MATLAB package for bifurcation analysis of delay differential equations. Technical Report TW-330, Department of Computer Science, K.U. Leuven, Leuven (2001)
5. Hale, J.K., Lunel, S.M.V.: Introduction to Functional Differential Equations. Springer, New York (1993)
6. Holt, R.D., Polis, G.A.: A theoretical framework for intraguild predation. Am. Nat. **149**, 745–764 (1997)
7. Hsu, S.-B., Ruan, S., Yang, T.-H.: Analysis of three species Lotka-Volterra food web models with omnivory. J. Math. Anal. Appl. **426**, 659–687 (2015)
8. Namba, T., Tanabe, K., Maeda, N.: Omnivory and stability of food webs. Ecol. Complex. **5**, 73–85 (2008)
9. Polis, G.A., Myers, C.A., Holt, R.D.: The ecology and evolution of intraguild predation: potential competitors that eat each other. Annu. Rev. Ecol. Syst. **20**, 297–330 (1989)
10. Shu, H., Hu, X., Wang, L., Watmough, J.: Delay induced stability switch, multitype bistability and chaos in an intraguild predation model. J. Math. Biol. **71**, 1269–1298 (2015)
11. Smith, H.: An Introduction to Delay Differential Equations with Applications to the Life Sciences. Springer, New York (2011)
12. Tanabe, K., Namba, T.: Omnivory creates chaos in simple food web models. Ecology **86**, 3411–3414 (2005)
13. Wang, Y., Wu, J., Xiao, Y.: A stage structured predator-prey model with time delays. Rocky Mountain J. Math. **38**, 1721–1743 (2008)
14. Yamaguchi, M., Takeuchi, Y., Ma, W.: Dynamical properties of a stage structured three-species model with intraguild predation. J. Comput. Appl. Math. **201**, 327–338 (2007)

# A Conceptual Model for the Pliocene Paradox

Brady Dortmans, William F. Langford and Allan R. Willms

**Abstract** In the Pliocene Epoch (5.3–2.6 million years ago), there was an abrupt cooling of the Arctic, from an ice-free to an ice-covered climate state. A simple conceptual mathematical model of Arctic climate is used to explore the potential role of forcing factors, such as $CO_2$ concentration and ocean heat transport to the Arctic, as well as nonlinear feedback mechanisms, such as ice-albedo feedback and water vapour feedback, in the climate change of the Pliocene Arctic. The mathematical model provides a plausible explanation for this abrupt climate change, involving both of these forcing factors and both of the nonlinear feedback mechanisms. The model also sheds light on the fact that modern general circulation models have been unable to reproduce this dramatic change in Arctic climate.

**Keywords** Climate change · Pliocene paradox · Slab model · Water vapour
Carbon dioxide

## 1 Introduction

Better understanding of climate changes that have occurred in the geological record of the Earth may enable us to predict climate change that will occur in the future. The Pliocene Epoch (5.3–2.6 MYa) was a time of dramatic climate change in the Arctic region on Earth. The Arctic cooled from ice-free to ice-covered, while the climate of the remainder of the planet changed relatively little. The major climate "forcing mechanisms" such as solar radiation, $CO_2$ concentration, Earth orbital parameters and geography were all very close to today's values. Therefore, it is a challenge

B. Dortmans (✉) · W. F. Langford · A. R. Willms
Department of Mathematics and Statistics,
University of Guelph, Guelph, ON N1G 2W1, Canada
e-mail: Brady.Dortmans@gmail.com

W. F. Langford
e-mail: wlangfor@uoguelph.ca

A. R. Willms
e-mail: awillms@uoguelph.ca

© Springer Nature Switzerland AG 2018
D. M. Kilgour et al. (eds.), *Recent Advances in Mathematical
and Statistical Methods*, Springer Proceedings in Mathematics & Statistics 259,
https://doi.org/10.1007/978-3-319-99719-3_31

for climate scientists to explain why the early Pliocene Arctic climate was so much warmer than today, even though the forcing mechanisms were little different from today. This question is known as the *Pliocene Paradox* [4]. Climate scientists have developed powerful computer models of weather and climate, known as General Circulation Models (GCM), which accurately reproduce today's climate. When a modern GCM is adjusted to the forcing mechanisms of the Pliocene, the predicted climate is little different from today's climate [4]. The conceptual model presented here explains the difficulty for GCM's to reproduce the warm Arctic climate of the early Pliocene and provides a simple resolution of the Pliocene Paradox.

In this paper we present a preliminary analysis of a conceptual model of Arctic climate, with emphasis on the role of greenhouse gases and ocean heat transport (OHT). The model is built on basic physical laws such as: the Stefan-Boltzmann law, Beer's law, the ideal gas equation, and the Clausius-Clapeyron equation. No weather data are used. The geometry of the Arctic is simplified to an absolute minimum. The atmosphere of the Arctic is represented as a column of unit cross-section, centred on the North Pole, with uniform temperature $T_A$. The surface temperature is $T_S$. These are the only two state variables in the model. Similar conceptual models have been studied by many authors, see [2, 3, 8, 9, 11] and further references therein. This paper extends previous uniform slab models, by investigating the interplay between two *climate forcing mechanisms* ($CO_2$ concentration and ocean heat transport) and two *climate feedback mechanisms* (ice-albedo feedback and water vapour feedback).

Rather than isolating the climate forcing and feedback parameters pertinent to the Pliocene itself, this model brackets the Pliocene conditions using published parameter values for the warm Eocene Epoch (56–34 MYa) [5, 12] and the pre-industrial modern era [6]. As the forcing parameters sweep from Eocene values to pre-industrial values, the model exhibits an abrupt change (bifurcation point or tipping point) in the climate state, homologous to what occurred in the Pliocene.

## 2  Conceptual Model of Arctic Climate

Only a summary of the mathematical model is presented here. For a complete derivation of the model, see [3]. The Arctic atmosphere is represented as a uniform column of air, of unit cross-section, vertically above the surface at the North Pole. The total mass of air in this uniform column is equal to the total mass of a (non-uniform) column of the actual atmosphere, from the surface to the tropopause, at the North Pole. This model is based on the model used in Payne et al. [9], modified as shown in Fig. 1. The symbols in Fig. 1 are defined in Table 1. The incoming solar radiation is denoted $F_S$, ocean heat transport is $F_O$ and atmospheric heat transport is $F_A$. The surface emits longwave radiation with intensity $I_S$, of which a fraction $\eta$ is absorbed by the greenhouse gases in the atmosphere. The atmosphere is assumed to emit longwave radiation with intensity $I_A$ upwards and downwards, with half going in each direction. The primary difference between our model and Payne's model is that the absorptivity of the greenhouse gases in our model are expressed as functions of the $CO_2$ concentration and the atmospheric temperature.

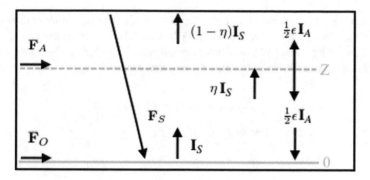

**Fig. 1** A visualization of the conceptual model. Symbols are defined in Table 1

**Table 1** Summary of variables and parameters used in the model. For details see [3]

| Variables | Symbol | Values |
|---|---|---|
| Mean temperature of the surface | $T_S$ | −50 to +20 °C |
| Infrared radiation from the surface | $I_S = \sigma T_S^4$ | 141 to 419 Wm$^{-2}$ |
| Mean temperature of the atmosphere | $T_A$ | −70 to 0 °C |
| Infrared radiation from the atmosphere | $I_A = \varepsilon \sigma T_A^4$ | 87 to 219 Wm$^{-2}$ |
| Parameters and Constants | Symbol | Values |
| Stefan-Boltzmann constant | $\sigma$ | $5.670 \times 10^{-8}$ Wm$^{-2}$K$^{-4}$ |
| Emissivity of dry air | $\varepsilon$ | 0.9 |
| Greenhouse gas absorptivity | $\eta$ | 0 to 1 |
| Absorptivity for $CO_2$ | $\eta_C$ | 0 to 1 |
| Absorptivity for $H_2O$ | $\eta_W$ | 0 to 1 |
| Ocean heat transport | $F_O$ | 20 to 60 Wm$^{-2}$ |
| Atmospheric heat transport | $F_A$ | 70 to 127 Wm$^{-2}$ |
| Absorption of solar radiation | $F_S$ | $(1 - \alpha)Q$ |
| Incident solar radiation at North Pole | $Q$ | 173.2 Wm$^{-2}$ |
| Molar concentration of $CO_2$ in ppm | $\mu$ | 270 to 600 ppm |
| Relative humidity of $H_2O$ | $\delta$ | 0 to 1 |
| Absorption coefficient for $CO_2$ | $k_C$ | 0.0474 m$^2$/kg |
| Absorption coefficient for $H_2O$ | $k_W$ | 0.016 m$^2$/kg |
| Warm surface Albedo for ocean | $\alpha_W$ | 0.04 |
| Cold surface Albedo for ice/snow | $\alpha_C$ | 0.7 |

In the model it is assumed that both the surface and the atmosphere are at equilibrium; that is, *energy in = energy out* for each, and the two temperatures $T_S$ and $T_A$ are determined by these two equilibrium equations. From Fig. 1, the energy balance equations for the surface and the atmosphere are, respectively,

$$0 = F_S + F_O + \frac{1}{2}I_A - I_S, \tag{1}$$

$$0 = F_A + \eta I_S - I_A. \tag{2}$$

## 2.1 Radiation Balance

It is assumed that the shortwave radiation from the sun passes through the atmosphere without being absorbed. At the surface, the amount of solar radiation absorbed $F_S$ is determined by the annually averaged intensity of solar radiation striking the surface, $Q$, and by the *albedo* of the surface, $\alpha$, which is the fraction of $Q$ reflected by the surface back into space. Thus

$$F_S = (1 - \alpha)Q. \tag{3}$$

The value of $Q$ at the North Pole is $Q = 173.2$ Wm$^{-2}$, see [3, 7]. Typical values of the albedo $\alpha$ are 0.6–0.9 for snow, 0.4 for ice, 0.2 for cropland and 0.1 or less for open ocean. In this paper, two values of $\alpha$ are used corresponding to whether the surface temperature is below or above freezing, that is

$$\alpha = \begin{cases} \alpha_c = 0.7 & \text{if } T_S \leq 273.15\,\text{K}, \\ \alpha_w = 0.04 & \text{if } T_S > 273.15\,\text{K}. \end{cases} \tag{4}$$

The emission of radiation from the atmosphere and surface is governed by the *Stefan-Boltzmann law*, that is

$$I_S = \sigma T_S^4, \quad \text{and} \quad I_A = \varepsilon \sigma T_A^4. \tag{5}$$

Here $\sigma = 5.670 \times 10^{-8}$ W m$^{-2}$ K$^{-4}$ is the Stefan-Boltzmann constant. The surface of the Earth acts as a black-body, so $\varepsilon = 1$ in $I_S$. However, the atmosphere is an imperfect black-body, with $\varepsilon = 0.9$ in $I_A$.

Substituting (3) and (5) into (1) and (2) gives the surface and atmosphere energy balance equations in terms of the two equilibrium temperatures $T_S$ and $T_A$:

$$0 = (1 - \alpha)Q + F_O + \frac{1}{2}\varepsilon \sigma T_A^4 - \sigma T_S^4, \tag{6}$$

$$0 = F_A + \eta \sigma T_S^4 - \varepsilon \sigma T_A^4. \tag{7}$$

## 2.2 Greenhouse Gases

The coefficient $\eta$ in Eqs. (2) and (7) represents the fraction of the outgoing radiation $I_S$ from the surface that is absorbed by the greenhouse gases in the atmosphere, also known as absorptivity. Then $(1 - \eta)$ is the fraction of the outgoing infrared radiation that escapes to space. Most previous conceptual models leave $\eta$ as a parameter, which is adjusted manually in the equation. In this paper, $\eta$ is expressed as a function of more fundamental physical parameters.

The two principal greenhouse gases are carbon dioxide $CO_2$ and water vapour $H_2O$. Because they act in different ways, we determine the absorptivities $\eta_C$, $\eta_W$ of $CO_2$ and $H_2O$ separately, and then combine their effects as

$$\eta = 1 - (1 - \eta_C)(1 - \eta_W). \tag{8}$$

Equation (8) simply states that the absorption done by $CO_2$ and water vapour is independent, so that the total fraction of radiation passing through the atmosphere is a product of the fractions that pass through the two gases individually. Other greenhouse gases have only minor influence and are ignored in this paper. Although it is well-known that $CO_2$ and $H_2O$ absorb the infrared radiation $I_S$ at specific wavelengths, in this paper the *grey gas approximation* [10] is used; that is, absorptivity is given as a single number averaged over the infrared spectrum.

The concentration of $CO_2$ in the atmosphere is usually expressed as a ratio $\mu$, in molar parts per million (ppm) of dry air. Today there is convincing evidence that $\mu$ is increasing due to human activity. The value before the industrial revolution was $\mu = 270$ ppm, but today $\mu$ is slightly above 400 ppm. To convert molar ppm to mass ppm one must multiply $\mu$ by the ratio of molar masses of $CO_2$ and dry air, $\frac{m_C}{m_A} \approx 1.52$ ($CO_2$ is about 50% heavier than air, which is primarily nitrogen gas $N_2$).

*Beer's law* [3] dictates that for the slab model with constant density, $\rho$, of $CO_2$, the radiation from the surface passing through this gas is $(1 - \eta_C)I_S = I_S e^{-k_C \rho Z}$, where $Z$ is the height of the troposphere and $k_C$ is the absorption coefficient for $CO_2$. The mass of a column of air, of unit cross-section, from surface to tropopause, is determined as $M_A = P_A/g$, where $P_A$ is the atmospheric pressure at the surface and $g$ is acceleration due to gravity. It follows that

$$\eta_C = 1 - \exp\left[-\frac{\mu}{10^6}\left(\frac{m_C}{m_A}\right)k_C M_A\right] \equiv 1 - \exp[-\mu \cdot G_1]. \tag{9}$$

These constants combine to give the greenhouse gas constant for $CO_2$ as $G_1 = 7.44 \times 10^{-4}$.

The absorptivity of water vapour in (8) can not be expressed as simply as is the case for $CO_2$ in (9), because the concentration of water vapour in the atmosphere is strongly dependent on temperature. There is a temperature-dependent maximum (saturated) value of $H_2O$ gas concentration, above which the water vapour condenses out of the atmosphere and falls as rain (or snow). This saturated value, usually expressed as partial pressure, is determined by the *Clausius-Clapeyron equation* [10]. The ratio of the actual partial pressure of $H_2O$ in the atmosphere to the saturated partial pressure (under any given conditions) is called *relative humidity* and denoted $\delta$, $0 \leq \delta \leq 1$. Using the Clausius-Clapeyron equation, the absorptivity of water vapour in the atmosphere at temperature $T$ has been determined in [3] as

$$\eta_W = 1 - \exp\left[-\delta k_W \frac{P_{sat}(T_R)}{g}\left[\frac{T_R}{T_A}\right]\exp\left(\frac{L_v}{R_W}\left[\frac{1}{T_R} - \frac{1}{T_A}\right]\right)\right]. \quad (10)$$

Here, $T_R$ is a reference temperature, which we take to be the freezing point of water, $273.15\,°K$, and $P_{sat}(T_R)/g$ is the mass of a column, with unit cross-section, of water vapour at the saturated partial pressure $P_{sat}(T_R)$. The absorption coefficient of water vapour is $k_W$ and the specific heat of vaporization is $L_v$. The above equations are simplified by non-dimensionalizing temperatures and forcing factors. Define

$$\tau_A = \frac{T_A}{T_R} \quad \tau_S = \frac{T_S}{T_R} \quad q = \frac{Q}{\sigma T_R^4} \quad fo = \frac{T_O}{\sigma T_R^4} \quad f_A = \frac{F_A}{\sigma T_R^4}, \quad (11)$$

then $\tau = 1$ is the freezing point of water and (10) simplifies to

$$\eta_W = 1 - \exp\left[-\delta\frac{G_2}{\tau_A}\exp\left(G_3\left[\frac{\tau_A - 1}{\tau_A}\right]\right)\right], \quad (12)$$

where the greenhouse gas constants for water vapour are $G_2 = 0.9969$, $G_3 = 17.899$. Combining all the above results, the energy balance equation for the surface is

$$\tau_S^4 = 0.5\varepsilon\tau_A^4 + (1 - \alpha)q + fo, \quad (13)$$

and the energy balance equation for the atmosphere may be written

$$\tau_S^4 = \frac{\varepsilon\tau_A^4 - f_A}{1 - \exp\left[-\mu \cdot G_1 - \delta\dfrac{G_2}{\tau_A}\exp\left(G_3\left[\dfrac{\tau_A - 1}{\tau_A}\right]\right)\right]}. \quad (14)$$

There are two state variables, $\tau_S$ and $\tau_A$, determined by these two equilibrium equations. There are four parameters of interest here, namely $\mu$, $\delta$, $\alpha$, $fo$, which we can vary independently to determine their effects on $\tau_S$ and $\tau_A$.

Due to space limitations, this paper presents a partial investigation of this model, which can display further interesting behaviours, including saddle-node bifurcations, temperature inversion and a "hot" equilibrium solution. For details see [3].

# 3 Application of the Model to the Pliocene Paradox

A dramatic climate change occurred in the Arctic during the Pliocene Epoch (5.3–2.6 MYa). For many years before the Pliocene, back to the Cretaceous Period and beyond, the Arctic was warm and ice-free. There is irrefutable evidence that the northernmost Arctic islands of present-day Canada supported a temperate rain forest during the Eocene (56–34 MYa), see [5, 12]. Ever since the Pliocene, the Arctic has had year-round ice cover. In this section, we use the conceptual model of Sect. 2 to explore possible mechanisms for this dramatic climate change, varying the parameters independently, to determine the influence of each on the behaviour.

We present the predictions of our model for three different scenarios. First we decrease $CO_2$ concentration in steps ($\mu = 800, 600, 400, 200$ ppm), while holding $\delta = 0$, $F_A = 100$ and $F_O$ constant. Then we add water vapour feedback, with decreasing $\mu$ as before. Finally, we vary ocean heat transport $F_O > 0$ in the model.

The pre-industrial modern value of $CO_2$ concentration has been established as $\mu = 270$ ppm [6]. The warmest part of the Cenozoic Era was the Eocene Epoch. Estimates of $CO_2$ concentration during the Eocene vary widely, in the range 350–1000 ppm, with a new consensus of 490 ppm reported in [12]. The model is used to explore the effects of decreasing $CO_2$ concentration from this Eocene value of 490 ppm to its pre-industrial value of 270 ppm.

## 3.1 Varying $CO_2$ Concentration Only

Fixing the relative humidity $\delta = 0$ and the ocean heat transport $F_O = 60$ W/m$^2$ allows us to examine the effects of varying $CO_2$ on the climate, see Fig. 2a. The blue lines represent the atmosphere energy balance Eq. (14) for increasing values of $CO_2$ concentration $\mu$, from left to right in the figure. The orange and magenta lines represent the surface energy balance Eq. (13), with a discontinuity across the dashed line at the freezing point $T_S = 273.15$ K ($\tau_S = 1$) due to the change in albedo there. Temperatures are shown in dimensionless units $\tau$, for convenience of interpretation. Each point of intersection of a blue line with an orange/magenta line is an equilibrium solution.

As $\mu$ varies, Fig. 2a shows that for $\mu$ greater than about 400 ppm there exist two distinct equilibrium solutions, one with $\tau_S > 1$ above freezing (on the magenta curve) and the other with $\tau_S < 1$ below freezing (on the orange curve); however, for values of $\mu$ less than about 400 ppm the warm equilibrium solution does not exist and only the frozen solution remains. Therefore, if the climate were in the warm state on the magenta curve, and the $CO_2$ concentration $\mu$ were to *decrease* sufficiently, this warm equilibrium state would disappear and the climate would cool abruptly to the ice-covered state on the orange curve.

## 3.2 Water Vapour Feedback

The inclusion of water vapour adds more non-linearity to the model, see Fig. 2b, where $\delta = 0.2$ and $F_O = 60$. The blue atmosphere energy balance curves represent the same levels of $CO_2$ concentration as in Fig. 2a, but they now bend further to the right. The transition from ice-free to ice-covered equilibrium solution still occurs as $\mu$ decreases, but for a smaller value of $\mu$ than in Fig. 2a; that is, approximately at $\mu = 360$ ppm. Thus, the warming effect of added water vapour as a greenhouse gas partially offsets the cooling effect of decreasing $CO_2$ concentration $\mu$.

## 3.3 Ocean Heat Transport

For most of the past few hundred million years, both the Arctic and the Antarctic were relatively warm and were free of ice-caps. In the mid-Cretaceous, the South Pole lay in open ocean waters and was heated by warm ocean currents of the South Pacific O-cean. Antarctica was surrounded by warm ocean waters and was ice-free at that time. Near the end of the Cretaceous period, the slow drift of the continent of Antarctica began to move it over the South Pole. Over the next 10–20 million years, Antarc-tica continued to drift until the South Pole was near the centre of Antarctica, and the Antarctic Circumpolar Circulation (ACC) began. The ACC is a cold ocean cur-rent, circulating around Antarctica, and isolating it from warm ocean currents to the North. As time passed, Antarctica cooled further and snow began to accumulate. The cooling of Antarctica was accelerated by ice-albedo feedback and water vapour feed-back. For about 30 million years prior to the Pliocene, the Antarctic was ice-capped

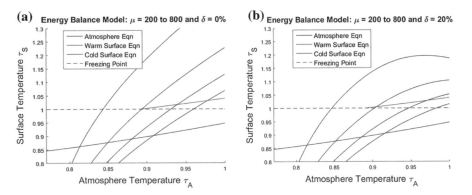

**Fig. 2** Energy Balance Equations with varying $CO_2$ concentration $\mu$. The blue curves represent the atmosphere equilibrium equation and the magenta/orange curves represent the surface equilibrium equation. From left to right, on the blue curves, $\mu$ is 200 ppm, 400 ppm, 600 ppm, 800 ppm. **a** No water vapour, $\delta = 0$. **b** $CO_2$ with water vapour, $\delta = 0.2$

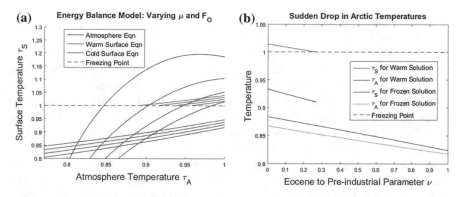

**Fig. 3** Energy balance with changing $CO_2$ and ocean heat transport $F_O$, and fixed $\delta = 0.2$. **a** Orange/magenta lines represent surface energy balance with $F_O = 60, 50, 40, 30$, respectively (moving downward in the figure). Blue curves represent atmospheric energy balance as in Fig. 2, with decreasing $CO_2$. **b** Equilibrium solutions with both $F_O$ and $\mu$ decreasing linear functions of the bifurcation parameter $\nu$, as defined in Eq. (15). There is a sudden drop in Arctic temperatures near $\nu = 0.273$, which corresponds to $\mu = 430$

while the Arctic remained ice-free. It is estimated that the total volume of ice on Antarctica today corresponds to a change in sea level of about 60 m [6].

The North Pole is situated in the Arctic Ocean, which is warmed by ocean currents (such as the Gulf Stream) bringing heat from the tropics. The gradual drop in sea level, due to growth of the Antarctic ice-cap, caused a decrease in ocean heat transport (OHT) to the Arctic, denoted $F_O$ in this paper. Continental drift also affected OHT. In the late Cretaceous, a land bridge formed between what is now North America and Asia, further reducing $F_O$. Paleoclimate estimates of OHT are difficult to obtain. Barron [1] estimated the OHT to the Arctic in the mid-Cretaceous to be $46.7\,\mathrm{Wm}^{-2}$ and gave today's value as $10.7\,\mathrm{Wm}^{-2}$. This provides a range of values for $F_O$ in our conceptual model.

From the Eocene Epoch to pre-industrial modern times, the concentration $\mu$ of $CO_2$ decreased (rising blue lines in Fig. 3a) and ocean heat transport, $F_O$, decreased (descending magenta/orange lines). Note that in Fig. 3a, for every choice of one blue (atmosphere) curve and one orange (cold surface) curve, there exists an intersection corresponding to an equilibrium solution below freezing. However, above the dashed freezing line $\tau_S = 1.0$ ($T_S = 273.15$ K), the intersection of the blue curve with the magenta curve disappears, as $\mu$ decreases and/or $F_O$ decreases. At this point, the ice-free Arctic climate, which had existed at least since the mid-Cretaceous, ceases to exist and is replaced by a frozen ice-capped Arctic climate on the orange curve.

Figure 3b introduces a "time surrogate" or bifurcation parameter $\nu$, with $0 \le \nu \le 1$, such that both $\mu$ and $F_O$ are linear functions of $\nu$ given by

$$\mu = 490 - 220\nu,$$
$$F_O = 60 - 30\nu,$$

$$(15)$$

so that $\nu = 0$ corresponds to the Eocene, and $\nu = 1$ corresponds to pre-industrial time. As seen in Fig. 3b, as $\nu$ increases (so both of $\mu$ and $F_O$ decrease), the ice-free surface equilibrium (on a magenta line) cools to the freezing point, at which the albedo $\alpha$ changes from $\alpha = \alpha_W$ to $\alpha = \alpha_C$ so that this equilibrium point disappears causing the surface temperature $\tau_S$ and the atmosphere temperature $\tau_A$ to drop to the frozen solution (orange and cyan lines). This jump occurs at forcing parameter values approximately $\mu = 430$ ppm and $F_O = 52$ W/m$^2$, close to estimated Pliocene conditions. One would not expect the values of $\mu$ and $F_O$ to vary linearly with time between the Eocene and the present, so the value $\nu \approx 0.273$ at which the jump takes place does not correspond to a specific time in the past. However, the model shows that this jump must occur at some point between the Eocene and present. Stability analysis performed in [3] shows that all the equilibrium solutions seen in Figs. 2 and 3 are *stable* in the dynamical systems sense.

## 4 Conclusions

The conceptual climate model presented in this paper predicts that, as the Earth's forcing parameters evolved slowly from the values of the Eocene (high $CO_2$ concentration $\mu$ and high ocean heat transport $F_O$) to today's values (lower $\mu$ and lower $F_O$), at some point in this evolution the climate of the Arctic changed abruptly from a warm surface ice-free state to a cold ice-capped state. This prediction is supported by the geological record, which shows that an abrupt cooling took place during the Pliocene Epoch. The model suggests that this abrupt Pliocene cooling was an inevitable consequence of the underlying climate mechanisms considered here.

This is not to say that the climate of the Earth cooled linearly from Eocene to modern conditions, as depicted in Fig. 3b. Neither can this extremely simple model be expected to give accurate quantitative predictions. All that can be inferred from this model is that, as the forcing parameters vary between Eocene and modern values, somewhere in that evolution there should be an abrupt cooling of the Arctic from ice-free to ice-capped.

Note that in the model the transition from warm (magenta) to frozen (orange) surface temperature is one-way only. Once on the frozen equilibrium branch, variation of the forcing parameters will not produce a transition back up to the warm equilibrium solution, see Fig. 3b. This suggests an explanation for the fact that GCM computations, originally designed to model today's climate, have failed to find a solution corresponding to the warm early Pliocene climate.

**Acknowledgements** The authors would like to thank J. Bassinger, D. Greenwood and G. Lewis for helpful discussions in the course of this work.

# References

1. Barron, E.J., Thompson, S.L., Schneider, S.H.: An ice-free Cretaceous? Results from climate model simulations. Science **212**, 10–13 (1981)
2. Budyko, M.I.: The effect of solar radiation variations on the climate of the Earth. Tellus XXI **5**, 611–619 (1968)
3. Dortmans, B.: A Conceptual Model of Climate Change Incorporating the Roles of Carbon Dioxide and Water Vapour as Greenhouse Gases. M.Sc. Thesis, Department of Mathematics and Statistics, University of Guelph, in preparation (2017)
4. Fedorov, A.V., Dekens, P.S., McCarthy, M., Ravelo, A.C., deMenocal, P.B., Barreiro, M., Pacanowski, R.C., Philander, S.G.: The Pliocene paradox (Mechanisms for a permanent El Niño). Science **312**, 1485–1489 (2006)
5. Greenwood, D.R., Basinger, J.F., Smith, R.Y.: How wet was the Arctic Eocene rain forest? Estimates of precipitation from Paleogene Arctic macrofloras. Geology **38**, 15–18 (2010)
6. IPCC, 2013: Climate Change 2013: The Physical Science Basis. In: Stocker, T.F., Qin, D., Plattner, G.-K., Tignor, M., Allen, S.K., Boschung, J., Nauels, A., Xia, Y., Bex, V., Midgley, P.M. (eds.) Contribution of Working Group I to the Fifth Assessment Report of the Intergovernmental Panel on Climate Change, 1535 p. Cambridge University Press, Cambridge (2013). Also available at http://www.ipcc.ch/
7. McGehee, R., Lehman, C.: A paleoclimate model of ice-albedo feedback forced by variations in Earth's orbit. SIAM J. Appl. Dynam. Sys. **11**, 684–707 (2012)
8. North, G.R., Cahalan, R.F., Coakley, J.A.: Energy balance climate models. Rev. Geophys. Space Phys. **19**, 91–121 (1981)
9. Payne, A.E., Jansen, M.F., Cronin, T.W.: Conceptual model analysis of the influence of temperature feedbacks on polar amplification. Geophys. Res. Lett. **42**, 9561–9570 (2015)
10. Pierrehumbert, R.T.: Principles of Planetary Climate. Cambridge University Press, Cambridge (2010)
11. Sellers, W.D.: A global climate model based on the energy balance of the earth-atmosphere system. J. Appl. Meteo. **8**, 392–400 (1969)
12. Wolfe, A.E., Reyes, A.V., Royer, D.L., Greenwood, D.R., Doria, G., Gagen, M.H., Siver, P.A., Westgate, J.A.: Middle Eocene $CO_2$ and climate reconstructed from the sediment fill of a subarctic kimberlite maar. Geology **45**, 619–622 (2017)

# First Order Versus Monod Kinetics in Numerical Simulation of Biofilms in Porous Media

**Harry J. Gaebler and Hermann J. Eberl**

**Abstract** We study a system of partial differential equations that model a macroscopic porous medium biofilm reactor. Solutions to the system are calculated numerically using the second order Uniformly accurate Central Scheme. We investigate and compare two different growth rate functions, first order and Monod kinetics. Although the reactor quickly becomes substrate limiting, a first order approximation of Monod kinetics leads to estimation errors in the reactor.

**Keywords** Balance laws · Porous media · Biofilms · Numerical simulation

## 1 Introduction

Biofilms are aggregates of microorganisms on immersed surfaces that occur in a variety of environments. In Environmental Engineering, biofilms create a foundation for microbial processes that can be utilized in wastewater treatment, soil remediation and the protection of ground water [1, 2, 10]. Biofilms play an important role in porous media, such as soils, which prompts the development of models for such an environment. In these systems, a growth substrate travels through the porous medium and biomass is produced through the consumption of such substrate. As the biofilm forms on the substratum, different forces influence its behaviour.

Perhaps the most important mechanism for modelling biofilm growth in porous media is the description of substrate flux into the biofilm. Some models describe substrate flux through empirical expressions [18], while others describe it using Fick's first law [1, 8, 11–13]. In the models described by [1, 11, 12], the substrate inside the biofilm is calculated as the solution to a two-point boundary value problem where the growth/consumption kinetics are described by the Monod equation [14].

H. J. Gaebler (✉) · H. J. Eberl
University of Guelph, 50 Stone Rd. E., Guelph, ON, Canada
e-mail: gaeblerh@uoguelph.ca

H. J. Eberl
e-mail: heberl@uoguelph.ca

© Springer Nature Switzerland AG 2018                                                  351
D. M. Kilgour et al. (eds.), *Recent Advances in Mathematical
and Statistical Methods*, Springer Proceedings in Mathematics & Statistics 259,
https://doi.org/10.1007/978-3-319-99719-3_32

The widely accepted kinetics for modelling microbial growth is the Monod equation, which expresses growth as a function of a limiting nutrient [5, 14, 15]. However, in regimes where substrate concentration is sufficiently low, Monod kinetics predict substrate utilization as a linear function dependent on substrate concentration [5]. The advantage of expressing microbial growth as a linear function rather than the Monod equation is that the simplified expression can be solved analytically. However, using a linear description when a full Monod description is more appropriate can lead to over estimations of substrate consumption [5].

The objective of this study is to investigate the difference between two different kinetics, linear and Monod, which govern the dynamics for substrate consumption inside the biofilm layer, and differences in biofilm and suspended bacteria growth inside a porous medium. Here, we utilize the model presented in [7] and adapt the growth kinetics accordingly. In [7], Gaebler and Eberl found, using Monod kinetics, that the system quickly becomes substrate limiting, which indicates that a linear approximation may be appropriate. The goal here is to determine if a simplified flux calculation can be utilized inside a substrate limiting porous medium reactor to reduce computational effort while still providing an accurate solution.

In Sect. 2 we present the porous medium biofilm model derived in [7], which is paired with different kinetics for the purpose of this study. In Sect. 3 we introduce a numerical method proposed by [9] and apply the method to solve the stiff system of partial differential equations. We describe the calculation of substrate flux into the biofilm for Monod kinetics and present the analytical solution for linear kinetics. In Sect. 4 simulations outlining the effect of different growth kinetics on the solution and flux calculations to the described system are reported and compared.

## 2 Mathematical Model

The derivation of the macroscopic model stems from the traditional mesoscopic one-dimensional Wanner-Gujer biofilm model described in [17]. The porous medium is described by identical, parallel, non-communicating flow channels of width $\varepsilon$. Each flow channel is divided into sub-intervals of length $\varepsilon$, in which the mesoscopic processes are described. These include hydrodynamics and transport of substrates in the reactor, biofilm and suspended bacteria growth in the pore space through consumption of a single, non-reproducing growth limiting substrate, attachment of suspended cells to the biofilm, detachment of biofilm cells, and cell lysis. Using a similar process as described in [1], the mesoscopic equations are up-scaled from the biofilm scale to the reactor scale (macroscale) by passing the limit as $\varepsilon \to 0$. The details of the derivation are given in [7] and yield a system of balance laws given by

$$\frac{\partial}{\partial t}\begin{pmatrix}(p-2\lambda)C\\(p-2\lambda)U\\\lambda\end{pmatrix}+\frac{\partial}{\partial x}\begin{pmatrix}QC\\QU\\0\end{pmatrix}=\begin{pmatrix}-2J(\lambda,C)-\frac{[p-2\lambda]}{Y_u}g(C)U\\2X_\infty d\lambda-2a[p-2\lambda]U+g(C)[p-2\lambda]U\\\frac{Y_l}{X_\infty}J(\lambda,C)-k_d\lambda-d\lambda+\frac{a}{X_\infty}[p-2\lambda]U\end{pmatrix},$$

(1)

where $C$, $U$, $\lambda$ respectively describe substrate concentration [g m$^{-2}$], suspended bacteria concentration [g m$^{-2}$], and relative biofilm thickness [$-$]. In this system, $g(C)$ represents the growth kinetics for suspended bacteria and $J(\lambda, C)$ represents the flux of substrate into the biofilm layer. For a complete derivation of the macroscopic model see [7]. All other parameter descriptions are given in Table 1.

Substrate flux into the biofilm layer is determined from the solution to the two-point boundary value problem

$$D\frac{d^2c}{dz^2}=f(c),\qquad\frac{dc}{dz}(0)=0,\qquad c(\lambda)=C,\qquad 0<z<\lambda,$$

(2)

where $f(c)$ describes how substrate is consumed inside the biofilm layer and $c = c(z)$ is the substrate concentration inside the biofilm. Flux of substrate into the biofilm is then obtained as

$$J(\lambda,C)=D\frac{dc}{dz}\Big|_\lambda.$$

(3)

**Table 1** Model parameter values used in simulations

| Parameter | Symbol | Value | Unit | Reference |
|---|---|---|---|---|
| Substrate inflow concentration | $C_0$ | 1.0 | g m$^{-2}$ | Assumed |
| Suspended bacteria inflow concentration | $U_0$ | 0.0 | g m$^{-2}$ | Assumed |
| Relative biofilm thickness at inflow | $\lambda_0$ | 0.0025 | $-$ | Assumed |
| Biomass density | $X_\infty$ | 100.0 | g m$^{-2}$ | [16] |
| Biofilm maximum growth rate | $\mu_\lambda$ | 6.0 | d$^{-1}$ | [16] |
| Biofilm half saturation constant | $\kappa_\lambda$ | 4.0 | g m$^{-2}$ | [16] |
| Biofilm yield coefficient | $Y_\lambda$ | 0.63 | $-$ | [16] |
| Suspended bacteria maximum growth rate | $\mu_u$ | 6.0 | d$^{-1}$ | [16] |
| Suspended bacteria half saturation constant | $\kappa_u$ | 4.0 | g m$^{-2}$ | [16] |
| Suspended bacteria yield coefficient | $Y_u$ | 0.63 | $-$ | [16] |
| Void fraction | $p$ | 0.5 | $-$ | Assumed |
| Biofilm natural cell death rate | $k_d$ | 0.4 | d$^{-1}$ | [16] |
| Detachment coefficient | $d$ | 0.5 | d$^{-1}$ | [1] |
| Attachment coefficient | $a$ | 0.3 | d$^{-1}$ | Assumed |
| Flow velocity | $Q$ | 0.05 | md$^{-1}$ | Assumed |
| Diffusion coefficient | $D$ | 10$^{-4}$ | m$^2$d$^{-1}$ | [16] |
| Reactor length | $L$ | 0.15 | m | Assumed |

We considered the consumption of substrate inside the biofilm layer to follow two different kinetics (i.e. linear kinetics and Monod kinetics), whereby the flux of substrate into the biofilm layer is determined from the solution of (2) with (3) where

$$ f_{linear}(c) = \frac{\mu_\lambda}{\kappa_\lambda} c \quad \text{or} \quad f_{Monod}(c) = \frac{\mu_\lambda c}{\kappa_\lambda + c}. $$

To study this system numerically, we use a variable transformation in order to investigate how system (1) progresses over time rather than space. The variable transformation is given by

$$ S := (p - 2\lambda)C, \quad W := (p - 2\lambda)U. \tag{4} $$

With the variable transformation (4), the system (1) is written as

$$ \frac{\partial}{\partial t} \begin{pmatrix} S \\ W \\ \lambda \end{pmatrix} + \frac{\partial}{\partial x} \begin{pmatrix} \frac{QS}{p-2\lambda} \\ \frac{QW}{p-2\lambda} \\ 0 \end{pmatrix} = \begin{pmatrix} -2J\left(\lambda, \frac{S}{p-2\lambda}\right) - \frac{1}{Y_u} g\left(\frac{S}{p-2\lambda}\right) W \\ 2X_\infty d\lambda - 2aW + g\left(\frac{S}{p-2\lambda}\right) W \\ \frac{Y_\lambda}{X_\infty} J\left(\lambda, \frac{S}{p-2\lambda}\right) - (k_d + d)\lambda + \frac{aW}{X_\infty} \end{pmatrix}. \tag{5} $$

## 3 Numerical Treatment

### 3.1 Discretization of the Partial Differential Equation with the Second Order Uniformly Accurate Central Scheme

Over the years many different numerical solvers have been proposed for hyperbolic systems. However, most of these schemes were developed for conservation laws (i.e. systems without any reaction terms). In this study we solve a system of the form

$$ u_t + (\hat{f}(u))_x = h(u). $$

Here $u$ represents the dependent variable, $\hat{f}(u)$ describes diffusion and $h(u)$ describes all reaction terms. Here $u$, $\hat{f}(u)$ and $h(u)$ are given by

$$ u = \begin{pmatrix} S \\ W \\ \lambda \end{pmatrix}, \quad \hat{f}(u) = \begin{pmatrix} \frac{SQ}{p-2\lambda} \\ \frac{WQ}{p-2\lambda} \\ 0 \end{pmatrix}, \quad h(u) = \begin{pmatrix} -2J\left(\lambda, \frac{S}{p-2\lambda}\right) - \frac{1}{Y_u} g\left(\frac{S}{p-2\lambda}\right) W \\ 2X_\infty d\lambda - 2aW + g\left(\frac{S}{p-2\lambda}\right) W \\ \frac{Y_\lambda}{X_\infty} J\left(\lambda, \frac{S}{p-2\lambda}\right) - (k_d + d)\lambda + \frac{aW}{X_\infty} \end{pmatrix}. $$

Due to the widely varying time scales between substrate depletion and biofilm growth, an appropriate solver for stiff balance equations is considered. We employ the *Uniformly accurate Central Scheme of Order 2* (UCS2) as proposed in [9].

UCS2 separates the reaction and transport terms and treats them in different manners. In order to deal with the stiffness of the system, the reaction terms are treated implicitly, while transport terms are treated explicitly. To guarantee that UCS2 is stable, the time step $\Delta t$ must satisfy a stability condition, given by,

$$\Delta t \leq \Delta x \frac{(p - 2 \max_j(\lambda_j))}{2Q}, \qquad \Delta x = L/N$$

where $j$ is the grid position, $\lambda_j$ is the relative biofilm thickness in the $j$th grid position, $L$ is the length of the reactor, and $N$ is the number of grid points.

UCS2 utilizes two predictor steps for the reaction terms and calculates intermediate time steps at $\Delta t/2$ and $\Delta t/3$. The predictor steps are given by

$$u_j^{n+1/2} = u_j^n - \frac{1}{2}\frac{\Delta t}{\Delta x}f_j' + \frac{\Delta t}{2}h\left(u_j^{n+1/2}\right), \tag{6}$$

$$u_j^{n+1/3} = u_j^n - \frac{1}{3}\frac{\Delta t}{\Delta x}f_j' + \frac{\Delta t}{3}h\left(u_j^{n+1/3}\right), \tag{7}$$

where $n$ is the time step, $j$ is the grid position and $f_j'/\Delta x$ is an appropriate derivative approximation for the diffusion function. In this study we approximate the derivative of the diffusion function using the min-mod function as a flux limiter as proposed in [9]. By using the min-mod function as a flux limiter, spurious oscillations due to high order spatial discretizations are avoided. Thus, the derivative of the diffusion function is therefore approximated by

$$f_j' = MM\left(\hat{f}_{j+1} - \hat{f}_j, \hat{f}_j - \hat{f}_{j-1}\right), \tag{8}$$

where MM denotes the min-mod function

$$MM(x, y) = \begin{cases} \text{sgn}(x)\min(|x|, |y|) & \text{if } \text{sgn}(x) = \text{sgn}(y), \\ 0 & \text{otherwise.} \end{cases}$$

The predictor steps are used to compute the solution to the system at the next time step at staggered grid points. The new time step solution is given by

$$u_{j+1/2}^{n+1} = \frac{1}{2}(u_j^n + u_{j+1}^n) + \frac{1}{8}(u_j' - u_{j+1}') - \frac{\Delta t}{\Delta x}\left(\hat{f}\left(u_{j+1}^{n+1/2}\right) - \hat{f}\left(u_j^{n+1/2}\right)\right)$$

$$+ \Delta t \left(\frac{3}{8}h\left(u_j^{n+1/3}\right) + \frac{3}{8}h\left(u_{j+1}^{n+1/3}\right) + \frac{1}{4}h\left(u_{j+1/2}^{n+1}\right)\right), \tag{9}$$

where $u_j'$ is analogous to (8).

This method can be computationally involved since it requires a system of non-linear equations to be solved for each of the predictor steps (6) and (7), as well as for the new time step calculation (9). We use for this Newton's Method (cf. [3, 6]) and compute the Jacobian using a finite difference approximation.

## 3.2 Calculation of the Substrate Flux for Monod Kinetics

The flux of substrate into the biofilm is calculated from the solution to the two-point boundary value problem (2). For Monod kinetics, the second order differential equation is broken into a system of two first order equations given by

$$x' = y, \quad y' = \frac{\mu_\lambda x}{\kappa_\lambda + x}, \tag{10}$$

with boundary conditions

$$x(\lambda) = C, \quad y(0) = 0, \tag{11}$$

where $C$ is the concentration of substrate at the aqueous-biofilm boundary.

To solve the system described by (10) and (11), we use a backward shooting method. To this end, we change the initial condition (11) to

$$x(\lambda) = C, \quad y(\lambda) = \beta_i. \tag{12}$$

The goal is to construct a sequence of $\beta_i$'s such that the solution to (10) with (12) satisfies condition (11). We use the bi-section method, which in each iteration step requires (10) with (12) to be solved, for which we use a time-adaptive error controlled Runge-Kutta 4/5 scheme [4]. Two stopping criteria are implemented for the bi-section method. We calculate the absolute differences between two successive $\beta_i$'s, as well as for each $\beta_i$ the corresponding $y(0)$. The algorithm is terminated once either of these values is smaller than a specified value. Finally the flux of substrate into the biofilm is obtained as

$$J(\lambda, C) = D \frac{dc}{dz}\bigg|_\lambda = D\beta_{sol},$$

where $D$ is the diffusion constant and $\beta_{sol}$ is the final value of $\beta_i$.

**Note**: For linear kinetics, the two-point boundary value problem simplifies to a linear second order differential equation that can be solved analytically. For a complete derivation of the linear flux see [7]. The linear macroscopic flux becomes

$$J(\lambda, C) = C \frac{\mu_\lambda}{\kappa_\lambda} \lambda.$$

## 3.3 Implementation

The numerical method was implemented in C and compiled and tested using gcc and Intel compilers (icc version 17.0.2, gcc version 5.0.0). Simulations were carried out on a standard Linux desktop workstation under Ubuntu 16.04. All plots were generated using MATLAB v. 8.6.0.267246 (R2015b).

## 3.4 Grid Refinement for Linear and Monod Kinetics

To check the convergence of the numerical method we carry out a standard grid refinement study. This is done by numerically calculating the solution of (5) at different grid resolutions and comparing these solutions to a true solution. Since we do not have the true solution to the system, we instead compare different grids (64, 128, 256, 512) to a much finer grid resolution (1024 grid points). The relative distance between the various solutions are calculated using relative errors based on three different norms $(l_1, l_2, l_\infty)$ as follows

$$Dist = \frac{||U - U_{1024}||}{||U_{1024}||}.$$

Since grid spacing varies depending on the number of grid points, only grid locations that appear in both the current and 1024 grid resolutions are considered.

In the grid refinement simulations the effect of suspended bacteria and attachment were considered, with all other parameter values listed in Table 1. The substrate inflow concentration was set to 1.0 [g m$^{-2}$], while the suspended bacteria inflow concentration was set to 0.0 [g m$^{-2}$]. In these simulations it was assumed there was an established biofilm with relative thickness 0.0025 [−] throughout the reactor. The results for linear and Monod kinetics are reported in Table 2.

In Table 2, we see for the $l_1, l_2$, and $l_\infty$ norm the relative distance between solutions decreases as the number of grid points increases. This suggests that the computed solution is converging as the grid resolution is refined. In all three cases, substrate concentration, suspended bacteria concentration, and relative biofilm thickness all have a low error at a grid resolution of 256 grid points. For this reason, further simulations are computed using a grid resolution of 256 points.

## 4 Comparison Between First Order and Monod Kinetics

We compare the solution values for substrate concentration, suspended bacteria concentration, and relative biofilm thickness between the solution calculated using linear kinetics and the solution calculated using Monod kinetics. Here the simulation con-

**Table 2** Relative distance between solutions with various grid resolutions for both linear and nonlinear kinetics inside the biofilm layer. All distances are calculated relative to the 1024 grid resolution

| # Points | $\|\cdot\|_1$ | $\|\cdot\|_2$ | $\|\cdot\|_\infty$ | $\|\cdot\|_1$ | $\|\cdot\|_2$ | $\|\cdot\|_\infty$ |
|---|---|---|---|---|---|---|
| *Substrate concentration (C)* | | | | | | |
| | Linear kinetics | | | Monod kinetics | | |
| 64 | $7.18 \times 10^{-4}$ | $3.27 \times 10^{-3}$ | $1.71 \times 10^{-2}$ | $1.27 \times 10^{-3}$ | $2.62 \times 10^{-3}$ | $1.35 \times 10^{-2}$ |
| 128 | $3.80 \times 10^{-4}$ | $1.91 \times 10^{-3}$ | $1.24 \times 10^{-2}$ | $6.30 \times 10^{-4}$ | $1.53 \times 10^{-3}$ | $1.01 \times 10^{-2}$ |
| 256 | $1.75 \times 10^{-4}$ | $9.71 \times 10^{-4}$ | $6.88 \times 10^{-3}$ | $2.80 \times 10^{-4}$ | $7.81 \times 10^{-4}$ | $5.68 \times 10^{-3}$ |
| 512 | $5.96 \times 10^{-5}$ | $3.90 \times 10^{-4}$ | $2.95 \times 10^{-3}$ | $9.59 \times 10^{-5}$ | $2.99 \times 10^{-4}$ | $2.45 \times 10^{-3}$ |
| *Suspended bacteria concentration (U)* | | | | | | |
| | Linear kinetics | | | Monod kinetics | | |
| 64 | $5.08 \times 10^{-3}$ | $2.32 \times 10^{-2}$ | $1.35 \times 10^{-1}$ | $5.25 \times 10^{-3}$ | $2.32 \times 10^{-2}$ | $1.36 \times 10^{-1}$ |
| 128 | $2.67 \times 10^{-3}$ | $1.36 \times 10^{-2}$ | $1.00 \times 10^{-1}$ | $2.75 \times 10^{-3}$ | $1.36 \times 10^{-2}$ | $1.00 \times 10^{-1}$ |
| 256 | $1.22 \times 10^{-3}$ | $6.90 \times 10^{-3}$ | $5.60 \times 10^{-2}$ | $1.25 \times 10^{-3}$ | $6.89 \times 10^{-3}$ | $5.58 \times 10^{-2}$ |
| 512 | $4.16 \times 10^{-4}$ | $2.60 \times 10^{-3}$ | $2.40 \times 10^{-2}$ | $4.29 \times 10^{-4}$ | $2.63 \times 10^{-3}$ | $2.39 \times 10^{-2}$ |
| *Relative biofilm thickness (λ)* | | | | | | |
| | Linear kinetics | | | Monod kinetics | | |
| 64 | $3.86 \times 10^{-5}$ | $1.75 \times 10^{-4}$ | $9.65 \times 10^{-4}$ | $4.58 \times 10^{-4}$ | $4.74 \times 10^{-4}$ | $1.07 \times 10^{-3}$ |
| 128 | $2.19 \times 10^{-5}$ | $1.03 \times 10^{-4}$ | $6.41 \times 10^{-4}$ | $2.15 \times 10^{-4}$ | $2.27 \times 10^{-4}$ | $6.43 \times 10^{-4}$ |
| 256 | $1.08 \times 10^{-5}$ | $5.16 \times 10^{-5}$ | $3.30 \times 10^{-4}$ | $9.39 \times 10^{-5}$ | $1.00 \times 10^{-4}$ | $3.21 \times 10^{-4}$ |
| 512 | $3.82 \times 10^{-6}$ | $1.89 \times 10^{-5}$ | $1.21 \times 10^{-4}$ | $3.18 \times 10^{-5}$ | $3.44 \times 10^{-5}$ | $1.18 \times 10^{-4}$ |

figuration is identical to the configuration outlined in Sect. 3.4 with parameter values given in Table 1. The difference in solutions are calculated as

$$U_{diff} = 2 \frac{U_{linear} - U_{Monod}}{|U_{linear} + U_{Monod}|}.$$

Figure 1a illustrates that as time increases the substrate concentration in the linear solution is less than the substrate concentration in the Monod solution. We see from Fig. 1d that the flux into the biofilm is larger for the linear solution than the Monod solution. This leads to the linear solution having a thicker biofilm at the inlet than in the Monod solution (Fig. 1c). With a larger biofilm thickness, we see in Fig. 1b that there is a higher concentration of suspended bacteria in the linear case, which can be contributed to both the linear growth of suspended and detachment from the thicker biofilm. Over time, for both suspended bacteria concentration and relative biofilm thickness, simulations illustrate that the difference first increases then decreases. Initially, substrate is abundant which allows the solutions to be controlled by the growth kinetics. However, as substrate becomes depleted, the growth of both the biofilm and suspended bacteria becomes limited causing the dynamics to be controlled by the balance between attachment and detachment.

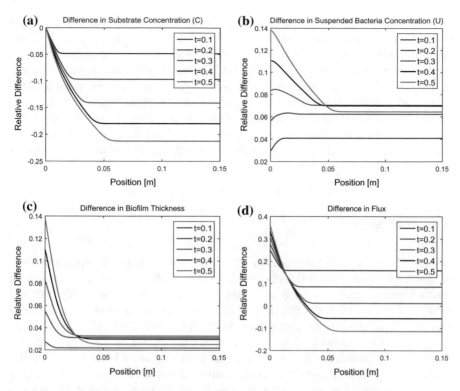

**Fig. 1** Solution difference of (5) with linear and nonlinear flux inside the biofilm layer. Parameter values reported in Table 1. Inflow concentration of substrate and suspended bacteria are $C_0 = 1.0$ [g m$^{-2}$] and $U_0 = 0.0$ [g m$^{-2}$] respectively

Simulations demonstrate a difference between the solution of (5) when different kinetics are considered. After 0.5 days there is up to a 21.20% difference in substrate concentration, 13.72% difference in suspended bacteria concentration, 13.75% difference in relative biofilm thickness, and 35.93% difference for flux of substrate into the biofilm. For both suspended bacteria concentration and relative biofilm thickness, the largest difference occurs at the inlet. Since substrate is not yet limiting, flux into the biofilm is over estimated by the linear kinetics. An over estimation of flux correspondingly results in a thicker biofilm. Since detachment is included in these simulations, a thicker biofilm increases the amount of biomass becoming detached resulting in a higher suspended bacteria concentration, which is seen in Fig. 1b. The largest difference for substrate concentration occurs near the end of the reactor. Since linear kinetics depletes the substrate concentration faster than Monod kinetics one would expect the largest difference to be at the end of the reactor. The flux of substrate into the biofilm also displays the same decreasing trend in Fig. 1d. Initially when there is abundant substrate, linear kinetics over estimate the flux into the biofilm. However, as time increases this over estimation causes the substrate to become depleted too early. We see in Fig. 1d that for $t = 0.4$ [days] and $t = 0.5$ [days] the difference in flux becomes negative. This is due to the rapid depletion of substrate by the linear kinetics before the reactor becomes substrate limiting.

Another major artifact of using different kinetics is its effect on computation time. By modelling the flux of substrate into the biofilm via Monod kinetics, the solution to the two-point boundary value problem becomes more complex and must be calculated numerically. This significantly increases computation time. When simulating the configuration described in Sect. 3.4 over a time period of 1.0 day, linear kinetics had a real time simulation of 0.617 s, while Monod kinetics had a real time simulation of 509.766 s, which marks a 826 fold increase.

# 5 Conclusion

Although linear kinetics is computationally faster and a good approximation of Monod kinetics in a concentration limiting regime, it may not be appropriate for a substrate limiting biofilm reactor. In the system described above, the reactor rapidly becomes substrate limiting. However, the inflow regime of the reactor is not substrate limiting, which causes an over estimation of substrate flux into the biofilm and changes the behaviour of the model. Initially, the over estimation causes a rapid decrease in substrate concentration and an increase in both suspended bacteria and biofilm thickness. Over time, substrate concentrations continue to decrease at a rate higher than Monod kinetics. Eventually the decrease caused by the linear kinetics results in an under estimation of substrate flux.

This study illustrates the importance of accurately modelling the flux of substrate into the biofilm. This process determines the decay of substrate, as well as the growth of the biofilm and suspended bacteria. In this study we see that although the reactor quickly becomes substrate limiting, it is important to describe the flux in the inflow regime by Monod kinetics to avoid estimation errors.

# References

1. Abbas, F., Eberl, H.: Investigation of the role of mesoscale detachment rate expressions in a macroscale model of a porous medium biofilm reactor. Int. J. Biomath. Biostats. **2**(1), 123–143 (2013)
2. Abbas, F., Sudarsan, R., Eberl, H.J.: Longtime behavior of one-dimensional biofilm models with shear dependent detachment rates. Math. Biosc. Eng. **9**(2), 215–239 (2012)
3. Burden, R.L., Faires, J.D.: Numerical Analysis. Brooks/Cole Publishing, Boston, MA (2010)
4. Chapra, S.C., Canale, R.P.: Numerical Methods for Engineers, 6th edn. McGraw-Hill, New York, NY (2010)
5. Corapcioglu, M.Y. (ed.): Advances in Porous Media, vol. 3. Elsevier, Amsterdam, The Netherlands (1993)
6. Epperson, J.F.: An Introduction to Numerical Methods and Analysis. Wiley, New York (2002)

7. Gaebler, H.J., Eberl, H.J.: A simple model of biofilm growth in a porous medium that accounts for detachment and attachment of suspended biomass and their contribution to substrate degradation. Eur. J. Appl. Math. (2018). https://doi.org/10.1017/S0956792518000189

8. Horn, H., Lackner, S.: Modeling of biofilm systems: a review. Adv. Biochem. Eng. Biotechnol. **146**, 53–76 (2014)

9. Liotta, S.F., Romano, V., Russo, G.: Central schemes for balance laws of reaction type. SIAM. J. Num. An. **38**(4), 1337–1356 (2000)

10. Logan, J.D.: Transport Modeling in Hydrogeochemical Systems. Springer, New York, NY (2000)

11. Mašić, A., Eberl, H.J.: Persistence in a single species CSTR model with suspended flocs and wall attached biofilms. Bull. Math. Biol. **75**(5), 1001–1026 (2012)

12. Mašić, A., Eberl, H.J.: On optimization of substrate removal in a bioreactor with wall attached and suspended bacteria. Math. Biosci. Eng. **11**(5), 1139–1166 (2014)

13. Muslu, Y.: Mass transfer and substrate utilization in biofilm reactors. J. Chem. Tech. Biotechnol. **57**, 127–135 (1993)

14. Rittmann, B.E., McCarty, P.L.: Environmental Biotechnology: Principles and Applications. McGraw-Hill, Boston, MA (2001)

15. Smith, H.L., Waltman, P.: The Theory of the Chemostat: Dynamics of Microbial Competition. Cambridge University Press, New York, NY (1995)

16. Wanner, O., Eberl, H.J., Morgenroth, E., Noguera, D.R., Picioreanu, C., Rittmann, B.E., van Loosdrecht, M.: Mathematical Modeling of Biofilms. IWA Publishing, London, UK (2006)

17. Wanner, O., Gujer, W.: A multispecies biofilm model. Biotechnol. Bioeng. **28**, 314–386 (1986)

18. Williamson, K., McCarty, P.L.: A model of substrate utilization by bacterial films. J. Water Pollut. Control Fed. **48**(1), 9–24 (1976)

# Predictability of Marine Population Trajectories Affected by Birth and Harvest Pulses

Anna S. J. Frank and Sam Subbey

**Abstract** Predicting future states of harvested marine populations requires an understanding of how intrinsic time delay processes and volatile phenomena (e.g., impulsive mortality) act in concert to alter the dynamic population trajectory. Separately, the effects (on population dynamics) of time-delays, and impulses, have been studied theoretically by several authors. This paper shows an example approach, where the effects of impulses and time-delays are integrated in the same modeling framework, to understand how they may alter the predictability of future population states. The paper uses a stage-structured, Impulsive-Delay-Differential-Equation (IDDE) model to describe a single species marine population system. It presents results based on numerical experiments.

**Keywords** Impulsive-Delay-Differential-Equations · Approximate entropy Unstable periodic orbits (UPOs) · Predictability · Birth and harvest impulses Marine population

## 1 Introduction

Impulses are momentous occurring perturbations in a system [13]. Such perturbations occur in ecological, biological, physical, medical and numerous other fields [7]. Specifically for marine populations, the effect of birth pulses has been studied in [26] using a population dynamics model. The authors concluded that regular impulsive

A. S. J. Frank (✉)
School of Pharmacy, University of Oslo, Postboks 1068, Blindern 0316 Oslo, Norway
e-mail: a.s.j.frank@farmasi.uio.no

A. S. J. Frank
Department of Biological Statistics and Computational Biology,
Cornell University, 1175 Comstock Hall, Ithaca 14853, USA

S. Subbey
Institute of Marine Research, PB-1870, 5817 Bergen, Norway
e-mail: samuel.subbey@imr.no

S. Subbey
Cornell University, 120 Fernow Hall, Ithaca 14853, USA

© Springer Nature Switzerland AG 2018
D. M. Kilgour et al. (eds.), *Recent Advances in Mathematical
and Statistical Methods*, Springer Proceedings in Mathematics & Statistics 259,
https://doi.org/10.1007/978-3-319-99719-3_33

birth events can lead to chaos. In [19], the authors considered the effect of periodically occurring impulses on biological systems, and concluded that under certain parameter conditions, impulsive events can lead to period-doubling cascades and eventually to chaos. The authors in [11] used a deterministic model that incorporates birth and harvest pulses, to study the effect of the impulses, using bifurcation analysis. The authors concluded that birth events add complexity to the existing system, and that the population dynamics are affected by the timing of the harvest impulses. For marine populations, known to exhibit complex dynamics, external impulses such as harvesting can destroy the system predictability [12].

Time delays in the system dynamics is an intrinsic characteristic of biological systems and networks. Such delays may have regulatory effects on the system dynamics and its trajectory. For instance, in neural networks, it has been shown (see [5]) that delays may initiate different rhythmic spatio-temporal patterns, and that delays are capable of altering the stability of such rhythmic patterns [9]. In predator-prey systems, delays influence system behavior through the introduction of repetitive and feedback cycles [4, 15, 27]. For marine populations in general, delays represent among others, resource regeneration times, maturation periods, feeding, and reaction times (see e.g., [13, 24]).

Whereas the effects of impulses, and time delays on the regulation of marine populations have been studied separately, lacking in the literature is a study of their combined effect on the population dynamics. This is perhaps due to the fact that each individual (impulse or time-delay) effect presents several dimensions of computational challenges. Close-form solutions for equations representing mathematical models that incorporate both effects may not exist, or the solutions may be intractable. A viable alternative is to study such combined effects, using a simulation approach.

This paper uses a numerical simulation approach to demonstrate how the combined effect of delays in inter-species relationships and, birth and harvest pulses may be investigated for complex population dynamic models. The emphasis is on how the combined effect regulates the predictability of the dynamics trajectory of a marine population. We use a mathematical model, defined by a system of Delay Differential Equation (DDE), to describe the dynamics of a hypothetical marine population. Using the time series of biomass from the mathematical model, we conduct predictability analysis of the system. We quantify the regularity of the system using the Approximation Entropy (ApEn) measure [21], and the predictability, based on the the the occurrence of Unstable Periodic Orbits (UPOs) [3] in the biomass trajectory. Finally, we compare the inference based on analysis of UPOs with two alternative methods for quantifying system predictability namely, the Maximum Lyapunov exponent (MLE) [29] and System Forecast Errors (SFE) [16]. This manuscript only considers constant impulses and time delays.

The article is organized in the following way. Section 2 gives a description of the mathematical model, while Sect. 3 presents a brief description of the metrics for quantifying predictability and other basic definitions, which are necessary for understanding the rest of the manuscript. Section 4 gives a brief description of the methodological approach, including a description of the base case and the numerical experiments to be performed. Simulation results presented in Sect. 5 are further discussed in Sect. 6, which also summarizes our main conclusions.

## 2 Model Description

This section presents equations to describe the marine population dynamics. The description uses the nomenclature in Table 1.

The base-case model $S_0$ is given by Eq. (1),

$$
S_0 \equiv \begin{cases}
\dot{z}(t) = f(z(t), \boldsymbol{\theta}) - a_x z(t) x(t), \\
\dot{x}(t) = \mu a_x z(t - \tau_1) \cdot x(t - \tau_1) - d_x x(t) - \delta x(t), \\
\dot{y}(t) = -d_y y(t) + \delta x(t - \tau_2),
\end{cases} \tag{1}
$$

with $f(z(t), \boldsymbol{\theta}) : \mathbb{R}_+ \mapsto \mathbb{R}_+$ is defined by (2),

$$
f(z(t), \boldsymbol{\theta}) = \frac{az(t)}{b + z(t)}, \ a \in \mathbb{R}_+, \ b \in \mathbb{R}_+. \tag{2}
$$

The resource-growth function in Eq. (2) is the Holling-II function [25]. The base-case model $S_0$, together with $f(z(t), \boldsymbol{\theta})$ in equation (2), correspond to the model in [10].

**Table 1** Nomenclature for the base-case model $S_0$ in Eq. (1)

| | |
|---|---|
| $z(t) \in \mathbb{R}_+, z(0) = 2.0$ | Resource biomass, and initial condition |
| $x(t) \in \mathbb{R}_+, x(0) = 1.0$ | Biomass of immature population, Initial condition |
| $y(t) \in \mathbb{R}_+, y(0) = 0.5$ | Biomass of mature population, Initial condition |
| $t \in \mathbb{R}$ | Simulation time |
| $\tau_i \in \mathbb{R}, i \in \{1, 2\}$ | Time delays |
| $f(z(t), \boldsymbol{\theta})$ | Resource-growth-function (Holling-II function) |
| $\boldsymbol{\theta} \in \mathbb{R}$ | Parameter-set of the resource-growth function $f(z(t), \boldsymbol{\theta})$ |
| $a_x = 1.6 \in \mathbb{R}_+$ | Resource uptake rate of the immature population (fixed parameter) |
| $\mu = 0.4 \in (0, 1)$ | Resource conversion rate into biomass (fixed parameter) |
| $d_x = 0.2 \in (0, 1), d_y = 0.15 \in (0, 1)$ | Mortality rate of $x(t)$, $y(t)$ (fixed parameter) |
| $\delta = 0.35 \in (0, 1)$ | Maturation rate (fixed parameter) |
| $B$ | Recruitment impulse on the immature population $x(t)$ |
| $H_x, H_y$ | Harvest impulses on $x(t)$, $y(t)$ |

The impulse functions (direction and degree) are defined by (3)–(5). The system is exposed to birth- $(B)$ and harvest $(H_x, H_y)$ impulses that satisfy (for $k \in \mathbb{Z}$ and $s \in \mathbb{Z}$):

$$x(k^+) = x(k^-) + B(k^-), \tag{3}$$

$$x(s^+) = x(s^-) + H_x(s^-), \tag{4}$$

$$y(s^+) = y(s^-) + H_y(s^-), \tag{5}$$

where the impulsive events on system $S_0$ are predefined at simulation steps $k \in \mathbb{Z}_+$ and $s \in \mathbb{Z}_+$. In (3), $k^+$ is the state, which occurs right after a birth impulse, while $k^-$ indicates a state just before an impulse takes place (similarly for harvest impulses at $s$ for (4) and (5)). We define:

$$B(k) = \alpha e^{-\beta y(k)} y(k), \quad \beta \in \mathbb{R}_+ \tag{6}$$

$$H_x(s) = h_x x(s), \quad h_x \in (0, 1), \tag{7}$$

$$H_y(s) = h_y y(s), \quad h_y \in (0, 1). \tag{8}$$

In the literature, the impulsive term $B$ is referred to as the *stock recruitment*, and the form in (6) is the Ricker function [26] representation.

## 3 Basic Definitions and Predictability Metrics

This section presents brief definitions of the UPOs and ApEn measures. In general, periodic orbits are defined by periodic visits along some close trajectory, where closeness is defined with respect to the neighborhood of the orbit, see [3]. Stable Period Orbits (SPO) are characterized by stable periodic cycling, i.e., with time, the system trajectories visit all points in a close neighborhood of the orbit and remain there for an infinite time period. This paper is concerned with the Unstable Periodic Orbits (UPOs), which are defined by Definition 1.

**Definition 1** *(UPO)* Periodic orbit characterized by transitory visits to trajectory points in close neighborhood of each of the periodic orbits, followed by *(random)* transition to new orbits.

Dynamical systems that are both sensitive to initial conditions and consist of an infinite number of UPOs are termed chaotic, [3]. In general, UPOs present the skeleton of chaotic attractors. The randomness in the motion on an attractor can be quantified as a function of the number of UPOs, and the random walk from UPO to UPO results in a stochastic process. The randomness of time series therefore provides another measure for chaos and, hence predictability [23] of a system. UPOs can also be used to approximate the *topological entropy*, which provides better insight into the underlying chaotic structure and dynamics [1, 2, 6, 14]. The topological entropy measures the complexity and growth rate of all periodic orbits [18]. However, it is a computational challenge to derive the topological entropy. A viable alternative is to use the ApEn, which we describe shortly, for the perturbed system in the numerical analysis.

Consider the $m$th delay coordinator $x(t) = \{u(t), \dots, u(t + m - 1)\}$, of the time series $u(t)_{t=1}^{N}$. The reconstructed phase space of the delay coordinator is given by $X_m(t) = \{x(1), \dots, x(n)\} \in \mathbb{R}^m$, with $n = N - m + 1$, (see [28]). Now let $x_i(t)$ be the $i$-th component of $x \in \mathbb{R}^m$, where $||.||_\infty$ is the usual $L^\infty$-norm on $\mathbb{R}^m$, and define

$$\Phi_m(r) = -\frac{1}{|X_m|} \sum_{x \in X_m} \log \left( \frac{|y \in X_m : ||x - y||_\infty \le r|}{|X_m|} \right). \tag{9}$$

In (9), $r$ is a similarity measure (quantifying the distance between two data points) that specifies the filtering level [28]. The bracket term under the summation sum is the average of points $x(i)$, $i \in \{1, \dots, n\}$, which fulfills the condition, and $|X_m| := N - m + 1$.

**Definition 2** (*ApEn*) Let (9) prevail. Then the ApEn for the time series $u(t)$ (for $t = 1, \dots, N$) is defined by (10).

$$ApEn(m, r, N) := \Phi_{m+1}(r) - \Phi_m(r), \tag{10}$$

with $ApEn(0, r, N) := \Phi_1(r)$ and $X_0 = \{\}$, i.e. empty.

The ApEn is a *logarithmic likelihood*, which estimates whether the closeness of regular patterns for $N$ observations in $m$-dimension is preserved in dimension $m + 1$ [21, 22]. An increase in the likelihood is thus indicative of a decrease in the ApEn value, and a preservation of the closeness property of the points.

### The Maximum Lyapunov Exponent

The Lyapunov exponent (LE) quantifies the sensitivity of a time series to changes in the initial conditions (that is, the local instability in a state space) [8, 17]. For two trajectories of a dynamical system separated in phase-space by $\delta_0$ at $t = 0$ and $\delta_t$ at some later time $t > 0$, and satisfying (11), $\lambda$ is the Lyaponov exponent. A rearrangement of (11) leads to (12).

$$\delta_t = \delta_0 e^{\lambda t}, \tag{11}$$

$$\lambda = \lim_{t \to \infty} \frac{1}{t} \ln \left( \frac{\delta_t}{\delta_0} \right). \tag{12}$$

Assume a number of points initially localized in a $d$-dimensional embedding space such that neighboring points are contained in a hyper-sphere at $t = 0$. Then at some $t > 0$, the hyper-sphere is stretched to a hyper-ellipsoid with the length of the $i$-th principal axis given by $\delta_i(t)$. Then there exists a spectrum of Lyapunov exponents (one for each principal axis) which can be calculated from a time series using (13).

$$\lambda_i = \lim_{t \to \infty} \frac{1}{t} \ln \left( \frac{\delta_i(t)}{\delta_0} \right). \tag{13}$$

Lyapunov exponents are independent of the initial condition; a property guaranteed by the Oseledets multiplicative ergodic theorem [20]. The maximum LE (MLE) is indicative of the predictability of the dynamical system. A positive MLE implies that small perturbations in the initial conditions may result in widely divergent results.

## 4 Methodological Approach

We first define a model consisting of a series of fixed impulses and parameters in the model $S_0$, defined by (1). We analyze the time series from this model to determine (i) the number of UPOs, and (ii) time series irregularity, based on the ApEn algorithm. The results from this model (UPOs and ApEn metrics) are used to define a classification scheme for all other simulation results. Deriving a good ApEn-measure for the time series $u(t)$ (for $t = 1, \ldots, N$) requires that $N > 10^3$ [21]. We therefore set $N = 3 \times 10^3$ for all simulations. Table 2 summarizes the input data for the base-case. For simplicity, we fix the value of $\tau_2$, and consider four instances of the sub-case defined by the delay size $\tau_1$. Next, we introduce four different sets of scenarios, where each scenario consists of constant levels of birth and harvest impulses, as well as the delay parameters in $S_0$. For each scenario, we keep the strength of the impulses $(B, H_x, H_y)$ constant. However, we consider two instances of the impulse frequency, (i.e., the number of perturbations per time interval), $I_f = 1$ and $I_f = 4$.

This paper follows the implementation in [16], in quantifying UPO, ApEn, and MLE metrics. Integration of the system of DDEs in (1) was performed on the Matlab computational platform.

## 5 Summary of Results from Numerical Experiments

This section describes a summary of simulation results. It presents the base-case analysis and classification scheme, which is used in assessing other simulation results. Table 3 summarizes the main results for all sub-cases. It shows the SFE (System Forecast Errors) for 500 iteration steps, MLEs, and the number, $N_p$, of UPOs with periods $p$. It also shows the ApEn-values for the filtering level $r$.

**Table 2** Input data for the base-case

| Parameter | a | b | $\alpha$ | $\beta$ | $h_x$ | $h_y$ | $\tau_1$ | $\tau_2$ |
|-----------|-----|-----|-----|-----|-----|-----|-----|-----|
| Value | 2.0 | 2.0 | 3.8 | 4.0 | 0.9 | 0.8 | $\{0.1, 0.4, 0.5, 0.63\}$ | 0.1 |

**Table 3** Results from the base-case analysis

|  | Base-case |  |  |  |
|---|---|---|---|---|
| $\tau_1$ | 0.10 | 0.40 | 0.50 | 0.63 |
| $p$ | 1 | 1 | 1 | 1 |
| $N_p$ | 2 | 1 | 1 | 3 |
| SFE | 0 | 0.3 | 0.9 | 1.2 |
| MLE | $\lambda_1 < 0$ | $\lambda_1 \approx 0$ | $\lambda_1 \approx 0$ | $\lambda_1 > 0$ |
| $\sigma$ | 0.096 | 0.12 | 0.16 | 0.24 |
| ApEn | [0.05, 0.03] | [0.00] | [0.00, 0.01] | [0.10, 0.15] |

**Table 4** Classification scheme based on the Base-case analysis. Nomenclature for the inference column: P/MP≡Periodic/Multi-periodic; and C/NC ≡ Chaotic/Non-chaotic

| Time series characterization | ApEn-threshold | Number UPOs | Inference | Predictability |
|---|---|---|---|---|
| Very irregular or Regular | ApEn> 0.1 | $N_p > 2$ | C/P/MP | No |
| Multi-periodic or Periodic | ApEn< 0.2 | $\max(N_p) = 2$ | P/MP/C/NC | Short-term |
| Very irregular or repetitive | ApEn< 0.1 | $N_p \leq 2$ | Regular | Yes |

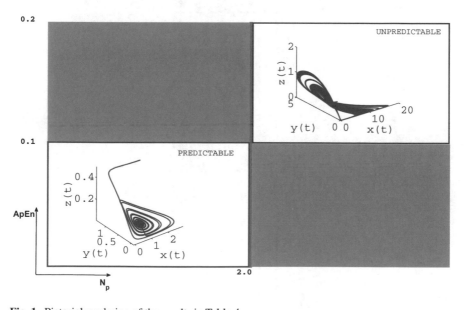

**Fig. 1** Pictorial rendering of the results in Table 4

The algorithm for the computation of ApEn follows directly from Definition 2. The implementation procedure for ApEn is according to [16], where computational details can also be obtained. The ApEn-algorithm yields confident values, when the

**Table 5** Results from scenario simulations

| Scenario | I ($I_f = 1$) | I ($I_f = 4$) | II ($I_f = 1$) | II ($I_f = 4$) | III ($I_f = 1$) | III ($I_f = 4$) | IV ($I_f = 1$) | IV ($I_f = 4$) |
|---|---|---|---|---|---|---|---|---|
| $p$ | 1 | 1 | 1 | 1 | 1 | 1 | 1 | 1 |
| $N_p$ | 1 | 1 | 1 | 1 | 3 | 4 | 9 | 9 |
| MLE | $\lambda_1 \leq 0$ | $\lambda_1 \leq 0$ | $\lambda_1 \leq 0$ | $\lambda_1 \leq 0$ | $\lambda_1 \geq 0$ | $\lambda_1 > 0$ | $\lambda_1 > 0$ | $\lambda_1 > 0$ |
| SFE | 0.60 | 0.47 | 0.67 | 0.55 | 0.95 | 0.88 | 0.70 | 0.73 |
| $\sigma$ | 0.02 | 0.05 | 0.07 | 0.07 | 0.14 | 0.13 | 0.34 | 0.33 |
| ApEn | [0.05, 0.06] | [0.05, 0.04] | [0.10, 0.14] | [0.06, 0.11] | [0.14, 0.19] | [0.13, 0.20] | [0.34, 0.33] | [0.44, 0.42] |

**Table 6** Scenario inference based classification scheme in Table 4

| Scenario | System observations | Inference |
|----------|--------------------|-----------|
| I | Regular patterns | Predictable system |
| II | Regular time series | Predictable, but high forecast errors |
| III | System is chaotic | System is unpredictable |
| IV | System is chaotic | System is unpredictable |

filter parameter $r \in [0.10\sigma, \ 0.25\sigma]$, with $\sigma$ being the *standard deviation* of the series being considered.

Based on the base-case simulation results in Table 3, we developed the scheme presented in Table 4, for classification of results from further simulation scenarios. The classification is based on the $N_p$ and ApEn-values. The table shows that the system can be expected to be predictable over a long time horizon, when the UPO$s <$ 2, and the ApEn$< 0.1$.

Figure 1 is a pictorial rendering of the results in Table 4, with marked (green) transition zone for when the system transitions from being predictable to unpredictable. The figure also shows the example simulation results of state variables for the dynamical system defined in (1). Table 5 summarizes the results from the scenario simulations discussed previously, where the cases are also defined (see Sect. 4). Combining the classification scheme in Table 4 and scenario simulation results from Table 5, leads to the inference Table 6.

# 6 Discussion and Conclusions

We have observed that the irregularity (i.e. high ApEn-value) in the time series is synchronous with occurrence of UPOs, and that both instances are dependent on the size of the time-delay. Changes in the impulsive frequency from $I_f = 1$ to $I_f = 4$ had an apparently marginal effect on the predictability. The number of UPOs, $N_p$, appeared to depend more on the impulse type, and less on the impulsive frequency. On the other hand, the ApEn-value seems to increase with an increase in the impulse frequency. As shown in [10], we could have also separated the dynamics into predictable and unpredictable systems, depending on a critical delay-value, which seemed to occur at approximately $\tau_1 = \tau^* = 0.4$.

A further observation is that the chaotic time series are connected to large time delays. Periodic and multi-periodic series, with medium delay values are short term predictable, while very regular series, which are consistent with small delay values, are predictable. In order to make inference about predictability of IDDE systems, the time-series regularity and the structure of the system attractor need to be considered, if delay-values are unknown.

The authors in [26] found out that stronger impulsive strength lead to faster movement into chaos. In the present analysis, we observed that the size of delays interferes with system predictability under constant impulsive strength – we could relate large delays to chaos, and small delays to stability. However, we can imply from [26] that delay-values of a system under increasing impulsive strength must be decreasing to maintain stability. Hence, under stronger impulses, dynamical systems will become chaotic also for small delays.

Of all considered instances, the delay-size was the most important factor regulating the dynamics of the IDDE system under constant impulsive strength, as its size dictated the motion on the attractor and the pattern of the time series, and hence predictability.

In terms of predictability, the MLE and the approach combining the concepts of ApEn-values and UPOs lead to the same conclusion. However, the results show that the latter approach adds another level of information over the MLE, as it allows for making inference about the degree of irregularity imposed on the system by the combined effect of impulses and system time-delays.

In this work, we have assumed that there is always food available. Thus resource issues such as food-competition, have not been considered. Though we, assumed that the strength of birth impulses is independent of population size, we have observed that stronger birth impulses lead to more complex dynamics, while harvest impulse-strength needed to be set quite high to observe an effect on the system. While these observations may be particular to the model formulation and choice of parameters, this must not be considered as a limitation to the results.

Indeed, the strength of this paper lies in demonstrating a simulation approach that allows for checking the combined effect of delays and impulsive phenomena on the stability and predictability of marine population trajectories.

Marine populations are usually split into juveniles and adults; the latter being contributors to birth pulses. Our results show that the time delay in resource availability and conversion to the juvenile biomass dictates the system predictability. Such delays may be caused by extended time for access resource due to, e.g. competition, or temporal shift in overlap between resource and juveniles (e.g. delayed zooplankton bloom). When this delay is below a threshold value, the population dynamics are predictable, as long as the birth and harvest pulses have insignificant fluctuations about average values. However when the resource dynamics change so that the time delay exceeds the threshold value, the population dynamics becomes chaotic. This is true even for cases where the resource biomass is large. Harvest rules must therefore consider the effects of resource feedback to the population dynamics when setting harvest levels or quotas. Because it is simulation-based, the framework presented in this paper can be easily adapted to empirical marine populations.

**Acknowledgements** The authors are grateful to Prof. Christina Kuttler for her useful comments.

# References

1. Auerbach, D., Cvitanović, P., Eckmann, J.P., Gunaratne, G., Procaccia, I.: Exploring chaotic motion through periodic orbits. Phys. Rev. Lett. **58**(23), 2387 (1987)
2. Balanov, A.G., Janson, N.B., Schöll, E.: Delayed feedback control of chaos: bifurcation analysis. Phys. Rev. E **71**(1), 016,222 (2005)
3. Boccaletti, S., Grebogi, C., Lai, Y.C., Mancini, H., Maza, D.: The control of chaos: theory and applications. Phys. Rep. **329**(3), 103–197 (2000)
4. Bocharov, G.A., Rihan, F.A.: Numerical modelling in biosciences using delay differential equations. J. Comput. Appl. Math. **125**(1), 183–199 (2000)
5. Coombes, S., Laing, C.: Delays in activity-based neural networks. Philos. Trans. R. Soc. Lond. A: Math. Phys. Eng. Sci. **367**(1891), 1117–1129 (2009)
6. Deane, J., Marsh, L.: Unstable periodic orbit detection for ODEs with periodic forcing. Phys. Lett. A **359**(6), 555–558 (2006)
7. Dishlieva, K.: Impulsive differential equations and applications. J. Appl. Comput. Math. **1**, e117 (2012)
8. Eckmann, J.P., Kamphorst, S.O., Ruelle, D., Ciliberto, S.: Liapunov exponents from time series. Phys. Rev. A **34**(6), 4971–4979 (1986)
9. Ermentrout, B., Ko, T.W.: Delays and weakly coupled neuronal oscillators. Philos. Trans. R. Soc. Lond. A: Math. Phys. Eng. Sci. **367**(1891), 1097–1115 (2009)
10. Frank, A.S.: Predictability of marine population trajectories-the effect of delays and resource availability. ESAIM: Proc. Surv. **57**, 23–36 (2017)
11. Gao, S., Chen, L.: The effect of seasonal harvesting on a single-species discrete population model with stage structure and birth pulses. Chaos, Solitons Fractals **24**(4), 1013–1023 (2005)
12. Glaser, S.M., Fogarty, M.J., Liu, H., Altman, I., Hsieh, C.H., Kaufman, L., MacCall, A.D., Rosenberg, A.A., Ye, H., Sugihara, G.: Complex dynamics may limit prediction in marine fisheries. Fish Fish. **15**(4), 616–633 (2014)
13. Gopalsamy, K.: Stability and Oscillations in Delay Differential Equations of Population Dynamics, vol. 74. Springer Science & Business Media, Berlin (2013)
14. Grebogi, C., Ott, E., Yorke, J.A.: Unstable periodic orbits and the dimensions of multifractal chaotic attractors. Phys. Rev. A **37**(5), 1711 (1988)
15. He, X.Z.: Stability and delays in a predator-prey system. J. Math. Anal. Appl. **198**(2), 355–370 (1996)
16. Hegger, R., Kantz, H., Schreiber, T.: Practical implementation of nonlinear time series methods: The tisean package. Chaos Interdisc. J. Nonlinear Sci. **9**(2), 413–435 (1999)
17. Kantz, H., Schreiber, T.: Nonlinear Time Series Analysis, vol. 7. Cambridge University Press, Cambridge (2004)
18. Lamb, J.: Entropy and chaos (Chap. 8), Lecture Notes in Dynamical Systems, 15 pp, Imperial College, London, UK (accessed March 2018)
19. Liu, X., Chen, L.: Complex dynamics of Holling type II Lotka-Volterra predator-prey system with impulsive perturbations on the predator. Chaos, Solitons Fractals **16**(2), 311–320 (2003)
20. Oseledec, V.I.: A multiplicative ergodic theorem. lyapunov characteristic numbers for dynamical systems. Trans. Moscow Math. Soc **19**(2), 197–231 (1968)
21. Pincus, S.M.: Approximate entropy as a measure of system complexity. Proc. Nat. Acad. Sci. **88**(6), 2297–2301 (1991)
22. Pincus, S.M., Goldberger, A.L.: Physiological time-series analysis: what does regularity quantify? Am. J. Physiol.-Heart Circulatory Physiol. **266**(4), H1643–H1656 (1994)
23. Pinto, P.R., Baptista, M., Labouriau, I.S.: Density of first Poincaré returns, periodic orbits, and Kolmogorov-Sinai entropy. Commun. Nonlinear Sci. Numer. Simul. **16**(2), 863–875 (2011)
24. Ruan, S.: Delay differential equations in single species dynamics. Delay Differ. Equ. Appl. **205**, 477–517 (2006)
25. Skalski, G.T., Gilliam, J.F.: Functional responses with predator interference: viable alternatives to the holling type II model. Ecology **82**(11), 3083–3092 (2001)

26. Tang, S., Chen, L.: Density-dependent birth rate, birth pulses and their population dynamic consequences. J. Math. Biol. **44**(2), 185–199 (2002)
27. Wang, W., Chen, L.: A predator-prey system with stage-structure for predator. Comput. Math. Appl. **33**(8), 83–91 (1997)
28. West, J., Lacasa, L., Severini, S., Teschendorff, A.: Approximate entropy of network parameters. Phys. Rev. E **85**(4), 046,111 (2012)
29. Wolf, A., Swift, J.B., Swinney, H.L., Vastano, J.A.: Determining lyapunov exponents from a time series. Physica D: Nonlinear Phenomena **16**(3), 285–317 (1985)

# Phage Therapy and Antibiotics for Biofilm Eradication: A Predictive Model

**Amjad Khan, Lindi M. Wahl and Pei Yu**

**Abstract** Bacteria that make up the complex physical structures known as biofilms can be 10–1000 fold more resistant to antibiotics than planktonic (free-living) bacteria. In this study we develop a mathematical model to analyze therapeutic techniques that have been proposed to reduce and/or eradicate biofilms, specifically, antibiotics and phage therapy. In this context, the biofilm can be understood as a group defense mechanism, such that the functional response of phages to the biofilm bacterial density is reduced as the biofilm approaches carrying capacity. To capture this mechanism we introduce the function $f(x) = \left(\kappa - \frac{x}{K}\right)x$, where $x$ is the biofilm density, $K$ is the biofilm carrying capacity and $1 < \kappa < 2$ is the group defense parameter. The model predicts that two therapeutic strategies of recent experimental interest (phage therapy followed by antibiotics, or antibiotics followed by phage therapy) can reduce but not eradicate the biofilm. In contrast, we predict that complete elimination of biofilm bacteria can be achieved by mechanisms that block the attachment of planktonic bacteria to the biofilm.

**Keywords** Biofilm · Antibiotics · Therapeutic technique · Phage therapy
Group defense · Equilibrium · Stability

## 1 Introduction

Bacteria are ubiquitous unicellular organisms, with critical importance in both human health and disease [1]. Bacteria can exist as planktonic (free-living) cells, or in complex communities known as biofilms. In the biofilm state, the bacterial colony is attached to a surface; within the biofilm each cell is sessile and surrounded by extra-

A. Khan · L. M. Wahl (✉) · P. Yu
Applied Mathematics, University of Western Ontario, London, Canada
e-mail: lwahl@uwo.ca

A. Khan
e-mail: akhan659@uwo.ca

P. Yu
e-mail: pyu@uwo.ca

© Springer Nature Switzerland AG 2018
D. M. Kilgour et al. (eds.), *Recent Advances in Mathematical
and Statistical Methods*, Springer Proceedings in Mathematics & Statistics 259,
https://doi.org/10.1007/978-3-319-99719-3_34

cellular polymeric substances (EPS), substances produced by bacteria in the colony that determine the physical and chemical properties of the biofilm [18]. Biofilms are responsible for a variety of problems in water distribution systems [11], the food industry [27], and medical treatment [8, 25]. Most importantly, biofilms have been implicated as a key factor in two-thirds of human infections [17].

Bacteria are able to rapidly develop resistance against agents employed to eradicate them. In particular, bacteria in a biofilm have been shown to increase resistance to antibiotics by factors of 10–1000 [9]. Amongst the reasons for enhanced resistance in the biofilm state is the EPS structure surrounding the biofilm colony, which can completely block the infiltration of antibiotics, and the presence of persister cells in the biofilm colony, which are in a metabolically inactive state and thus protected from antibiotic action [9].

The goal or reducing or eradicating biofilm populations has been the focus of research over many years, and there has been much experimental work in this regard [8, 12, 14]. Many agents have been employed for this purpose, which include but are not limited to natural inhibitors of biofilm, for example honey [21], drugs (antibiotics, biofilm-degrading components) [23, 24], bacteriophages and phage-derived enzymes [2, 5, 13] or combinations of some of these [7]. While phage therapy has been proposed as possibly the most effective of these agents, phages alone may not be sufficient to completely eradicate a biofilm [2]. Most recently, experimental work demonstrated that using phage therapy first, followed by antibiotics, maximized the killing of bacteria in an established biofilm.

In this article, we develop a mathematical model to study these therapeutic strategies in detail. In Sect. 2, we develop the model, tracking biofilm and planktonic bacteria in two linked compartments. In Sect. 3, we explore therapeutic strategies including: phage followed by antibiotics; antibiotics followed by phage; and a novel strategy we propose which may have the potential to eradicate the biofilm. In Sect. 4, we derive some conclusions from our analysis.

# 2   Mathematical Model

We model the interaction between bacteria and bacteriophages (viruses that infect bacteria) using an established predator-prey approach [22]. Our model considers cells of a single bacterial species in either a biofilm or planktonic compartment. The model studies the population dynamics of biofilm cells, $B$, planktonic cells, $P$ and phage, $V_B$ and $V_P$, in the biofilm and planktonic compartments respectively. The parameters of the model are described as follows.

The bacterial populations (biofilm or planktonic) are modeled as cell densities per unit volume, cells/cm$^3$. The biofilm population can increase logistically with a maximum growth rate $r$, but is limited by a fixed number of available attachment sites in the biofilm matrix, given by carrying capacity $K_B$ cells/cm$^3$. Similarly, planktonic bacteria can grow logistically with maximum growth rate $r$ but are limited by carrying capacity $K_P$. The planktonic bacteria join the biofilm at rate $\mathscr{A}(B, P)$ and biofilm bacteria leave the biofilm with detachment rate $\mathscr{D}(B, P)$. It has been shown that T4 can diffuse fairly through biofilm channels [10]; in the model, phages enter the biofilm compartment at rate $p$ and leave at rate $q$. In addition, as described above, bacteria in a mature biofilm present substantial resistance to bacteriophages. The expression $f(B) V_B$ gives the number of adsorption events per unit time in the biofilm, where $f(B)$, the phage response function, will model this group defense mechanism. The number of adsorption events per unit time in the planktonic compartment is given by $g(P) V_P$, where $g(P)$ is the phage response function in the absence of group defense. We neglect the time delay between infection and lysis and assume that each adsorption event instantaneously produces $b$ daughter phages, resulting in new $bf(B) V_B$ and $b g(P) V_P$ bacteriophages in the biofilm and planktonic compartments respectively. Bacteriophage are cleared or denatured at rate $c$. These assumptions yield the following system:

$$\frac{dB}{dt} = r\left(1 - \frac{B}{K_B}\right) B - f(B)V_B + \mathscr{A}(P, B) - \mathscr{D}(B, P)$$

$$\frac{dP}{dt} = r\left(1 - \frac{P}{K_P}\right) P - g(P)V_P - \mathscr{A}(P, B) + \mathscr{D}(P, B)$$

$$\frac{dV_B}{dt} = bf(B)V_B - cV_B + pV_P - qV_B$$

$$\frac{dV_P}{dt} = bg(P)V_P - cV_P + qV_B - pV_P. \qquad (1)$$

We note that the attachment and detachment rates, $\mathscr{A}(B, P)$ and $\mathscr{D}(B, P)$, satisfy $\mathscr{A}(B, 0) = 0$ and $\mathscr{D}(0, P) = 0$. More generally, system (1) can also be considered as a two-patch predator-prey model, with group defense acting in one patch only, as illustrated in Fig. 1.

**Fig. 1** In patch-1 there is no group defense mechanism whereas in patch-2, group defense offers prey some degree of protection from predators. The dashed line indicates the protective cover around patch-2 (the EPS structure of the biofilm)

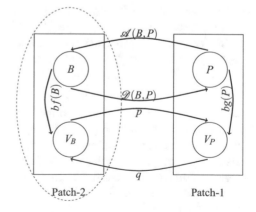

# 3   Therapeutic Strategies

Recent experimental work has addressed approaches for minimizing or eradicating bacterial biofilms [7]. In particular, Chaudhry et al. compared two therapeutic strategies: applying antibiotics and then phages, or applying the same two agents in the reverse order. Treatment with phages first followed by antibiotics resulted in maximum killing of biofilm bacteria. Here we predict that although these strategies can indeed reduce the biofilm, neither strategy can eradicate the biofilm completely.

## 3.1   Using Antibiotics First and then Phages

Given that planktonic bacteria are many-fold more sensitive to antibiotics than biofilm bacteria, we assume that an appropriate antibiotic is administered such that planktonic bacteria can be effectively eliminated before phage therapy. We also assume that $\mathscr{A}(B, P) = \mathscr{D}(B, P)$. After the application of antibiotic we will arrive at the following system

$$
\frac{dB}{dt} = r\left(1 - \frac{B}{K_B}\right)B - f(B)V_B
$$
$$
\frac{dV_B}{dt} = bf(B)V_B - cV_B. \tag{2}
$$

This is a standard predator-prey system with group defense, as studied in [6, 15, 28, 30]. In particular, $f(B)$ must satisfy $f(0) = 0$, $f(B) > 0$ for all $B > 0$, and if there exists a constant $M > 0$, such that $f'(B) > 0$ if $B < M$ and $f'(B) < 0$ if $B > M$, then the system models group defence [15]. The function $f(B) = \frac{mB}{\alpha B^2 + \beta B + 1}$, called the Holling Type-IV or the Monod-Haldane function, was introduced in [4] and satisfies these properties. System (2) has been previously studied with the above functional response for $\beta > -2\sqrt{\alpha}$ [19, 30], and with $f(B) = \alpha e^{-\beta B}$ [29].

In this study, we consider biofilm bacteria that cannot exceed their carrying capacity, such that $B \leq K_B$ at all times. Hence we replace the property $f(B) > 0$ for all $B > 0$ by $f(B) > 0$ for all $0 < B \leq K_B$. To model this phenomenon, we propose a relatively simple functional response $f(B) = \alpha\left(\kappa - \frac{B}{K_B}\right)B$. The rationale for this function is similar to the rationale underpinning logistic growth: we assume that as the biofilm population approaches carrying capacity, the ability of phage to penetrate the biofilm is reduced, linearly. The resulting functional response has the same properties as that of $f(B)$ defined in [29, 30] for $0 < B \leq K_B$. Here $\alpha$ is proportional to the adsorption rate of phages to bacteria, $1 < \kappa < 2$ is the group defense parameter, and $K_B$ is the carrying capacity of the biofilm bacteria. A convenient feature of this model is that the group defense mechanism can be controlled through the parameter $\kappa$; $\kappa = 1$ corresponds to a perfect group defense mechanism (no phage adsorption when the biofilm is at carrying capacity) and $\kappa = 2$ corresponds to the absence of effective group defense ($f(B)$ increasing on $0 < B \leq K_B$).

System (2) has a maximum of four equilibria. Two boundary equilibria are: $E_0 = (0, 0)$, which represents the complete extinction of biofilm bacteria and phages; and $E_{K_B} = (K_B, 0)$, which represents the extinction of phages while the biofilm bacteria reaches carrying capacity. In addition, two positive equilibria are: $E_{\mu_1} = (\mu_1, \mathcal{F}(\mu_1))$ and $E_{\mu_2} = (\mu_2, \mathcal{F}(\mu_2))$ subject to some conditions of existence. Here $\mathcal{F}(B) = \dfrac{r\left(1-\frac{B}{K_B}\right)}{\alpha\left(\kappa-\frac{B}{K_B}\right)}$ and $\mu_1$ and $\mu_2$ are solutions to the equation $\hat{f}(B) = \hat{c}$, where $\hat{f}(B) = \left(\kappa - \frac{B}{K_B}\right) B$ and $\hat{c} = \frac{c}{b\alpha}$ and $\mu_1 < \frac{\kappa K_B}{2} < \mu_2 < K_B$. The existence of the two positive equilibria $E_{\mu_1}$ and $E_{\mu_2}$ depend on the positioning of the prey isocline $V_B = \mathcal{F}(B)$ and predator isoclines $B = \mu_1$ and $B = \mu_2$. As we increase $\hat{c}$ in the interval $(0, \hat{c}_m)$, $\mu_1$ and $\mu_2$ become closer to each other; when $\hat{c} = \hat{c}_m$ the two equilibria coincide and we get $E_{\mu_1} = E_{\mu_2} = \left(\frac{\kappa K_B}{2}, \frac{r\left(1-\frac{\kappa}{2}\right)}{\alpha\left(\kappa-\frac{\kappa}{2}\right)}\right)$. Equilibria and their existence can be summarized in the following theorem.

**Theorem 1** *System (2) has four equilibria $E_0$, $E_{K_B}$, $E_{\mu_1}$ and $E_{\mu_2}$ if $\hat{c} \in (\hat{c}_m, \hat{c}_M)$, three equilibria $E_0$, $E_{K_B}$ and $E_{\mu_1}$ if $\hat{c} \in (0, \hat{c}_m)$, three equilibria $E_0$, $E_{K_B}$ and $E_{\mu_1} = E_{\mu_2} = E_\mu = \left(\frac{\kappa K_B}{2}, \frac{r\left(1-\frac{\kappa}{2}\right)}{\alpha\left(\kappa-\frac{\kappa}{2}\right)}\right)$ if $\hat{c} = \hat{c}_M$, only two equilibria $E_0$ and $E_{K_B}$ if $\hat{c} > \hat{c}_M$, where $\hat{c} = \frac{c}{b\alpha}$, $\hat{c}_M = \frac{\kappa^2}{4} K_B$ and $\hat{c}_m = (\kappa - 1)K_B$.*

### 3.1.1 Stability Analysis

It can be easily shown that $E_0 = (0, 0)$ has eigenvalues $\lambda_1 = r > 0$, $\lambda_2 = -c < 0$ showing that $E_0 = (0, 0)$ is a saddle point. The equilibria $E_{K_B} = (K_B, 0)$ has $\lambda_1 = -r$, $\lambda_2 = b\alpha(\hat{c}_m - \hat{c})$, as eigenvalues, showing that $E_{K_B}$ is an attractive node, if $\hat{c} > \hat{c}_m$, and is a saddle point if $\hat{c} < \hat{c}_m$. To study the stability of the other two equilibria, if they exist, we write the model (2) as

$$\frac{dB}{dt} = f(B)\left(\mathcal{F}(B) - V_B\right)$$
$$\frac{dV_B}{dt} = bf(B)V_B - cV_B. \tag{3}$$

The eigenvalues for $E_{\mu_1}$ are $\lambda_{1,2} = \frac{\xi_1 \pm \sqrt{\xi_1^2 - 4\Delta_1}}{2}$, where $\xi_1 = f(\mu_1)\mathcal{F}'(\mu_1)$ is the trace of Jacobian matrix of (3) at $E_{\mu_1}$. Since $\mathcal{F}'(B) < 0$, hence $\xi_1 < 0$ and $\Delta_1 = b\alpha^2 \mu_1\left(\kappa - \frac{\mu_1}{K_B}\right)\left(\kappa - \frac{2\mu_1}{K_B}\right)$ is the determinant of the Jacobian matrix at $E_{\mu_1}$. As $\mu_1 < \frac{\kappa K_B}{2}$, hence $\Delta_1 > 0$. This demonstrates that $E_{\mu_1}$ is an attracting focus. Similarly, the eigenvalues corresponding to $E_{\mu_2}$ are $\lambda_{1,2} = \frac{\xi_2 \pm \sqrt{\xi_2^2 - 4\Delta_2}}{2}$, where $\xi_2 = f(\mu_2)\mathcal{F}'(\mu_2) < 0$ is the trace of Jacobian matrix at $E_{\mu_2}$ and $\Delta_2 =$

$b \alpha^2 \mu_2 \left( \kappa - \frac{\mu_2}{K_B} \right) \left( \kappa - \frac{2\mu_2}{K_B} \right) < 0$ is the determinant of the Jacobian matrix at $E_{\mu_2}$.
We conclude that $E_{\mu_2}$ is a saddle point. Since only one equilibrium corresponds to
the extinction of biofilm bacteria, and it is a saddle point for all feasible parameter
values, we conclude that complete eradication of the biofilm is not possible using
this therapeutic strategy. This conclusion is consistent with the view, as discussed in
an extensive review [3], that phage action is not sufficient for complete eradication
of biofilms.

## 3.2   Using Phages First and then Antibiotics

In order to understand phage therapy, we return to model (1), approximating the
complicated processes of attachment and detachment by simpler functions to gain
tractability. Specifically, we assume biofilm bacteria detach at constant per capita
rate $n$; this assumption has a long history in the literature, extending back to Freter's
influential research on bacterial colonization of the intestinal tract [16, 20]. We further
assume that planktonic bacteria attach at constant per capita rate $m$. In Freter's original
biofilm model, attachment is also proportional to the number of planktonic bacteria,
but is further restricted by the number of available "wall attachment sites" [16]. In
our model, we restrict biofilm *growth* by the number of attachment sites, $K_B$, but
take a linear attachment rate. Since $B$ and $P$ are densities (cells per unit volume),
the net transfer of cells between compartments must be scaled, yielding $\mathscr{A}(B, P) = \left( \frac{vol_P}{vol_B} \right) m P$ and $\mathscr{D}(B, P) = \left( \frac{vol_B}{vol_P} \right) n B$, where $vol_B$ and $vol_P$ are the volumes of
the biofilm and planktonic compartments respectively. After the substitution of these
function into system (1), it can be shown by direct calculation that the resulting
system has three equilibrium solutions: the trivial equilibrium, an equilibrium with
both classes of bacteria only, and the all-existing equilibrium (exact expressions
omitted for brevity). Out of these equilibria the only equilibrium which corresponds
to the complete eradication of biofilm bacteria is $E_0$. It can be shown by a direct
calculation that this equilibrium $E_0$ is a saddle point for all feasible parameter values.
This demonstrates that phage therapy will not eradicate the biofilm. Since the biofilm
bacteria are resistant to antibiotics, we can conclude that even phage therapy followed
by antibiotics will not remove the biofilm.

## 3.3   A Novel Therapeutic Strategy: Blocking Attachment

The model developed here allows us to address the following question: is there a
therapeutic strategy, *in principle*, that could eradicate the biofilm? Since attachment
of planktonic bacteria is critical to biofilm maintenance, we investigated the model
assuming this attachment is negligible, and phage therapy is also applied. In this
case it can be shown by direct calculations that system (1), with the substitutions

$\mathscr{A}(B, P) = 0$ and $\mathscr{D}(B, P) = \left(\frac{vol_B}{vol_P}\right) n B$, has five equilibrium solutions:

$$
\begin{aligned}
E_0 &: (B, P, V_B, V_P) = (0, 0, 0, 0) \\
E_1 &: (B, P, V_B, V_P) = (0, K_P, 0, 0) \\
E_2 &: (B, P, V_B, V_P) = \left(0, \frac{c(c+p+q)}{\alpha b(c+q)}, \frac{M p r}{b a^2 (c+q)^2 K_P}\left(\frac{vol_P}{vol_B}\right), \frac{M r}{b a^2 K_P}\right), \qquad (4)\\
E_3 &: (B, P, V_B, V_P) = (B^*, P^*, 0, 0), \\
E_4 &: (B, P, V_B, V_P) = \left(B^{**}, P^{**}, V_B^{**}, V_P^{**}\right),
\end{aligned}
$$

where
$$
M = bq\alpha K_P - c(c + p + q - b\alpha K_P). \qquad (5)
$$

Three of these equilibria, $E_0$, $E_1$ and $E_2$, represent complete eradication of the biofilm. The equilibria $E_0$ and $E_1$ exist for any positive parameter values, while $E_2$ exists only for $M \geq 0$, i.e. $\alpha \geq \frac{c(c+p+q)}{b K_P(c+q)}$. The equilibrium $E_0$ is a saddle point for all feasible values of parameters. The equilibrium $E_1$ is asymptotically stable if $n > r$ and $\alpha < \frac{c(c+p+q)}{b K_P(c+q)}$. This implies that if the detachment rate is greater than the birth rate of bacteria in the biofilm and adsorption rate is less than $\frac{c(c+p+q)}{b K_P(c+q)}$, then elimination of biofilm bacteria is possible; in particular, planktonic bacteria will reach their carrying capacity and there will be no biofilm or planktonic viruses. Using the Hurwitz criterion, it can be shown that the equilibrium $E_2$ is stable if $M > 0$, i.e. $\alpha > \frac{c(c+p+q)}{b K_P(c+q)}$ (which guarantees its existence), and $n > \max(0, \bar{N}_1)$, where

$$
\bar{N}_1 = r - \frac{r \kappa p (\frac{vol_P}{vol_B}) M}{b a (c + q)^2 K_P}.
$$

If $\bar{N}_1$ is negative, the conditions for elimination of the biofilm become $n > 0$ and $\alpha > \frac{c(c+p+q)}{b K_P(c+q)}$. Thus, the model predicts that biofilm eradication is possible if the attachment of planktonic bacteria to the biofilm, $\mathscr{A}(B, P)$ can be blocked. Although an analysis of realistic numerical parameter values is outside the scope of this contribution, we note that the rate at which the biofilm could be eliminated depends on the difference between the logistic growth rate, $r$, and the loss rate of biofilm $(f(B)V_B - \mathscr{D}(B, P))/B$.

## 4   Summary and Conclusions

Biofilm formation starts with the attachment of planktonic (free-living) bacteria to a surface. As these bacteria become sessile and start producing the extracellular matrix (EPS) which defines the biofilm, other bacteria from the planktonic state continue to attach. In this way the bacteria develop a colony that can minimize the infiltration of antibacterial agents. In particular, antibiotics are often ineffective against biofilms, both due to the extracellular structure and the presence of persister cells, which are metabolically inactive. Phages (viruses that infect bacteria) offer the most promising alternative strategy for removing biofilms. Some phages such as T4 can easily infiltrate the EPS structure and can also infect and kill persister cells [18].

A range of experimental studies have shown that phages, antibiotics or other agents alone are not enough to eradicate a biofilm completely, hence a combination of these agents is typically recommended [7, 26]. In this study we derive a mathematical model which predicts that a combination of antibiotics and phage therapy cannot eradicate a biofilm, whether applied as antibiotics followed by phage, or in the reverse order, as studied in [7].

In Sect. 3.3, we investigate a novel, hypothetical therapeutic strategy. In particular, we demonstrate that if further attachment of planktonic bacteria to the biofilm can be blocked (even if the biofilm is already mature), complete elimination of the biofilm is possible using phages. After eliminating the biofilm, antibiotics can be used to eliminate any remaining planktonic bacteria. This result suggests that blocking attachment, perhaps by blocking EPS production, is a promising avenue for biofilm eradication. Interestingly, the genetic pathways associated with quorum sensing may in fact be the targets of several natural biofilm inhibitors [21].

Mathematically, the model we derive is a two-patch predator-prey system with group defense by the prey in one patch. Our analysis was made tractable by proposing a simple, novel functional response describing group defense. While this function is invalid (becomes negative) for biofilm densities that exceed an upper bound, in reality physical constraints limit the density of cells in biofilms, and this limitation did not impede analysis. We expect that this functional form may have further uses in the study of group defense mechanisms, particularly when other aspects of the model become more complex.

# References

1. Abedon, S.T. (ed.): Bacteriophage Ecology: Population Growth, Evolution, and Impact of Bacterial Viruses. Cambridge University Press, Cambridge (2008)
2. Abedon, S.T.: Ecology of anti-biofilm agents I: antibiotics versus bacteriophages. Pharmaceuticals **8**(3), 525–558 (2015a)
3. Abedon, S.T.: Ecology of anti-biofilm agents II: bacteriophage exploitation and biocontrol of biofilm bacteria. Pharmaceuticals (Basel) **8**(3), 559–589 (2015b)
4. Andrews, J.F.: A mathematical model for the continuous culture of microorganisms utilizing inhibitory substrates. Biotechnol. Bioeng. **10**(6), 707–723 (1968)
5. Azeredo, J., Sutherland, I.W.: The use of phages for the removal of infectious biofilms. Curr. Pharm. Biotechnol. **9**(4), 261–266 (2008)
6. Broer, H.W., Naudot, V., Roussarie, R., Saleh, K.: A predator-prey model with non-monotonic response function. Regul. Chaotic Dyn. **11**, 155–165 (2006)
7. Chaudhry, W.N., Concepcin-Acevedo, J., Park, T., Andleeb, S., Bull, J.J., Levin, B.R.: Synergy and order effects of antibiotics and phages in killing Pseudomonas aeruginosa biofilms. PLOS ONE **12**(1), e0168615 (2017)
8. Ciofu, O., Rojo-Molinero, E., Maci, M.D., Oliver, A.: Antibiotic treatment of biofilm infections. APMIS **125**(4), 304–319 (2017)

9. Davies, D.: Understanding biofilm resistance to antibacterial agents. Nat. Rev. Drug Discovery **2**(2), 114–122 (2003)
10. Doolittle, M.M., Cooney, J.J., Caldwell, D.E.: Tracing the interaction of bacteriophage with bacterial biofilms using fluorescent and chromogenic probes. J. Ind. Microbiol. **16**(6), 331–341 (1996)
11. Douterelo, I., Husband, S., Loza, V., Boxall, J.: Dynamics of biofilm regrowth in drinking water distribution systems. Appl. Environ. Microbiol. **82**(14), 4155–4168 (2016)
12. Feng, G., Cheng, Y., Wang, S.-Y., Borca-Tasciuc, D.A., Worobo, R.W., Moraru, C.I.: Bacterial attachment and biofilm formation on surfaces are reduced by small-diameter nanoscale pores: how small is small enough? NPJ Biofilms Microbiomes **1**, 201522 (2015)
13. Fernndez, L., Gonzlez, S., Campelo, A.B., Martnez, B., Rodrguez, A., Garca, P.: Low-level predation by lytic phage phiIPLA-RODI promotes biofilm formation and triggers the stringent response in Staphylococcus aureus. Sci. Rep. **7**, 40965 (2017)
14. Fleming, D., Rumbaugh, K.P.: Approaches to dispersing medical biofilms. Microorganisms **5**(2), 15 (2017)
15. Freedman, H.I., Wolkowicz, G.S.K.: Predator-prey systems with group defence: the paradox of enrichment revisited. Bull. Math. Biol. **48**(5–6), 493–508 (1986)
16. Freter, R., Brickner, H., Fekete, J., Vickerman, M.M., Carey, K.E.: Survival and implantation of *Escherichia coli* in the intestinal tract. Infect. Immun. **39**(2), 686–703 (1983)
17. Fux, C.A., Stoodley, P., Hall-Stoodley, L., Costerton, J.W.: Bacterial biofilms: a diagnostic and therapeutic challenge. Expert Rev. Anti-Infective Ther. **1**(4), 667–683 (2003)
18. Harper, D.R., Parracho, H.M.R.T., Walker, J., Sharp, R., Hughes, G., Werthn, M., Lehman, S., Morales, S.: Bacteriophages and biofilms. Antibiotics **3**(3), 270 (2014)
19. Jiang, J., Yu, P.: Multistable phenomena involving equilibria and periodic motions in predator-prey systems. Int. J. Bifurcat. Chaos **27**(03), 1750043 (2017)
20. Jones, D., Kojouharov, H.V., Le, D., Smith, H.: The Freter model: a simple model of biofilm formation. J. Math. Biol. **47**(2), 137–152 (2003)
21. Lee, J.-H., Park, J.-H., Kim, J.-A., Neupane, G.P., Cho, M.H., Lee, C.-S., Lee, J.: Low concentrations of honey reduce biofilm formation, quorum sensing, and virulence in *Escherichia coli* O157:H7. Biofouling **27**(10), 1095–1104 (2011)
22. Lenski, R.E.: Dynamics of interactions between bacteria and virulent bacteriophage. In: Advances in Microbial Ecology, pp. 1–44. Springer, Boston, MA. (1988). https://doi.org/10.1007/978-1-4684-5409-3_1
23. Lynch, A.S., Abbanat, D.: New antibiotic agents and approaches to treat biofilm-associated infections. Expert Opin. Ther. Pat. **20**(10), 1373–1387 (2010)
24. Mu, H., Tang, J., Liu, Q., Sun, C., Wang, T., Duan, J.: Potent antibacterial nanoparticles against biofilm and intracellular bacteria. Sci. Rep. **6**, 18877 (2016)
25. Omar, A., Wright, J.B., Schultz, G., Burrell, R., Nadworny, P.: Microbial biofilms and chronic wounds. Microorganisms **5**(1), 9 (2017)
26. Ryan, E.M., Alkawareek, M.Y., Donnelly, R.F., Gilmore, B.F.: Synergistic phage-antibiotic combinations for the control of *Escherichia coli* biofilms in vitro. FEMS Immunol. Med. Microbiol. **65**(2), 395–398 (2012)
27. Van Houdt, R., Michiels, C.: Biofilm formation and the food industry, a focus on the bacterial outer surface. J. Appl. Microbiol. **109**(4), 1117–1131 (2010)
28. Wolkowicz, G.: Bifurcation analysis of a predator-prey system involving group defence. SIAM J. Appl. Math. **48**(3), 592–606 (1988)
29. Xiao, D., Ruan, S.: Global analysis in a predator-prey system with nonmonotonic functional response. SIAM J. Appl. Math. **61**(4), 1445–1472 (2001)
30. Zhu, H., Campbell, S.A., Wolkowicz, G.S.K.: Bifurcation analysis of a predator-prey system with nonmonotonic functional response. SIAM J. Appl. Math. **63**(2), 636–682 (2002)

# A Simple Model of Between-Hive Transmission of Nosemosis

**Nasim Muhammad and Hermann J. Eberl**

**Abstract** We present a simple metapopulation extension of a mathematical model of Nosemosis for the between-hive transmission of the disease in an apiary. The transmission of the disease between neighbouring colonies is modeled by impulsive transfer of pathogens. The model is studied in computer simulations. Our results illustrate how the disease, starting from a single colony, can spread and lead to drastic reduction in the bee population in the apiary, even in the subcritical case.

**Keywords** Honeybee · Mathematical model · Nosema
Between-hive transmission

## 1 Introduction

The Western honeybee (*Apis mellifera*) plays an important role in agriculture, both for the production of honey and wax but also for its use as managed pollinators. They are estimated to pollinate one third of Canadian food crops, corresponding to an economic value to Canadian agriculture of over $2 billion annually [17]. Any major decline of the pollinating population, therefore, can have a dramatic impact on biodiversity, ecosystems and related economic activities.

In recent years beekeepers have reported huge losses of colonies, which can manifest themselves in the form of Colony Collapse Disorder or Wintering Losses. The exact causes for this phenomenon are unclear, but it is now widely assumed that it is the multifactorial interplay of several stressors, each of which independently

N. Muhammad
Mohawk College and McMaster University, 1280 Main Street West,
Hamilton, ON L8S 0A3, Canada
e-mail: nasimm@mcmaster.ca

H. J. Eberl (✉)
University of Guelph, 50 Stone Rd E, Guelph, ON N1G 2W1, Canada
e-mail: heberl@uoguelph.ca

© Springer Nature Switzerland AG 2018
D. M. Kilgour et al. (eds.), *Recent Advances in Mathematical and Statistical Methods*, Springer Proceedings in Mathematics & Statistics 259,
https://doi.org/10.1007/978-3-319-99719-3_35

could be sub-critical, that might be responsible. Important among those stressors are parasites and diseases of the honeybee.

To aid in understanding the role of honeybee diseases, several mathematical models have been introduced, either for generic diseases [2, 3, 11] or for specific diseases such as the Acute Bee Paralysis Virus, the Deformed Wing Virus, Nosemosis, Varroatosis, or American Foulbrood, e.g. [8, 9, 13, 14, 16, 20]. These models draw on the well-developed machinery of Mathematical Epidemiology and combine them with models for honeybee population dynamics; in may cases they are based on [10]. These disease modeling studies have in common that they focus on a single, isolated, colony. In many beekeeping operations, however, several hives are maintained in close proximity. This introduces the possibility for disease transfer from one colony to others.

Our objective is to present a first such model for the spread of a disease in an apiary. We focus on Nosemosis, a honeybee disease caused by the microsporidians *Nosema apis* and *N. ceranae*. Although some authors have suggested that nosema might be a causative agent of colony failure [7], more commonly it is assumed to be a subcritical disease that weakens colonies but does not by itself lead to colony loss. The reduction in colony strength is primary due to the shorter life span of infected older foraging bees. The primary route of transmission within a hive is through defecation of spores by infected bees and subsequent ingestion by healthy bees, e.g. during hive cleaning activities, primarily in early Spring, cf. [13] and the references therein. The transfer of the disease between hives in an apiary is not well understood. It has been suggested that this might happen during hive maintenance, e.g. hive cleaning or transferring of contaminated combs, splitting and uniting contaminated hives, but also by drifting of infected bees to neighbouring hives [4, 5].

## 2   Mathematical Model

Our mathematical model is a metapopulation extension of the nosemosis model for in-hive transmission that was introduced and described in more detail in [13]. The main assumptions are that the worker bees in each colony are divided into two casts, hive bees that are responsible for cleaning and nursing duties, and forager bees. Each of these two casts is sub-divided into infected and susceptible sub-groups. The recruitment rates for hive bees to become foragers, as well as possible reversion from foraging to hive duties are state dependent. Infected hive bees become infected foragers, susceptible hive bees become susceptible foragers and *vice versa*. The transmission of the disease is assumed to be indirect: infected bees deposit nosema spores in the hive by defecation. Susceptible bees become infected when they ingest these spores, e.g. during hive cleaning activities. Infected forager have a shorter life expectation than healthy foragers. Newly emerging worker bees are assumed to be not infected. As is common in most models of honeybee population and disease dynamics, e.g. [2, 9, 11, 14, 20], we assume that the queen is not affected by the disease. Drones are neglected, also in agreement with these studies.

Newly introduced is here the transmission of the disease between colonies. This could be by movement of infected individuals into neighbouring hives, or, and this is the route that we describe here, by transfer of spores between neighbouring hives. We assume that this happens at most at a few discrete events per year during hive maintenance operations. To model such discrete interventions we follow the framework that was set up in [15] to describe discrete events in a continuous honeybee disease model. Our model for the $i$th hive, $i = 1, \ldots, N$ reads

$$\dot{H}_0^i = \beta(t)\frac{(Z^i)^n}{\kappa(t)^n + (Z^i)^n} - \sigma_1(t)H_0^i + \sigma_2(t)\frac{F^i}{Z^i}F_0^i - \eta_0(t)H_0^i$$
$$-\alpha(t)H_0^i\frac{E^i}{\lambda(t) + E^i}, \tag{1}$$

$$\dot{H}_1^i = -\sigma_1(t)H_1^i + \sigma_2(t)\frac{F^i}{Z^i}F_1^i - \eta_1(t)H_1^i + \alpha(t)H_0^i\frac{E^i}{\lambda(t) + E^i}, \tag{2}$$

$$\dot{F}_0^i = \sigma_1(t)H_0^i - [\sigma_2(t)\frac{F^i}{Z^i} + \phi_0(t)]F_0^i, \tag{3}$$

$$\dot{F}_1^i = \sigma_1(t)H_1^i - [\sigma_2(t)\frac{F^i}{Z^i} + \phi_1(t)]F_1^i, \tag{4}$$

$$\dot{E}^i = \gamma(t)H_1^i - \delta(t)E^i - \tilde{\alpha}(t)H^i\frac{E^i}{\lambda(t) + E^i} \tag{5}$$

where

$$H^i := H_0^i + H_1^i, \qquad F^i := F_0^i + F_1^i, \qquad Z^i := H^i + F^i \tag{6}$$

Here, $H_0^i$, $H_1^i$ are the susceptible and infected hive bee sub-populations and $F_0^i$, $F_1^i$ are the susceptible and infected forager sub-populations in the $i$th hive. By $E^i$ we denote the environmental disease potential, i.e. a measure for the contamination with the pathogen. We assume that transmission of spores between hives only happens in the beginning of Spring during hive maintenance. For this discrete event, we update the environmental potential value of the $k$th hive ($E^k$) at times $t_j$, $j = 1, 2 \ldots$ as follows:

$$E^k(t_j) := \lim_{t \to t_j^-} \left( [1 - \xi^k p] * E^k(t) + p \sum_{i \in \Omega^k} E^i(t) \right) \tag{7}$$

where $\xi^k$ is the number of neighbours of the $k$th hive and $p$ the percentage of spores exchanged between neighbouring hives. The first term on the right of Eq. (7) represents the amount of spores left after transferring to neighbouring hives and the second term for the amount of spores placed in $k$th hive from its grid neighbourhood $\Omega^k$, which is dependent on the hive arrangement in the apiary and the location of the hive.

We assume for simplicity that the parameters describing honeybee population and disease dynamics are the same in each hive. The model parameters and their default values used in our simulations are described in Table 1. For a more detailed explanation we refer the reader to [13]. All parameters are time-dependent, non-

**Table 1** Definition of model parameters and their values used in the simulations, from [13]

| Parameter | Symbol | Unit | Spring | Summer | Fall | Winter | References |
|---|---|---|---|---|---|---|---|
| Max. eclosion rate | $\beta$ | Bees/days | 500 | 1500 | 500 | 0 | [20] |
| Brood maintenance coefficient | $\kappa$ | Bees | 8000 | 12,000 | 8000 | 6000 | [14] |
| Base recruitment rate | $\sigma_1$ | 1/days | 0.25 | 0.25 | 0.25 | 0 | [10] |
| Max. feedback rate | $\sigma_2$ | 1/days | 1.5 | 1.5 | 1.5 | 1.5 | [13] |
| $H_0$ death rate | $\eta_0$ | 1/days | 0 | 0 | 0 | 0.00649 | [18] |
| $H_1$ death rate | $\eta_1$ | 1/days | 0 | 0 | 0 | 0.00649 | [18] |
| $F_0$ death date | $\phi_0$ | 1/days | 0.08511 | 0.08511 | 0.08511 | 0 | [1] |
| $F_1$ death date | $\phi_1$ | 1/days | 0.16936 | 0.16936 | 0.16936 | 0 | [1, 6] |
| Infection rate | $\alpha$ | 1/days | 0.55 | 0.12 | 0.24 | 0 | [12] |
| Spore deposition rate | $\gamma$ | $\frac{\text{env.pot.}}{\text{bees} * \text{days}}$ | $0.2061\gamma_w$ | $0.2835\gamma_w$ | $0.2527\gamma_w$ | $\gamma_w$ | [13] |
| Spore viability decay rate | $\delta$ | 1/days | 0.006570 | 0.023300 | 0.015683 | 0 | [13] |
| Spore uptake rate | $\tilde{\alpha}$ | $\frac{\text{env.pot.}}{\text{bees} * \text{days}}$ | 0.14 | 0.14 | 0.14 | 0.14 | [13] |
| Half saturation const. for E. potential | $\lambda$ | $\frac{\text{env.pot.}}{\text{days}}$ | 10,000 | 10,000 | 10,000 | 10,000 | [13] |
| Hill exponent disease transmission | n | – | 2 | 2 | 2 | 2 | [13] |
| Parameter | p | – | 1% | – | – | – | Assumed |

negative, and assumed to be periodic with periods of one year to reflect seasonal changes in honeybee population dynamics. In Table 1 we give average parameter values for each season.

Even for the single hive model, the results that were obtainable by analytical techniques in [13] were limited. Therefore, we study the model in computer simulations. To this end it was implemented in R using the package deSolve [19]. To take advantage of the multi-core architecture of modern computers a coarse grain parallelisation approach was taken, mapping hives to cores using the packages doParallel and Foreach [21]. Simulations were run on a Lenovo ThinkServer RD650 with 256G of RAM and 16 cores/32 threads in 2 sockets, with 122TB hard drives. The CPUs are Intel Xeon(R) E5-2640 v3 @ 2.60GHz.

In our simulations we assume that the first day of spring is the first day of the year. Initially, the model Eqs. (1)–(6) are integrated for the first three seasons with initial values $H_0(0) = 10^4$, $H_1(0) = 0$, $F_0(0) = 10^4$, $F_1(0) = 0$, and $E(0) = 0$. To simulate the onset of the disease, we perturb the disease free solution by increasing $H_1$ to 10 on the first day of the first Winter.

## 3   Simulations

### 3.1   Apiary Set-up

We consider here for simplicity beehives that are placed in a rectangular grid of size $N_1 \times N_2$. These beehives are labeled from 1 to $N = N_1 \cdot N_2$ using lexicographical ordering, $k = k(i, j) := N_2(i - 1) + j$, $i = 1, \ldots, N_1$, $j = 1, \ldots, N_2$. For disease transmission between hives we consider the Moore neighbourhood, i.e. for a hive $k$ at an interior location $(i, j)$, all 8 neighbour hives are affected ($\xi^k = 8$), for a hive in a corner $\xi^k = 3$, etc. In the simulations presented below we chose $N_1 = 6, N_2 = 5$, representing a medium sized bee yard.

### 3.2   Base Case Simulation

We first examine a base case with no disease. In this scenario all hives are identical. The simulation results are shown in Fig. 1. In the absence of nosema, the colony very quickly reaches a healthy periodic solution, as shown in Fig. 1. Since no disease is introduced, the colony only contains healthy hive bees and healthy forager bees. The populations fluctuate with the seasons as expected. The colony population peaks towards the end of Summer and reaches a minimum near the end of Winter. Foragers return to the hive in Winter, increasing hive bee populations. This effect is reversed at the beginning of Spring.

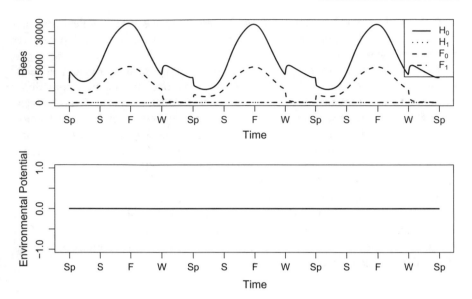

**Fig. 1** Base case simulation of the model (1)−(6) without disease

### 3.3 Disease Propagation Between Hives

Two simulations were conducted to investigate the effect of the position of infected hives on bee population and the spread of spores in an apiary. Initially, Hive #01 (a corner hive) was infected in one simulation and Hive #13 (a center hive) in the other one, whereas all other hives are assumed to be initially pathogen free. It was reported in [13] for the single hive scenario that the population does not die but reaches an endemic periodic solution with moderate spore uptake $\tilde{\alpha} = 0.15$ and low spore deposition $\gamma_\omega = 0.1$. We used the same values for $\tilde{\alpha}$ and $\gamma_\omega$ with between-hive disease transmission of $p = 1\%$. The results are presented in Figs. 2, 3, 4, 5 and 6.

Figure 2 shows the behavior of the environmental pathogen reservoirs of two typical hives that are placed farthest away from each other in an apiary. Hive #01 is infected in the first year of simulation whereas the remaining hives were initially disease free. The disease quickly establishes itself. The data collected during the simulation shows that the maximum value of reservoirs Hive#01 and Hive#30 reach to 372.9 and 372.6 respectively and occurs on the same 10568th day (29 years and 12 days). The propagation of the disease is slow, taking many years. This is made more quantitative in Table 2 in which the times are reported at which pathogens reach 5, 100 and 300 levels. Hive #30 reaches to 300 level in 24 years and 5 days whereas Hive #01 in 3 years and 10 days.

As mentioned above, the simulation scenario is sub-critical in the sense that disease infestation does not lead to colony failure but to weaker colonies. We calculate the percent short fall of the apiary's population by taking the ratio of the average

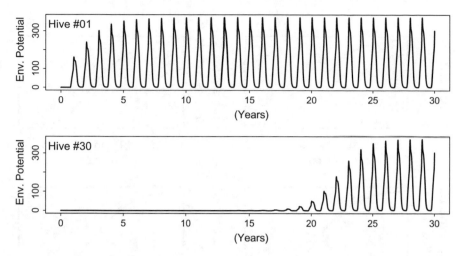

**Fig. 2** Behavior of Environmental Reservoirs for Hive #01 (initially infected) and Hive #30 with $\tilde{\alpha} = 0.14$, $\gamma_\omega = 0.1$ and $p = 1\%$

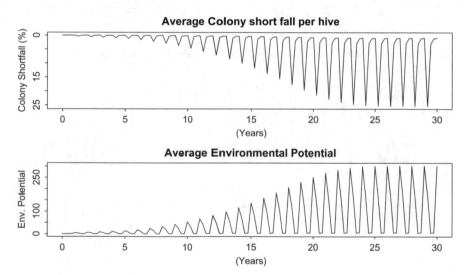

**Fig. 3** Simulation results showing average population shortfall and average environmental potential with $\tilde{\alpha} = 0.14$, $\gamma_\omega = 0.1$, and $p = 1\%$ when Hive #01 was infected

population in the apiary with the disease free population (base case simulation). This is shown in Fig. 3, indicating a rather drastic effect of the disease on the number of bees in the apiary, which in these simulations drops by 25%. To further investigate this, we report four data points at the beginning of each season for every year in Fig. 4. It shows that the populations' shortfall at the beginning of season is 1% in Spring, 3% in Fall and Winter, and 25% in Summer. Thus although the disease intensity is

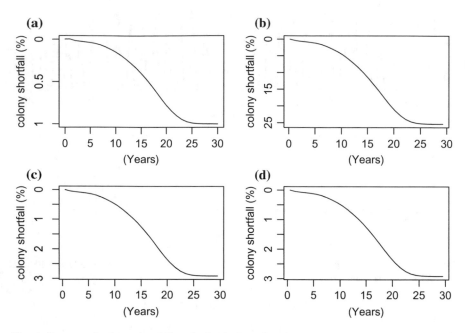

**Fig. 4** Percent of colony shortfall at the beginning of each season, **a** Spring **b** Summer **c** Fall **d** Winter

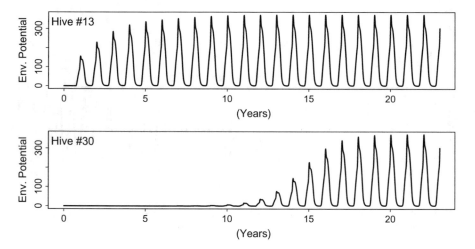

**Fig. 5** Behavior of Environmental Reservoirs for Hive #13 (initially infected) and Hive #30 with $\tilde{\alpha} = 0.14$, $\gamma_\omega = 0.1$ and $p = 1\%$

strongest in Spring when cleaning activities primarily take place, cf. [13], it becomes most noteworthy in Summer when the colonies are strongest.

We repeat the above simulations assuming now that the hive approximately in the centre of the apiary is the initially infected one. Changing the location of initial

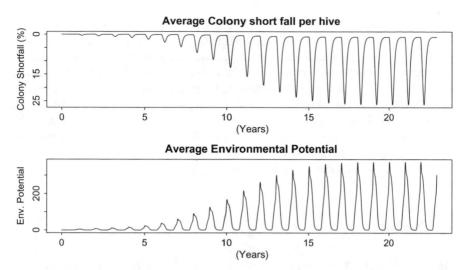

**Fig. 6** Simulation results showing average population shortfall and average environmental potential with $\tilde{\alpha} = 0.14$, $\gamma_\omega = 0.1$, and $p = 1\%$ when Hive #13 was infected

**Table 2** Approximate time at which pathogen spore levels 5, 100 and 300 are obtained for the simulation of Fig. 2

| Env. reservoir level | 5 | 100 | 300 |
|---|---|---|---|
| Hive #01 (days) | 282 | 358 | 1102 |
| Hive #30 (days) | 6547 | 7653 | 8741 |
| Time difference (years-days) | 17y 77d | 20y 15d | 20y 359d |

**Table 3** Approximate time at which pathogen spore levels 5, 100 and 300 are obtained for the simulation of Fig. 5

| Env. reservoir level | 5 | 100 | 300 |
|---|---|---|---|
| Hive #13 (days) | 282 | 358 | 1462 |
| Hive #30 (days) | 3640 | 5094 | 6190 |
| Time difference (years-days) | 9y 82d | 13y 4d | 12y 360d |

disease outbreak has two primary effects: If the infection originates in a hive in the centre, it will have spread faster across the entire apiary than if it originates on the boundary, i.e one will expect a faster spread of the disease. Secondly, in this scenario, from the location of first outbreak the disease is transmitted into 8 neighbouring sites on the Moore neighbourhood, whereas in the previous scenario it had only 3 neighbours on the grid. Therefore it can be expected that both the diseases spreads in more directions but also leads to a faster reduction in the original location. Figure 5 shows the pathogen levels in Hives #13 (location of initial outbreak) and #30 (the hive furthest removed). The levels of contamination that are reached are the same as in the previous scenario, but the disease spreads across the apiary faster, see also Table 3 for more quantitative data. Noteworthy is here that in this case it takes longer for the disease to reach $E = 300$ in the site of first outbreak than in the previous scenario; this is an effect of having more neighbours into which pathogens are initially distributed. The level of population shortfall across the apiary, as per Fig. 5 is similar to the previous scenario, i.e. the longterm effect of the disease outbreak in a single hive on the overall apiary does not depend on the location of the outbreak. However, the time that it takes for the disease to spread across the yard does.

## 4 Conclusion

Most models of the dynamics of honeybee diseases are concerned with individual colonies. However, most apiaries operate several hives in one location which provides an opportunity for pathogens to spread between colonies. We presented here a simple metapopulation model to simulate such a scenario for Nosemosis. Our simulations suggest that the spread of a sub-critical nosema infection that originates in a single hive across an apiary can lead to a drastic shortfall in the total bee population, which has immediate consequences for both pollination performance and honey production.

A key assumption in our model, which obviously affects simulation results, was that the disease spreads between hives by propagation of the pathogen at few occasions during the year. In reality the transmission of the disease in an apiary is not well understood and it is possible that, depending on the disease under question, several mechanisms might be responsible. Under this light, our results cannot be understood as quantitative predictions. However, they highlight the importance of further investigations of the effect of between-hive disease transmission. They raise the question, to which extent the observations made here carry over to other transmission mechanisms, and how sensitive they are with respect to the parameters that describe those.

## References

1. Becerra-Guzmán, F., Guzmán-Novoa, E., Correa-Benítez, A., Zozaya-Rubio, A.: Length of life, age at first foraging and foraging life of Africanized and European honey bee (*Apis mellifera*) workers, during conditions of resource abundance. J. Apicult. Res. **44**(4), 151–156 (2005)
2. Betti, M.I., Wahl, L.M., Zamir, M., Rueppell, O.: Effects of infection on honey bee population dynamics: a model. PloS One **9**(10), e110237 (2014)
3. Betti, M.I., Wahl, L.M., Zamir, M.: Reproduction number and asymptotic stability for the dynamics of a honey bee colony with continuous age structure. Bull. Math. Biol. **79**(7), 1586–1611 (2017)

4. Fries, I.: Comb replacement and Nosema disease (*Nosema apis* Z.) in honey bee colonies. Apidologie **19**, 343–354 (1988)
5. Free, J.B.: The drifting of honey-bees. J. Agric. Sci. **51**, 294–306 (1958)
6. Goblirsch, M., Huang, Z.Y., Spivak, M., Amdam, G.V.: Physiological and behavioral changes in honey bees (*Apis mellifera*) induced by Nosema ceranae infection. PloS One **8**(3), e58165 (2013)
7. Higes, M., Martn-Hernndez, R., Garrido-Bailn, E., Garca-Palencia, P., Meana, A.: Detection of infective Nosema ceranae (Microsporidia) spores in corbicular pollen of forager honeybees. J. Invertebr. Pathol. **97**, 76–78 (2008)
8. Jatulan, E.O., Rabajant, J.F., Banaay, C.G.B., Fajardo Jr., A.C., Jose, E.C.: A mathematical model of intra-colony spread of American foulbrood in European honeybees (*Apis mellifera* L.). Plos One **10**(12), e0143805 (2015)
9. Kang, Y., Blanco, K., Davis, T., Wang, Y., DeGrandi-Hoffman, G.: Disease dynamics of honeybees with Varroa destructor as parasite and virus vector. Math. Biosc. **275**, 71–92 (2016)
10. Khoury, D.S., Myerscough, M.R., Barron, A.B., Marshall, J.A.R.: A quantitative model of honey bee colony population dynamics. PloS One **6**(4), e18491 (2011)
11. Kribs-Zaleta, C.M., Mitchell, C.: Modeling colony collapse disorder in honeybees as a contagion. Math. Biosc. Eng. **11**(6), 1275–1294 (2014)
12. Lacey, B.: A two year study of Nosema ceranae in Ontario. Ont. Bee J. **33**(2), 14–16 (2014)
13. Petric, A., Guzman-Novoa, E., Eberl, H.J.: A mathematical model for the interplay of Nosema infection and forager losses in honey bee colonies. J. Biol. Dyn. **11**(S2), 348–378 (2017)
14. Ratti, V., Kevan, P.G., Eberl, H.J.: A mathematical model of the honeybeevarroa destructor-acute bee paralysis virus system with seasonal effects. Bull. Math. Biol. **77**(8), 1493–1520 (2015)
15. Ratti, V., Kevan, P.G., Eberl, H.J.: A discrete-continuous modeling framework to study the role of swarming in a honeybee-Varroa destrutor-virus system. In: Belair, J. (ed.) Mathematical and Computational Approaches in Advancing Modern Science and Engineering, pp. 299–308. Springer, Berlin (2016)
16. Ratti, V., Kevan, P.G., Eberl, H.J.: A mathematical model of forager loss in honeybee colonies infested with Varroa destructor and the acute bee paralysis virus. Bull. Math. Biol. **79**(6), 12181253 (2017)
17. Statistical Overview of the Canadian Honey and Bee Industry and the Economic Contribution of Honey Bee Pollination 2013–2014. http://www.agr.gc.ca/resources/prod/doc/pdf/1453219857143-eng.pdf
18. Sakagami, S.F., Fukuda, H.: Life tables for worker honeybees. Res. Pop. Ecol. **10**(2), 127–139 (1968)
19. Soetaert, K., Petzoldt, T., Setzer, R.W.: Solving differential equations in R: package deSolve. J. Stat. Softw. **33**(9), 1–25 (2010)
20. Sumpter, D.J.T., Martin, S.J.: The dynamics of virus epidemics in varroa-infested honey bee colonies. J. Animal Ecol. **73**(1), 51–63 (2004)
21. Weston, S., Calaway, R.: Getting Started with doParallel and foreach. https://cran.r-project.org/web/packages/doParallel/vignettes/gettingstartedParallel.pdf (2017)

# Spreading of Nearshore Effluent Discharges on Eroded Sloping Sandy Beaches

Anton Purnama, Huda A. Al-Maamari and E. Balakrishnan

**Abstract** A far field modeling study is presented to evaluate the effect of erosion of a sloping sandy beach upon the mixing and dispersion of the effluent discharges from a multiport diffuser. The two-dimensional advection-diffusion equation with multiple point sources is analytically solved and illustrated graphically by plotting contours of solution to replicate the interaction and merging of the nearshore effluent discharged plumes in coastal waters. The compounded shoreline concentration is asymptotically approximated and used as an environmental impact measure to assess how well the effluent plumes are diluted downstream. It is found that the significant increase in maximum concentration value due to erosion can be reduced by adding more ports and extending the diffuser pipe. The result demonstrates that a modern marine outfall system equipped with multiport diffusers does produce lower potential environmental impacts.

**Keywords** Advection diffusion equation · Far field model
Multiport diffuser · Sea outfall · Shoreline concentration

## 1  Introduction

It is widely accepted that the environmental effects of discharging pretreated wastewater through an effective and well design long sea outfall system which terminates in multiport diffusers could be kept to a minimum [1, 2]. A multiport diffuser is a linear structure consisting of many closely spaced ports or nozzles designed to discharge a series of effluent jets and rapidly dilute the effluent stream [3–5]. For nearshore

A. Purnama (✉) · H. A. Al-Maamari · E. Balakrishnan
Sultan Qaboos University, PO Box 36, Muscat Al-Khod PC 123, Oman
e-mail: antonp@squ.edu.om

H. A. Al-Maamari
e-mail: s23298@student.squ.edu.om

E. Balakrishnan
e-mail: balak@squ.edu.om

© Springer Nature Switzerland AG 2018
D. M. Kilgour et al. (eds.), *Recent Advances in Mathematical and Statistical Methods*, Springer Proceedings in Mathematics & Statistics 259,
https://doi.org/10.1007/978-3-319-99719-3_36

discharges, as the water depth is gradually decreasing towards the shoreline, it is observed in the far field that the bent-over effluent plumes are spreading towards the shoreline and may cause concentration build-up to higher levels in the coastal waters [6–9].

Physically, the coastal area is a dynamic region where land and sea meet. In some places, it takes the form of a sloping sandy beach, but in other places it is a mountainous coast with rocky sea cliffs. The process of a sandy beach erosion is complicated due to the inherently nature of sediment fluid interaction in the nearshore, and the sandy beaches are actively adjusting their form to an equilibrium profile in response to incident waves [10], winds and storms [11], and sea level rise also exacerbates beach erosion [12]. Erosion is causing sediment to move alongshore and/or drift out to sea.

The simple empirical power law for the equilibrium beach profile is given by $h = Ay^n$, where $h$ is the water depth, $A$ is the scale parameter, and $y$ is the offshore distance [13, 14]. This formula was found by fitting (stable) beach profiles, and agreed well with data obtained from the experiments in the laboratory. The value of $A = 0.1$ was suggested in [15, 16], but different values were reported for the power law: $n = 2/3$ in [13, 14, 17], $n = 0.78$ in [18] and $n = 4/5$ in [16].

Owing to the unpredicted nature of the sea, a full understanding of the integrated shoreline evolution and dispersion process of effluent discharges are not yet known, and the mathematical models has been widely used for assessing the environmental impacts of marine effluent discharges [19–21]. While the far field modelling in this paper involves drastic simplifications, key physical mixing and dispersion processes are represented, and thus the analytical solution remains useful in providing a qualitative understanding and in suggesting general behaviour of the marine outfall effluent discharge plumes [22–24]. In terms of the practical applicability, it is well recognized that the far field models can be applied as a tool to perform quick preliminary worst-case assessments. If this easy-to-apply assessment indicates no significant impacts, no further action is needed and the use of more sophisticated and time-consuming integrated three-dimensional shoreline evolution, hydrodynamic and water quality modeling can be avoided.

## 2   Advection-Diffusion Equation for Multiport Diffusers

As we are mainly concerned with the effect of variations in the beach profile, the coastline is considered to be straight and the sea wide, and the far field outfall's effluent discharges plume is assumed to be vertically well-mixed. We model the seabed depth as $h(y) = my^n$ $(0 < n \leq 1)$ [7, 8, 24]. As illustrated in Fig. 1, when $n = 1$ the profile is known as the (non-eroded) sloping sandy beach with slope $m$. The beach profiles due to bed erosion are represented by $n < 1$.

The longshore (drift) current is assumed to be steady with a speed $U$ and remains in the $x$-direction parallel to the beach at all times. The dispersion mechanisms are represented by eddy diffusivities, and diffusion in the $x$-direction is neglected, as the

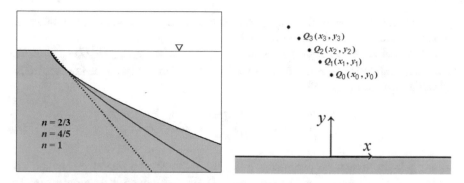

**Fig. 1** Cross-section profile of eroded sloping sandy beach (left), and diagram of multiple point sources to represent a multiport diffuser (right)

effluent plumes in steady currents become very elongated in the $x$-direction [25, 26]. The variations in the $y$-direction of drift current $U$ and coefficient of dispersivity $D$ are assumed as the power functions only of water depth $h$, where $U$ is proportional to $h^{1/2}$ and $D$ to $h^{3/2}$, respectively. These scalings are appropriate for a turbulent shallow-water flow over a smooth bed [6, 26]. Other complexities such as tidal motions, density and temperature are ignored.

Without loss of generality, we represent the single outfall (port) discharging an effluent stream at a constant rate $Q_0$ as a point source at the end of the outfall pipeline $(x_0 = 0, y_0 = \alpha h_0)$, where $h_0$ is an arbitrary reference water depth. As illustrated in Fig. 1, for multiport diffusers with $N$ ports (in addition to the single outfall), the first port discharges at a rate $Q_1$ as a point source at $(x_1 = -\ell h_0, y_1 = (\alpha + d)h_0)$; the second port discharges at a rate $Q_2$ as a point source at $(x_2 = -2\ell h_0, y_2 = (\alpha + 2d)h_0)$; and so on, where $d$ is the outfall's (offshore) and $\ell$ (along the shore) separation distances. So that the $k$th port discharges at a rate $Q_k$ is represented by a point source at $(x_k, y_k)$, where $x_k = -k\ell h_0, \ y_k = (\alpha + kd)h_0$ with $k = 0, 1, 2, \ldots N$.

Details on the mathematical derivation for the case of a non-eroding sloping sandy beach are given in published papers [6, 8, 9], and since the extension for eroded sandy beach can easily be done, to avoid repetition, these lengthy derivations are omitted. By applying the superposition principle $c(x, y) = \sum_{k=0}^{N} c_k(x, y)$, the two-dimensional advection-diffusion equation for effluent concentration $c_k(x, y)$ from a point source at $(x_k, y_k)$ is given by

$$\frac{\partial}{\partial x}(hUc_k) - \frac{\partial}{\partial y}\left(hD\frac{\partial c_k}{\partial y}\right) = Q_k\delta(x + x_k)\delta(y - y_k), \tag{1}$$

with the boundary condition $hD\partial c_k/\partial y = 0$ at the shoreline $y = 0$, and since the concentration is ultimately dissolved at far distance, $c_k(x, y) \to 0$ as $y \to \infty$. We note $\delta(*)$ is the Dirac delta function.

First, by removing the delta functions, the equation is solved separately for all $x \geq x_k$ in the two regions $0 \leq y < y_k$ and $y > y_k$, and the solutions are then connected by the matching condition at $y_k = (\alpha + kd)h_0$. Since no concentration is lost or produced anywhere other than being released from the point source, the solutions must also satisfy $\int_0^\infty hU c_k(x, y)\, dy = Q_k$.

In terms of dimensionless quantities $c_k(x, y) = c_{k*}(x_*, y_*) Q_0 / h_0^2 U_0$, $x = x_* h_0$, $y = y_* h_0$, and setting $U = U_0 y_*^{1/2}$, $D = D_0 y_*^{3/2}$, and by applying the Laplace transform, the equation to be solved is

$$y_* \frac{d^2 \overline{c_{k*}}}{dy_*^2} + (n + \frac{3}{2}) \frac{d\overline{c_{k*}}}{dy_*} - p\lambda \overline{c_{k*}} = 0, \tag{2}$$

where $p$ is the transform parameter, and $\lambda = h_0 U_0 / D_0$ the model parameter. On writing $\overline{c_{k*}}(p, y_*) = y_*^{-v/2} u(z)$ with $z = 2\sqrt{\lambda p y_*}$, the equation is reduced to the modified Bessel's equation of order $v = n + 1/2$.

The exact solution is obtained using the inversion of the Laplace transform, and after summing for all concentrations $c_{k*}$ from the $N + 1$ ports, we obtain

$$c_{N*}(x_*, y_*) = \sum_{k=0}^{N} \frac{\lambda q_k}{m(x_* + k\ell)\left([\alpha + kd]y_*\right)^{v/2}} \times$$
$$\exp\left(-\frac{\lambda[y_* + \alpha + kd]}{x_* + k\ell}\right) I_v \left(\frac{2\lambda \sqrt{[\alpha + kd]y_*}}{x_* + k\ell}\right), \tag{3}$$

where $q_k = Q_k / Q_0$ with $\sum_{k=0}^{N} q_k = 1$. Note that for a multiport diffuser with $N$ ports, the total effluent discharged is distributed equally, and so each port discharges at a constant rate of $q_k = 1/(N + 1)$.

For nearshore discharges, the appropriate measure for assessing the potential impact of marine effluent discharges would be the shoreline concentration values. In the limit as $y_* \to 0$ and by replacing the modified Bessel function of the first kind $I_v(*)$ by its asymptotic form, we obtain the compounded shoreline concentration

$$c_{N*}(x_*, 0) \approx \frac{1}{m\Gamma(n + 3/2)} \sum_{k=0}^{N} q_k \left(\frac{\lambda}{x_* + k\ell}\right)^{n+3/2} \exp\left(-\frac{\lambda[\alpha + kd]}{x_* + k\ell}\right), \tag{4}$$

where $\Gamma(*)$ is the Gamma function.

## 3 Single Outfall Discharges

Sea outfalls are built predominantly on the sloping sandy beaches [1]. For the quantitative illustration of the solutions, the value of $m = 0.1$ will be used in the subsequent calculations and plots.

## 3.1 Non-eroding Sloping Sandy Beaches

Since $n = 1$, the exact solution for a single outfall ($k = 0$) discharge is given by

$$c_{0*}(x_*, y_*) = \frac{\lambda}{mx_*}\left(\frac{1}{\alpha y_*}\right)^{3/4} \exp\left(-\frac{\lambda[y_* + \alpha]}{x_*}\right) I_{3/2}\left(\frac{2\lambda\sqrt{\alpha y_*}}{x_*}\right). \qquad (5)$$

The contour plots of the solution for $\alpha = 20$ are shown in Fig. 2 for two different values of $\lambda = 0.2$ and $\lambda = 0.4$. The larger the values of $\lambda$, the more elongated the far field effluent discharge plumes. In coastal waters, larger values of $\lambda$ are mostly due to a stronger drift current $U_0$ with less dispersivity $D_0$. As anticipated, the concentration contours are deflected and turning towards the beach, and thus, a higher build-up in concentration will occur close to the beach.

The concentration at the beach for a point source discharge reduces to

$$c_{0*}(x_*, 0) = \frac{1}{m\Gamma(5/2)}\left(\frac{\lambda}{x_*}\right)^{5/2} \exp\left(\frac{-\lambda\alpha}{x_*}\right). \qquad (6)$$

As plotted in Fig. 3(left), it has a maximum value of $c_{1m} = \frac{1}{m\Gamma(5/2)}\left(\frac{5}{2\alpha e}\right)^{5/2}$ at $x_{1*} = 2\lambda\alpha/5$. From the first column of Table 1, the maximum value for $\alpha = 20$ is reduced by 43% when the outfall pipe is extended to $\alpha = 25$, and by more than 64% when $\alpha = 30$. This result shows and agrees with the standard practice of building a longer

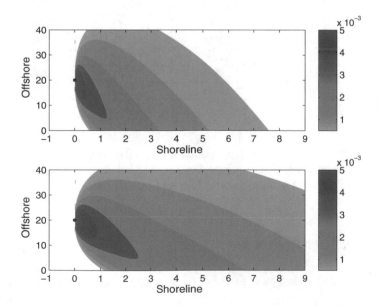

**Fig. 2** Concentration for a point source for $\lambda = 0.2$ (top) and $\lambda = 0.4$ (bottom)

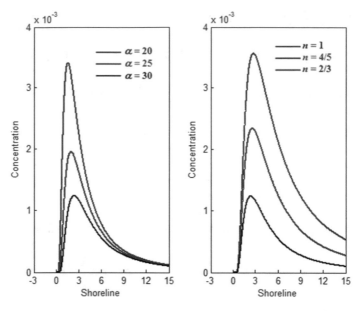

**Fig. 3** Concentration at the beach for $\lambda = 0.2$ on a sloping sandy beach (left), and an eroded sandy beach at $\alpha = 30$ (right)

**Table 1** Maximum concentration values $c_{nm} \times 10^{-3}$

| $\alpha$ | $n = 1$ | $n = 0.9$ | $n = 0.8$ | $n = 2/3$ |
|---|---|---|---|---|
| 20 | 3.4112 | 4.5035 | 5.9397 | 8.5766 |
| 25 | 1.9527 | 2.6361 | 3.5553 | 5.2886 |
| 30 | 1.2379 | 1.7019 | 2.3375 | 3.5628 |
| 35 | 0.8420 | 1.1756 | 1.6397 | 2.5511 |
| 40 | 0.6030 | 0.8532 | 1.2061 | 1.9102 |
| 45 | 0.4492 | 0.6431 | 0.9199 | 1.4800 |

outfall in order to meet the standard regulatory criterion "does not exceed a certain level of concentration anywhere along the beach" to control public health risks in the areas where coastal waters are used for recreational purposes.

## 3.2 Eroded Sandy Beaches

For eroded sandy beaches ($n < 1$), the maximum value of concentration at the beach is given by $c_{nm} = \frac{1}{m\Gamma(n+3/2)}\left(\frac{n+3/2}{\alpha e}\right)^{n+3/2}$, which occurs at $x_{n*} = \lambda\alpha/(n + 3/2)$. As shown in Fig. 3(right) for $\alpha = 30$, the seabed erosion increases substantially the shoreline's concentration level. From Table 1, this increase persists and is getting larger even for longer outfall lengths. A maximum value for $\alpha = 40$ on non-eroding sloping sandy beaches with $n = 1$ is increased by more than double on the eroded sandy beaches with $n = 4/5$, and by more than three-fold when $n = 2/3$. This suggests that extending the outfall pipe alone may not be enough to overcome the beach erosion.

## 4 Multiport Diffusers Discharges on Eroded Sandy Beaches

Economically, it is cheaper to install a multiport diffuser at the end of the outfall pipeline rather than extending the outfall length. Note that both values of $d$ and $\ell$ are small compared to $\alpha$. For example, in Barka desalination plant's multiport diffusers [4], $\ell h_0 = 3.75$ m and $d h_0 = 6.5$ m which are much shorter than that of the outfall pipe length $\alpha h_0 = 650$ m.

The contours of the solution for five ports ($N = 4$) are reproduced graphically in Fig. 4 for $\lambda = 0.3$ with $\alpha = 30, d = 0.5$ and $\ell = 0.3$. The effluent plumes from these ports are immediately merged as they are released, and for $x_* > 0$ the combined plumes appear to be spreading as one. This supports the concept that a multiport diffuser will rapidly dilute effluent discharge in coastal waters and improve the mixing of effluent plumes substantially.

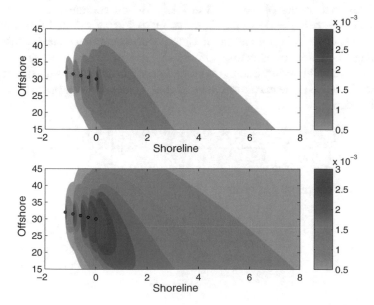

**Fig. 4** Merging concentrations for five point sources for $n = 1$ (top) and $n = 0.8$ (bottom)

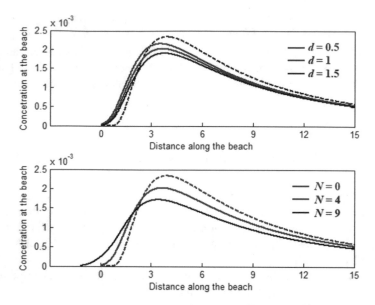

**Fig. 5** Compounded concentration at the beach for discharges from multiport diffusers

Next, for eroded sandy beaches with $n = 0.8$, the compounded concentration at the beach for five ports ($N = 4$) is shown in Fig. 5(top) for $\lambda = 0.3$ with $\alpha = 30$ and $\ell = 0.3$ for three values of $d = 0.5$, 1 and 1.5. The concentration at the beach for a single outfall with $d = 0$ and $\ell = 0$ is also plotted using a dotted line. Similarly, for $d = 1$ as shown in Fig. 5(bottom), the smaller concentration value is achieved by increasing the number of ports to 10 ($N = 9$).

For the quantitative illustration on eroded sandy beaches, by substituting $x_* + k\ell \approx \lambda\alpha/(n + 3/2)$, the maximum value of compounded concentration at the beach is estimated as

$$c_{Nm} \approx \frac{1}{m\Gamma(n + 3/2)} \sum_{k=0}^{N} \frac{1}{N+1} \left(\frac{n+3/2}{\alpha}\right)^{n+3/2} \exp\left[-\left(\frac{n+3/2}{\alpha}\right)(\alpha + kd)\right].$$

(7)

Linearization in term of $d/\alpha$ gives

$$\frac{c_{Nm}}{c_{nm}} \approx \sum_{k=0}^{N} \frac{1}{N+1}\left[1 - (n+3/2)\frac{kd}{\alpha} + \frac{(n+3/2)^2}{2}\left(\frac{kd}{\alpha}\right)^2 - \frac{(n+3/2)^3}{6}\left(\frac{kd}{\alpha}\right)^3 + \cdots\right].$$

(8)

Finally, after summing for $N$ ports, we obtain

$$\frac{c_{Nm}}{c_{nm}} \approx 1 - \frac{(n+3/2)}{2} N \frac{d}{\alpha} + \frac{(n+3/2)^2}{12} N(2N+1) \left(\frac{d}{\alpha}\right)^2$$
$$- \frac{(n+3/2)^3}{24} N^2(N+1) \left(\frac{d}{\alpha}\right)^3 + \cdots . \qquad (9)$$

Note that, the values of $\ell$ are in the range $0 < \ell < \frac{\lambda d}{n+3/2}$.

For comparison with that of the sloping sandy beach maximum value for a point source, the ratio of maximum values for $n < 1$ is given by

$$\frac{c_{nm}}{c_{1m}} = \frac{\Gamma(5/2)}{\Gamma(n+3/2)} \left(\frac{2n+3}{5}\right)^{5/2} \left(\frac{2n+3}{2\alpha e}\right)^{n-1} . \qquad (10)$$

The last term increases significantly larger for $\alpha > 1.25$. As shown in Fig. 6(left), for long sea outfalls $\alpha > 10$, the maximum concentration value is more than double that of the non-eroding sloping sandy beach value for a relatively small erosion represented by $n > 0.7$.

As shown in Fig. 6(right) and from Table 2, we noted that as the number of ports $N$ increases and $\alpha$ gets longer, the maximum concentration at the beach gets smaller than that of the single point source value $c_{nm}$. Finally, using the maximum values from Tables 1 and 2 for $\alpha = 30$, we can estimate for the eroded sandy beaches with $n = 0.8$ the ratio of maximum values $c_{N=14m}/c_{1m}$ is about 1.466 for $d = 1$ and reduces to 0.861 for $d = 1.5$.

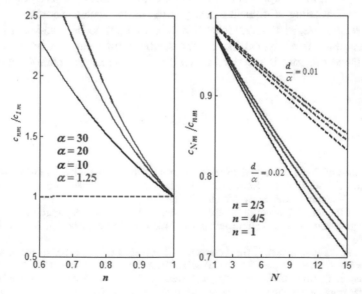

**Fig. 6** Ratio of maximum values $c_{nm}/c_{1m}$ for a point source (left) and $c_{Nm}/c_{nm}$ for multiple point sources (right)

**Table 2** Maximum concentration values $c_{nm} \times 10^{-3}$ when $\alpha = 30$

|       | $n = 1$ |         | $n = 0.8$ |         | $n = 2/3$ |         |
| ----- | ------- | ------- | --------- | ------- | --------- | ------- |
| $N$   | $d = 1$ | $d = 1.5$ | $d = 1$ | $d = 1.5$ | $d = 1$ | $d = 1.5$ |
| 4     | 1.0550  | 0.9789  | 2.0168    | 1.8808  | 3.0994    | 2.9012  |
| 9     | 0.8720  | 0.7356  | 1.6913    | 1.4489  | 2.6244    | 2.2689  |
| 14    | 0.7189  | 0.5130  | 1.4189    | 1.0662  | 2.2259    | 1.7208  |
| 19    | 0.5732  | 0.2349  | 1.1665    | 0.6232  | 1.8621    | 1.1153  |

# 5   Conclusion

The analytical solution of an advection-diffusion equation on eroded sloping sandy beaches with multiple point sources is used to study the interaction and merging effluent discharge plumes from a multiport diffuser, using a simple model of changing seabed depth profile as the power functions of distance from the beach. The diffuser-induced concentration at the beach is then formulated, and based on the maximum concentration values, it is found that building a longer sea outfall alone will not be enough to suppress the effect of seabed erosion. Installing a multiport diffuser at the end of the outfall's long pipeline to enhance dilution of the effluent discharges in the coastal waters reduces significantly the effect of erosion [24].

The inclusion of the seabed erosion on the mathematical models for assessing the environmental impacts of outfall's effluent discharges has never been reported before. Thus, the proposed far field mathematical model can be regarded as the first (analytical) model application for evaluating the effect of eroded sloping sandy beaches on spreading of effluent discharges in coastal waters. Shoreline erosion is a complex process, and a significant simplification has to be made as a first step toward building an analytical model. The simple (empirical) power law of depth with distance offshore is the right choice for complexity in obtaining the model solution.

# References

1. Institution of Civil Engineers (ICE): Long Sea Outfalls. Thomas Telford, London (2001)
2. Roberts, P.J.W., Tian, X.: New experimental techniques for validation of marine discharge models. Environ. Model. Softw. **19**, 691–699 (2004)
3. Jirka, G.H.: Integral model of turbulent buoyant jets in unbounded stratified flows. Part 2. Plane jet dynamics resulting from multiport diffuser jets. Environmental. Fluid Dyn. **6**, 43–100 (2006)
4. Purnama, A., Al-Barwani, H.H., Bleninger, T., Doneker, R.L.: CORMIX simulations of brine discharges from Barka plants, Oman. Desalin. Water Treat. **32**, 329–338 (2011)
5. Bleninger, T., Jirka, G.H.: Modelling and environmentally sound management of brine discharges from desalination plants. Desalination **221**, 585–597 (2008)

6. Kay, A.: The effect of cross-stream depth variations upon contaminant dispersion in a vertically well-mixed current. Estuar. Coast. Shelf Sci. **24**, 177–204 (1987)
7. Al-Barwani, H.H., Purnama, A.: Re-assessing the impact of desalination plants brine discharges on eroding beaches. Desalination **204**, 94–101 (2007)
8. Al-Barwani, H.H., Purnama, A.: Analytical solutions for brine discharge plumes on a sloping beach. Desalin. Water Treat. **11**, 2–6 (2009)
9. Purnama, A.: Merging effluent discharge plumes from multiport diffusers on a sloping beach. Appl. Math. **3**, 80–85 (2012)
10. Yates, M.L., Guza, R.T., O'Reilly, W.C.: Equilibrium shoreline response: observations and modelling. J. Geophys. Res. **114**, C09014, 16 (2009)
11. Dissanayake, P., Brown, J., Karunarathna, H.: Impacts of storm chronology on the morphological changes of the Formby beach and dune system, UK. Nat. Hazards Earth Syst. Sci. **15**, 1533–1543 (2015)
12. Pilkey, O.H., Cooper, J.A.G.: Society and sea level rise. Science **303**, 1781–1782 (2004)
13. Bruun, P.: Sea level rise as a cause of shore erosion. J. Waterways. Harbors Div. ASCE **88**, 117–130 (1962)
14. Bruun, P.: Review of conditions for use of the Bruun rule of erosion. Coast. Eng. **7**, 77–89 (1983)
15. Bernabeu, A.M., Medina, R., Vidal, C.: Wave reflection on natural beaches: an equilibrium profile model. Estuarine Coast. Shelf Sci. **57**, 577–585 (2003)
16. Wang, H., Toue, T., Dette, H.H.: Movable bed modeling criteria for beach profile response. In: Proceedings of 22nd ICCE, ASCE, Delft, The Netherlands (1990)
17. Dean, R.G.: Equilibrium beach profile: characteristics and applications. J. Coast. Res. **7**, 53–84 (1991)
18. Vellinga, P.: Beach and dune erosion during storm surges. J. Coast. Eng. **6**, 361–389 (1982)
19. Signell, R.P., Jenter, H.L., Blumberg, A.F.: Predicting the physical effects of relocating Boston's sewage outfall. J. Estuarine, Coast. Shelf Sci. **50**, 59–72 (2000)
20. Macqueen, J.F., Preston, R.W.: Cooling water discharges into a sea with a sloping bed. Water Res. **17**, 389–395 (1983)
21. Palomar, P., Losada, I.J.: Impacts of brine discharge on the marine environment. Modelling as a predictive tool. In: Schorr, M. (ed.) Desalination, Trends and Technologies, pp. 279–310. InTech Open Access Publisher, Rijeka, Crotia (2011)
22. Chin, D.A., Roberts, P.J.W.: Model of dispersion in coastal waters. J. Hydraul. Eng. **111**, 12–28 (1985)
23. Wood, I.R.: Asymptotic solutions and behavior of outfall plumes. J. Hydraul. Eng. **119**, 553–580 (1993)
24. Purnama, A., Al-Maamari, H.A., Balakrishnan, E.: Optimal outfall systems for nearshore effluent discharges on eroded sandy beaches. J. Coupled Syst. Multiscale Dyn. **5**, 217–224 (2017)
25. Ostendorf, D.W.: Longshore dispersion over a flat beach. J. Geophys. Res. **87**, 4241–4248 (1982)
26. Smith, R.: Longitudinal dispersion of buoyant contaminant in a shallow channel. J. Fluid Mech. **78**, 677–688 (1976)

# Part VI
# Mathematical Modelling in Medical and Health Sciences

# Using Social Media to Improve Knowledge Sharing among Healthcare Practitioners

Haitham Alali

**Abstract** *Aim* This paper aims to explore and analyse how findings from social media literature can inform healthcare researchers and providers, particularly in the subject of online healthcare social groups, one of the most promising knowledge sharing approaches in healthcare. *Methods* This paper conducted a systematic review of the social media literature. The Leximancer software "Lexi-Portal Version 4" was used to analyse 298 studies. The Leximancer software exposed a group of relational themes that supported the interpretative content analysis undertaken. *Results* Two primary findings stand out in the social media literature: The social networking and communication among healthcare practitioners is crucial for maximizing the group work behaviour, besides, social media contribute to research, practice, develop professionalism, and knowledge sharing, particularly within healthcare services. *Conclusions* Overall, this paper found that social media has a long and rich history of research in knowledge sharing that offers useful tools to healthcare practitioners. Healthcare practitioners may benefit from participating in healthcare knowledge sharing social media platforms by attaining knowledge that enhances their ability to effectively contribute issues and dilemmas faced in the healthcare profession.

**Keywords** Social media · Knowledge sharing · Healthcare
Web 2.0 technologies · Leximancer

## 1 Introduction and Background

Social media is considered as an interactive channel that can support applications and features that are part of knowledge management systems. Social Media as an communicating network was developed in the last years, to facilitate knowledge sharing activities. Typically, healthcare practitioners can easily adapt to computer-mediated collaborative activities and different types of social media and build a

H. Alali (✉)
Amman Arab University, Amman, Jordan
e-mail: h.alali@aau.edu.jo

© Springer Nature Switzerland AG 2018                                               411
D. M. Kilgour et al. (eds.), *Recent Advances in Mathematical
and Statistical Methods*, Springer Proceedings in Mathematics & Statistics 259,
https://doi.org/10.1007/978-3-319-99719-3_37

'virtual' social space [1, 2] on a variety of social media platforms, such as Facebook, Twitter, YouTube, online forums and WordPress. Such social spaces, also referred to as online communities of practice, are among the best places for healthcare practitioners to engage in healthcare knowledge sharing because they face the same challenges; share common interests; and engage in similar occupational practices [1–3].

Social media supports bothsynchronous and asynchronous communication [4]. Clark and Brennan [5, p. 229] have characterised various components that communication media might provide: audibility "A and B can communicate through speaking to each other", visibility "A and B are visible to each other", Co-presence "A and B share the same environment", co-temporality "B receives at roughly the same time as A presents, i.e. synchronous communication". Moreover, reviewability "B can review A's message", revisability "A can revise messages for B", simultaneity "A and B can send and receive at once and simultaneously", and sequentiality "A's and B's turns cannot get out of sequence as in asynchronous communication" [6].

In spite of the rapid diffusion of the use of social media and knowledge management across organizations, so far, the little research has been carried out on the use, design, and the outcomes of the social media in the healthcare literature [7–10]. Knowledge sharing literature has primarily dealt with general case studies of knowledge sharing initiatives in the organizations and conceptual models i.e. SECI knowledge creation model [11, 12]. Accordingly, there is no broadly accepted model that encompasses critical aspects of efficient knowledge sharing to examine this phenomenon in the healthcare sector, and more specifically, among members in healthcare social groups [8, 10, 13]. Hence, there is a necessity to explore the social media literature and provide more information on the way they support the success of knowledge sharing among healthcare practitioners. Therefore, the available social media literature should be explored to identify the primary dimensions and concepts that contribute to the success of healthcare social groups [14].

The dimensions and its related factors that determine the acceptance of healthcare social groups might support healthcare organizations in various ways, such as providing suggestions to improve the design, implementation, usage, and operation of online healthcare social groups [3, 15]. Moreover, the main concepts of online healthcare social groups might improve the decision-making process regarding KM project investments and online healthcare social media tools, and instruments that can serve as benchmarks for further measurement and improvement of online healthcare social groups [1, 16]. The missing gap that should be overcome by further research is to be identified by the literature review [14, 17].

Theoretically, Wenger et al. [18], have reported that the broad implementation of online social groups in different industries (i.e. marketing, information technology, and education) has so far achieved high levels of success. Nevertheless, the number of studies that assessed online social groups in the healthcare sector is still limited [19, 20]. Moreover, those studies are mainly descriptive. Hence, the purpose of this work is to review the literature online healthcare social groups. Furthermore, the aim of the study is to explore and analyse the primary dimensions and concepts that contribute to understand the online healthcare social groups.

## 2    Methods

In order to conduct a comprehensive analysis of the literature related to social media in healthcare, the researcher looked for the cited research from 2005 to 2018 in different databases; "health informatics", "information systems", and "social science" databases, including EBSCO, Science direct, Taylor, ProQuest, Sage, Wiley, Emerald, Pub Med, Springer Link, and the ACM. Further articles were incorporated using Google Scholar and Yahoo search engines. A wide range of keywords were used i.e. "electronic", "virtual", "online", "web-base", "communities of practice", "network", "social networks", "forum", "Facebook", "social media", "LinkedIn", "group", and "healthcare". Nevertheless, the search keywords with similar meaning are combined by "OR" and the keywords that are required to be combined with other keywords are paired by "AND and NOT" Boolean operators.

As revealed in Fig. 1 there were several steps of the selection process. First, the initial screening of titles and abstracts identified 1023 relevant studies. When duplicates were removed, 1001 references were kept. Further 276 articles were excluded because their research aims were not relevant. Nevertheless, in the cases of doubt regarding the exclusion, the decision was to keep the article for further evaluation. Subsequently, all full articles were read, irrelevant studies were excluded, and lastly, 298 studies were kept to be analysed by Leximancer software.

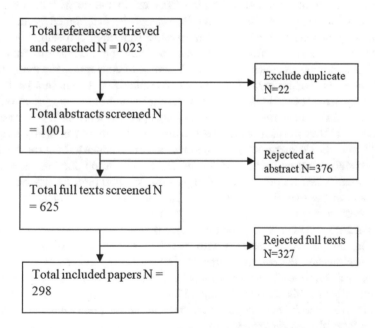

**Fig. 1** Identification of articles for analysis of using social media to improve knowledge sharing among healthcare practitioners

Leximancer is an emergent instrument used in the analysis of textual data with a purpose to map out the underlying themes within the textual data [21, 22]. The Leximancer software "Lexi-Portal Version 4" [23], is a data-mining software, was used to analyse 298 articles. This software is used for the automatic extraction of the major themes and concepts from the data. It represents a mechanism for automatic, unbiased, and objective discovery of the concepts. It is crucial for the content analysis, as it can manage massive amounts of textual information and it is highly reliable in revealing the conceptual and semantic relations of the concepts in the content [21]. Moreover, the results analysis is given in a visual form as well. This software is excellent in providing interpretative judgment about the nature of the content, and it provides reliable results [21, 22]. The software was used to reveal the primary themes and concepts from all selected articles.

## 3 Content Analysis

As depicted in Fig. 2, the concepts map of the previous studies was created depending on the thematic analysis by Lexi-Portal Version 4. Once Leximancer analyses a document, the documents key words and phrases are tallied, parsed and compared with the Leximancer internal dictionary. After that, Leximancer selects and extracts the most common phrases and words, the 'themes' of the document. Next, Leximancer once more classifies these themes into categories determined by their lexical meanings and their use within the text. Themes that show similar meaning or are used together several times within a document become 'concepts', which form the starting point of the Leximancer concept map, the closeness of concepts in the map suggests that two concepts appear in similar conceptual contexts [21]. Within a Leximancer concept map, a number of indicators are present that support the interpretation of the data [21]. In Leximancer, the brightness of a concept is associated with the frequency of the data, in other words, the brighter the concept, the more frequently it appears in the documents. Furthermore, the brightness of links relates to how frequently the two associated concepts occur in close proximity within the documents. Only the most dominant lines are presented with a purpose to avoid unnecessary cluttering.

The dots in the map indicate the concepts, and the circles indicate the themes and how each concept is associated to other concepts. The previous studies of social media in healthcare mainly adopted two major themes: *networking* and *content*; the *networking* theme has intersection with *healthcare*, *Facebook*, *social importance* and *users*. However, the *content* theme has intersection with *knowledge*, *data*, and *research*; besides, there is an emphasis on *use* behaviour of the social media tools including online healthcare social groups. The map also illustrates how *social media* contribute to *research, practice*, develop *professionalism*, and *knowledge sharing*, particularly within *healthcare* services.

The lists of words in Fig. 3 are the top-ranked words from trained thesaurus entries for the central concepts and its frequency in the literature. Fig. 3 shows that the key themes were derived from all articles were mainly focusing on; *knowledge*

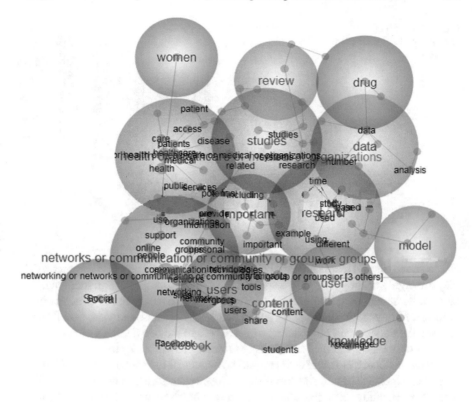

**Fig. 2** Concept map of key themes and concepts in literature

*sharing* 23%, *network* 20%, *healthcare* 15%, *social interaction* 14%, *social media* 13%, *members* 9%, and *technology* 6%. These results suggest that healthcare sector as a knowledge-based institutions, is paying more attention to the professionals' experiences, skills, and knowledge as the main vital asset. The shared purpose across various worldwide health institutions is to develop a successful knowledge sharing tools that are inexpensive and available for all healthcare practitioners and even for patients [15, 24, 25].

Nowadays, social media penetrating every possible aspect of people's lives fuelled by Twitter, Facebook, LinkedIn, Skype and other services, and by the enabling applications and hardware such as tablets, phones, and telecommunication devices. In addition to, the second generation of online platforms "Web 2.0 applications" including blogs, wikis, tagging, RSS feeds, social bookmarking and collaborative real-time editing. These platforms are technologies used widely for social networking to serve online collaboration and sharing of user-generated content. Mobile sociable technologies, Web 2.0 technologies, and social applications are enablers in health and health care from external sources and within the healthcare organizations, benefits to the healthcare administration and practitioners. ... Parcell [25, P. 68] stated, "to be connected to the people who have the knowledge is more important than capturing

**Fig. 3** Counts and
percentage of key themes in
literature

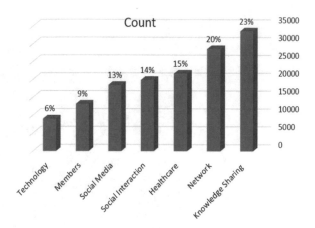

all the knowledge". Healthcare practitioners do not need to formulate advance skills; they are highly acknowledged in a specific area such as management, medicine, and laboratory. Social media supports the engagement of diverse groups of actors in the process of knowledge sharing. As evidenced in the content analysis, social media allowed the patients and other actors to get access to the perspectives of people who live in different geographical locations to interact in a virtual space.

Social media in healthcare sector could be beneficial to groups and countries who face challenges, adversity, and turbulence. Despite the fact that many people live a wealthy and healthy life in few countries, many countries around the world still suffer from the challenges of poverty, disease, or their geographical borders and even language constraints. Telecommunication technologies including mobile applications, web 2.0 technologies, smart devices and social media that are motivating new healthcare models where providers and patients be capable to join simultaneously in online social space that facilitate real-time communications and support patients to obtain a superior role for forming and improving the quality of healthcare services.

## 4   Limitations

This paper only reviewed articles published in a 13 years period, and books or book chapters published during that time were excluded because of access permissions and downloading difficulties. The search was limited to articles whose titles included at least one keyword. The results of this analysis are limited to the articles that retrieved from "health informatics", "information systems", and "social science" databases as discussed in methods section, therefore, the results of this paper are limited to the social media in healthcare. As a result of these limitations, the search process may have missed a few related articles. Nevertheless, this paper is confident that the analysis outcomes would not have been changed in any considerable way by adding any articles that did not included the search. Consequently, this paper confident that the adopted approach was the most suitable for this study, especially when there is a massive amount of articles on a specific topic.

## 5   Conclusion and Future Research

Interestingly, the two themes (*networking* and *content*) highlighted in the content analysis outcomes are clearly linked, reflecting the interrelated nature of the social media with the knowledge shared among healthcare practitioners and patients. Healthcare practitioners may benefit from participating in healthcare knowledge sharing groups by attaining knowledge that enhances their ability to effectively contribute the issues and dilemmas faced in the healthcare profession. Enhancing their problem solving skills and confidence to resolve dilemmas when they arise; becoming familiar with an online healthcare social groups where assistance may be sought concerning problems/issues faced in the workplace; providing access to expertise; and allowing for pleasurable experiences, meaningful participation and a sense of belonging in an online healthcare social groups.

Healthcare practitioners and patients need more than information from healthcare. They also need knowledge sharing and social interaction. Consequently, healthcare organizations should transform themselves to become social enablers, as a result, patients can collect, learn from, voice their concerns, and share their views, in order to improve the quality of healthcare services. There is an urgent need to increase awareness of social media tools and its potential capabilities in knowledge sharing and healthcare services, and a need to empirically investigate this phenomenon to inform superior use of social media in healthcare sector.

## References

1. Wasko, M.M.L., Faraj, S.: Why should I share? Examining social capital and knowledge contribution in electronic networks of practice. MIS Q. **29**(1), 35–57 (2005)
2. Wasko, M.M.L., Teigland, R., Faraj, S.: The provision of online public goods: examining social structure in an electronic network of practice. Decis. Support Syst. **47**(3), 254–265 (2009)
3. Tseng, F.-C., Kuo, F.-Y.: A study of social participation and knowledge sharing in the teachers' online professional community of practice. Comput. Educ. **72**, 37–47 (2014)
4. McNurlin, B., Sprague, R.: Supporting Collaboration. Book of Information Systems Management in Practice, 7th edn. Pearson Prentice Hall, Upper Saddle River (2006)
5. Clark, H.H., Brennan, S.E.: Grounding in communication. Perspect. Socially Shared Cogn. **1991**(13), 127–149 (1991)
6. IJsselsteijn, W., van Baren, J., and van Lanen, F.: Staying in touch: social presence and connectedness through synchronous and asynchronous communication media. Hum.-Comput. Interact.: Theory Pract. (Part II) **2**(924), e928 (2003)
7. Alavi, M., Leidner, D.E.: Review: knowledge management and knowledge management systems: conceptual foundations and research issues. MIS Q. **25**(1), 107–136 (2001)

8. Alali, H.: Virtual communities of practice success in healthcare sector: a comparative review. In: Advances in Human Factors and Ergonomics in Healthcare, pp. 141–153. Springer, Cham (2017)
9. Alali, H., Salim, J.: Success dimensions of the online healthcare communities of practice. In: Towards an evaluation framework. In: Social Media Mobile Technologies for Healthcare p. 16 (2014)
10. Alali, H., Salim, J.: Virtual health communities of practice success factors: towards taxonomy and a framework. Int. J. Web Based Communities 12, 180–194 (2016)
11. Hahn, J., Subramani, M.R.: A framework of knowledge management systems: issues and challenges for theory and practice. In: A Framework of Knowledge Management Systems: Issues and Challenges for Theory and Practice, pp. 302–312. Australia (2000)
12. Lee, K., Lee, S., Kang, I.: KMPI: measuring knowledge management performance. Inf. Manage. 42(3), 469–482 (2005)
13. Jung, Y., Hur, C., Jung, D., Kim, M.: Identifying key hospital service quality factors in online health communities. J. Med. Internet Res. 17(4) (2015)
14. Kankanhalli, A., Tan, B.C.Y.: Knowledge management metrics: a review and directions for future research. Int. J. Knowl. Manage. 1(3), 20–32 (2005)
15. Pablos, A.: WHO meeting on knowledge translation in global health: a link to policy and action. Proceedings of Knowledge Management and Health, 10–12 Oct 2005
16. Alali, H., Salim, J.: Theoretical and empirical investigation of "Virtual Communities of Practice" success in health care services at rural areas. In: Proceedings of RICTD 2010, Kedah, Malaysia, 23rd– 25th November 2010
17. Fernandez, I., Gonzalez, A., Sabherwal, R.: Knowledge Management, Solutions. Technology. Prentice-Hall Inc., Upper Saddle River (2004)
18. Wenger, E., McDermott, R., Snyder, W.: Cultivating Communities of Practice: A Guide to Managing Knowledge. Harvard University Press, Boston (2002)
19. Alali, H., Salim, J.: Conceptual Model of "Virtual Communities of Practice" Success in Health Care: A Literature Review, pp. 1–10 (2011)
20. Alali, H., Salim, J.: Virtual communities of practice: the role of content quality and technical features to increase health care professionals' satisfaction. J. Theor. Appl. Inf. Technol. 54, 269–275 (2013)
21. Crofts, K., Bisman, J.: Interrogating accountability: an illustration of the use of Leximancer software for qualitative data analysis. Qual. Res.n Acc. Manage. 7(2), 180–207 (2010)
22. Sotiriadou, P., Brouwers, J., Le, T.-A.: Choosing a qualitative data analysis tool: a comparison of NVivo and Leximancer. Ann. Leisure Res. 17(2), 218–234 (2014)
23. Jeffrey, B.: Between-group behaviour in health care: gaps, edges, boundaries, disconnections, weak ties, spaces and holes. a systematic review. BMC Health Serv. Res. 10, 330 (2010)
24. Pablos-Mendez, A., Chunharas, S., Lansang, M.A., Shademani, R., Tugwell, P.: Bulletin of the World Health: Knowledge Translation in Global Health. World Health Organization (2005)
25. Parcell, G.: The Bulletin Interview with Geoff Parcell. World Health Organization (2005)

# Model Based Economic Assessment of Avian Influenza Vaccination in an All-in/All-out Housing System

Meagan Coffey, Hermann J. Eberl and Amy L. Greer

**Abstract** We formulate a dynamic predictive model for the progression of avian influenza in an all-in/all-out broiler housing system, accounting also for flock vaccination measures. In this model we assume that the route of transmission is indirect: infected individuals shed the virus in the barn environment, susceptible individuals acquire it when they come in contact with the pathogen. The vaccination measures are assumed to be imperfect, in the sense that some birds might receive full protection, whereas other might enter a latent stage without progressing to the symptomatic stage, and a third group might not receive protection at all. The information provided by the dynamic model is then used to estimate economic loss incurred due to an avian influenza outbreak in the barn. We find, under the assumptions made in our analysis, that the loss per bird decreases as flock size increases and terminal bird weight increases. We also find that for small flocks vaccination might not be able to prevent financial loss, whereas for larger flocks, flock vaccination can turn losses into profit. Crucial in this analysis is the relationship between vaccination cost and efficacy, about which, however, currently little information is available.

**Keywords** All-in/all-out housing system · Avian influenza · Broiler Mathematical model · Vaccincation

M. Coffey · H. J. Eberl (✉)
Department Mathematics and Statistics, University of Guelph,
50 Stone Rd E, Guelph, ON N1G2W1, Canada
e-mail: heberl@uoguelph.ca

M. Coffey
e-mail: mcoffey@uoguelph.ca

A. L. Greer
Department Population Medicine, University of Guelph,
50 Stone Rd E, Guelph, ON N1G2W1, Canada
e-mail: agreer@uoguelph.ca

© Springer Nature Switzerland AG 2018                                                    419
D. M. Kilgour et al. (eds.), *Recent Advances in Mathematical
and Statistical Methods*, Springer Proceedings in Mathematics & Statistics 259,
https://doi.org/10.1007/978-3-319-99719-3_38

# 1 Introduction

Avian influenza, a subtype of the influenza A virus, developed as a highly pathogenic infectious disease in the 1980s causing mass mortalities in the poultry industry [3]. The virus is zoonotic and can spread from domesticated and wild avian hosts to humans as well as other mammals. Sixteen different haemagglutinin subtypes exist of varying levels of pathogenicity (H1–H16) [15]. Strains of low pathogen avian influenza present mild clinical symptoms, such as decreased appetite and egg production, or can be completely asymptomatic with no disease induced mortality [2]. Highly pathogenic strains show moderate to severe clinical symptoms (i.e. swelling, coughing, sneezing, and diarrhea) and have a varied mortality rate ranging from 5 to 100% [13]. H5 and H7 have been shown to have the highest pathogenicity and to be the most fatal to domestic poultry [13, 20]. Their case fatality can range from 20 to 100% of birds, causing it to be one of the most important infections in the poultry industry [1, 3]. The primary route of transmission of avian influenza is indirect: infected animals shed the virus with bodily fluids into the environment. Susceptible individuals acquire the infection, at a certain rate/probability when they come in contact with the deposited pathogens [18].

Domestic poultry in North America are layer chickens, broiler chickens, and turkeys that are produced for food consumption either through egg or meat production [2]. Each type of poultry is raised in unique housing systems, across which bird-bird interaction can vary greatly. The type and intensity of interaction between individuals affect disease dynamics within a population. Broiler is a term used to describe chickens being raised for meat consumption [7]. In North America, these birds are most often kept in open housing systems where all birds are free to roam anywhere in an enclosed barn [7]. Due to the short lifespan of these birds, typically between 30 and 45 days [2], most production systems use an all-in-all-out strategy. All birds are of the same age. They enter an empty barn at day 0 and they all leave the barn for processing at the same time [7]. The population dynamics of these broiler chickens are very unnatural due to their short lifespan and housing system. They are seldom studied in relation to disease dynamics.

The avian influenza vaccine is a tool that can be used to help decrease the presence of avian influenza pathogens, and decrease the number of infected individuals in a domestic bird population [8]. Its main purpose is to protect against clinical symptoms and death, reduce pathogen shedding by infected individuals, prevent transmission of disease through contact between individuals, increase disease resistance, and provide 20 or more weeks of protection [19].

Economical considerations play a key role in guiding practices and regulations in the poultry industry. The loss of a flock of broilers can be financially devastating to a farm. Highly pathogenic strains of avian influenza are considered to be very detrimental to domestic poultry flocks [6]. Prevention measures such as biosecurity practices and vaccinations can also be very costly to individual farmers, so the long term economic benefit is small, especially if the chance of avian influenza infection is small. Disease outbreaks play an important role on production profits, but even the public knowledge of the presence of disease can lead to a profit loss [2].

**Table 1** Summary of avian influenza models in the literature

| Cite | Author | Humans in model | Bird type in model | Model type | Location | Intervention | Time frame | Transmit Type |
|------|--------|-----------------|--------------------|------------|----------|--------------|------------|----------------|
| [12] | Iwami et. al. | Yes | Combined | SI-SIR | Japan | Isolation | Infinite | Direct |
| [11] | Gumel | Yes | Wild and domestic | SI-SI | Canada | Isolation | Infinite | Direct |
| [5] | Chong et. al. | Yes | Combined | SI-SIR | China | Isolation and vaccination | Infinite | Direct |
| [23] | Xiao et. al. | Yes | Domestic | SI-SEIR | China | None | Infinite | Direct |
| [4] | Chong and Smith | No | Domestic | SIR | China | Isolation | Infinite | Direct |
| [9] | Gulbudak and Martcheva | No | Domestic | SIR | USA | Culling | Infinite | Direct |
| [24] | Zhai et. al. | No | Combined | SIR | China | None | Infinite | Direct |
| [21] | Thiuthad et. al. | No | Domestic | SIS | Thailand | None | Infinite | Direct and indirect |
| [14] | Nickbakhsh et. al. | No | Domestic | SIR | UK | Metapopulation | Infinite | Direct and indirect |
| [10] | Gulbudak and Martcheva | No | Domestic | SEIS | USA | Vaccination and culling | Infinite | Direct |
| [22] | Vaidya and Wahl | No | Wild | SIR | Canada | Vaccination | Infinite | Direct and indirect |

Based on a predictive model of high pathogenic avian influenza disease dynamics in broiler operations we develop a framework that might aid in investigating whether flock vaccination is economically worthwhile.

Several mathematical models for avian influenza can be found in the literature, some of which are summarized in Table 1. Some of these models include disease control interventions, such as isolation, or vaccination. These models, however, cannot be readily adopted for the situation of all-in/all-out broiler housing systems. Many of them focus on zoonotic aspects with a focus on human populations, and do not distinguish between wild and domestic birds. The existing model studies focus on longterm asymptotic dynamics, whereas it is important in the context of all-in/all-out housing systems to account for finite time termination. Virtually all existing models use generic, direct mass-action disease transmission, either in SI or SEI fashion. This does not adequately reflect the disease transmission in closed broiler housing, where the predominant route of transmission is indirect: infected birds shed pathogens into the environment through bodily fluids, and it is the environment that acts as the reservoir of infection for susceptible birds. The first step in our study, therefore, is the formulation of a predictive mathematical model for the spread avian influenza in a broiler barn.

## 2   Mathematical Model

### 2.1   Disease Dynamics and Vaccination

Our mathematical model will be based on the following assumptions

1. The farm operations considered include thousands of birds, large enough for a continuous description by ODE models. All broilers are free to roam within a room/building, therefore having equal likelihood to contact any other bird and the shared environment, and equal likelihood of contracting the disease.
2. All broilers that enter the barn at day 0 are of the same age. No broilers are introduced after initial time. Broiler death by natural causes accounts for less than 1% of population overall [2] and is neglected.
3. Broilers only become infected through contact with pathogens in the environment. The rate of infection is dependent on the pathogen concentration in the environment. Exposed and infected individuals contribute to the disease reservoir by shedding the pathogen through bodily fluids [22].
4. The pathogen will lose viability in the reservoir at some rate when not in a host [20]. Pathogens can also be externally removed from the environment during facility maintenance operations.
5. Susceptible birds that acquire the pathogen become exposed (infected but asymptomatic); exposed birds become infected (infected and symptomatic).
6. A flock can be vaccinated upon entering the barn at day 0 and no birds are vaccinated after this time [7]. Some birds will receive full protection, whereas

others are only imperfectly protected or receive no protection at all. Infection rates are the same for non-vaccinated susceptible and imperfectly vaccinated [2]. Imperfectly vaccinated birds can become exposed but exposed vaccinated birds will not become infected.

7. An imperfectly protected broiler that becomes exposed will shed the disease at an equal or lesser rate than the unvaccinated counterpart [2].

The mathematical model is formulated in terms of the dependent variables non-vaccinated susceptible birds $S$, imperfectly vaccinated susceptible birds $S_v$, non-vaccinated exposed birds $E$, imperfectly vaccinated exposed birds $E_v$, infected birds $I$, perfectly vaccinated birds $R_v$, and pathogens in environment $P$. We have

$$\dot{S} = -\frac{\gamma P S}{1 + P} \tag{1}$$

$$\dot{E} = \frac{\gamma P S}{1 + P} - \lambda E \tag{2}$$

$$\dot{I} = \lambda E - \delta I \tag{3}$$

$$\dot{P} = \alpha I + \beta (E + E_v) - \nu P \tag{4}$$

$$\dot{S_v} = -\frac{\gamma P S_v}{1 + P} \tag{5}$$

$$\dot{E_v} = \frac{\gamma P S_v}{1 + P} \tag{6}$$

$$\dot{R_v} = 0 \tag{7}$$

where we assume a hyperbolic force of infection to account for saturation effects in highly contaminated barns. All parameters in this model are non-negative. Their meaning is summarized in Table 2, where also default values are given that have been obtained from the literature and that will be used in our simulations below.

The dynamic model is completed by initial conditions

$$S(0) = (1 - \xi_S - \xi_R)N, \quad E(0) = 0, \quad I(0) = 0, \quad P(0) = p,$$

$$S_v(0) = \xi_S N, \quad E_v(0) = 0, R_v(0) = \xi_R N$$

**Table 2** Disease dynamics parameters and the values used in our study with references

| Parameter | Units | Definition | Value | Citation |
|---|---|---|---|---|
| $\gamma$ | $day^{-1}$ | Infection rate | 0.4 | [11] |
| $\lambda$ | $day^{-1}$ | Incubation period | 1.4 | [2] |
| $\delta$ | $day^{-1}$ | Death rate | 0.06 | [12] |
| $\alpha$ | $day^{-1}$ | Infectious shedding rate | 0.3 | [22] |
| $\beta$ | $day^{-1}$ | Exposed shedding rate | $\leq \alpha$ | [2] |
| $\nu$ | $day^{-1}$ | Cleaning/Degradation rate | Varied | Assumed |

where $N$ is the size of the flock, $\xi_R$ the fraction of birds that are perfectly vaccinated, $\xi_S$ the fraction of imperfectly vaccinated birds. We require $0 \leq \xi_S, 0 \leq \xi_R, \xi_S + \xi_R \leq 1$.

Using the next generation matrix approach one finds for the submodel describing the disease progression without vaccination intervention as $R_0 = \sqrt{\frac{N}{\nu}\left(\frac{\beta}{\lambda} + \frac{\alpha}{\delta}\right)}$, indicating that pathogens must be removed much fast, relative to their deposition, from the envrionment in order to suppress disease manifestation.

## 2.2 Economic Analysis

To conduct an economic analysis of avian influenza vaccination, we determine the loss $L$ to a farm associated with an infected barn. It is the sum of several components: Costs independent of the number of birds $\Omega$ include cost of a building, electricity, farm hands, etc. Costs dependent on current population size include food expenses. Broilers are on a strict food plan and food intake is heavily monitored. The cost of food per day is represented by $\varphi$. The cost of vaccination is assumed to be dependent on the efficacy of the vaccine, represented by function $v(e)$, where efficacy $e$ is defined as $\xi_S + \xi_R$. In our simulations we assume $\xi_S = \xi_R$. Finally, to offset loss, the surviving and healthy birds, $R_v, S, S_v, E, E_v$ can be sold into the market at some price. This income is dependent on weight and the number of surviving birds $N - I(t) - R(t) = R_v + S + S_v + E + E_v$, where $R$ denotes the number of individuals that died form the disease, given by $R(t) = \delta \int_0^t I(t)dt$. The expected weights of the birds dependent on age, $\kappa(t)$, is obtained from [7]. The price per lb is represented by $\rho$. All parameters and their values are represented in Table 3. Overall the equation to represent loss is as follows:

$$L(N, e, t) = \Omega + \varphi \int_0^t (N - R(\tau))d\tau + N(v(e)) - \rho\kappa(t)(N - R(t) - I(t))$$

(8)

where $L$ depends on the number of birds initially in the flock $N$, the efficacy of the vaccine $e$, and the age $t$ at which the birds are sold.

**Table 3** Estimated parameter values for economic analysis equations

| Parameter | Units | Definition | Value | Citation |
|---|---|---|---|---|
| $\Omega$ | Dollars | Upfront costs | 5000 | [16] |
| $\varphi$ | Dollars/bird * day | Food cost | 1.49 | [16] |
| $\rho$ | Dollars/lb | Profit | 1.11 | [2] |
| $v(e)$ | Dollars/bird | Vaccine cost | Assumed | – |
| $\kappa(t)$ | lbs | Bird weight | Time dependent | [7] |

## 3   Results

An illustrative simulation of the disease model is depicted in Fig. 1. The parameters are as described in Table 2 and $\beta = 0.2$, $\nu = 0.3$, $\xi_S = \xi_R = \frac{1}{3}$. The susceptible group is monotonically decreasing from 10,000 birds to 0 by day 18. Over half of the population is removed from the susceptible bird population by day 3. The exposed group is increasing until it reaches its peak of 1626 exposed individuals at day 3, then is decreasing until the population reaches 0 at day 21. The infected group increases until it reaches its peak of approximately 7088 on day 7 and decreases after that. The infected class reaches 1129 by the 40th day. The environmental potential increases first and declines eventually. The vaccinated susceptible individuals, $S_V$, have the same result to the susceptible individuals. The vaccinated susceptible group is monotonically decreasing from 10,000 to 0 by day 18 with over half of the population removed by day 3. The vaccinated exposed individuals, $E_v$, are much different than the exposed individuals. The exposed susceptible group is monotonically increasing from 0 to 10,000 by day 18. The completely vaccinated group $R_v$ remains constant at 10,000 individuals.

In Fig. 2 we plot the financial loss per bird $L(N, e, t)/N$ for various population sizes $N$, as a function of efficacy $e$ for termination at day $t = 25$ and at day $t = 40$, without accounting for the cost of vaccination. The cost for vaccination is independent of the state variables and is a function that depends only on the efficacy of the vaccination $e$. To obtain the total loss, this (unknown) function is added to the data reported in Fig. 2 *a posteriori*. When $L/N$ becomes negative, a loss turns to a profit.

The more efficient vaccination is, the smaller the loss per bird. The larger the population size $N$, the smaller the loss per bird. In the case of termination at $t = 25$

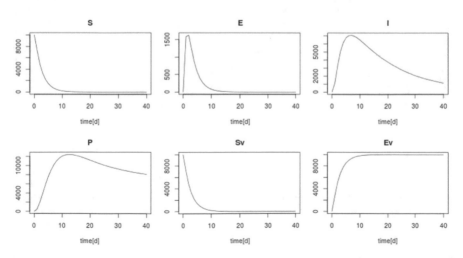

**Fig. 1** Illustrative simulation of vaccine model, Eqs. (1)–(7), with initial conditions (10,000, 0, 0, 0.001, 10,000, 0, 10,000) over 40 days. $R_v$ remains constant (data not shown)

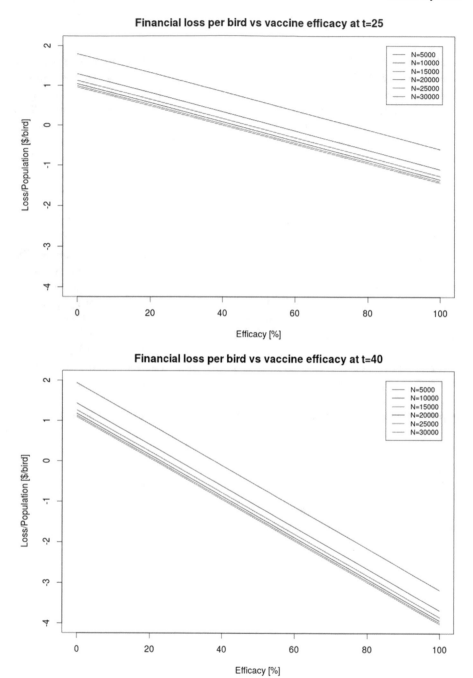

**Fig. 2** Financial loss per bird $L(N, e, t)/N$ for various population sizes $N$, plot versus efficacy $e$ for termination at day $t = 25$ (top) and day $t = 40$, without accounting for vaccination cost, $v(e) = 0$

we find that for the smallest population size tested, $N = 5000$, even a 100% effective vaccine does not yield a profit. However, the larger the population size in the barn, the smaller is the loss per bird. For larger populations the loss turns negative at an efficacy level of approximately 60%. At larger termination ages, the loss per bird turns negative, i.e. a profit is achieved, at an vaccination efficacy of $e = 40\%$ and already at an efficacy level of 20% for larger populations.

That the curves in Fig. 2 are straight lines is reflective of the observation in Fig. 1 that the state variables describing consumable birds $S$, $E$, $S_V$, $E_V$ reach their steady state values quickly, before the termination age. The parameter set used in our simulations describes a highly pathogenic strain that causes an epidemic in the broiler barn. For milder strains with slower disease progression and lower mortality, these loss curves can be nonlinear.

It is important to note that these curves are lower bounds on the actual loss, that is obtained if the costs of vaccination $v(e)$ are taken into account as well. Vaccintation costs per bird are usually between $0.50 and $3.40 [17], but a relationship between cost and efficacy is not known. It seems reasonable to assume that more efficient vaccines are more expensive, and that zero-efficacy (i.e. no vaccination) does not incur cost. To illustrate how accounting for vaccination cost affects loss and/or profit, we assume $v(e) = e^2$ and plot the corresponding data in Fig. 3. The actual loss data are a superposition of the linear curve previously obtained and a nonlinear curve

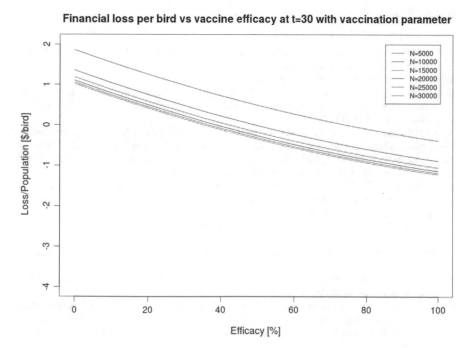

**Fig. 3** Finanical loss per bird versus efficacy at day 40 with vaccination cost $e^2$

determined by vaccine price, which can be substantial relative to the other costs incurred. Although the lower estimates in Fig. 2 (bottom) suggest that a profit can be made even for vaccines with moderate efficacy, the price to be paid for highly effective vaccines can invalidate these results.

## 4 Conclusion

Economic considerations are important in disease control of avian influenza in broiler production in an all-in/all-out housing system. The question how the cost of vaccination affects profitability depends both on the efficacy of the vaccine, and on the virulence and pathogenecity of the strain, which determine the time course of disease progression. A dynamic model that accounts for the effect of vaccination can be used to estimate the population size up to the time when the flock leaves the barn. Using this information the costs of operation as well as the income can be estimated. Together these two pieces of information give a lower bound on the loss incurred by an avian influenza outbreak. To obtain more accurate estimates the relationship between vaccine cost and efficacy must be known.

## References

1. Agusto, F.B., Gumel, A.B.: Qualitative dynamics of lowly-and highly-pathogenic avian influenza strains. Math. Biosci. **243**(2), 147–162 (2013)
2. Aphis, U.: Avian Influenza Disease (2016)
3. Brugh, M., Perdue, M.L.: Emergence of highly pathogenic virus during selective chicken passage of the prototype mildly pathogenic chicken/pennsylvania/83 (h5n2) influenza virus. Avian Dis. **35**, 824–833 (1991)
4. Chong, N.S., Smith, R.J.: Modelling avian influenza using filippov systems to determine culling of infected birds and quarantine. Nonlinear Anal.: Real World Appl. **24**, 196–218 (2015)
5. Chong, N.S., Tchuenche, J.M., Smith, R.J.: A mathematical model of avian influenza with half-saturated incidence. Theor. Biosci. **133**(1), 23–38 (2014)
6. der Goot, J.A.V., Koch, G., Jong, M.C.M.D., Boven, M.V.: Quantification of the effect of vaccination on transmission of avian influenza (h7n7) in chickens. Proc. Natl. Acad. Sci. U. S. A. **102**(50), 18141–18146 (2005)
7. Donald, J.O.: Environmental Management in the Broiler Breeder Rearing House. Aviagen Inc (2005)
8. For Animal Health, W.O.: Avian Influenza Vaccination. World Organization for Animal Health (2007)
9. Gulbudak, H., Martcheva, M.: Forward hysteresis and backward bifurcation caused by culling in an avian influenza model. Math. Biosci. **246**(1), 202–212 (2013)
10. Gulbudak, H., Martcheva, M.: A structured avian influenza model with imperfect vaccination and vaccine-induced asymptomatic infection. Bull. Math. Biol. **76**(10), 2389–2425 (2014)
11. Gumel, A.B.: Global dynamics of a two-strain avian influenza model. Int. J. Comput. Math. **86**(1), 85–108 (2009)
12. Iwami, S., Takeuchi, Y., Liu, X.: Avian-human influenza epidemic model. Math. Biosci. **207**(1), 1–25 (2007)

13. Mo, I.P., Brugh, M., Fletcher, O.J., Rowland, G.N., Swayne, D.E.: Comparative pathology of chickens experimentally inoculated with avian influenza viruses of low and high pathogenicity. Avian Dis. **41**, 125–136 (1997)
14. Nickbakhsh, S., Matthews, L., Reid, S.W.J., Kao, R.R.: A metapopulation model for highly pathogenic avian influenza: implications for compartmentalization as a control measure. Epidemiol. Infect. **142**(9), 1813–1825 (2014)
15. Nili, H., Asasi, K.: Natural cases and an experimental study of h9n2 avian influenza in commercial broiler chickens of iran. Avian Pathol. **31**(3), 247–252 (2002)
16. Of Ontario, C.F.: Chicken Farmers of Ontario (2016)
17. Peyre, M., Choisy, M., Sobhy, H., Kilany, W.H., Gely, M., Tripodi, A., Dauphin, G., Saad, M., Roger, F., Lubroth, J., Jobre, Y.: Added value of avian influenza (h5) day-old chick vaccination for disease control in egypt. Avian Dis. **60**, 245–252 (2016)
18. Rohani, P., Breban, R., Stallknecht, D.E., Drake, J.M.: Environmental transmission of low pathogenicity avian influenza viruses and its implications for pathogen invasion. Proc. Natl. Acad. Sci. **106**(25), 10365–10369 (2009)
19. Swayne, D.E.: Principles for vaccine protection in chickens and domestic waterfowl against avian influenza. Ann. N. Y. Acad. Sci. **1081**(1), 174–181 (2006)
20. Swayne, D.E., Suarez, D.L.: Highly pathogenic avian influenza. Revue Scientifique et Technique-office International des Epizooties **19**(2), 463–475 (2000)
21. Thiuthad, P., Manoranjan, V.S., Lenbury, Y.: Analytical solutions for an avian influenza epidemic model incorporating spatial spread as a diffusive process. East Asian J. Appl. Math. **5**(2), 150–159 (2015)
22. Vaidya, N.K., Wahl, L.M.: Avian influenza dynamics under periodic environmental conditions. SIAM J. Appl. Math. **75**(2), 443–467 (2015)
23. Xiao, Y., Sun, X., Tang, S., Wu, J.: Transmission potential of the novel avian influenza a (h7n9) infection in mainland china. J. Theor. Biol. **352**, 1–5 (2014)
24. Zhai, Y., Xiong, Y., Ma, X., and Bai, H.: Global hopf bifurcation analysis for an avian influenza virus propagation model with nonlinear incidence rate and delay. In Abstract and Applied Analysis (2014)

# Estimating the Crossover Point of a Fuzzy Willingness-to-Pay/Accept for Health to Support Decision Making

Michał Jakubczyk

**Abstract** Selecting health technologies to finance with public money requires juxtaposing their cost and health gains. Determining the exact values of willingness-to-pay/willingness-to-accept (WTP/WTA) may be difficult and considered unethical. As a solution, both may be treated as fuzzy sets. Then, a crossover-point (CP) of a fuzzy WTP is such a value that a decision maker is just as convinced as unconvinced it is worth paying for a unit of health (analogously for fuzzy WTA). In this fuzzy approach, I motivate why health technologies should be compared using CPs. I introduce three statistical methods of assessing the CP based on random-samples, survey data: using hypothesis testing, Bayesian hierarchical modelling, and frequentist estimation. I use the previously published dataset for Poland and show how the methods may be employed. The results suggest no (significant) difference in CPs for fuzzy WTP and WTA, but more stochastic uncertainty regarding the latter. The estimation methods can be used to assess the fuzzy preferences in other decision problem contexts.

**Keywords** Willingness to pay/accept · Crossover point · Fuzzy set

## 1 Introduction

To decide whether to finance a health technology (HT) with public money, its medical benefits and cost must be juxtaposed. This requires, explicitly or implicitly, valuing life, i.e. determining the willingness-to-pay (WTP) for a unit of health (e.g. a quality-adjusted life year, QALY). Determining WTP feels difficult and apparently is, noting the variability of published results see [1, 8]. The variability is not surprising, in view of the non-market nature of health and no preference-forming experience (health *services* are bought, not health itself). A belief that the societally wanted WTP can be set precisely and used in the cost-effectiveness analysis is, thus, a naïveté.

M. Jakubczyk (✉)
Decision Analysis and Support Unit, SGH Warsaw School of Economics,
Al. Niepodległości 162, 02-554 Warsaw, Poland
e-mail: michal.jakubczyk@sgh.waw.pl

© Springer Nature Switzerland AG 2018
D. M. Kilgour et al. (eds.), *Recent Advances in Mathematical and Statistical Methods*, Springer Proceedings in Mathematics & Statistics 259,
https://doi.org/10.1007/978-3-319-99719-3_39

The thresholds used in practice may reflect the convenience of predefined rules, e.g. triple annual gross domestic product per capita in Poland, see [6]; of benchmark technologies [7]; or of round numbers, e.g. $50,000, see [10]. Moreover, an ethical component emerges: refusing a treatment due to cost of QALY exceeding the WTP by $1 sounds inhumane and repudiates the readiness to define a threshold. It seems more natural to adopt a gradually diminishing acceptance when cost per QALY increases. This property invokes the use of fuzzy sets, invented to represent not complete membership or acceptance [13].

Jakubczyk and Kamiński [4], onwards J&K, suggested treating WTP and willingness-to-accept (WTA, for effect-reducing, cost-saving alternatives) as fuzzy sets, discussing the case of comparing two HTs. Jakubczyk [5] considered more than two alternatives, but only effect-increasing ones. In the present paper, I further the analysis. First, I propose and motivate a new decision making rule that can be used for both effect-increasing and reducing HTs. Then, as the major contribution, I introduce three statistical methods to estimate the parameters of fuzzy WTP/WTA, whose results can be subsequently used to choose one of the alternatives. I illustrate the estimation methods using the J&K's dataset.

## 2   Comparing Decision Alternatives with Fuzzy Net Benefit

In this section, I first briefly introduce the cost-effectiveness analysis (CEA) of HTs. Then, I define the fuzzy WTP, WTA, and net benefit (of a health technology), following ideas of J&K. Finally, I propose a decision making rule in the fuzzy context.

### 2.1   Standard (Crisp) Cost-Effectiveness Analysis

The decision maker has $n$ HTs, $A_1, \ldots, A_n$, to choose from. Each $A_i$ is characterized by expected (across a population of possible patients) effect, $e_i$, and cost, $c_i$, $A_i = (e_i, c_i)$. For simplicity, I neglect the estimation error: $(e_i, c_i)$ is known. The $e_i$ and $c_i$ are measured relative to some *status quo* (a current standard, a lack of treatment, etc.). Whether this null option may be chosen (by not choosing any $A_i$) does not affect the results (as discussed below). A possible approach to CEA is to calculate the net benefit (NB) of each $A_i$ (in monetary terms):

$$NB_i = e_i \times \text{WTP} - c_i, \tag{1}$$

(WTA would be used for $e_i < 0$) and to find $i$ that maximizes the NB.[1] Obviously, the problem lies in determining the WTP (WTA).

---

[1]In applied CEA it is more common to calculate the incremental cost-effectiveness ratios and compare them with WTP, algebraically equivalent to maximizing NB [5].

## 2.2 Fuzzy Willingness-to-Pay/Accept, Fuzzy Net Benefit

As motivated in the Introduction, the decision maker may find it difficult to determine WTP and WTA precisely. Thus, I redefine both as fuzzy sets: fuzzy WTP/WTA (fWTP/fWTA). In this, I follow J&K's idea with one difference: J&K derived fWTP/fWTA from the fuzzy preference relation, being a primitive of their model. I treat fWTP/fWTA as primitives.

**Definition 1** *Fuzzy WTP, fWTP, (fuzzy WTA, fWTA)* is a fuzzy set with an upper semi-continuous, non-increasing (non-decreasing) membership function, $\mu_{\text{fWTP}} : \mathbb{R} \to [0, 1]$ ($\mu_{\text{fWTA}} : \mathbb{R} \to [0, 1]$), such that $\mu_{\text{fWTP}}(0) = 1$ ($\mu_{\text{fWTA}}(0) = 0$).

I interpret $\mu_{\text{fWTP}}(x) = m$ to denote that the decision maker is convinced to degree $m$ that paying additional $x$ for a unit of effect is acceptable ($\mu_{\text{fWTA}}(x) = m$ is interpreted symmetrically). No relation between fWTP and fWTA is assumed a priori, and their selected characteristics are estimated and compared below. Then, for each $A_i$, I define the fuzzy NB.

**Definition 2** For any decision alternative $A = (e, c)$, define *fuzzy net benefit (fNB)*— a fuzzy set with membership function:

$$\mu_{\text{fNB}(A)}(x) = \begin{cases} \mu_{\text{fWTA}}(\frac{c+x}{e}), \text{ for } e < 0, \\ \mathbf{1}_{(-\infty, -c]}(x), \text{ for } e = 0, \\ \mu_{\text{fWTP}}(\frac{c+x}{e}), \text{ for } e > 0. \end{cases} \tag{2}$$

$\mu_{\text{fNB}(A)}(x)$ measures the conviction that using $A$ is equivalent to the monetary gain of $x$ (would be acceptable even if costed $x$ more). Following the assumptions on fWTP/fWTA, $\mu_{\text{fNB}(A)}(x)$ is non-increasing and upper-semi continuous. In Fig. 1, I present an example how fNBs might look. To make comparing HTs easier, I define

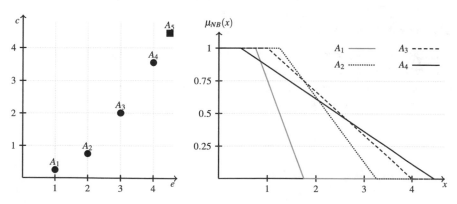

**Fig. 1** The available technologies in cost-effectiveness plane (left): $A_1 = (1, 0.25)$, $A_2 = (2, 0.75)$, $A_3 = (3, 2)$, $A_4 = (4, 3.55)$, and $A_5 = (4.5, 4.45)$. Their respective fNB membership functions (right), when $\mu_{\text{fWTP}}$ decreases linearly from 1 to 0 in [1; 2] interval (fNB($A_5$) not drawn)

the right-boundary of $\alpha$-cuts of fNB: $\tau_A(\alpha) = \sup\{x \in \mathbb{R} : \mu_{\text{fNB}(A)}(x) \geq \alpha\}$, for $\alpha \in ]0, 1]$, and $\tau_A(0) = \sup_{\alpha \in ]0,1]}\{\tau_A(\alpha)\}$. $\tau_A(\alpha)$ can be interpreted as the largest value that the decision maker would agree with conviction $\alpha$ that using $A$ is worth.

## 2.3 Decision Making Rule

Jakubczyk [5] suggested to choose HTs by maximizing the measure of set of $\alpha$s in $[0, 1]$ that a given HT, $A_i$ maximizes $\tau_{A_i}(\alpha)$. In Fig. 1 (when $A_5$ is ignored) that would be technology $A_4$, as it maximizes the $\tau_A(\alpha)$ for all $\alpha < 0.45$, and the remaining technologies maximize $\tau_A(\alpha)$ for shorter intervals. That approach, however, violates the independence of irrelevant alternatives: adding $A_5$ to the menu would switch the choice to $A_3$, previously available but not chosen.

For the above reason, I propose to base the choice of $A_i$ by maximizing the $\tau_{A_i}(0.5)$ ($A_3$ in Fig. 1, irrespectively of whether $A_5$ is being considered), denoted by CfNB$_i$ (crossover fNB) for brevity. When considering crisp NBs, typically such $i^*$ is selected that maximizes $NB_{i^*}$. In our case, fNBs are sets; hence, the analogy would be to select $i^*$ that results in the greatest (including all others) set. The following proposition states why maximizing CfNB$_i$ does just that in a sense of weak inclusion of fuzzy sets, see def. of [2].[2]

**Proposition 1** *Consider n HTs, $A_i = (e_i, c_i)$. If $A_{i^*}$ maximizes $CfNB$, then (i) fNB$_{i^*}$ weakly includes, to degree 0.5, fNB$_i$ for any i not maximizing CfNB, and (ii) fNB$_i$ weakly includes fNB$_{i^*}$ at maximum to degree 0.5. Formally:*

$$\inf_{x \in \mathbb{R}} \max\left(\mu_{\text{fNB}(A_{i^*})}(x), 1 - \mu_{\text{fNB}(A_i)}(x)\right) \geq \frac{1}{2},$$

$$\inf_{x \in \mathbb{R}} \max\left(\mu_{\text{fNB}(A_i)}(x), 1 - \mu_{\text{fNB}(A_{i^*})}(x)\right) \leq \frac{1}{2}.$$

*Moreover, two implications hold.*

- *If $\mu_{\text{fWTP}}$ and $\mu_{\text{fWTA}}$ are strictly decreasing where they take values from within $(0, 1)$ interval, then the above inequalities are strict.*
- *If $\mu_{\text{fWTP}}$ and $\mu_{\text{fWTA}}$ are continuous, then all CfNB-maximizing options, say $i^*$ and $i^{**}$, weakly include each other to the same degree.*

---

[2]This approach can also be seen (not pursued formally, for brevity) as applying the Orlovsky-score [11]: maximizing the degree to which a given alternative is not dominated by others.

# 3   Estimation of the Crossover Point

When maximizing CfNB (i.e. applying a decision making rule defined in the previous section), it is most convenient to estimate the upper bound of the 0.5-cut of fWTP and fWTA (i.e. the crossover point of fWTP/fWTA, CP). In the present section, I propose three methods of assessing these values based on random samples. First, I briefly introduce the dataset used for illustrative purposes. Then, I introduce the methods along with presenting their results.

## 3.1   *Data*

I use the data collected by J&K: 27 respondents in Poland (5 removed due to inconsistencies) answered with a 5-level Likert scale if they consider paying/saving $\lambda$ for an additional/lost unit of health (in QALY) as acceptable, for various $\lambda$s. The reader is referred to the original publication for more details. Figure 2 presents the responses (WTP part only, for brevity) for various $\lambda$s (horizontal axis, hundreds of 000s PLN/QALY). The horizontal bars span the $\lambda$s for which the middle level was used by an individual. For other levels, the circle area is proportional to the number of answers. Black lines depict jumps across the middle answer.

The small sample size lowers the precision of the estimates obtained below (e.g. the credible intervals are quite large). Still, the present paper should be treated more as a conceptual one. Importantly, the methods introduced below can be used to any, similarly collected (but larger) dataset.

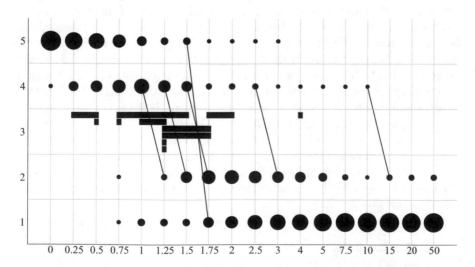

**Fig. 2**  Survey results for WTP, values in horizontal axis in hundreds of 000s of PLN/QALY, answers (vertical axis) from a 5-level Likert scale (1—definitely disagree, 5—definitely agree). Horizontal bars represent individuals, circles—the fraction of respondents, lines—jumps across the middle option

## 3.2 Assessing the CP for fWTP/fWTA via Hypothesis Testing

I assume that for each $\lambda \in \mathbb{R}_+$ there is an (unknown) average conviction in the population, $\mu_{fWTP}(\lambda)$.[3] The sought for estimand, CP, is defined as $\mu_{WTP}(CP) = 0.5$. I assume that the values of $\mu_{fWTP,i}(CP)$ for every individual, $i$ (index added, for clarity), are drawn from a common, symmetric distribution, and so are the responses in the Likert scale. Hence, for each $\lambda$, I test $H_0 : CP = \lambda$ by testing the symmetry of the Likert answers. I use the test proposed by [3] (with $H_2$ alternative, according to their notation). Mann-Whitney test could be used (vs a vector of 3s); with no impact on the conclusions in the present data, but in general Dykstra test uses more information, differentiating between Likert levels 1/2 (4/5).

For WTP the test does not reject $H_0$ for $\lambda = 125$ ($p^* = 0.0612$) and $\lambda = 150$ ($p^* = 0.6313$), while e.g. for $\lambda = 100$ or $\lambda = 175$ the test yields $p^* = 0.0001$ and $p^* = 0.0028$, respectively. For WTA, the test does not reject $H_0$ for $\lambda = 150$ ($p^* = 0.1994$), $\lambda = 175$ ($p^* = 0.2532$), $\lambda = 200$ ($p^* = 0.166$), $\lambda = 250$ ($p^* = 0.1308$), and $\lambda = 300$ ($p^* = 0.0849$). The conclusions (which $H_0$ to reject) do not change if a one-sided test is used. As the inference is conducted separately for each $\lambda$, there is no need to correct for multiple hypothesis.

## 3.3 Data Transformation for Bayesian/Frequentist Estimation

In the remaining two approaches I consider a cross-over range (CR): a range of $\lambda$s for which the decision maker selected (would have selected) the middle Likert answer. Identifying CRs from the data requires some transformation and assumptions, described below for WTP (analogous for WTA). Firstly, even if the respondent did not use the middle option, I still assume it would be used for $\lambda$ equal to the average of the greatest $\lambda$ with options 4 or 5 selected and the lowest $\lambda$ with 1 or 2. Secondly, I assume CR's lower endpoint as the mean of the greatest $\lambda$ with options 4 or 5 and the lowest $\lambda$ with 3 (directly selected or inferred); analogously for the upper endpoint.[4] The assumptions suffice to calculate CRs for WTP; in case of WTA, two respondents used only options 1 & 2, and one respondent only option 3, for all $\lambda$s, thwarting the calculation. All three were removed, as they, in principle, disagree with sacrificing effectiveness to make savings, while the methods developed here accept such trade-offs (and aim to quantify them); hence, should not be based on the opinions in such a fundamental disagreement.

---

[3]The explanation is done for WTP, but refers to WTA *mutatis mutandis*.
[4]Example 1: if the respondent selected option 4 for $\lambda = 100$, option 3 for $\lambda = 125$ and $\lambda = 150$, and option 2 for $\lambda = 175$, then $CR = [112.5; 162.5]$. Example 2: if the respondent selected option 4 for $\lambda = 100$ and immediately switched to option 2 for $\lambda = 125$, then $CR = [106.25; 118.75]$.

In the calculations below, log of λs were used,[5] for three reasons. Firstly, the distribution of the middles of the non-logged CRs was skewed, and statistical methods typically work on non-skew data better. Secondly, the length of CR is positively correlated with the location (for non-logs). Intuitively, the respondents thinking about large amounts allow larger tolerance in absolute terms (and λs were sparser for large values). It is more convenient to model the respondents uncertainty in relative terms, not to have to model the relation between the CR's middle and length, and this is automatically done with logs. Thirdly, with logs the results do not change whether WTP/WTA are taken as PLN/QALY or QALY/PLN; not the case with original data (arithmetic and geometric means differing).

## 3.4 Hierarchical Bayesian Modelling

I assume the following data generating process. Each of $k$ respondents, indexed by $j \in \{1, \ldots, m\}$, has a single, *true*, log of CP value, denoted $\eta_j$, drawn from a common distribution $N(\eta, \xi^2)$.[6] The respondent does not precisely perceive own $\eta_j$, only the bounds, $l_j$ and $u_j$, $l_j = \eta_j - \Delta'_j$ and $u_j = \eta_j + \Delta''_j$, where $\Delta'_j$, $\Delta''_j$ are independent random variables from a single (for every $j$), exponential distribution, $\text{Exp}(\kappa)$. Non-informative prior distributions were used to define $\eta$ (normal distribution, $N(0, 100)$), $\xi^{-2}$ and $\kappa$ (for both, the gamma distribution, with mean equal to 1 and variance equal to 100).

Then, $l_j$ and $u_j$ are observed as the lower/upper endpoints of CR (logs), and the distribution of observables is based on parameters $(\eta, \xi, \kappa)$. The independence of $\Delta$s reflects the unpredictability of misjudging one's CP. Using the exponential distribution has two nice consequences: (1) knowing that one's CP is misjudged upwards by at least some amount does not change the distribution of by how much *more* it is misjudged; (2) the resulting distribution of $\Delta'_j / (\Delta'_j + \Delta''_j)$ is uniform. Both reflect a conservative approach assuming no regularity how CP is imperfectly perceived.

The model was estimated with MCMC in JAGS/R (10,000 burn-in iterations, 50,000 of actual iterations, thinning 5). The mean of the posterior was taken as the estimate, and percentiles 2.5 and 97.5% as boundaries of the 95% credible interval (CrI). In result, for WTP the estimate of $\exp(\eta)$ equals 145.68, 95%CrI $= (106.99; 197.95)$, while for WTA it amounts to 162.29 and $(115.78; 228.15)$, respectively.

---

[5] 1 PLN/QALY added, to avoid $\ln(0)$.

[6] Taking the logs, conveniently, allows using a normal distribution, as the non-log CR are bounded by zero from below.

## 3.5 A Meta-analytic Approach with Bootstrap

I assume the random effects model: respondents differ in terms of their *true* log CP, denoted by $\eta_j$, drawn from a $N(\eta, \xi^2)$. I use the same symbols as in the previous subsection, as intuitions are identical. In the frequentist approach here, $\eta$ is the true, unknown parameter of interest (with no probability distribution). I assume the precision for each $j$ is given by the length of CR and the observed CR ($[l_j, u_j]$) is uniformly distributed, subject to $\eta_j \in [l_j, u_j]$. Then $m_j = {}^{(l_j + u_j)}/_2$ is uniformly distributed around $\eta_j$ with variance ${}^{(u_j - l_j)^2}/_{12}$, and $m_j$ is an unbiased point estimate of $\eta_j$ for every $j$. I use the inverse-variance weighted average to calculate the point estimate $\hat{\eta}$, accounting for random effects, using standard formulae see, e.g. [12]. As the distribution of estimated $\hat{\eta}$ is not normal, I assess the 95%confidence interval (CI) for $\eta$ via bootstrapping: (i) re-sample the set of respondents (to account for sampling error), (ii) for each re-sampled respondent generate a new $m_j^*$ from a uniform distribution $[l_j, u_j]$, (iii) keep the length of CR, (iv) calculate the $\hat{\eta}^*$ in this bootstrap sample (inverse-variance, random effects), (v) repeat for 10,000 bootstrap samples and take percentiles 2.5 and 97.5% to define the 95%CI.

For WTP the $\exp(\hat{\eta}) = 153.57$, $95\%CI = (121.19; 202.89)$. For WTA, respectively, 163.29 and (120.94; 225.13). No bias prevails: mean bootstrap results equal 154.26 and 163.03 for WTP and WTA, respectively (close to the meta-analysis results). Notice, that assuming the normal distribution of the standard error in the meta-analysis would yield more narrow (and probably overly optimistic) 95%CI: (130.57; 180.61) and (135.03; 197.47), respectively.

## 3.6 Summary of the Results

Table 1 juxtaposes the—reassuringly consistent—results. The CP for WTP/WTA exceeds the official threshold in Poland (130,002 PLN/QALY as of 1st Sept, 2017, and 111,381 PLN/QALY in the time the survey was run). CP for WTA seems no greater than for WTP, but all methods suggest there is more uncertainty for WTA.

The statistical testing requires fewest assumptions (e.g. no specific distribution assumed) and its results do not require (or change with) any transformation of $\lambda$s. Hypothesis testing works on complete data, while other methods require some han-

**Table 1** Estimation results for the indecisiveness point (in 000s PLN/QALY) along with 95% confidence or credible (depending on context) interval (95%CI)

| Method | Willingness-to-pay | Willingness-to-accept |
|---|---|---|
| Hypothesis testing | Not rejected for 125, 150 | Not rejected for 150–300 |
| Bayesian modelling (95%CrI) | 145.7, (107.0; 197.9) | 162.3, (115.8; 228.1) |
| Meta-analysis (95%CI) | 153.6, (121.2; 202.9) | 163.3, (120.9; 225.1) |

dling of the respondents not crossing the middle Likert option. Adding extremely undecided respondents (selecting the middle option) would change the results of the last two methods, while are effectively ignored by hypothesis testing.

The last two methods require using the middle option to account for possibly wide CR (otherwise the intra-respondent uncertainty regarding the location of CP could be underestimated). The hypothesis testing can be used with or without the middle level, irrespectively how it is worded (e.g. *neither/nor* or *I don't know*, as long as it is symmetric). Making the middle answer more inclusive does not prevent hypothesis testing, but may reduce the power. Matell [9] showed that using more (odd number of) levels decreases the frequency of selecting the middle option, hence all the methods might profit from using a greater than five, odd number of levels.

No method required an interval interpretation of the Likert scale. In the hypothesis testing the assumption is made, however, that options 1 & 2 are symmetrical counterparts of 5 & 4 (not a strong assumption, as wording is symmetrical).

The usefulness of hypothesis testing depends most heavily on the design of the questionnaire, as the conclusions can be drawn only for $\lambda$s included, but obviously using more $\lambda$s would be tiresome. Another downside is that not rejecting $H_0$ does not denote accepting it in statistical parlance. Also, all the non-rejected $\lambda$s have to be treated identically with no telling which are more likely to represent CP. Bayesian approach produces a posteriori distributions, easy to use in sensitivity analysis. It could also account for covariates and explain part of the heterogeneity between the respondents.

The hypothesis testing allows for $\mu_{\text{fWTP}}(x) = 0.5$ ($\mu_{\text{fWTA}}(x) = 0.5$) for a range of, not a single, $x$. The remaining two methods would have to be somehow adopted.

# 4  Conclusion

Health technologies can also be compared when WTP and WTA are treated as fuzzy set: the recommended decision making rule uses the crossover point of the fuzzy WTP/WTA. This value can be assessed based on simple surveys (i.e. Likert based) in random samples using several approaches. The results of the approaches are consistent (for the present dataset), and the crossover point for WTP and WTA seems not to differ. This finding suggests that the WTP-WTA disparity should be redefined and rechecked in the fuzzy-set context.

**Proofs**

*Proof* (Proposition 1) Proving the first part. Take any $x \in (\text{CfNB}_i, \text{CfNB}_{i*})$ (the interval is non-empty), $\mu_{\text{fNB}(i)}(x) \leq 1/2 \leq \mu_{\text{fNB}(i*)}(x)$; using the monotonicity of $\mu_{\text{fNB}}$ (for $i^*$, $i$) yields the result. Proving the first bullet implication: take any $x \in (\text{CfNB}_i, \text{CfNB}_{i*})$ (again, exists), $\mu_{\text{fNB}(i)}(x) < 1/2 < \mu_{\text{fNB}(i*)}(x)$, and use monotonicity again. Proving the last bullet. First consider $e_{i*} \neq 0 \neq e_{i**}$, and so $\mu_{\text{fNB}}$ are continuous for $i^*$, $i^{**}$. Then $\mu_{\text{fNB}(i*)}(x) = \mu_{\text{fNB}(i**)}(x) = 1/2$, and the rest follows from monotonicity. Now consider $e_{i*} = 0 = e_{i**}$, then fNBs are equal, crisp numbers (with upper semi-continuous, step membership functions, jumping from 1 to 0), and so weakly include each other to the degree 1. Finally consider $e_{i*} \neq 0 = e_{i**}$. $\mu_{\text{fNB}(i*)}$ is continuous and monotonic, and fNB$_{i**}$ is a crisp number. It easily follows (considering $x = \text{CfNB}_{i*}$) that fNB$_{i*}$ weakly includes fNB$_{i**}$ to the degree $1/2$. Approaching this $x$ from right yields the weak inclusion to the same degree.

**Acknowledgements** The research was financed by the funds obtained from National Science Centre, Poland, granted following the decision number DEC-2015/19/B/HS4/01729.

# References

1. Bellavance, F., Dionne, G., Lebeau, M.: The value of a statistical life: a meta-analysis with a mixed effects regression model. J. Health Econ. **28**(2), 444–464 (2009)
2. Dubois, D., Prade, H.: Fuzzy Sets and Systems: Theory and Applications. Academic Press, New York (1980)
3. Dykstra, R., Kochar, S., Robertson, T.: Likelihood ratio tests for symmetry against one-sided alternatives. Ann. Inst. Stat. Math. **47**(4), 719–730 (1995)
4. Jakubczyk, M., Kamiński, B.: Fuzzy approach to decision analysis with multiple criteria and uncertainty in health technology assessment. Ann. Oper. Res. **251**, 301–324 (2017)
5. Jakubczyk, M.: Using a fuzzy approach in multi-criteria decision making with multiple alternatives in health care. Multiple Criteria Decis. Making **10**, 65–81 (2015)
6. Jakubiak-Lasocka, J., Jakubczyk, M.: Cost-effectiveness versus cost-utility analyses: what are the motives behind using each and how do their results differ?–a Polish example. Value Health Reg. Issues **4C**, 66–74 (2014)
7. Lee, C., Chertow, G., Zenios, S.: An empiric estimate of the value of life: updating the renal dialysis cost-effectiveness standard. Value Health **12**(1), 80–87 (2009)
8. Lindhjem, H., Navrud, S., Braathen, N., Biausque, V.: Valuing mortality risk reductions from environmental, transport, and health policies: a global meta-analysis of stated preference studies. Risk Anal. **31**(9), 1381–1407 (2011)
9. Matell, M., Jacoby, J.: Is there an optimal number of alternatives for Likert-scale items? effects of testing time and scale properties. J. Appl. Psychol. **56**(6), 506–509 (1972)
10. Neumann, P., Cohen, J., Weinstein, M.: Updating cost-effectiveness–the curious resilience of the $50,000-per-QALY threshold. N. Engl. J. Med. **371**(9), 796–797 (2014)
11. Orlovsky, S.: Decision-making with a fuzzy preference relation. Fuzzy Sets Syst. **1**, 155–167 (1978)
12. Whitehead, A.: Meta-Analysis of Controlled Clinical Trials, 1st edn. Wiley (2002)
13. Zadeh, L.: Fuzzy sets. Inf. Control **8**, 338–353 (1965)

# Fuzzy Approach to Elicitation
# of Preferences for Health States

Bogumił Kamiński and Michał Jakubczyk

**Abstract** Eliciting people's preferences for health states is crucial to understand what society values and support public decision making in healthcare. Thought experiments are used to assign utilities to health states but the lack of actual experience may result in the preferences being vague. Based on previously published studies, we model the disutilities of health worsening using fuzzy numbers. In our model, we define a new interval-arithmetic operator to differentiate between two alternatives being compared by looking into a single criterion (e.g. how much mobility is reduced in two states being compared) or trading off several criteria (e.g. mobility worsening vs increasing pain). We use a large dataset from a discrete choice experiment to estimate the parameters of our model. We find that (i) imprecision should indeed be handled differently for within-criterion and between-criteria comparisons, (ii) large imprecision leads to a more erratic behaviour in choice experiments, (iii) the type of time unit used matters little in comparing health states with duration.

**Keywords** Fuzzy preferences · Health state utility · QALY
Discrete choice experiment

## 1 Introduction

Numerous decision problems in real life involve multiple goals; hence, people have to trade-off individual criteria. If decision makers lack adequate experience with past choices, they may find it difficult, only vaguely understanding the importance of individual criteria.

B. Kamiński (✉) · M. Jakubczyk
Decision Analysis and Support Unit, SGH Warsaw School of Economics,
Al. Niepodległości 162, 02-554 Warsaw, Poland
e-mail: bogumil.kaminski@sgh.waw.pl

M. Jakubczyk
e-mail: michal.jakubczyk@sgh.waw.pl

© Springer Nature Switzerland AG 2018                                441
D. M. Kilgour et al. (eds.), *Recent Advances in Mathematical
and Statistical Methods*, Springer Proceedings in Mathematics & Statistics 259,
https://doi.org/10.1007/978-3-319-99719-3_40

In particular, people rarely directly choose between health states (at best they choose between unhealthy pleasures and health or free time and health improvement). At the same time, understanding preferences for health states is crucial to measuring health gains and supporting public decisions what health technologies to finance. The health measure used to support such decisions must combine the longevity of life with health-related quality of life, which introduces the first two criteria to trade-off. We must additionally make the notion of quality of life operational; typically, the EQ-5D-5L[1] descriptive system is used see [6]. In this system, a health state is described using five attributes[2]: mobility, self-care, usual activities, pain/discomfort, and anxiety/depression, always considered in this ordering. In each dimension, a person can be at one of five levels (1–5): simplifying, no problems (denoted by value 1) to extreme problems (denoted by value 5).[3] A health state can then be briefly coded as a five-tuple of digits (the ordering of dimensions as above); e.g. 11111 denotes the best possible health state (in the EQ-5D-5L descriptive system), 55555 denotes the worst possible health state, and 11131 denotes the state in which one feels moderate pain/discomfort but otherwise experiences no health problems.[4]

The description of health state presented above adds two sources of imprecision. Firstly, the notion of, say, self-care is vague (what activities are included?). Various people may understand it differently, and a single person may be unsure how to understand it (e.g. what counts as self care, rather than mobility?) and, thus, what importance to attach to it. Secondly, how the verbal description of levels is interpreted is subjective too (e.g. where does the boundary between slight and moderate problems lie?).

The above difficulties are particularly visible for choosing between health states, but can be observed in many multiple-criteria problems (for example, related to other intangible goods like clean environment or safety). Imprecision and gradualness in preferences can be modelled using fuzzy sets [14]. Jakubczyk and Golicki [7] showed how to use fuzzy set concepts to account for imprecision when eliciting utility for health states with a time trade-off method; Jakubczyk et al. [9] and Kamiński and Jakubczyk [10] did it for the other dominant elicitation method: discrete choice experiment (DCE).

In the present paper, we further the methodology presented by [10], based on the following motivation (made more formal in the next section). A person might find it problematic to compare 11141 and 11114, i.e. the disutility of severe pain/discomfort (fourth attribute at level 4) and the disutility of severe anxiety/depression (fifth attribute at level four). The same person may find it difficult to compare 11141 and 11115, while the choice between 11114 and 11115 is obvious. Hence, within-

---

[1] https://euroqol.org/eq-5d-instruments/.

[2] In the health preference research literature using EQ-5D-5L, the attributes are typically referred to as *dimensions*, and we use this terminology in the present paper.

[3] Previously, EQ-5D-3L system was widely used, in which three levels were available in every dimension see [3]. Readers with interest in other descriptive systems can have a look at a study by [11].

[4] Again, to align with the health preference research literature we do not write this 5-tuple as a vector, e.g. [1, 1, 1, 1, 3].

criterion comparisons are easier than between-criteria ones. Less trivially: a person may find it easier to compare 11115 with 11314 than 11115 with 11341, because the first comparison requires thinking about two criteria only.[5] The former choice can be framed as asking oneself: *'is setting usual activities at level 3 as bad as deteriorating anxiety/depression dimension from level 4 to level 5'*; the latter requires a more complex framing. Hence, if fuzzy utilities are attached to level-criterion combination, then the comparisons (subtracting the fuzzy numbers) must differentiate between comparisons within or between the criteria. We formalize this idea in the present paper.

In the next section we introduce a model of preferences we consider. How the choices are made accounts for the difference between inter or intra-criteria analysis, as described above. We then estimate the parameters of the model based on an actual dataset and discuss the results. We show possible further directions of research in the last section.

## 2 Model of Preferences

Consider two health states $A$ and $B$ described in the EQ-5D-5L descriptive system, where $A$ lasts for $T_A$ and $B$ for $T_B$ (various time units are used in the paper). Our objective is to derive the probability that option $A$ is chosen over option $B$ by a respondent. Our approach can be summarized in the following steps:

(a) assign a fuzzy number to each health dimension, i.e. each attribute describing a decision alternative (to be used in the assessment of both considered options, $A$ and $B$);
(b) for each attribute, calculate the advantage/disadvantage of option $A$ over $B$ (accounting for the duration of health problems); the result of this comparison is a fuzzy number for every attribute separately; this analysis over individual dimensions allows us to treat the within-criterion comparisons differently;
(c) aggregate the fuzzy comparisons for all dimensions to get the comparison of considered options $A$ and $B$ as fuzzy numbers;
(d) crispify this fuzzy number to calculate the probability of choice of option $A$ over option $B$.

The key innovation in our approach is that we allow the comparisons *within a single criterion* (within one EQ-5D-5L dimension) to be simpler for the respondent than *between criteria* (between dimensions). Standard fuzzy number arithmetic is commutative and associative so it would be impossible to distinguish such effect in steps (b) and (c) of the above procedure. Therefore in this text we introduce a novel notion of subtraction of fuzzy numbers (in step b) that allows distinguishing the above

---

[5]We neglect possible interactions between criteria both in this motivation, and in the general framework below. Omitting the interactions is a generally an accepted approach to modelling EQ-5D-5L data (in a crisp approach), but could obviously be studied in further research.

two types of comparisons. In Sect. 4, we show that the empirical data confirm our assumptions (i.e. it is easier for the respondents to compare states within dimension than between dimensions).

In this section, we first present the model of disutilities attached to EQ-5D-5L dimensions as fuzzy numbers. Then, we show how two fuzzy numbers representing health states should be subtracted, accounting for the possibility that the same criteria are worsened. Third, we present how to crispify the fuzzy preferences to get the probability of choosing one of the alternatives. Sections 2.1 and 2.3 follow the model by Kamiński, B., Jakubczyk [10].

## 2.1 Disutility of a Health State

We consider a choice between two health states, $A$ or $B$, lasting for $T_A$ or $T_B$ time units, respectively. The variable $d_i^A$ denotes the level of dimension $i$ ($i = 1, \ldots, 5$) for state $A$. $T_A$ and $T_B$ can be measured in different units, which is reflected in the formulas below.

Each dimension, $i = 1, \ldots, 5$, is associated with a fuzzy number, $\widetilde{DU}_i$, measuring its importance. We interpret $\widetilde{DU}_i$ as a fuzzy disutility of level 5 in dimension $i$, where we interpret the utility of a health state in a sense of the QALY model [2]. In the present paper, we trivially assume $\widetilde{DU}_i$ is rectangular and normal: the membership function takes value 1 in the interval $[l_i, h_i]$ and 0 otherwise. In other words, there is a set of numbers that the respondent accepts as disutilities of setting dimension $i$ to level 5 (membership function equal to 1) and the respondent rejects any other number as a disutility (membership function equal to 0). We still treat and interpret $\widetilde{DU}_i$ as a fuzzy number for three reasons: (i) in future research our assumptions may be relaxed and fractional membership can be used (i.e. there may be numbers that the respondent only partially accepts as disutilities of worsening $i$ to level 5), (ii) we want to directly refer to and develop arithmetic of fuzzy numbers, thus, we discuss our work in this context, and (iii) our interpretation of $\widetilde{DU}_i$ is easiest in the epistemic (rather than ontic) sense, and the distinction is stressed more in the fuzzy set context [4, 13, 15].

The relative (to level 5) importance of levels 2, 3, 4 is given as crisp weights $w_{i,j}$, where $i$ denotes the dimension and $j = 2, 3, 4$ denotes the level. To simplify formulas, we set $w_{i,1} = 0$ and $w_{i,5} = 1$. In future, separate fuzzy numbers for the combinations of dimensions and levels could be defined (and this fact motivates our approach, as discussed below).

The utility of living in $A$ for time $T_A$ is given as a fuzzy number

$$\widetilde{U}(A, T_A) = \tau_{\text{unit}(A)} \times T_A \times \left(1 - \sum_{i=1,\ldots,5} w_{i,d_i^A} \times \widetilde{DU}_i\right), \tag{1}$$

where unit($A$) is the time unit $T_A$ is measured in (days, weeks, months, or years, coded as 1–4, respectively), and $\tau_k > 0$ are the scaling factors to reflect the (subjectively perceived by the decision maker) duration of the units.

If $A$ denotes being dead comparisons vs dead are often used to anchor the utility values to an interpretable scale, see [12], then $T_A$ is irrelevant and $\widetilde{U}(A, T_A)$ amounts to a crisp 0 (i.e. only value 0 has a membership function equal to 1).

## 2.2 Comparing Two Health States

The difference in utilities of $(A, T_A)$ and $(B, T_B)$ is given by the difference $\widetilde{U}(A, T_A) - \widetilde{U}(B, T_B)$ both defined by Eq. (1), after reorganization:

$$\tau_{\text{unit}(A)}(T_A - T_B) + \tau_{\text{unit}(A)} \sum_{i=1,\dots,5} \left( w_{i,d_i^B} \times T_B \times \widetilde{DU}_i \boxminus w_{i,d_i^A} \times T_A \times \widetilde{DU}_i \right),$$

(2)

where we use the fact that in our dataset $A$ and $B$ with identical time units are compared. The operator $\boxminus$ is introduced in the equation to allow for a particular form of within-criterion comparisons motivated in the introduction and is explained formally below.

In Eq. (2), we decomposed the differences in utilities into two sources: the duration of life (the first term), and the accumulated (over time) stream of disutility (the second term, notice the reversal of $A$ and $B$) due to health problems (further decomposed into individual dimensions).

Because the fuzzy numbers are fully represented as intervals (1-cuts), interval arithmetic applies. The multiplication of a fuzzy number, $[a, b]$, by a crisp number, $[c, c]$, yields a fuzzy number $[ac, bc]$ (we use the fact that we only multiply by positive numbers: relative level weights or duration). Obviously $[a, a] \times [c, c] = [ac, ac]$. Adding two intervals works as follows: $[a, b] + [c, d] = [a + c, b + d]$ (possibly for degenerate intervals).

Standard subtraction of fuzzy numbers increases the imprecision (as measured by the length of $\alpha$-cuts) of the result, as compared to the imprecision of the minuend and subtrahend. In case of intervals, that would lead to the following formula: $[a, b] - [c, d] = [a - d, b - c]$, with the length of the result being the sum of the starting lengths. In Eq. (2), the disutilities from individual dimensions are considered one by one. For this reason, we introduce a new operator, $\boxminus$, to be explained below, that can generalize regular subtraction to account for the possible smaller imprecision of within criteria comparisons.

For example, the interpretation of $\widetilde{DU}_1 = [0.2, 0.4]$ is that the decision maker cannot rule out any value from the interval $[0.2, 0.4]$ as the possible (crisp) disutility of worsening mobility to level 5. Assume $w_{1,4} = 0.5$, i.e. the relative gravity of level 4 in mobility equal 0.5. Then the disutility of mobility at level 4 is given as $[0.1, 0.2]$. Standard subtraction would yield $[0.2, 0.4] - [0.1, 0.2] = [0, 0.3]$. The imprecision of $\widetilde{DU}_1$ as reflected by the length of $[0.2, 0.4]$ is due to the decision maker being unsure how important mobility is (perhaps because they have never experienced reduced mobility) or what counts as mobility (and, for example, what as self-care). Still, when comparing two levels of mobility, substantial part of this uncertainty cancels out. If the decision maker gains more experience (or can get more insight into own preferences by longer introspection) and updates own beliefs so that the disutility of level is $[0.35, 0.4]$, then we expect that the disutility of level 4 to be shorter and closer to its previous upper bound, 0.2, too. Reflecting that effect requires, imprecisely speaking, to subtract the high values of the subtrahend from the high values of the minuend.

For the above reason, we propose to replace the standard $-$ with $\boxminus$, so defined that $[a, b] \boxminus [c, d]$ is an interval $[e, f]$, where:

$$e = \frac{(a + b) - (c + d)}{2} - \frac{\max(b - a, d - c) + \kappa \times \min(b - a, d - c)}{2}, \quad (3)$$

$$f = \frac{(a + b) - (c + d)}{2} + \frac{\max(b - a, d - c) + \kappa \times \min(b - a, d - c)}{2}, \quad (4)$$

for some parameter $\kappa \in [-1, 1]$.

Notice that $\kappa = 1$ results in regular subtraction of fuzzy numbers. On the other hand, $\kappa = -1$ results in the formula $[a, b] \boxminus [c, d] = [\min(a - c, b - d), \max(a - c, b - d)]$, as wanted (this is equivalent to taking $\widetilde{DU}_i$ out of the parenthesis in Eq. (2)). The value of $\kappa$ is subject to estimation, and can demonstrate whether the effect of within-criterion comparisons is present.

## 2.3 Choosing Between Two Health States

Based on the previous subsection, the difference in utilities of two compared alternatives, $(A, T_A)$ and $(B, T_B)$, is given as an interval, which we denote by $[L_\Delta, H_\Delta]$. Then, we define the ancillary score, $\pi$,

$$\pi = \frac{1}{1 + \exp\left(-(H_\Delta + L_\Delta)/2\right)}. \quad (5)$$

In this way, we transform the advantage of one alternative over another into the $\pi \in [0, 1]$ interval, to facilitate interpreting the gain in terms of probabilities.[6]

We want to account for the fact that a larger difference between $L_\Delta$ and $H_\Delta$ denotes larger imprecision in the assessment of the difference in utility between the alternatives. We assume that a larger imprecision may dilute the preferences, i.e. drag the probability of one alternative being chosen towards 50%. Specifically, we take:

---

[6]Such a logit formula is often used in health preference research in modelling the discrete choice experiments, see [8].

$$\Theta = (H_\Delta - L_\Delta)/2, \tag{6}$$

and we define the resulting probability of $(A, T_A)$ being chosen as

$$P = \frac{\pi - 0.5}{1 + \omega\Theta} + 0.5, \tag{7}$$

where $\omega$ is a parameter to be estimated. For $\omega = 0$ there is no impact of imprecision on preferences. Additionally for $\pi = 0.5$ we see that $P = 0.5$ independent from $\omega$. In short, the transformation

$$P: \pi \rightarrow \left[0.5 - \frac{0.5}{1 + \omega\Theta}, 0.5 + \frac{0.5}{1 + \omega\Theta}\right]$$

squashes $\pi$ towards 0.5, and the higher the value of $\omega$ or $\Theta$ the stronger the squashing is.

## 3 Data and Estimation Process

We use the same dataset as [10], produced during a modelling competition described by Jakubczyk et al. [8]. In our approach, there are 31 parameters to be estimated: five pairs for dimension importance, 15 weights $w_{i,j}$, four $\tau$s, $\kappa$, and $\omega$.

The data set consists of 81,480 stated preferences over pairs of health states for 1560 different combinations of pairs health states. We will denote a unique pair health states as $((A_i, T_{A_i}), (B_i, T_{B_i}))$, where $i \in \{1, 2, \ldots, 1560\}$. For every $i$, we have an information how many responses in total were given, denoted as $n_i$, how many respondents chose state $(A_i, T_{A_i})$, denoted as $a_i$. Obviously, the number of times $(B_i, T_{B_i})$ was chosen amounts to $b_i = n_i - a_i$. We let $P_{A,i}$ denote the probability that $(A_i, T_{A_i})$ was chosen, and similarly $P_{B,i}$ denotes the probability that $(B_i, T_{B_i})$ was chosen. The probabilities $P_{A,i}$ and $P_{B,i}$ are calculated using the formula described in Sect. 2.

We used maximum-likelihood to obtain the estimates of the model parameters. The formula for maximized log-likelihood is:

$$\sum_{i=1}^{1560} a_i \ln(P_{A_i}) + b_i \ln(P_{B_i}).$$

The optimization process was performed using the Nelder-Mead method and was implemented in Julia [1]. The optimization procedure used the penalty method, to ensure that $\kappa \in [-1, 1]$, $l_i \le h_i$, $\omega \ge 0$ and $0 \le w_{1,j} < w_{2,j} < w_{3,j} \le 1$.

We calculate 95% confidence intervals (CIs) of parameters based on 200 bootstrap replicates of the estimation process.

# 4 Results

The estimation results are presented in Tables 1, 2 and 3, containing the information on the importance of individual dimensions, relative level importance, and other parameters, respectively.

For the estimated parameters the following constraints were binding. Firstly, condition $l_i \leq h_i$ for $i$ equal to 1 and 2. This result is quite intuitive, as we can expect that regarding mobility and self care people have good understanding of the dimension meaning (hence, importance) and have low uncertainty in the assessment of the disutility. Still, in another dataset or under some other specification, we might expect some non-degenerate intervals, denoting some imprecision.

Secondly, in the anxiety/depression dimension, the disutility of levels 4 and 5 was estimated as equal: the respondents cannot really say the difference between extreme

**Table 1** Results: dimensions importance (bounds of the interval defining the disutility)

| Dimension | $l_i; h_i$ | 95%CI($l_i$); 95%CI($h_i$) |
|---|---|---|
| Mobility ($i = 1$) | 0.3927; 0.3927 | [0.3513, 0.4357]; [0.3567, 0.4381] |
| Self-care ($i = 2$) | 0.3845; 0.3845 | [0.3410, 0.4203]; [0.3481, 0.4402] |
| Usual activities ($i = 3$) | 0.2663; 0.3569 | [0.1911, 0.3357]; [0.2893, 0.4380] |
| Pain/discomfort ($i = 4$) | 0.5622; 0.6822 | [0.4713, 0.6175]; [0.5846, 0.8263] |
| Anxiety/depression ($i = 5$) | 0.3776; 0.5544 | [0.2987, 0.4275]; [0.4964, 0.6459] |

**Table 2** Results: relative level importance

| Level | Dimensions | | | | |
|---|---|---|---|---|---|
| | Mobility | Self-care | Usual activities | Pain/discomfort | Anxiety/depression |
| $1^a$ | 0.0000 | 0.0000 | 0.0000 | 0.0000 | 0.0000 |
| 2 | 0.1877 | 0.0418 | 0.3610 | 0.1127 | 0.2248 |
| 3 | 0.2469 | 0.1275 | 0.4279 | 0.2104 | 0.4474 |
| 4 | 0.6929 | 0.6049 | 0.8765 | 0.7198 | 1.0000 |
| $5^a$ | 1.0000 | 1.0000 | 1.0000 | 1.0000 | 1.0000 |

$^a$ by definition

**Table 3** Results: other parameters

| Parameter | Value | 95% CI |
|---|---|---|
| $\tau_1$ | 0.1492 | [0.1301, 0.1719] |
| $\tau_2$ | 0.4544 | [0.4017, 0.5281] |
| $\tau_3$ | 0.4376 | [0.3851, 0.5319] |
| $\tau_4$ | 0.4813 | [0.4175, 0.5701] |
| $\kappa$ | −0.2922 | [−0.6900, 0.2096] |
| $\omega$ | 0.7871 | [0.5253, 1.6544] |

and severe anxiety/depression. Again, this is unsurprising as the reversals between levels 4 and 5 were observed in the past in the last two dimensions (see [5], we do not observe this effect for pain/discomfort in our data, however).

Most of the estimation results were stable (as measured by 95% CIs). The only two parameters that have relatively uncertain estimates are $\kappa$ and $\omega$. However, in both cases the uncertainty of the estimate does not significantly influence the qualitative conclusions drawn from the results. Firstly, $\kappa$ is much lower than 1 which means that within-criterion comparisons are simpler than between-criteria ones, and thus new $\boxminus$ operator introduced in this paper proves useful: when we are comparing two imprecisely-perceived alternatives we must account for the source of imprecision and how much this imprecision may overlap (hence, cancel out in the comparison).

Secondly $\omega$ is significantly greater than zero, so we can observe the effect that the more difficult the comparison is (the more fuzziness is present) the more erratic responses we can expect.

The estimated values of $\tau$ are quite surprising. The values $\tau_2 - \tau_4$ are practically identical, suggesting that it is the number of units rather than the actual length (that also results from the type of unit) matters for preferences. More research is needed to understand it fully; in particular, DCE with mixed units would be useful in this respect (e.g. months vs. years).

## 5   Final Remarks

We have shown that using fuzzy (interval) approach to modeling the preferences for health states is possible, adding to the current literature, e.g. [7], [9], or [10]. The central contribution of the present paper is proposing a new operator $\boxminus$, that can differentiate between within- and between-criteria comparisons, and showing that in actual data this operator is useful (i.e. estimated $\kappa$ is well below 1). Further research is required to fully define $\boxminus$ in the context of more general fuzzy numbers. Another line of further research is to account for imprecisely-perceived weights of levels.

More datasets are needed to understand how time is perceived in DCE involving health states with duration (but that was not the goal of the present study). Due to the lack of preformed preferences, the respondents may be very fragile to framing effect, and the selection of time unit may greatly impact how the alternatives are perceived. Still, in the present dataset, the time could be modeled using non-linear transformations to account for discounting. That could also impact the estimate of the relative impact of the time units used.

There is nothing particular about health states as decision alternatives studied in the present paper; hence, the ideas we introduced can well be used in other settings when available alternatives are compared with respect to several criteria, each evaluated at several levels. Obviously, using the $\boxminus$ operator makes sense for criteria with at least three levels, when non-degenerate intervals are being subtracted.

In the present study, we drew conclusions based on the point estimates and 95% CIs; in the future research, an attempt can be made to confirm if the imprecision modelling improves the predictive validity of the models [8].

**Acknowledgements** The research was financed by the funds obtained from National Science Centre, Poland, granted following the decision number DEC-2015/19/B/HS4/01729.

# References

1. Bezanson, J., Edelman, A., Karpinski, S., Shah, V.B.: Julia: a fresh approach to numerical computing. SIAM Rev. **59**, 65–98 (2017)
2. Bleichrodt, H., Wakker, P., Johannesson, M.: Characterizing QALYs by risk neutrality. J. Risk. Uncertainty **15**, 107–114 (1997)
3. Brooks, R., De Charro, F.: EuroQol: the current state of play. Health Policy **37**, 53–72 (1996)
4. Couso, I., Dubois, D.: Statistical reasoning with set-valued information: Ontic vs. epistemic views. Int. J. Approximate Reasoning **55**, 1502–1518 (2014)
5. Craig, B., Pickard, A., Rand-Hendriksen, K.: Do health preferences contradict ordering of EQ-5D labels? Qual. Life Res. **24**, 1759–1765 (2015)
6. Herdman, M., Gudex, C., Lloyd, A., Janssen, M., Kind, P., Parkin, D., Bonsel, G., Badia, X.: Development and preliminary testing of the new five-level version of EQ-5D (EQ-5D-5L). Qual. Life Res.: Int. J. Qual. Life Aspects Treat. Care Rehabil. **20**, 1727–1736 (2011)
7. Jakubczyk, M., Golicki, D.: Estimating the fuzzy trade-offs between health dimensions with standard time trade-off data. In: Kacprzyk, J., Szmidt, E., Zadrozny, S., Atanassov, K.T., Krawczak, M. (eds.) Advances in Fuzzy Logic and Technology 2017 pp. 266–277. Springer International Publishing (2018)
8. Jakubczyk, M., Craig, B., Barra, M., Groothuis-Oudshoorn, C., Hartman, J., Huynh, E., Ramos-Goñi, J., Stolk, E., Rand-Hendriksen, K.: Choice defines value: a predictive modeling competition in health preference research. Value Health **21**, 229–238 (2017)
9. Jakubczyk, M., Kamiński, B., Lewandowski, M.: Eliciting fuzzy preferences towards health states with discrete choice experiments. In: Berger-Vachon, C., Gil Lafuente, A.M., Kacprzyk, J., Kondratenko, Y., Merigó, J.M., Morabito, C.F. (eds.) Complex Systems: Solutions and Challenges in Economics, Management and Engineering: Dedicated to Professor Jaime Gil Aluja, pp. 131–147. Springer International Publishing (2018)
10. Kamiński, B., Jakubczyk, M.: Comparing the crisp and fuzzy approaches to modelling preferences towards health states. Multiple Criteria Decis. Making **12**, 75–89 (2017)
11. McDonough, C., Grove, M., Tosteson, T., Lurie, J., Hilibrand, A., Tosteson, A.: Comparison of EQ-5D, HUI, and SF-36-derived societal health state values among spine patient outcomes research trial (SPORT) participants. Qual. Life Res. **14**, 1321–1332 (2005)
12. Rowen, D., Brazier, J., Van Hout, B.: A comparison of methods for converting DCE values onto the full health-dead QALY scale. Med. Decis. Making **35**, 328–340 (2015)
13. Yager, R.: Set-based representations of conjunctive and disjunctive knowledge. Inf. Sci. **41**, 1–22 (1987)
14. Zadeh, L.: Fuzzy sets. Inf. Control **8**, 338–353 (1965)
15. Zadeh, L.: PRUF–a meaning representation language for natural languages. Int. J. Man-Mach. Stud. **10**, 395–460 (1978)

# Optimal Control of Breast Cancer: Investigating Estrogen as a Risk Factor

S. I. Oke, M. B. Matadi and S. S. Xulu

**Abstract** Breast cancer is the most common cancer in women both in the developed and underdeveloped world. In this paper, the dynamics of breast cancer disease is modeled in the presence of two control strategies. The model describes evolution of the cancer in the body system when anti-cancer drugs and ketogenic-diet are implemented as control strategies against the tumor cells. We analysed the necessary and sufficient conditions, optimality and transversality conditions using Pontryagin Maximum Principle. We conclude through numerical simulations that estrogen level need to be monitored and combination of the two control is the best to reduce tumor-size and toxicity side effects.

**Keywords** Breast cancer · Optimal control · Maximum principle · Ketogenic diet

## 1 Introduction

Cancer occurs as a result of mutations, or abnormal changes in the genes responsible for regulating the growth of cells and keeping them healthy. The genes in each cell's nucleus, acts as the control room of each cell. Cancer prevalence has been on the increase due to an aging and growing World population, as well as the choices of cancer-causing lifestyle and behaviours such as alcohol, smoking, Hormone Replacement Therapy (HRT) [1]. Cancer is a leading cause of morbidity and mortality worldwide, yet much is still unknown about its mechanism of establishment and destruction. According to World Health Organization report [2], approximately 14.1 million new cancer were diagnosed (excluding non-melanoma skin cancer cases) and 8.2 million cancer-related deaths were recorded. The same report indicated that more than 60% of cancer cases occurred in Africa, Asia, Central and South America. These regions account for over 60% of all documented cancer mortality.

S. I. Oke (✉) · M. B. Matadi · S. S. Xulu
Department of Mathematical Sciences, University of Zululand, Private Bag X1001,
KwaDlangezwa 3886, South Africa
e-mail: segunoke2016@gmail.com

© Springer Nature Switzerland AG 2018

451

D. M. Kilgour et al. (eds.), *Recent Advances in Mathematical
and Statistical Methods*, Springer Proceedings in Mathematics & Statistics 259,
https://doi.org/10.1007/978-3-319-99719-3_41

It is predicted that 13 million death will erupt worldwide by the year 2030 [2]. However, Sub-Saharan Africa recorded the highest morbidity (25.5%) and mortality (23.2%) of all breast cancer cases in women globally [2].

The present study will focus on breast cancer which is common among women due to hormonal imbalance *estrogen* as one of the risk factors that is responsible for tumor growth in the breast. The biological implications of mathematical models concerning tumor-normal competition and breast cancer dynamics have been previously studied by number of authors such as [3–8]. Most notably, [6] investigated the effects of excess estrogen on breast cancer dynamics with an addition of an immune cell compartment to model the body's natural response on tumor growth. The authors were able to established equilibrium points as well as both local and global stability conditions. The aim of this paper is to study an optimal control model of breast cancer by considering two control measures, such as: anti-cancer drugs and ketogenic-diet as form of treatments.

Similarly, [5] worked on anti-angiogenic therapy as a therapeutic technique in cancer therapy to prevent the development of tumor through the supply of blood needed for the tumor growth. The authors further used geometric optimal control theory which enabled a further analysis to complete the solution. However, for each of these models in [5, 9] complete mathematical analysis of the strategy of optimal control was done. The authors further applied optimal control only to contain one interval where generally available inhibitors are subject to at maximum dose for the model.

Chemotherapy is the use of therapeutic drugs such as Tamoxifen to destroy malignant tumor cells. However, chemotherapy is known to have side effects and it is also very expensive when it is used alone to combat cancer cells [10]. Recently, combination of ketogenic diet and chemotherapy is proposed to have a synergistic potency in the treatment and control of tumor cells [11]. Ketogenic diet is a diet which is rich in triglyceride (fats or lipids) and low in protein and carbohydrate. In addition, in the body ketogenic diet. metabolised into free-fatty acid which is used as a source of energy by the cells due to little or no glucose postprandial. Cancer cells lack glucose to survive due to ketogenic-diet. Recently [8], an extension of this work was done by the same authors. The authors analyzed the stabilities of the model to get equilibria points,using Routh-Hurwitz method to established basic reproduction number, Uncertainty and sensitivity analysis and the existence of an optimal control were also considered.

We carried out detailed qualitative optimal control analysis of the resulting model and found the necessary conditions for optimal control of the breast cancer using Pontryagin's Maximum Principle [12] in order to determine optimal strategies for combating the tumor growth and metastasis.

Our goal are: first to investigate the model under the assumption that:

- the control measures are constants ( that is use of anti-cancer drugs and ketogenic diet)

- set up an optimal control problem relatively to the model. In order to achieve this, we used the following control parameters: anti-cancer drugs ($u_1$), ketogenic diet ($u_2$) as time dependent variables.

The organization of the paper is as follows, in Sect. 2, we formulated a model consisting of ordinary differential equations that describes the dynamics of breast cancer and the underlying assumption. In Sect. 3, we employed Pontryagin's Maximum Principle to investigate analysis of control strategies and to determine the necessary conditions for the optimal control of the disease. In Sect. 4, we discussed the existence of the optimal control system for the model and characterization of optimal control using Pontryagin's Maximum Principle [12]. In Sect. 5, we showed and discuss the simulation results.

## 2 Model Formulation

We developed our model by assuming logistic (Verhulst) growth of cell population and basis competition between normal cells and tumor cells. We considered the immune cells compartment to comprise of Natural Killer cells (NK) and $CD8^+$ T-cells as in [6] and we used similar equation to model the immune response dynamic by introducing immune booster (ketone bodies) and to check the efficacy of anti-cancer drug.

We adapted estrogen equation as presented in a model by Pinho et al. [13]. Pinho and Coworker [13], considered that a chemotherapy agent as continuously infused into the body engulfed by different cell populations and natural death can occur. We handled excess estrogen in a similar way and assumed that it is saturated daily through birth control (constant source rate) $(1 - k)$ which was introduced to serve as anti-cancer drug efficacy (e.g Tamoxifen) in order to bind estrogen receptors positive ($ER_+$) and to reduce excess estrogen from promoting tumor growth [14].

In this study, we reflected on the model that splits the entire population P(t) of cells of the human breast tissues at any given period of time (t) into four compartments known as:

$$
\begin{aligned}
\frac{dN}{dt} &= N \left( \alpha_1 - \mu_1 N - \phi_1 T \right) - (1 - k) \left( \lambda_1 N E \right) \\
\frac{dT}{dt} &= T \left( \alpha_2 d - \mu_2 T \right) - \gamma_2 M T - \mu_5 T + (1 - k) \left( \lambda_1 N E \right) \\
\frac{dM}{dt} &= s\beta + \frac{\rho M T}{\omega + T} - \gamma_3 M T - \mu_3 M - \left( (1 - k) \frac{\lambda_3 M E}{g + E} \right) \\
\frac{dE}{dt} &= (1 - k) \epsilon - \mu_4 E
\end{aligned}
\tag{1}
$$

where; $N(t) =$ Normal cells, $T(t) =$ Tumor cells, $M(t) =$ Immune response, $E(t) =$ Estrogen.

## 3 Optimal Control

Control variable was introduced into system (1) time dependent treatment efforts $u_1(t)$ and preventive measures $u_2(t)$ as control to curtail the spread of cancerous cells in the body system. Thus system (1) becomes

$$
\begin{aligned}
\frac{dN}{dt} &= N(\alpha_1 - \mu_1 N - \phi_1 T N) - (1 - u_1(t))(\lambda_1 N E) \\
\frac{dT}{dt} &= (1 - u_2(t)) T(\alpha_2 - \mu_2 T - \gamma_2 M - \mu_5) + (1 - u_1(t))(\lambda_1 N E) \\
\frac{dM}{dt} &= s\beta + \frac{\rho M T}{\omega + T} - \gamma_3 M T - \mu_3 M - \left((1 - u_1(t))\frac{\lambda_3 M E}{g + E}\right) \\
\frac{dE}{dt} &= (1 - u_1(t))\epsilon - \mu_4 E
\end{aligned}
\tag{2}
$$

Where;
$u_1(t)$ is the treatment effort using anti-cancer drugs by the patient
$u_2(t)$ is the time preventive control using ketogenic-diet in order to starve cancer cells.

### 3.1 Extension of System (2) to Optimal Control Problem

In the previous section, the controls on disease (ketogenic-diet, immune booster and anti-cancer treatment) are considered as constants hence no cost determination is taken care of which will be incurred in their implementation. In this section, we formulated a corresponding optimal control problem for the model in system (2) considering the ketogenic diet and chemotherapy as control interventions to minimize the cancer prevalence and corresponding economic burden. Optimal control technique has been used successfully to determine the relevant control strategy with optimal cost [15]. A few of the studies relevant to control problem are described in the following [15–18].

The system (2) which involves a system of coupled non-linear differential equation and two controls will be introduced with initial conditions given at $t = 0$.

### 3.2 The Associated Interaction of Normal Cells and Tumor Cells:

As tumor formation rate increases due to DNA damaging by excess estrogen, the tumor cells population increases as the density of normal cells population (that is prone to be cancerous), we implemented a measure that reduced the interaction by $(1 - u_1(t))$, where $u_1(t)$ measures the level of successful treatment efforts, which has practical advantages in the reduction of the cancer prevalence during the dead-free tumor or co-existing free tumor metastasis. The control variable $u_1(t)$ denoted the use of anti-cancer drugs which are alternative preventive measures to minimize the growth or eliminate tumor from the body system, such as: the use of Tamoxifen or Taxol = Paclitaxel.

### 3.2.1  Ketogenic Diet to Tumor Cells Population:

The ketogenic diet to tumor cells $u_2$ is chosen at time dependent control intervention as $u_2(t)$. A control variable that represents the level of ketogenic diet in which a cancer patient is placed on is $u_2(t)$. Ketogenic diet will aid the starvation of tumor from receiving necessary nutrient and glucose from the body system. It follows that the growth rate of the tumor population will be reduced by a factor $(1 - u_2(t))$. $u_2$ also serves as measures for level of successful prevention (personal protection efforts) [19–27]. Thus, our main objective is to investigate the optimal way for the control policies which minimized the economic load as well as disease prevalence.

### 3.2.2  Determination of the Total Cost

We first determined the total cost incurred due to implementation of control policies and burden of breast cancer which eventually will be minimized in this study. Therefore, weighted sum of the total cost incurred is described as follow:

(i) Cost incurred due to breast cancer: is the weighted cost due to opportunity lost of the cancer patient [15] and given as:

$$\int_0^{T_f} (A_1 T(t) + A_2 E(t)) \, dt \tag{3}$$

many factors are responsible for the opportunity loss e.g loss in efficiency due to sickness, loss of manpower, loss realised in searching for treatment and protection, patient caring etc [28].

(ii) Cost incurred in treatment: this is the cost that provides treatment to tumor cells population during the metastasis stage and is given as:

$$\int_0^{T_f} \left( \frac{1}{2} A_3 u_1^2(t) \right) dt \tag{4}$$

the total weighted cost incurred in treatment includes the costs of efforts made on treatment process, scanning through mammography or X-rays, cost of

medication, diagnosis charges, cost of admission in the hospital during the
period of providing treatment.

(iii) Cost incurred in ketogenic diet: the weighted sum of cost realised in ketogenic
diet nutritions which includes the cost of restricted diet that will starve tumor
cells from getting necessary nutrient from the body system is given as:

$$\int_0^{T_f} \left( \frac{1}{2} A_4 u_2^2(t) \right) dt \tag{5}$$

Based on the state of severity and effect of treatment on tumor cells population, we
considered a nonlinear relationship between cost, efforts made on ketogenic diet and
treatments.

Hence, we define the control problem as per the above discussion for control
policies and cost incurred. Thus, the objective function which has to be minimized is:

$$J_1(u_1, u_2) = \int_0^{T_f} \left( A_1 T(t) + A_2 E(t) + \frac{1}{2} A_3 u_1^2(t) + \frac{1}{2} A_4 u_2^2(t) \right) dt \tag{6}$$

$\min_{J_1(u_1,u_2)} (u_1, u_2 \in U)$     $U = \{u_1(t) \ \& \ u_2(t) : 0 \leqslant u_1(t) \leqslant u_{1max}, 0 \leqslant u_2(t) \leqslant u_{1max}, t \in [0, T_f]\}$ and $u_1$ and $u_2$ are Lebesgue measurable subject to the model
system (2):

$$\frac{dN}{dt} = N\alpha_1 - \mu_1 N^2 - \phi_1 TN - (1 - u_1(t))(\lambda_1 NE)$$

$$\frac{dT}{dt} = (1 - u_2(t)) T\alpha_2 - \mu_2 T^2 - \gamma_2 MT - \mu_5 T + (1 - u_1(t))(\lambda_1 NE)$$

$$\frac{dM}{dt} = s\beta + \frac{\rho MT}{\omega + T} - \gamma_3 MT - \mu_3 M - \left( (1 - u_1(t)) \frac{\lambda_3 ME}{g + E} \right) \tag{7}$$

$$\frac{dE}{dt} = (1 - u_1(t)) \epsilon - \mu_4 E$$

follow the initial conditions $N(0) \geqslant 0$, $T(0) \geqslant 0$, $M(0) \geqslant 0$, & $E(0) \geqslant 0$.

The objective function $J_1$ represents the total cost incurred as a result of application of control plans and breast cancer burden. However, the temporal cost is
measured by the integrand.

$$L(N, T, M, E, u_1, u_2) = A_1 T(t) + A_2 E(t) + \frac{1}{2} A_3 u_1^2(t) + \frac{1}{2} A_4 u_2^2(t) \tag{8}$$

Where $A_1$, $A_2$, $A_3$ & $A_4$ are positive weight constants related with the cost in unit
effort and also balance the units integrand. For convenience, we consider $u_1(t) = u_1$ & $u_2(t) = u_2$.

## 3.3 Analysis of Optimal Control

We applied Pontryagin's Maximum Principle [12], to characterize the optimal control pair $u_1^*$ & $u_2^*$ in the following results.

**Theorem 1** *Given optimal control variables $u_1^*$ & $u_2^*$ and $N^*$, $T^*$, $M^*$ & $E^*$ are corresponding optimal state variables of the control system (6) and (7). Then there exists adjoint variables*
$\theta = (\theta_1, \theta_2, \theta_3, \theta_4) \in \Re_+^4$ *that satisfies the following equations.*

$$\frac{d\theta_1}{dt} = 2\theta_1 \mu_1 N + \phi_1 \theta_1 T + (\theta_1 + \theta_2)(1 - u_2(t))\lambda_1 E - \alpha_1 \theta_1$$

$$\frac{d\theta_2}{dt} = -A_1 + \theta_1 \phi_1 N + \theta_2 (2T\mu_2 + \gamma_2 M + \mu_5 - \alpha_2(1 - u_2)) + \theta_3 \left(\gamma_3 M - \frac{\rho \omega M}{(\omega + T)^2}\right)$$

$$\frac{d\theta_3}{dt} = \theta_2 \gamma_2 T - \rho \theta_3 T + \gamma_3 \theta_3 T + \mu_3 \theta_3 + \theta_3 \left((1 - u_1)\frac{\lambda_1 E}{g + E}\right)$$

$$\frac{d\theta_4}{dt} = -A_2 + (\theta_1 - \theta_2)(1 - u_1)\lambda_1 N - \theta_3 \left((1 - u_1)\frac{\lambda_3 M g}{(g + E)^2}\right) - \theta_4 \mu_4$$

$$\tag{9}$$

*with transversality conditions*
$\theta_1(T_f) = \theta_2(T_f) = \theta_3(T_f) = \theta_4(T_f) = 0$
*The corresponding optimal controls $u_1^*$ & $u_2^*$ are given as,*

$$u_1^* = min\left\{max\left\{0, \frac{1}{A_3}\left(\theta_2\lambda_1 N^* E^* + \theta_3\epsilon - \theta_1\lambda_1 N^* E^* - \frac{\theta_3\lambda_3 M^* E^*}{g + E^*}\right)\right\}, u_{1max}\right\}$$

$$\tag{10}$$

*and*

$$u_2^* = min\left\{max\left\{0, \frac{1}{A_4}\left(\theta_2\alpha_2 T^*\right)\right\}, u_{2max}\right\} \tag{11}$$

*Proof* Let $u_1^*$ & $u_2^*$ be the given optimal control functions and $N^*$, $T^*$, $M^*$ & $E^*$ be the corresponding optimal state variables of the system (7) which minimizes the cost functional or objective (6). Then by Pontryagin's Maximum Principle [12], there exists adjoint variables $\theta_1, \theta_2, \theta_3,$ & $\theta_4$ which satisfies the following equations:

$$\frac{d\theta_1}{dt} = -\frac{\partial H}{\partial N}, \quad \frac{d\theta_2}{dt} = -\frac{\partial H}{\partial T}, \quad \frac{d\theta_3}{dt} = -\frac{\partial H}{\partial M}, \quad \frac{d\theta_4}{dt} = -\frac{\partial H}{\partial E}$$

with transversality conditions
$\theta_1(T_f) = \theta_2(T_f) = \theta_3(T_f) = \theta_4(T_f) = 0$
where H is the Hamiltonian and defined as:

$$H(N, T, M, E, u_1, u_2, \theta) = L(N, T, M, E, u_1, u_2) + \theta_1 N' + \theta_2 T' + \theta_3 M' + \theta_4 E'$$

$$\tag{12}$$

$$H = \begin{cases} A_1T(t) + A_2E(t) + \frac{1}{2}A_3u_1^2(t) + \frac{1}{2}A_4u_2^2(t) \\ +\theta_1\left(N\alpha_1 - \mu_1N^2 - \phi_1TN - (1 - u_1(t))\,(\lambda_1NE)\right) \\ +\theta_2\left((1 - u_2(t))\,T\alpha_2 - \mu_2T^2 - \gamma_2MT - \mu_5T + (1 - u_1(t))\,(\lambda_1NE)\right) \\ +\theta_3\left(s\beta + \frac{\rho MT}{\omega+T} - \gamma_3MT - \mu_3M - \left((1 - u_1(t))\,\frac{\lambda_3ME}{g+E}\right)\right) \\ +\theta_4\left((1 - u_1(t))\,\epsilon - \mu_4E\right) \end{cases}$$

from the optimality condition, we have
$\frac{\partial H}{\partial u_1} = 0$, at $u_1 = u_1^*$ and $\frac{\partial H}{\partial u_2} = 0$, at $u_2 = u_2^*$ which implies that,

$$0 = \frac{\partial H}{\partial u_1} = A_3u_1 + \theta_1\lambda_1NE - \theta_2\lambda_1NE + \theta_3\frac{\lambda_3ME}{g+E} - \theta_4\epsilon \tag{13}$$

$$0 = \frac{\partial H}{\partial u_1} = A_4u_2 - \theta_2\alpha_2T \tag{14}$$

Hence, we obtain (see [29])

$$u_1^* = \frac{1}{A_3}\left\{\theta_1\lambda_1NE + \theta_4\epsilon - \theta_1\lambda_1NE - \theta_3\frac{\lambda_3ME}{g+E}\right\} \tag{15}$$

$$u_2^* = \frac{1}{A_4}\left\{\theta_2\alpha_2T\right\} \tag{16}$$

Thus we have, (15) and (16).
By standard control arguments involving the bounds on the controls, we conclude

$$u_1^* = \begin{cases} 0 & \text{if } \frac{1}{A_3}\left(\theta_1\lambda_1NE + \theta_4\epsilon - \theta_1\lambda_1NE - \theta_3\frac{\lambda_3ME}{g+E}\right) < 0 \\ \frac{1}{A_3}\left(\theta_1\lambda_1NE + \theta_4\epsilon - \theta_1\lambda_1NE - \theta_3\frac{\lambda_3ME}{g+E}\right) \\ \quad \text{if } 0 \leqslant \frac{1}{A_3}\left(\theta_1\lambda_1NE + \theta_4\epsilon - \theta_1\lambda_1NE - \theta_3\frac{\lambda_3ME}{g+E}\right) \leqslant 1 \\ 1 & \text{if } \frac{1}{A_3}\left(\theta_1\lambda_1NE + \theta_4\epsilon - \theta_1\lambda_1NE - \theta_3\frac{\lambda_3ME}{g+E}\right) > 1 \end{cases}$$

and

$$u_2^* = \begin{cases} 0 & \text{if } \frac{1}{A_4}\left(\theta_2\alpha_2T^*\right) < 0 \\ \frac{1}{A_4}\left(\theta_2\alpha_2T^*\right) & \text{if } 0 \leqslant \frac{1}{A_4}\left(\theta_2\alpha_2T^*\right) \leqslant 1 \\ 1 & \text{if } \frac{1}{A_4}\left(\theta_2\alpha_2T^*\right) > 1 \end{cases}$$

However, we discuss the numerical solution of the optimality system and the corresponding results of varying the optimal controls $u_1$ & $u_2$ the parameter choices, and the interpretations from various cases.

# 4　Numerical Simulation and Discussion

In this section, we numerically investigated the effect of the optimal control strategies on breast cancer using estrogen as a risk factor. We investigated the process of one or both control strategies for minimal cost and breast cancer burden treatments on economy. The optimal control is acquired by solving the optimality system of four ordinary differential equations from the state variables and adjoint system. An iterative scheme is used to solve the optimality system. All the numerical simulations executed in MAPLE 18. We employed the forward-backward scheme method, beginning with an initial guess for optimal controls and solve the optimal state system forward in time and after that solved the adjoint state system backward in forward using finite difference scheme in MAPLE. The two controls were then updated by using a convex combination of the previous controls as well as the characterization (15) and (16). The entire process is repeated until the values of the unknown at the previous iterations are closed to the one at the current iteration [12, 29]. A mathematical modeling of breast cancer in the presence of ketogenic diet and chemotherapy as a control for tumor metastasis is designed.

Outcomes obtained without control are compared to those from the different strategies applied simultaneously. For numerical analysis, the weight factors used are $A_1 = 20, A_2 = 150, A_3 = 15, A_4 = 50$. The values used here were intended only for theoretical purposes to investigate the effect of various control practices. For example, $A_1$ & $A_2$ represented weight cost due to opportunity loss of the breast cancer patient, $A_3$ is the weighted cost for providing treatment (chemotherapy) to reduce or eliminate tumor cells growth in the body system. $A_4$ is the cost incurred during restricted diet ( ketogenic diet) that starved tumor cells from getting necessary nutrient and glucose from the body system. All control variables were constrained between zero and one ($0 \leqslant u_i(t) \leqslant 1, \ i = 1, 2$) when control is set to zero, it implies that there is no therapy apply and when it is one, the maximum control therapy or strategy is invested.

Figure 1, represents the tumor cells population (T) with and without control for different values of $u_1$ and $u_2$. In the absence of control, the tumor cells population (solid red line) is increase in less than Twenty days until all the normal cells crowd-out in the breast. In the presence of controls, the (dash green line) shows that the tumor growth or metastasis is being hindered due to the combination of the treatment and tumor cells population drastically reduced. Similarly, Fig. 2 represents the number or level of estrogen (E) in the body with and without controls for different values of $u_1$ and $u_2$. When there are no controls, the estrogen level reach maximum level in Hundred days while in the presence of controls (solid green line), the estrogen level reduced drastically. Figure 3 shows the effectiveness of ketogenic-diet parameter

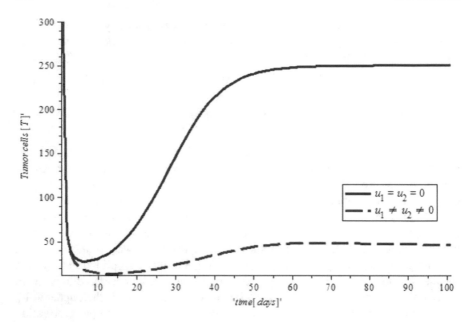

**Fig. 1** Simulation result of the model (7), showing Tumor cells population against Time with and without control

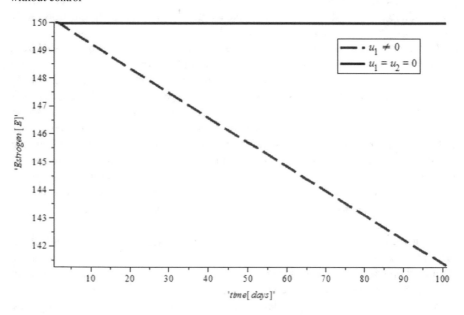

**Fig. 2** Simulation result of the model (7), showing Estrogen Level and Immune response against Time with and without control

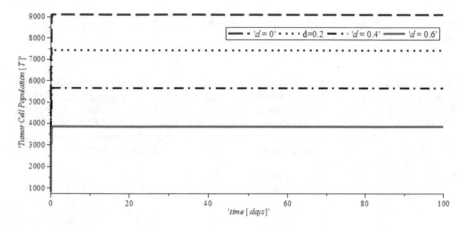

**Fig. 3** The variation of proportion of Tumor cell population for different for different values of $d$ with other parameters fixed

using values. Thus, for us to avoid *ketoacidosis*, ketogenic-diet parameter should not go above $d = 0.6$.

## 5  Conclusions

Breast cancer pose immense economic burden which particularly includes opportunity loss, health care related expenditures, losses due to mortality and dependent's care, and loss of work etc. Also, the costs for implementing control interventions such as medicine, ketogenic diet among others. are involved. Thus for policy makers, it is not only significant to control the tumor cells metastasis but also to minimize the overall cost incurred over a specified time period. An ample choice for a control policy to evaluate a single control intervention or multiple control interventions depend on availability of resources.

The dynamics of breast cancer disease is described here by a four-compartment deterministic model where classes differ from one another such as: Normal cells, Tumor cells, Immune response and Estrogen. They are considered together with two control strategies implemented to reduce the number of tumor cells and cost of treating breast cancer. The results show that optimal control of breast cancer is possible through ketogenic-diet (nutritional diet) and anti-cancer drugs. The combination of those control strategies is needed for better results. However, support to the implementation of the control strategies against breast cancer should be encouraged to reduce the burden of the disease on the economy of the countries. This study has its limitation.

The weights on cost considered here are for illustrative reasons. The realistic outcomes will be obtained if data on the cost of the implementation of control strategies are available. Hence, authors in the future work will consider cost-effectiveness of the breast cancer disease.

**Acknowledgements** The corresponding author appreciate National Research Foundation (NRF), South Africa for the grant towards my Ph.D.; Grant Number: 109824. The authors also acknowledges the support of Research Office of University of Zululand for providing the funds for attending AMMCS2017, Canada. The authors are grateful to Adeniyi Michael (LASPOTECH, Nigeria) and Alex Adekiya (Unizulu) for their useful comments in the preparation of the manuscript. The authors are grateful to the anonymous Reviewers and the Handling Editor for their constructive comments, which have enhanced the paper.
**Conflicts of Interest:** The authors declare no conflicts of interest.

# References

1. Jemal, A., Bray, F., Center, M.M., Ferlay, J., Ward, E., Forman, D.: Global cancer statistic. Cancer J. Clin. **61**(2), 6990 (2011)
2. World Health Organization. Global Action Plan for the Prevention and Control on NCDs (2014)
3. Agusto, F.B.: Optimal chemoprophylaxis and treatment control strategies of a tuberculosis transmission model. World J. Modell. Simul. **5**(3), 163–173 (2009)
4. Ding, C., Tao, N., Zhu, Y.: A mathematical model of Zika virus and its optimal control. In: Control Conference (CCC), 2016 35th Chinese, pp. 2642–2645. IEEE (2016)
5. Ledzewicz, U., Schttler, H.: Antiangiogenic therapy in cancer treatment as an optimal control problem. SIAM J. Control Optim. **46**(3), 1052–1079 (2007)
6. Chipo, M., Sorofa, W., Chiyaka, E.T.: Assessing the effects of estrogen on the dynamics of breast cancer. Computation and Mathematical Methods in Medicine (2012)
7. Nana-Kyere, S., Ackora-Prah, J., Okyere, E., Marmah, S., Afram, T.: Hepatitis B optimal control model with vertical transmission. Appl. Math. **7**(1), 5–13 (2017)
8. Oke, S.I., Matadi, M.B., Xulu, S.S.: Optimal control analysis of a mathematical model for breast cancer. Math. Comput. Appl. **23**(2), 21 (2018)
9. Swierniak, A., Ledzewicz, U., Schattler, H.: Optimal control for a class of compartmental models in cancer chemotherapy. Int. J. Appl. Math. Comput. Sci. **13**(3), 357–368 (2003)
10. Allen, B.G., Bhatia, S.K., Anderson, C.M., Eichenberger-Gilmore, J.M., Sibenaller, Z.A., Mapuskar, K.A., Schoenfeld, J.D., Buatti, J.M., Spitz, D.R., Fath, M.A.: Ketogenic diets as an adjuvant cancer therapy: history and potential mechanism. Redox Biol. **2**, 963–970 (2014)
11. Champ, C.E., Palmer, J.D., Volek, J.S., Werner-Wasik, M., Andrews, D.W., Evans, J.J., Glass, J., Kim, L., Shi, W.: Targeting metabolism with a ketogenic diet during the treatment of glioblastoma multiforme. J. Neuro-Oncol. **117**(1), 125–131 (2014)
12. Pontryagin, L.S.: Mathematical Theory of Optimal Processes. CRC Press (1987)
13. Pinho, S.T.R.D., Freedman, H.I., Nani, F.: A chemotherapy model for the treatment of cancer with metastasis. Math. Comput. Modell. **36**(7–8), 773–803 (2002)
14. American Cancer Society. Breast Cancer (2013)
15. Kumar, A., Srivastava, P.K.: Vaccination and treatment as control interventions in an infectious disease model with their cost optimization. Commun. Nonlinear Sci. Numer. Simul. **44**, 334–343 (2017)
16. Gaff, H.D., Schaefer, E., Lenhart, S.: Use of optimal control models to predict treatment time for managing tick-borne disease. J. Biol. Dyn. **5**(5), 517–530 (2011)
17. Nannyonga, B., Mwanga, G.G., Luboobi, L.S.: An optimal control problem for ovine brucellosis with culling. J. Biol. Dyn. **9**(1), 198–214 (2015)
18. Okosun, K.O., Smith, R.: Optimal control analysis of malaria-schistosomiasis co-infection dynamics. Math. Biosci Eng.: MBE **14**(2), 377–405 (2017)

19. An, J., Tzagarakis-Foster, C., Scharschmidt, T.C., Lomri, N., Leitman, D.C.: Estrogen receptor $\beta - selective$ transcriptional activity and recruitment of coregulators by phytoestrogens. J. Biol. Chem. **276**(21), 17808–17814 (2001)
20. Coddington, E.A. Levinson, N.: Theory of Ordinary Differential Equations. Tata McGraw-Hill Education (1955)
21. Ding, C., Sun, Y., Zhu, Y.: A schistosomiasis compartment model with incubation and its optimal control. Math. Methods Appl. Sci. **40** (2017)
22. Fleming, W.H., Rishel, R.: Optimal deterministic and stochastic control. MATH, Applications of Mathematics. Springer Berlin (1975)
23. Fuqua, S.A., Wiltschke, C., Zhang, Q.X., Borg, Castles, C.G., Friedrichs, W.E., Hopp, T., Hilsenbeck, S., Mohsin, S., OConnell, P., Allred, D.C.: A hypersensitive estrogen $receptor - \alpha$ mutation in premalignant breast lesions. Cancer Res. **60**(15), 4026–4029 (2000)
24. Oesterreich, S., Zhang, P., Guler, R.L., Sun, X., Curran, E.M., Welshons, W.V., Osborne, C.K., Lee, A.V.: Re-expression of estrogen receptor $\alpha$ in estrogen receptor $\alpha - negative$ MCF-7 cells restores both estrogen and insulin-like growth factor-mediated signaling and growth. Cancer Res. **61**(15), 5771–5777 (2001)
25. Kimmel, M., Swierniak, A.: Control theory approach to cancer chemotherapy: Benefiting from phase dependence and overcoming drug resistance. In: Tutorials in Mathematical Biosciences III, pp. 185–221. Springer, Berlin, Heidelberg (2006)
26. House, S.W., Warburg, O., Burk, D., Schade, A.L.: On respiratory impairment in cancer cells. Science **124**(3215), 267–272 (1956)
27. Warburg, O.: On the origin of cancer cells. Science **123**(3191), 309–314 (1956)
28. Gaff, H., Schaefer, E.: Optimal control applied to vaccination and treatment strategies for various epidemiological models. Math. Biosci. Eng.: MBE **6**(3), 469–492 (2009)
29. Lenhart, S., Workman, J.T.: Optimal Control Applied to Biological Models. CRC Press (2007)

# Part VII

# Mathematics and Computation in Finance, Economics, and Social Sciences

# Dynamical Analysis of a Modified Prey-Predator Model for Venture Capital Investment

Letetia Mary Addison, Balswaroop Bhatt and David Owen

**Abstract** The Lotka-Volterra predator-prey model for population dynamics between prey and predator species, has been an important model in Biology for many years. Most recently, it has been used to explain the relationship between Venture Capital investment opportunities and the experience of the investors, which represent the prey and predator respectively. Our work extends this model to include a modification with two investment opportunities available to the venture capitalist. The dynamics of the system are investigated via analytical work and numerical simulations to obtain bifurcation points which affect the stability of the system. Results are presented numerically and graphically. In our study, parameters related to returns to investment experience, investment handling time, rate of conversion of investment opportunities and depreciation of investment experience have threshold values where the system switches from stable to unstable. The stability regions for each of these parameters display suitable ranges. This provides investors with guidance to invest only when these parameters are within the stability regions.

**Keywords** Prey-Predator · Venture capital · Stability · Bifurcations

## 1 Introduction

Venture Capital (VC) has developed into an important intermediary in financial markets, providing capital to firms that might otherwise have difficulty attracting financing [10]. Venture Capitalists (VCs) are wealthy investors who invest capital in

L. M. Addison (✉) · B. Bhatt · D. Owen
Department of Mathematics and Statistics, Faculty of Science and Technology, The University of the West Indies, St. Augustine Campus, St. Augustine, Trinidad and Tobago, Republic of Trinidad and Tobago
e-mail: letetia.addison@sta.uwi.edu; letetia.addison@gmail.com

B. Bhatt
e-mail: bal.bhatt@sta.uwi.edu

D. Owen
e-mail: drowentt@yahoo.com

© Springer Nature Switzerland AG 2018
D. M. Kilgour et al. (eds.), *Recent Advances in Mathematical and Statistical Methods*, Springer Proceedings in Mathematics & Statistics 259,
https://doi.org/10.1007/978-3-319-99719-3_42

start-up companies in hopes of high returns in the long run. VCs receive most of their funding from foundations with large amounts of capital, pension funds and endowments. According to [25], VC investors play a crucial role in incubating new firms by supplying them with VC. Research in [10] stated that the first true VC firm was American Research and Development, which consisted of a small group of business leaders who made risky investments for emerging technological companies in World War II. Since then, VC has been a vastly growing industry.

Previous research has considered its role in different aspects: [15] examined the innovation VC provided in terms of higher patenting rates while [5] assessed the geographical impact on the performance of VC firms. Several papers [7, 8, 14] have also examined methods to estimate risk and returns for private equity investment. These papers use methods such as the Capital Asset Pricing Model (CAPM) and Generalized Method of Moments (GMM) model, which mainly use statistical techniques to estimate the risk and return parameters for an investment.

Some papers have also explored the idea of the experience of VCs as it relates to the success of their investment. The idea here is that it is preferable to have a measure of experience that is specific to the match between the VCs and the entrepreneur [23]. Their research investigates this idea using the theory of a two-sided matching model involving Bayesian inference and Markov Chain Monte Carlo Methods. The findings are that investments by the most experienced investors are twice as likely to result in public offerings as investments by the least experienced investors [23].

Consequently, the impact of experience of investors on the investment has been examined extensively over the years. However, few papers have applied a prey-predator modelling approach to investigate investment dynamics. Research in [3] considered an endogenous idea to partially explain investment behavior. Here, the greater the level of VC investment, the greater the depletion of unexploited investment opportunities. They observed that VC investments in industry have similar cyclical patterns associated with the traditional biological Lotka-Volterra [16, 26] prey-predator model, with the investors acting like predators and the opportunities are similar to prey.

In addition, investment opportunities may borrow other analogous ideas from ecology such as herding and competition [13, 22]. Predators may also have the ability to switch to the abundant prey species in order to sustain the particular eco-system at hand [1, 12, 19]. The paper by [4] discussed the mathematical implications of prey switching [24] and its effects on economic and environmental sustainability in two situations: oil drilling and whale hunting.

Our paper applies this idea of prey-switching to VC investment in order to see its effects on the system and ultimately, the sustainability of investment. The prey-predator VC investment model is extended to include two sets of investment opportunities available to VCs from two different industries. The original model is improved with logistic growth in the prey opportunities and a switching mechanism [24], which allows VCs the optimal choice among investments. The introduction of these ideas into a VC model has not been studied thus far.

Hence, the aim of this work is to demonstrate the ideas of a prey-predator modelling to investigate the dynamics of a modified version of the Venture Capital investment model. The stability of the system is presented analytically and Hopf bifurcations for parameters are investigated numerically. Simulations are performed to study the behaviour of the system through time series graphs. Parameters representing returns to investment experience, investment handling time, rate of conversion of investment opportunities and depreciation of investment experience have bifurcation values where the system switches from stable to unstable. We recommend that the investor should invest only when these parameters are in the stable regions.

## 2 The Model

The following model is a modified version of the Venture Capital Investment model by [3]. A Rosenzweig and MacArthur [20] form of the original Lotka-Volterra [16, 26] predator-prey model is used with a more reasonable assumption of logistic growth rates in the prey populations. Consider a system of two investment opportunities available to a single VC investor. There is a switching mechanism where the VCs can switch to the investment which has the most profitable opportunities available.

$$
\frac{dP_1}{dt} = \rho_1 P_1 \left(1 - \frac{P_1}{K_1}\right) - \alpha_1 r_1(P) X^{\beta_1} P_1,
$$
$$
\frac{dP_2}{dt} = \rho_2 P_2 \left(1 - \frac{P_2}{K_2}\right) - \alpha_2 r_2(P) X^{\beta_2} P_2, \tag{1}
$$
$$
\frac{dX}{dt} = c_1 \alpha_1 r_1(P) X^{\beta_1} P_1 + c_2 \alpha_2 r_2(P) X^{\beta_2} P_2 - \delta X,
$$

where

$$
r_i(P) \equiv r_i(P_1, P_2) = \frac{1}{f_i(P_1, P_2)}, \qquad i = 1, 2, \tag{2}
$$
$$
f_1(P_1, P_2) = 1 + \frac{\gamma_2 P_2}{P_1},
$$
$$
f_2(P_1, P_2) = 1 + \frac{\gamma_1 P_1}{P_2}.
$$

PREY: $P_1$ and $P_2$ represent the investment opportunities available from the first and second industries respectively,
PREDATOR: $X$ represents the VCs experience measured via the size of the VC funds, where

$$
P_1, P_2, X \geq 0
$$

Parameters used in the model are all non-negative. For $i = 1, 2$:

$\alpha_i$  investment parameter for investment opportunities in industry $i$,
$\beta_i$  returns to experience for investment opportunities in industry $i$,
$\gamma_i$  handling time for investment opportunities in industry $i$,
$\rho_i$  natural growth rate of investment opportunities in industry $i$,
$c_i$  rate of conversion of VC funds into opportunities in industry $i$ funds,
$\delta$  depreciation rate of experience (death rate of VC fund),
$V_i$  a modified Cobb - Douglas [6] Investment function for opportunities in industry $i$ where $V = a_i r_i(P) X^{\beta_i} P_i$,
$r_i$  a functional response of the Venture Capitalists to the investment opportunities in industry $i$. It contains a built-in switching mechanism to switch [24] to the more profitable opportunity depending on the function, $f_i (P_1, P_2)$.

The assumptions of this model follow those outlined by [3]. The VCs experience in a particular company or industry is proportional to the profitability of the investment projects in that industry. The number of available projects also affects profitability of VC investments. It is also assumed that there is risk neutrality between investments and exogenous factors are ignored.

These ideas allow for less complication in the idea of the analysis and computations. In addition to these, we also incorporate additional mathematical assumptions, following those outlined in [2]:

**Assumption 1**  Each predatory function $r_i (P_1, P_2)$, $i = 1, 2$, is smooth and positive with a Taylor expansion about $(P_1^*, P_2^*)$ where $(P_1^*, P_2^*, X^*)$ is an equilibrium point of the system.

**Assumption 2**  The predatory functions $r_i (P_1, P_2)$, $i = 1, 2$, give the Venture Capitalist the ability to switch predation to the industry which has the larger number of investment opportunities between them. The following conditions hold:

1. $P_1 \gg P_2, r_1 (P_1, P_2) \to 1$ and $r_2 (P_1, P_2) \to 0$,
2. $P_1 \ll P_2, r_1 (P_1, P_2) \to 0$ and $r_2 (P_1, P_2) \to 1$.

Therefore, when there is a larger number of opportunities available in the first industry, the VC switches to make the investment in this industry and vice versa.

## 2.1  Existence of Positive Interior Equilibrium Point(s)

In order to find the steady state solutions of the equations in the original system, set each equation to zero. This gives:

$$\frac{dP_1}{dt} = \rho_1 P_1 \left(1 - \frac{P_1}{K_1}\right) - \alpha_1 r_1(P) X^{\beta_1} P_1 = 0, \tag{3}$$

$$\frac{dP_2}{dt} = \rho_2 P_2 \left(1 - \frac{P_2}{K_2}\right) - \alpha_2 r_2(P) X^{\beta_2} P_2 = 0, \tag{4}$$

$$\frac{dX}{dt} = c_1 \alpha_1 r_1(P) X^{\beta_1} P_1 + c_2 \alpha_2 r_2(P) X^{\beta_2} P_2 - \delta X = 0. \tag{5}$$

The system may have more than one positive interior equilibrium point. Let one such interior equilibrium point be $E = (P_1^*, P_2^*, X^*)$. For simplicity, the superscripts have been dropped in calculations. In order to find this point, set $P_1 = \overline{P}P_2$, where $\overline{P} > 0$ and after this substitution into $r_i(P_1, P_2)$, we get $r_i(\overline{P}P_2, P_2)$ and take this as $r_i$ (for $i = 1, 2$) in calculations.

Using Eqs. (3) and (4) and solving for $X$ respectively gives:

$$X = \left(\frac{\rho_1 (K_1 - \overline{P}P_2)}{\alpha_1 r_1 K_1}\right)^{\frac{1}{\beta_1}} \tag{6}$$

and

$$X = \left(\frac{\rho_2 (K_2 - P_2)}{\alpha_2 r_2 K_2}\right)^{\frac{1}{\beta_2}}. \tag{7}$$

Equating (6) and (7) give the following equation which must be satisfied by $\overline{P}$ and $P_2$:

$$(\alpha_2 r_2 K_2)^{\frac{1}{\beta_2}} \left(\rho_1 (K_1 - \overline{P}P_2)\right)^{\frac{1}{\beta_1}} = (\alpha_1 r_1 K_1)^{\frac{1}{\beta_1}} (\rho_2 (K_2 - P_2))^{\frac{1}{\beta_2}} \tag{8}$$

Also using (6) and (7), since $X$ must be positive (since it represents real populations), then the following inequalities must be satisfied:

$$\rho_1 (K_1 - \overline{P}P_2) > 0 \tag{9}$$

and

$$\rho_2 (K_2 - P_2) > 0. \tag{10}$$

Substituting Eqs. (6) and (7) into (5), another equation involving $\overline{P}$ and $P_2$ is:

$$c_1 \frac{\rho_1 (K_1 - \overline{P}P_2)}{r_1 K_1} \overline{P}P_2 + c_2 \frac{\rho_2 (K_2 - P_2)}{r_2 K_2} P_2 - \delta \left(\frac{\rho_2 (K_2 - P_2)}{\alpha_2 r_2 K_2}\right)^{\frac{1}{\beta_2}} = 0 \tag{11}$$

Solving Eqs. (8) and (11) for $\overline{P} > 0$, $P_2 > 0$, where the conditions in (9) and (10) hold, then $\overline{P}$ and $P_2$ are obtained. Hence, $P_1$ is found using the equation $P_1 = \overline{P}P_2$ and using either Eq. (6) or (7), $X$ can be found. This gives the equilibrium point, $E$.

We may thus write the following Lemma, resuming the use of the superscript, *, to depict the positive steady state values:

**Lemma 1** *The positive equilibrium point $E = (P_1^*, P_2^*, X^*)$ of the system in (1) exists and represents real populations if $\overline{P} > 0$ and $P_2 > 0$ are solutions to the equations (8) and (11) and satisfy the inequalities in (9) and (10).*

## 2.2  Stability Analysis of Positive Interior Equilibrium Point

The stability of the interior equilibrium point is discussed by examining the equilibrium point, $E = (P_1^*, P_2^*, X^*)$. The equations in system (1) are linearized using the substitutions:

$$P_1 = P_1^* + u, \tag{12}$$
$$P_2 = P_2^* + v, \tag{13}$$
$$X = X^* + w, \tag{14}$$

where $u$, $v$ and $w$ are small perturbations about the equilibrium point. Assuming Taylor's Theorem, all terms are expanded about the equilibrium point, while neglecting higher order terms of $u$, $v$ and $w$.

The characteristic equation has the form:

$$P(\lambda) = \lambda^3 + a_1\lambda^2 + a_2\lambda + a_3 = 0 \tag{15}$$

For stability, it is necessary for the eigenvalues, $\lambda$ in (15) to have negative real parts. These conditions are satisfied by the Routh-Hurwitz [11, 21], which states that a stable equilibrium occurs if and only if

$$a_1 > 0, \qquad a_3 > 0, \qquad a_1a_2 - a_3 > 0 \tag{16}$$

**Theorem 1** *Given an equilibrium point $E = (P_1^*, P_2^*, X^*)$ satisfying the equations in system (1), then once Lemma 1 holds, E exists and is stable if and only if (16) holds.*

### 2.2.1  Hopf Bifurcation Analysis

The existence of this type of bifurcation can be explored by applying the Hopf Bifurcation Theorem [9, 17] to the original system in (1). It is important to verify the traversality condition at a critical value $\mu = \mu^*$:

$$Re\left(\frac{d\lambda_i}{d\mu}\right)_{\mu=\mu^*} \neq 0, \qquad\qquad i = 1, 2. \qquad\qquad (17)$$

The system has a family of periodic solutions where the critical value, $\mu^*$, is the Hopf bifurcation point. Due to the complex nature of the system in symbolic form, the Hopf bifurcation points are found for a particular parameter set analytically using the Routh-Hurwitz criteria and then verified numerically.

## 3  Numerical Simulation Results and Discussion

The aim of the simulation study is to observe the effect of variation of parameter values on the stability of the system for the simulated dataset shown in Table 1. The stability of the dataset was examined with the positive interior equilibrium point as the initial value with slight perturbation. Then, each parameter was varied individually, while keeping others constant.

The Routh-Hurwitz criteria in Theorem 1 was used to analytically find Hopf bifurcation point(s), that is, values where the system exhibited a change in stability for the particular parameter. Table 2 shows the stability intervals for the system with respect to the variation of parameters for the simulated dataset shown in Table 1, which produced a change in stability of the system.

Time series graphs were generated using [18] for the system for one case of the parameter $c_1$ in stable and unstable intervals in Figs. 1 and 2 respectively, which verify the analytical results. It is possible to generate similar graphs for all the parameters in Table 2. This analysis allows an investor to study the parameter sets which would produce stable or unstable investments.

Parameters representing returns to investment experience, investment handling time, rate of conversion of investment opportunities and depreciation of investment experience experience Hopf bifurcation values, where the system switches stability. The investors must invest only when the parameters are within the stable regions.

Otherwise, if these parameters have values in the unstable regions it indicates that investors will experience losses or fluctuations in their investments. These recommendations can assist investors, not only in VC but also in the stock market, to use these bifurcation parameter thresholds to make more secure investments.

**Table 1**  Parameter values for simulated dataset[a]

| $\alpha_1$ | $\alpha_2$ | $\rho_1$ | $\rho_2$ | $\beta_1$ | $\beta_2$ | $K_1$ | $K_2$ | $\gamma_1$ | $\gamma_2$ | $c_1$ | $c_2$ | $\delta$ |
|---|---|---|---|---|---|---|---|---|---|---|---|---|
| 1 | 1 | 0.5 | 0.7 | 0.9 | 0.9 | 10 | 10 | 1 | 1 | 3.5 | 0.5 | 0.5 |

[a]Equilibrium point (0.27, 0.38, 1.18)

**Table 2** Stability/instability intervals for the system when each parameter in the simulated dataset in Table 1 is varied individually. The regions of stability are represented by (S) whereas the unstable regions are represented by (U). The Hopf bifurcation point for a parameter is the value which induces a qualitative change in the stability of the system

| Parameter | Stable (S)/Unstable (U) interval | Hopf bifurcation point/s |
|---|---|---|
| $\beta_1$ | $0 \le \beta_1 < 0.959$ (S) | 0.959 |
| | $0.959 \le \beta_1 < 29.680$ (U) | |
| $\beta_2$ | $0 \le \beta_2 < 0.943$ (S) | 0.943 |
| | $0.943 \le \beta_2 < 29.637$ (U) | |
| $\gamma_1$ | $0 \le \gamma_1 < 0.376$ (S) | 0.376 |
| | $0.376 \le \gamma_1 < 0.512$ (U) | 0.512 |
| | $0.512 \le \gamma_1 \le 30.484$ (S) | |
| $\gamma_2$ | $0 \le \gamma_2 < 3.589$ (S) | 3.589 |
| | $3.589 \le \gamma_2 < 19.416$ (U) | 19.416 |
| | $19.416 \le \gamma_2 \le 30.106$ (S) | |
| $c_1$ | $0 \le c_1 < 4.778$ (S) | 4.778 |
| | $4.778 \le c_1 < 32.431$ (U) | |
| $c_2$ | $0 \le c_2 < 0.268$ (U) | 0.268 |
| | $0.268 \le c_2 < 29.655$ (S) | |
| $\delta$ | $0 \le \delta < 0.269$ (S) | 0.269 |
| | $0.269 \le \delta < 29.286$ (U) | |

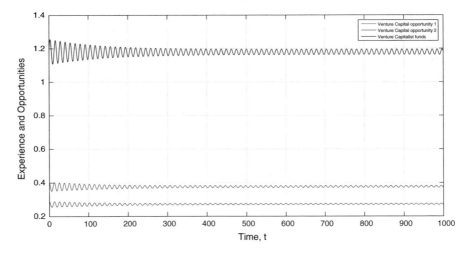

**Fig. 1** Time series graphs for two investment opportunities, $P_1$ (blue line), $P_2$ (red line) and VCs experience, $X$ (black line), measured in terms of their investment funds (black line). Parameters are from a stable (S) case from Table 2 where $\alpha_1 = 1, \alpha_2 = 1, \rho_1 = 0.5, \rho_2 = 0.7, \beta_1 = 0.9, \beta_2 = 0.9, K_1 = 10, K_2 = 10, \gamma_1 = 1, \gamma_2 = 1, c_1 = 3.5, c_2 = 0.5, \delta = 0.5$. The bifurcation parameter here is $c_1$, with a value of 3.5. Both sets of investment opportunities, as well as the experience of VCs in the system co-exist, with stable equilibrium over time for this dataset. This is an ideal eco-system for VCs to invest in the two opportunities since neither of them, nor the VCs experience, are depleted

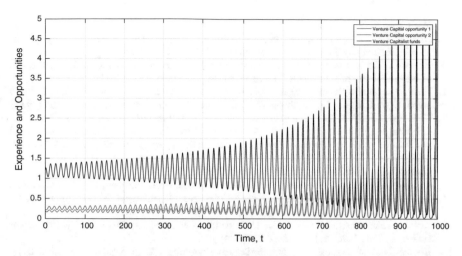

**Fig. 2** Time series graphs for two investment opportunities, $P_1$ (blue line), $P_2$ (red line) and VCs experience, $X$ (black line), measured in terms of their investment funds (black line). Parameters depict an unstable (U) case from Table 2 where $\alpha_1 = 1, \alpha_2 = 1, \rho_1 = 0.5, \rho_2 = 0.7, \beta_1 = 0.9, \beta_2 = 0.9, K_1 = 10, K_2 = 10, \gamma_1 = 1, \gamma_2 = 1, c_1 = 5.5, c_2 = 0.5, \delta = 0.5$. The bifurcation parameter here is $c_1$, with a value of 5.5. The investment opportunities as well as the VCs experience co-exist with unstable equilibrium over time. There exists large, increasing fluctuations over time for the VCs experience. For a particular set of opportunities, the VCs experience may increase or decrease drastically, eventually approaching zero as the oscillations increase. This may not be an ideal case for investment, hence it is unstable

## 4  Conclusion

The use of the prey-predator model enhances the investment of VCs. It provides a guide into the dynamics of the system which can be used to study the stability of the system for different parameter sets. The stability ranges are essential tools to provide advice to investors about the threshold bifurcation values which would cause their investment to become unstable and incur losses to their funds. The model is not meant to replace existing models but is a means of partially explaining the complex endogenous nature of the VC investment.

**Acknowledgements**  The authors thank the AMMCS International Conference 2017 for the opportunity to present this work and to Springer for its publication.

## References

1. Ajraldi, V., Venturino, E.: Stabilizing effect of prey competition for predators exhibiting switching feeding behavior. WSEAS Trans. Biol. Biomed. **5**, 65–74 (2008)
2. Bhatt, B.S., Owen, D.R., Jaju, R.P.: On the effect of switching, predation and harvesting on systems consisting of one predator and two prey species which live in different habitats. J.

Math. Res. **3**, 12–21 (2011)
3. Brander, J.A., De Bettignies, J.-E.: Venture capital investment: the role of predator–prey dynamics with learning by doing. Econ. Innov. New Technol. **1**, 1–19 (2009)
4. Bravo, G., Tamburino, L.: Are two resources really better than one? Some unexpected results of the availability of substitutes. J. Environ. Manag. **92**, 2865–2874 (2011)
5. Chen, H., et al.: Buy local? The geography of venture capital. J. Urban Econ. **67**, 90–102 (2010)
6. Cobb, C.W., Douglas, P.H.: A theory of production. The Am. Econ. Rev. **18**, 139–165 (1928)
7. Cochrane, J.H.: The risk and return of venture capital. J. Financ. Econ. **75**, 3–52 (2005)
8. Driessen, J., Lin, T.-C., Phalippou, L.: A new method to estimate risk and return of non traded assets from cash flows: the case of private equity funds. J. Financ. Quantit. Anal. **47**, 511–535 (2012)
9. Gandolfo, G.: Economic Dynamics. Springer, Berlin (2010)
10. Gompers, P., Lerner, J.: The venture capital revolution. J. Econ. Perspect. **15**, 145–168 (2001)
11. Hurwitz, A.: Ueber die Bedingungen, unter welchen eine Gleichung nur Wurzeln mit negativen reellen Theilen besitzt. Mathematische Annalen **46**(2), 273–284 (1895)
12. Khan, Q.J.A., Balakrishnan, E., Wake, G.C.: Analysis of a predator–Prey system with predator switching. Bull. Mat. Biol. **66**, 109–123 (2004)
13. Khanna, N., Mathews, R.D.: Can herding improve investment decisions? RAND J. Econ. **42**(1), 150–174 (2001)
14. Korteweg, A., Sorensen, M.: Risk and return characteristics of venture capital-backed entrepreneurial companies. Rev. Financ. Stud. **23**(10), 3738–3772 (2010)
15. Kortum, S., Lerner, L.: Assessing the contribution of venture capital to innovation. RAND J. Econ. **31**(4), 674–692 (2000)
16. Lotka, A.J.: Elements of Physical Biology. Williams and Wilkins, Baltimore (1925)
17. Marsden, J.E., McCracken, M.: The Hopf Bifurcation and its Applications. Springer, New York (1976)
18. MATLAB Version 7.10.0. The MathWorks Inc., Natick, Massachusetts (2011)
19. Matsuda, H., et al.: Switching effect on the stability of the prey-predator system with three trophic levels. J. Theor. Biol. **122**(3), 251–262 (1986)
20. Rosenzweig, M.L., MacArthur, R.H.: Graphical representation and stability conditions of predator-prey interactions. Am. Nat. **97**(895), 209–223 (1963)
21. Routh, E.J.: A Treatise on the Stability of a Given State of Motion: Particularly Steady Motion. Macmillan, London (1877)
22. Scharfstein, D.S., Stein, J.C.: Herd behavior and investment. Am. Econ. Rev. **80**(6), 465–479 (1990)
23. Sorenson, M.: How smart is smart money? A two-sided matching model of venture capital. J. Financ. **62**(6), 2725–2762 (2007)
24. Tanski, M.: Switching effects in prey-predator system. J. Theor. Biol. **70**(3), 263–271 (1978)
25. Ueda, M.: Banks versus venture capital: project evaluation, screening, and expropriation. J. Financ. **59**(2), 601–621 (2004)
26. Volterra, V.: Variazioni e fluttuazioni del numero dindividui in specie animali conviventi. Mem. Acad. Lincei Roma **2**, 31–113 (1926)

# Modelling Asynchronous Assets with Jump-Diffusion Processes

## Yuxin Chen and Roman N. Makarov

**Abstract** In this paper, we present a new multivariate jump-diffusion model for modelling financial securities that have missing or asynchronous data in time series of historical prices. The proposed model allows us to analyze a portfolio that combines a high-activity asset such as a market index (or an exchange-traded fund tracking a market index) and several low-activity assets. The model is constructed in such a way that low-activity assets correlate with each other only implicitly through the high-activity asset price process. To calibrate the model, we first estimate parameters of a high-activity asset and then estimate parameters for each low-activity asset by conditioning on the parameters of the high-activity asset. Here, we assume that the jump component follows a compound Poisson process, which is the same for all asset price processes. Two jump-size distributions are considered: the normal and the double-exponential probability distributions. We use the maximum likelihood method to estimate model parameters for different time-series datasets. The new models are compared with the model based on a multivariate Geometric Brownian motion.

**Keywords** Jump-diffusion · Asset pricing · Model calibration · Missing data
Maximum likelihood estimation

## 1 Introduction

There exist many low-activity assets that are not traded frequently on financial markets, which causes missing data for some dates. As a result, daily trading information for such asset may be no available. However, many investors may be willing to combine high- and low-activity assets in order to diversify their portfolios.

Y. Chen · R. N. Makarov (✉)
Wilfrid Laurier University, Waterloo, ON, Canada
e-mail: rmakarov@wlu.ca

Y. Chen
e-mail: chen1110@mylaurier.ca

© Springer Nature Switzerland AG 2018                                477
D. M. Kilgour et al. (eds.), *Recent Advances in Mathematical and Statistical Methods*, Springer Proceedings in Mathematics & Statistics 259,
https://doi.org/10.1007/978-3-319-99719-3_43

The objective of this paper is to introduce a new class of multivariate models, which allow for simulating an ensemble of low-activity assets. Since infrequently trading assets have missing and asynchronous data in time series of historical prices, the main feature of the model proposed in this paper is the possibility to estimate parameters for each asset price process despite the lack of historical data.

Very often, the dynamics of a financial market as a whole can be well described using one index such as S&P 500, which is widely regarded as the best single gauge of large-cap U.S. equities. Such an index can be used to describe the systemic behaviour of a market. For other assets, the return is then given by a combination of asset-specific and systemic components. To be more specific, we use a jump-diffusion process to model the log-value of the index and then introduce the same jump component in diffusions describing log-values of other assets. Our approach is somewhat similar to the capital asset pricing model (CAPM), where the expected asset return is given by a sum of a systemic (market) risk premium and a company-specific risk premium.

## 2 Multi-Asset Price Model

Let $S_0$ denote a high-activity asset such as a market index, and $S_i$ with $i = 1, 2, \ldots, n$ represent low-activity assets. The price of asset $S$ at time $t$ is denoted by $S(t)$. Suppose that for the high-activity asset, we have daily trading information for all time points $t_0, t_1, \ldots, t_m$ where $t_j = jh$ with $h > 0$ and $j = 0, 1, \ldots, m$. However, due to the low-frequency trading, prices of $S_1, S_2, \ldots, S_n$ are only available for selected dates when assets had been traded on. Hence, for each low-activity asset, we only have partial trading information for particular dates, whereas data for the other time points are missing.

In our project, we assume that the high-activity asset price follows a jump-diffusion process, and the strong solution under a real-world probability measure is as follows:

$$
S_0(t) = S_0(0) \exp\left( \left( \mu_0 - \frac{\sigma_0^2}{2} \right) t + \sigma_0 \left( W_0(t) + \sum_{j=1}^{N_\lambda(t)} Q_j \right) \right), \quad t \geq 0 \quad (1)
$$

where $\mu_0$ and $\sigma_0 > 0$ are constant, $\{Q_i\}_{i \geq 1}$ is a sequence of independent and identically distributed (iid) random variables with mean $\mu_J$ and variance $\sigma_J^2$, $\{N_\lambda(t)\}_{t \geq 0}$ is a Poisson process with intensity $\lambda$, and $\{W_0(t)\}_{t \geq 0}$ is Brownian motion. We assume that $\{Q_i\}, \{N_\lambda(t)\}$ and $\{W_0(t)\}$ are jointly independent. Here, all stochastic processes and random variables are defined on the same filtered probability space.

From the strong solution (1), we can derive the following stochastic differential equation (SDE) for the high-activity asset:

$$\frac{dS_0(t)}{S_0(t-)} = \mu_0 dt + \sigma_0 dW_0(t) + d\left(\sum_{j=1}^{N_\lambda(t)} (e^{\sigma_0 Q_j} - 1)\right). \tag{2}$$

For the case where all $Q_j$, $j \geq 1$ are zero, the strong solution and the SDE are respectively changing to

$$S_0(t) = S_0(0) \exp\left((\mu_0 - \frac{\sigma_0^2}{2})t + \sigma_0 W_0(t)\right), \tag{3}$$

$$dS_0(t) = S_0(t) \cdot (\mu_0 dt + \sigma_0 dW_0(t)). \tag{4}$$

Clearly, it is a Gaussian case without jumps.

For the $n$ low-activity assets, we assume the following strong solutions:

$$S_i(t) = S_i(0)e^{\left(\mu_i - \frac{\sigma_i^2}{2}\right)t + \sigma_i\sqrt{1-\rho_i^2}W_i(t) + \sigma_i\rho_i\left(W_0(t) + \sum_{j=1}^{N_\lambda(t)} Q_j\right)}, \quad t \geq 0 \tag{5}$$

where $\mu_i$, $\sigma_i > 0$ and $\rho_i \in (-1, 1)$ with $i = 1, 2, \ldots, n$ are constant and Brownian motions $W_0, W_1, \ldots, W_n$ are jointly independent. We use the same compound Poisson process to model jumps in the market index and the low-activity assets. Thus, all asset price processes can have a jump at the same time only and jump sizes for different assets are proportional to the same random variable.

The SDE for low-activity asset $i = 1, 2, \ldots, n$ can be found using Itô's formula:

$$\frac{dS_i(t)}{S_i(t-)} = \mu_i dt + \sigma_i\left(\sqrt{1-\rho_i^2}dW_i(t) + \rho_i dW_0(t)\right) + d\left(\sum_{j=1}^{N_\lambda(t)} (e^{\sigma_i\rho_i Q_j} - 1)\right). \tag{6}$$

The log-values $X_0(t) = \ln S_0(t)$, $X_i(t) = \ln S_i(t)$ for $i = 1, 2, \ldots, n$ are given by

$$X_0(t) = X_0(0) + \left(\mu_0 - \frac{\sigma_0^2}{2}\right)t + \sigma_0\left(W_0(t) + \sum_{j=1}^{N_\lambda(t)} Q_j\right), \quad t \geq 0, \tag{7}$$

$$X_i(t) = X_i(0) + \left(\mu_i - \frac{\sigma_i^2}{2}\right)t + \sigma_i\left(W_i(t)\sqrt{1-\rho_i^2} + \rho_i\left(W_0(t) + \sum_{j=1}^{N_\lambda(t)} Q_j\right)\right). \tag{8}$$

The strong solutions in (7) and (8) allow us to find the correlation coefficients between the log-returns $R_i(t) = \ln(S_i(t)/S_i(0)) = X_i(t) - X_i(0)$ with $i = 0, 1, 2, \ldots, n$:

$$\text{Corr}(R_i(t), R_0(t)) = \widehat{\rho}_i \equiv \rho_i\sqrt{\frac{1 + \lambda\sigma_J}{1 + \lambda\sigma_J\rho_i^2}} \quad \text{for } i \geq 1,$$

$$\text{Corr}(R_i(t), R_j(t)) = \widehat{\rho}_i\,\widehat{\rho}_j \quad \text{for } i, j \geq 1 \text{ with } i \neq j.$$

It is clear that $|\widehat{\rho}_i| \leq 1$ for all $i$ and $|\widehat{\rho}_i| < 1$ if $|\rho_i| < 1$. Moreover, it is not difficult to prove that the correlation matrix $\{\text{Corr}(R_i(t), R_j(t))\}_{1 \leq i,j \leq n}$ is a positive definite matrix provided that $|\rho_i| < 1$ holds for all $i$.

Two types of jump-size distributions are considered in this paper. The first one is the normal distribution $\text{Norm}(\mu_J, \sigma_J^2)$. This jump-diffusion model for asset prices with normally-distributed jump sizes is known in the literature as the Merton model [4]. The density of the jump amplitude is given by

$$\phi_Q(x) = \frac{1}{\sqrt{2\pi\sigma_J^2}} \exp\left(-\frac{(x-\mu_J)^2}{2\sigma_J^2}\right). \tag{9}$$

The second case is the Kou model [3] with double-exponential jump sizes. The density of the jump amplitude is

$$\phi_Q(x) = \frac{p_1}{\eta_1} \exp\left(\frac{x}{\eta_1}\right) I_{\{x<0\}} + \frac{p_2}{\eta_2} \exp\left(\frac{-x}{\eta_2}\right) I_{\{x\geq0\}} \tag{10}$$

where $\eta_1$ and $\eta_2$ are positive constants; the probabilities $p_1$ and $p_2$ of negative and positive jumps, respectively, satisfy $0 < p_1 < 1, 0 < p_2 < 1$ and $p_1 + p_2 = 1$. The condition $\eta_2 > 1$ is required to ensure that $E[e^Q] < \infty$. The jump amplitude $Q$ has mean $\mu_J = -p_1\eta_1 + p_2\eta_2$ and variance $\sigma_J^2 = p_1((\mu_J + \eta_1)^2 + \eta_1^2) + p_2((\mu_J - \eta_2)^2 + \eta_2^2)$.

## 3 Estimation of High-Activity Asset Parameters

The maximum likelihood estimation (MLE) is a commonly used method to estimate parameters of asset price models. To select values for the model parameters we need to maximize the likelihood function, which is defined as a joint density function for assets values.

For the high-activity asset $S_0$, the log-returns are iid, so we can apply the MLE method to estimate $\mu_0, \sigma_0, \lambda$ as well as parameters of the jump-amplitude distribution. To speed up our calculations, we use the multinomial maximum likelihood estimation (MMLE) method [1, 2]. Assume that we have all historical daily prices for the high-activity asset $S_0$, and hence we can calculate daily log-returns $\ln(S_0(t_j)/S_0(t_{j-1}))$ for all $j = 1, 2, \ldots, m$. Let $\phi(x; \mathbf{v})$ and $\Phi(x; \mathbf{v})$ denote, respectively, the probability density function (PDF) and the cumulative distribution function (CDF) of daily log-returns of the high-activity asset with parameter vector $\mathbf{v}$. The MMLE algorithm is as follows:

Step 1: Sort $m$ historical daily log-returns into $n_{bin}$ bins and get the sample frequency $f_k^{(s)}$ for each bin $k = 1, 2, \ldots, n_{bin}$

Step 2: Maximize the objective function:

$$\ell(\mathbf{v}) = \sum_{k=1}^{n_{bin}} [f_k^{(s)} \ln(f_k(\mathbf{v}))] \to \max_{\mathbf{v}}$$

Here $f_k(\mathbf{v})$ is the theoretical frequency for the model distribution with parameter vector $\mathbf{v}$ given by

$$f_k(\mathbf{v}) = m \int_{B_k} \phi(x; \mathbf{v}) dx = m\big(\Phi(b_k; \mathbf{v}) - \Phi(b_{k-1}; \mathbf{v})\big)$$

where $B_k = [b_{k-1}, b_k]$ is the $k$th bin.

To calculate the theoretical frequencies, we use a first-order approximation. That is, we assume that no more than one jump happens in any day. Assuming that there are 250 trading days per year, the duration of one (trading) day is equal to $h = \frac{1}{250}$. The probability distribution function for the daily log-return $\ln(S_0(t + h)/S_0(t))$ is then approximated as follows:

$$\Phi(x) \approx \frac{p_0}{p_0 + p_1} \Phi^{(0)}(x) + \frac{p_1}{p_0 + p_1} \Phi^{(1)}(x)$$

where $p_k = e^{-\lambda h}(\lambda h)^k / k!$ is the probability of having $k$ jumps during a time interval of length $h$ and $\Phi^{(k)}(x)$ is the CDF of the log-return given that $k$ jumps occur.

For the Merton model, we have

$$\Phi^{(k)}(x) = \mathcal{N}\left(x; (\mu_0 - \frac{\sigma_0^2}{2})h + k\mu_J, \sigma_0^2 h + k\sigma_J^2\right), \quad k = 0, 1, 2, \ldots$$

where $\mathcal{N}(x; a, b^2)$ is the CDF of the normal distribution with mean $a$ and variance $b^2$.

For the Kou model, we have the following two cases. If no jump happens, the probability distribution function of a log-return is

$$\Phi^{(0)}(x) = \mathcal{N}\left(x; (\mu_0 - \frac{\sigma_0^2}{2})h, \sigma_0^2 h\right).$$

Under the assumption that only one jump happens, we have:

$$\Phi^{(1)}(x) = \mathcal{N}\left(x, (\mu_0 - \frac{\sigma_0^2}{2})h, \sigma_0^2 h\right)$$
$$+ p_1 \cdot \exp\left(\frac{x - v_1}{\eta_1}\right) \cdot \mathcal{N}\left(-x; -(\mu_0 - \frac{\sigma_0^2}{2})h + \sigma_0^2 h/\eta_1, \sigma_0^2 h\right)$$
$$- p_2 \cdot \exp\left(\frac{-(x - v_2)}{\eta_2}\right) \cdot \mathcal{N}\left(x; (\mu_0 - \frac{\sigma_0^2}{2})h + \sigma_0^2 h/\eta_2, \sigma_0^2 h\right)$$

where $v_i = (\mu_0 - \sigma_0^2/2)h - \frac{\sigma_0^2 h}{2\eta_1}$ with $i = 1, 2$.

## 4   Estimation of Low-Activity Asset Parameters

Since all low-activity assets are dependent on the high-activity asset, we can estimate the parameters for each low-activity asset once we have estimated all parameters of the high-activity asset. Select one low-activity asset and let $i$ be its index with $i = 1, 2, \ldots, n$. Assume that for this low-activity asset we know $\hat{m} + 1$ historical values at times $\hat{t}_0, \hat{t}_1, \ldots, \hat{t}_{\hat{m}}$. For simplicity, we omit the hat accent above $t$'s and $m$ in what follows. Introduce the following notations:

$$Z_j = \ln S_0(t_j), \quad X_j = \ln S_i(t_j), \quad \text{and} \quad M_j = W_0(t_j) + \sum_{k=1}^{N_\lambda(t_j)} Q_k$$

for $j = 0, 1, 2, \ldots, m$. Using the strong solutions in (7) and (8), we have

$$Z_j = Z_{j-1} + \left(\mu_0 - \frac{\sigma_0^2}{2}\right)(t_j - t_{j-1}) + \sigma_0 \left(M_j - M_{j-1}\right), \tag{11}$$

$$X_j = X_{j-1} + \left(\mu_i - \frac{\sigma_i^2}{2}\right)(t_j - t_{j-1})$$
$$+ \sigma_i \left[\rho_i \left(M_j - M_{j-1}\right) + \sqrt{1 - \rho_i^2}\left(W_i\left(t_j\right) - W_i\left(t_{j-1}\right)\right)\right]. \tag{12}$$

After reorganizing Eq. (11), we have

$$M_j - M_{j-1} = \frac{Z_j - Z_{j-1} - \left(\mu_0 - \frac{\sigma_0^2}{2}\right)(t_j - t_{j-1})}{\sigma_0}. \tag{13}$$

Combine Eqs. (12) and (13) to obtain

$$X_j = X_{j-1} + \left(\mu_i - \frac{\sigma_i^2}{2}\right)h_j + \sigma_i \rho_i \frac{Z_j - Z_{j-1} - \left(\mu_0 - \frac{\sigma_0^2}{2}\right)h_j}{\sigma_0} \tag{14}$$

$$+ \sigma_i \sqrt{1 - \rho_i^2}\left(W_i\left(t_j\right) - W_i\left(t_{j-1}\right)\right). \tag{15}$$

where $h_j = t_j - t_{j-1}$. As we can see, $X_j$ conditional on $X_{j-1}$ and $\tilde{Z}_j = Z_j - Z_{j-1}$ follows a normal distribution, and there is no jump part in the equation for $X_j$. The joint probability function of $X_j$ and $Z_j$ conditional on $X_{j-1}$ and $Z_{j-1}$ is as follows:

$$p_{X_j, Z_j | X_{j-1}, Z_{j-1}} \left( X_j, Z_j \mid X_{j-1}, Z_{j-1} \right)$$
$$= p_{Z_j | Z_{j-1}} \left( Z_j \mid Z_{j-1} \right) \times p_{X_j | X_{j-1}, \widetilde{Z}_j} \left( X_j \mid X_{j-1}, \widetilde{Z}_j \right)$$
$$= p_{Z_j | Z_{j-1}} \left( Z_j \mid Z_{j-1} \right) \times \frac{1}{\sqrt{2\pi \sigma_i^2 h_j \left( 1 - \rho_i^2 \right)}}$$

$$\cdot \exp \left( - \frac{\left[ X_j - X_{j-1} - \left( \mu_i - \frac{\sigma_i^2}{2} \right) h_j - \frac{\sigma_i \rho_i \widetilde{Z}_j}{\sigma_0} + \frac{\sigma_i \rho_i \left( \mu_0 - \frac{\sigma_0^2}{2} \right) h_j}{\sigma_0} \right]^2}{2\sigma_i^2 \left( 1 - \rho_i^2 \right) h_j} \right)$$

where $p_{Z_j | Z_{j-1}}$ is the transition PDF for $\ln S_0(t)$. The conditional likelihood function for low-activity asset $i$ is as follows:

$$L_i \left( \mathbf{X} \mid \mathbf{Z} \right) = \prod_{j=1}^m p_{X_j | X_{j-1}, \widetilde{Z}_j} \left( X_j \mid X_{j-1}, \widetilde{Z}_j \right)$$

$$= \sigma_i^{-m} (2\pi)^{-\frac{m}{2}} \prod_{j=1}^m h_j^{-\frac{1}{2}} \left( 1 - \rho_i^2 \right)^{-\frac{m}{2}} \prod_{j=1}^m e^{-\left( \sum_{j=1}^m \frac{D_j^2}{h_j} \right) \frac{1}{2\sigma_i^2 \left( 1 - \rho_i^2 \right)}}$$

$$= \sigma_i^{-m} (2\pi)^{-\frac{m}{2}} \left( 1 - \rho_i^2 \right)^{-\frac{m}{2}} \prod_{j=1}^m h_j^{-\frac{1}{2}} e^{-\left( \sum_{j=1}^m \frac{D_j^2}{h_j} \right) \frac{1}{2\sigma_i^2 \left( 1 - \rho_i^2 \right)}} \qquad (16)$$

where $d_0 = \frac{\mu_0 - \frac{\sigma_0^2}{2}}{\sigma_0}$, $D_j = X_j - X_{j-1} - (\mu_i - \frac{\sigma_i^2}{2})h_j - \frac{\sigma_i \rho_i \widetilde{Z}_j}{\sigma_0} + \sigma_i \rho_i h_j d_0$. In the formula for $L_i$, we can omit the PDFs $p_{Z_j | Z_{j-1}}$ since the likelihood function is conditional on values of $S_0$.

In order to estimate the model parameters, let us introduce new variables:

$$u^2 = \sigma_i^2 (1 - \rho_i^2), \qquad v = \sigma_i \rho_i, \qquad w = \mu_i - \frac{\sigma_i^2}{2}.$$

Differentiate the log-likelihood function (16) w.r.t. $u$, $v$, $w$ and equate the derivatives to zero. Solving the obtained system, we get the following solution:

$$u^2 = \frac{\sum_{j=1}^m \left( \widetilde{X}_j - h_j w - \frac{\widetilde{Z}_j}{\sigma_0} v + d_0 v h_j \right)^2 / h_j}{m}$$

$$v = \frac{(c - (\Delta X \Delta Z / \Delta t)) \sigma_0}{b^2 - (\Delta Z)^2 / \Delta t}$$

$$w = \frac{\Delta X b^2 - \Delta Z c + \widetilde{\mu}_0 \Delta t c - \widetilde{\mu}_0 \Delta X \Delta Z}{\Delta t \left( b^2 - \Delta Z / \Delta t \right)}$$

where $\widetilde{X}_j = X_j - X_{j-1}$, $\Delta t = \sum_{j=1}^{m} h_j = t_m - t_0$, $\Delta X = \sum_{j=1}^{m} \widetilde{X}_j = X_m - X_0$, $\Delta Z = \sum_{j=1}^{m} \widetilde{Z}_j = Z_m - Z_0$, and $\widetilde{\mu_0} = \mu_0 - \frac{\sigma_0^2}{2}$. The parameters $a$, $b$, and $c$ are

$$a^2 = \sum_{j=1}^{m} \frac{\widetilde{x}_j^2}{h_j}, \qquad b^2 = \sum_{j=1}^{m} \frac{\widetilde{Z}_j^2}{h_j}, \qquad c = \sum_{j=1}^{m} \frac{\widetilde{Z}_j \widetilde{x}_j}{h_j}.$$

We can now obtain $\sigma_i$, $\mu_i$, $\rho_i$ as follows:

$$\sigma_i = \sqrt{u^2 + v^2}, \qquad \rho_i = \frac{v}{\sqrt{u^2 + v^2}}, \qquad \mu_i = w + \frac{u^2 + v^2}{2}.$$

It can be proved that this solution is a global maximum of the likelihood function (16).

The procedure described in this section is repeated for every low-activity asset one by one. In doing so, we use the important property of the proposed model that low-activity assets, $S_1, S_2, \ldots, S_n$, are conditionally independent given values of $S_0$.

## 5  Numerical Results

We performed two numerical tests, for which historical daily close values of Canadian and U.S. equity ETFs and respective market indices were retrieved from a Bloomberg terminal.

In the first test, we used data collected from the Canadian equity market during the time period July 11, 2014 to July 11, 2015. The S&P/TSX60 Composite Index was used as the high-activity asset $S_0$. We chose 10 low-frequently trading Canadian ETFs with the following tickers: FHG, QRD, FGM, ZEL, RLE, PZC, FPR, RHF, XMY, HXQ. The trading frequency for low-activity assets varies from once a week to once a month.

Parameters of the high-activity asset model with jumps were estimated using the multinomial maximum likelihood estimation. The two jump-diffusion processes, namely, the Merton model and the Kou model, were compared with the Gaussian case without jumps (see Table 1). After estimating parameters of $S_0$, we estimated parameters for each low-activity asset price process $S_i$ with $i = 1, 2, \ldots, 10$. Our method was robust for assets with various trading activities. As we can see in Table 2, the results were consistent for all three models.

**Table 1** High-activity asset parameters for the three models

| Gaussian | $\mu_0$ | $\sigma_0$ | | | | | |
|---|---|---|---|---|---|---|---|
| | −0.0036 | 0.1422 | | | | | |
| Merton model | $\mu_0$ | $\sigma_0$ | $\mu_J$ | $\sigma_J$ | $\lambda$ | | |
| | 0.052 | 0.1339 | −0.0058 | 0.021 | 3.289 | | |
| Kou model | $\mu_0$ | $\sigma_0$ | $\eta_1$ | $\eta_2$ | $\lambda$ | $p_1$ | $\mu_J$ | $\sigma_J$ |
| | 0.116 | 0.133 | 0.0095 | 7.56 | 7.413 | 0.975 | 0.178 | 1.67 |

**Table 2** Low-activity assets parameters

| ETF | Kou Model | | | Merton Model | | | Gaussian | | |
|-----|-----------|-----------|-----------|--------------|-----------|-----------|----------|-----------|-----------|
|     | $\mu$ | $\sigma$ | $\rho$ | $\mu$ | $\sigma$ | $\rho$ | $\mu$ | $\sigma$ | $\rho$ |
| FHG | -0.0440 | 0.0157 | -0.8786 | -0.0373 | 0.0158 | -0.8800 | -0.0314 | 0.0165 | -0.8915 |
| QRD | -0.0821 | 0.0353 | -0.3153 | -0.0767 | 0.0353 | -0.3172 | -0.0720 | 0.0355 | -0.3348 |
| FGM | 0.2009 | 0.0376 | -0.7752 | 0.2150 | 0.0377 | -0.7774 | 0.2274 | 0.0392 | -0.7955 |
| ZEL | 0.0184 | 0.0035 | 0.0526 | 0.0183 | 0.0035 | 0.0529 | 0.0182 | 0.0035 | 0.0562 |
| RLE | 0.1363 | 0.0555 | 0.7289 | 0.1167 | 0.0557 | 0.7313 | 0.0996 | 0.0576 | 0.7514 |
| PZC | -0.0329 | 0.0195 | 0.1184 | -0.0340 | 0.0195 | 0.1192 | -0.0350 | 0.0195 | 0.1265 |
| FPR | 0.0231 | 0.0560 | 0.9810 | -0.0052 | 0.0564 | 0.9813 | -0.0284 | 0.0598 | 0.9834 |
| RHF | -0.1604 | 0.0286 | 0.0122 | -0.1605 | 0.0286 | 0.0123 | -0.1607 | 0.0286 | 0.0130 |
| XMY | 0.1758 | 0.0267 | 0.8377 | 0.1649 | 0.0269 | 0.8395 | 0.1554 | 0.0281 | 0.8539 |
| HXQ | -0.0216 | 0.0303 | 0.7408 | -0.0324 | 0.0304 | 0.7431 | -0.0419 | 0.0315 | 0.7628 |

**Table 3** Tickers and names of low-activity assets selected from the U.S. equity ETFs

| Ticker | Full name |
| --- | --- |
| VBK | Vanguard Small Cap Growth ETF |
| VHT | Vanguard Healthcare ETF |
| MINT | PIMCO Enhanced Short Maturity Strategy Fund |
| VOE | Vanguard Mid-Cap Value ETF |

In the second numerical example, we used the Kolmogorov–Smirnov (K–S) test to verify whether the jump-diffusion models fit the historical data better than the diffusion model (the Gaussian case). We gathered another dataset with the S&P500 equity index used as the high-activity asset. To perform the K–S test, we need daily information. Hence, as low-activity assets we used four U.S. equity ETFs with high trading activity (see Table 3). The dataset collected from the U.S. equity market covers the period from September 18, 2015 to September 18, 2017.

The K–S statistic quantifies a distance between the empirical distribution function of the sample and the CDF of the reference distribution. Thus, it allows us to compare how well different reference distributions fit the empirical distribution function for a given sample data.

For a given set of $n$ iid observations, $x_1, x_2, \ldots, x_n$, the empirical distribution function $F_n(x)$ is defined as

$$F_n(x) = \frac{1}{n} \sum_{i=1}^{n} I_{\{x_i \leq x\}}$$

where $I$ denotes an indicator function. The Kolmogorov–Smirnov statistic for a given reference CDF $F(x)$ is

$$D_n = \sup_x |F_n(x) - F(x)|$$

The K–S test is a hypothesis test with the null hypothesis $H_0: F(x) = F_0(x)$. Thus, a larger value of the K–S statistic means a larger difference between the empirical distribution and the reference distribution.

In this paper, we compared three reference distributions of daily log-returns: the Gaussian case with normally distributed log-returns as well as the Kou model and the Merton model of jump-diffusion processes. Since, the model parameters have been estimated per annum, we need to convert them into daily values to perform the K–S test.

Firstly, we calculated the K–S statistic for the S&P/TSX60 Composite Index from the first numerical example. The K–S statistic for the model without jumps is 0.0593 with the $p$-value equal to 0.0558. For the Kou model we have $D_n = 0.0582$ and $p$-value $= 0.0639$, and for the Merton model we have obtained $D_n = 0.0542$

**Table 4** The K–S statistics for the high-activity index S&P500 and four low-activity assets

|        | Gaussian | Merton model | Kou model |
|--------|----------|--------------|-----------|
| S&P500 | 0.11603  | 0.11579      | 0.11529   |
| VBK    | 0.05177  | 0.05092      | 0.05081   |
| VHT    | 0.05680  | 0.05655      | 0.05667   |
| MINT   | 0.17633  | 0.17457      | 0.17402   |
| VOE    | 0.07196  | 0.07104      | 0.05013   |

and $p$-value $= 0.1007$. The second best model is the Merton model. So, both jump-diffusion models outperform the Gaussian model.

Secondly, we calculated K–S statistics for the S&P500 index and four U.S. equity ETFs. The results, which are reported in Table 4, supports the hypothesis that jump-diffusion models provide a better fit.

**Acknowledgements** R. Makarov wishes to acknowledge the generous support of the NSERC Discovery Grant program.

# References

1. Hanson, F.B., Westman, J.J., Zhu, Z.: Multinomial maximum likelihood estimation of market parameters for stock jump-diffusion models. Contemp. Math. **351**, 155–170 (2004)
2. Hanson, F.B., Zhu, Z.: Comparison of market parameters for jump-diffusion distributions using multinomial maximum likelihood estimation. In: 43rd IEEE Conference on Decision and Control, 2004, CDC, vol. 4, pp. 3919–3924. IEEE (2004)
3. Kou, S.G.: A jump-diffusion model for option pricing. Manage. Sci. **48**(8), 1086–1101 (2002)
4. Merton, R.C.: Option pricing when underlying stock returns are discontinuous. J. Fin. Econ. **3**(1–2), 125–144 (1976)

# Efficient Hedging in Bates Model Using High-Order Compact Finite Differences

**Bertram Düring and Alexander Pitkin**

**Abstract** We evaluate the hedging performance of the scheme developed in
B. Düring, A. Pitkin, "High-order compact finite difference scheme for option pricing in stochastic volatility jump models", 2017. We compare the scheme's hedging
performance to standard finite difference methods in different examples. We observe
that the new scheme achieves fourth-order convergence, outperforming a standard,
second-order central finite difference approximation in all our experiments.

**Keywords** Option pricing · Hedging · High-order compact finite differences
Stochastic volatility jump model · Bates model

## 1 Introduction

The Bates model [1] can be considered as the market standard in financial option
pricing applications. It combines the positive features of stochastic volatility and
jump-diffusion models. In this model the option price is given as the solution of a
partial integro-differential equation (PIDE), see e.g. [2].

In [4] we have presented a new high-order compact finite difference scheme
for option pricing in Bates model. The implicit-explicit scheme is based on the
approaches in Düring and Fournié [3] and Salmi et al. [5]. The scheme is fourth
order accurate in space and second order accurate in time. It requires only one initial
$LU$-factorisation of a sparse matrix to perform the option price valuation. Due to its
structural similarities with standard second-order finite difference schemes it can be
employed to upgrade existing implementations in a straightforward manner to obtain
a highly efficient option pricing code.

B. Düring (✉) · A. Pitkin
Department of Mathematics, University of Sussex, Pevensey II, Brighton BN1 9QH, UK
e-mail: bd80@sussex.ac.uk

A. Pitkin
e-mail: a.h.pitkin@sussex.ac.uk

© Springer Nature Switzerland AG 2018

489

D. M. Kilgour et al. (eds.), *Recent Advances in Mathematical
and Statistical Methods*, Springer Proceedings in Mathematics & Statistics 259,
https://doi.org/10.1007/978-3-319-99719-3_44

In the present work we evaluate the hedging performance of the scheme derived in [4]. We compare the scheme's hedging performance to standard finite difference methods where the new scheme outperforms a standard discretisation, based on a second-order central finite difference approximation, in all our experiments.

This article is organised as follows. In the next section we recall Bates model for option pricing and the related PIDE. We refer here to the [4] paper for the derivation of the *implicit-explicit high-order compact finite difference scheme* which we adapt and implement to conduct the numerical experiments. Section 3 is devoted to the computation of the so-called *Greeks* and the evaluation of the scheme's hedging performance in two examples of hedged portfolios.

## 2   The Bates Model

The Bates model [1] is a stochastic volatility model which allows for jumps in returns. Within this model the behaviour of the asset value, $S$, and its variance, $\sigma$, is described by the coupled stochastic differential equations,

$$dS(t) = \mu_B S(t)dt + \sqrt{\sigma(t)}S(t)dW_1(t) + S(t)dJ,$$

$$d\sigma(t) = \kappa(\theta - \sigma(t)) + v\sqrt{\sigma(t)}dW_2(t),$$

for $0 \leqslant t \leqslant T$ and with $S(0), \sigma(0) > 0$. Here, $\mu_B = r - \lambda\xi_B$ is the drift rate, where $r \geqslant 0$ is the risk-free interest rate. The jump process $J$ is a compound Poisson process with intensity $\lambda \geqslant 0$ and $J + 1$ has a log-normal distribution $p(\tilde{y})$ with the mean in $\log(\tilde{y})$ being $\gamma$ and the variance in $\log(\tilde{y})$ being $v^2$, i.e. the probability density function is given by

$$p(\tilde{y}) = \frac{1}{\sqrt{2\pi}\,\tilde{y}v}e^{-\frac{(\log \tilde{y}-\gamma)^2}{2v^2}}.$$

The parameter $\xi_B$ is defined by $\xi_B = e^{\gamma+\frac{v^2}{2}} - 1$. The variance has mean level $\theta$, $\kappa$ is the rate of reversion back to mean level of $\sigma$ and $v$ is the volatility of the variance $\sigma$. The two Wiener processes $W_1$ and $W_2$ have constant correlation $\rho$.

### 2.1   Partial Integro-Differential Equation

By standard derivative pricing arguments for the Bates model, we obtain the PIDE

$$\frac{\partial V}{\partial t} + \frac{1}{2}S^2\sigma\frac{\partial^2 V}{\partial S^2} + \rho v\sigma S\frac{\partial^2 V}{\partial S\partial \sigma} + \frac{1}{2}v^2\sigma\frac{\partial^2 V}{\partial \sigma^2} + (r - \lambda\xi_B)S\frac{\partial V}{\partial S} + \kappa(\theta - \sigma)\frac{\partial V}{\partial \sigma}$$

$$- (r + \lambda)V + \lambda\int_0^{+\infty} V(S\tilde{y}, v, t)p(\tilde{y})\,d\tilde{y},$$

which has to be solved for $S, \sigma > 0, 0 \leq t < T$ and subject to a suitable final condition, e.g. $V(S, \sigma, T) = \max(K - S, 0)$, in the case of a European put option, with $K$ denoting the strike price.

Through the following transformation of variables

$$x = \log S, \quad \tau = T - t, \quad y = \frac{\sigma}{v} \quad \text{and} \quad u = \exp(r + \lambda)V$$

we obtain

$$u_\tau = \frac{1}{2}vy \left( \frac{\partial^2 u}{\partial x^2} + \frac{\partial^2 u}{\partial y^2} \right) + \rho vy \frac{\partial^2 u}{\partial x \partial y} - \left( \frac{1}{2}vy - r + \lambda \xi_B \right) \frac{\partial u}{\partial x}$$
$$+ \kappa \frac{(\theta - vy)}{v} \frac{\partial u}{\partial y} \lambda \int_{-\infty}^{+\infty} \tilde{u}(x + z, y, \tau) \tilde{p}(z) \, dz,$$

which is now posed on $\mathbb{R} \times \mathbb{R}^+ \times (0, T)$, with $\tilde{u}(z, y, \tau) = u(e^z, y, \tau)$ and $\tilde{p}(z) = e^z p(e^z)$. The problem is completed by suitable initial and boundary conditions, which for a European put option are:

$$u(x, y, 0) = \max(1 - \exp(x), 0), \quad x \in \mathbb{R}, \ y > 0,$$
$$u(x, y, t) \to 1, \quad x \to -\infty, \ y > 0, \ t > 0,$$
$$u(x, y, t) \to 0, \quad x \to +\infty, \ y > 0, \ t > 0,$$
$$u_y(x, y, t) \to 0, \quad x \in \mathbb{R}, \ y \to \infty, \ t > 0,$$
$$u_y(x, y, t) \to 0, \quad x \in \mathbb{R}, \ y \to 0, \ t > 0.$$

## 2.2 Implicit-Explicit High-Order Compact Scheme

For the discretisation, we replace $\mathbb{R}$ by $[-R_1, R_1]$ and $\mathbb{R}^+$ by $[L_2, R_2]$ with $R_1, R_2 > L_2 > 0$. We consider a uniform grid $Z = \{x_i \in [-R_1, R_1] : x_i = ih_1, \ i = -N, ..., N\} \times \{y_j \in [L_2, R_2] : y_j = L_2 + jh_2, \ j = 0, ..., M\}$ consisting of $(2N + 1) \times (M + 1)$ grid points with $R_1 = Nh_1$, $R_2 = L_2 + Mh_2$ and with space step $h := h_1 = h_2$ and time step $k$. Let $u_{i,j}^n$ denote the approximate solution of (2) in $(x_i, y_j)$ at the time $t_n = nk$ and let $u^n = (u_{i,j}^n)$.

For the numerical solution of the PIDE we use the implicit-explicit high-order compact (HOC) scheme presented in [4]. The implicit-explicit discretisation in time is accomplished through an adaptation of the Crank-Nicholson method which includes an explicit treatment for the integral operator. The scheme is fourth-order accurate in space and second-order accurate in time. We refer to [4] for the details of the derivation of the scheme and the implementation of the initial and boundary conditions.

If not mentioned otherwise, we use the following default parameters in our numerical experiments: $\kappa = 2, \theta = 0.01, \rho = -0.5, v = 0.1, r = 0.05, \lambda = 0.2, \gamma = -0.5$.

## 3  The Greeks

The so-called *Greeks* are the partial derivatives of the option price with respect to independent variables or parameters. These quantities represent the market sensitivities of options. Practitioners use these quantities to gain an insight into the effects of different market conditions on an options price and furthermore to develop hedging strategies against unfavourable changes in a portfolio of assets.

### 3.1  Vega

Vega measures the sensitivity of the option price with respect to changes in the volatility of the underlying asset, with the volatility given by the square root of the variance, $\sqrt{\sigma}$, i.e.

$$\text{Vega} = \frac{\partial V}{\partial(\sqrt{\sigma})}.$$

We examine whether the higher-order convergence achieved in the option price will also be represented in the vega of the option. Vega is calculated from the option price $V(S, \sigma, t)$, while the order of the scheme is maintained by using a fourth-order approximation formula (Fig. 1).

$$\text{Vega} = \frac{\partial V}{\partial(\sqrt{\sigma})} = \frac{\partial y}{\partial(\sqrt{\sigma})} \frac{\partial V}{\partial y}$$

$$\text{Vega}_{i,j}^{n} = \frac{2\sqrt{\sigma}_j}{v} \left( \frac{\partial V}{\partial y} \right)_{i,j}^{n} = \frac{2\sqrt{\sigma}_j}{v} \frac{V_{i,j-2}^{n} - 8V_{i,j-1}^{n} + 8V_{i,j+1}^{n} - V_{i,j+2}^{n}}{12h}$$

We conduct a numerical study to evaluate the rate of convergence of vega. We refer to both the $l_2$-norm error $\epsilon_2$ and the $l_\infty$-norm error $\epsilon_\infty$ with respect to a numerical reference solution on a fine grid with $h_{\text{ref}} = 0.025$. By fixing the parabolic mesh ratio $k/h^2$ we expect these errors to converge as $\epsilon = Ch^m$ for some constants $m$ and $C$. We generate a double-logarithmic plot of $\epsilon$ against $h$ which should be asymptotic to a straight line with slope $m$, with $m$ being the experimentally determined order of the scheme.

As a tool for comparison we perform the same numerical study using a standard second-order central difference scheme. The results of these experiments are seen in Figs. 2 and 3. We observe here that the experimentally determined convergence rates match well the theoretical order of each scheme. The errors at coarse grid, $h = 0.4$, are comparable, while on finer grids the high-order compact scheme gives orders of magnitude better accuracy on the same grids, achieving convergence rates of about fourth order.

**Fig. 1** Vega of European put option priced under the Bates model with parameters: Strike $K = 100$, time to expiry $T = 0.5$

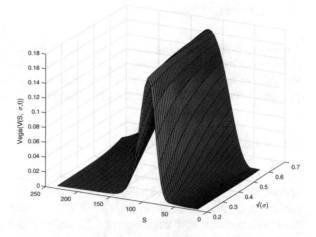

**Fig. 2** Convergence of $l_2$-error of the vega of a European put option priced under the Bates model with parameters: Strike $K = 100$, time to expiry $T = 0.5$

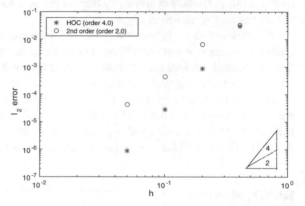

**Fig. 3** Convergence of $l_\infty$-error of the vega of a European put option priced under the Bates model with parameters: Strike $K = 100$, time to expiry $T = 0.5$

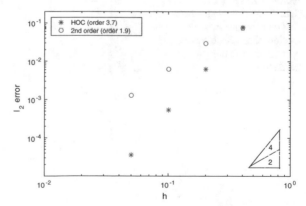

## 3.2 Hedging Vega

As with all financial trading, options are subject to risk and managing this risk is key to success. One method of managing risk is to establish a hedge against the implied volatility of the underlying asset. This is achieved by creating a vega neutral option position, which will be not be sensitive to fluctuations in volatility.

### 3.2.1 Hedging Example 1

An investment fund holds a long position in a non dividend paying stock, XYZ, which is currently trading at \$135. The investment fund wishes to secure an income from the position and writes some put options for XYZ with strike \$100. The investment fund now has a position with negative vega. To hedge this vega risk the investment fund creates a ratio vertical put spread by buying put options with strike \$150, creating a payoff diagram as shown in Fig. 4.

We propose that using the HOC scheme the investment fund can utilise the high-order convergence in vega to achieve a more accurate vega hedge when constructing the ratio spread. To measure this we compare the ratio used for each mesh size, $h$, with the fine reference grid and examine the resulting percentage error.

The results for the high-order scheme and those for a comparative second-order scheme are shown in Table 1. The high-order scheme significantly outperforms the second-order scheme at all mesh-sizes, suggesting that when entering a large position the HOC scheme will lead to a significant improvement in the vega hedge.

**Fig. 4** Payoff for ratio vertical put spread, examples include a 1:2 spread, where the trader writes two put options then goes long one put option with a higher strike price

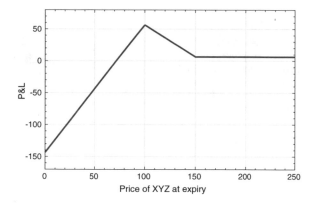

**Table 1** Percentage error in vega hedge ratio

| Scheme | Mesh-size | Percentage error | Scheme | Mesh-size | Percentage error |
|---|---|---|---|---|---|
| HOC | 0.4 | 33.3138 | Second-order | 0.4 | 62.0312 |
| HOC | 0.2 | 6.7519 | Second-order | 0.2 | 33.0638 |
| HOC | 0.1 | 0.6251 | Second-order | 0.1 | 7.4073 |
| HOC | 0.05 | 0.0400 | Second-order | 0.05 | 1.5364 |

## 3.3 Gamma

Gamma is the second derivative of the option price with respect to the underlying asset. Gamma measures the rate of change in an option's delta, providing information on the convexity of the option's value in relation to the price of the underlying asset,

$$\Gamma = \frac{\partial^2 V}{\partial S^2}.$$

We calculate gamma using the option price $V(S, \sigma, t)$. To maintain the order of the scheme we use a fourth-order approximation formula (Fig. 5).

$$\Gamma = \frac{\partial^2 V}{\partial S^2} = \frac{\partial^2 x}{\partial S^2} \frac{\partial^2 V}{\partial x^2}$$

$$\Gamma_{i,j}^n = \frac{1}{S_i^2} \left( \frac{\partial^2 V}{\partial x^2} \right)_{i,j}^n = \frac{1}{S_i^2} \frac{V_{i-2,j}^n - 16V_{i-1,j}^n + 30V_{i,j}^n - 16V_{i+1,j}^n + V_{i+2,j}^n}{12h^2}$$

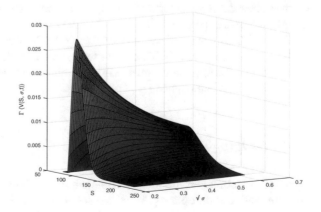

**Fig. 5** Gamma of European put option priced under the Bates model with parameters: Strike $K = 100$, time to expiry $T = 0.5$

**Fig. 6** Convergence of $l_2$-error of gamma of a European put option priced under the Bates model with parameters: Strike $K = 100$, time to expiry $T = 0.5$

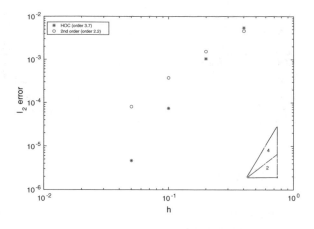

**Fig. 7** Convergence of $l_\infty$-error of gamma of a European put option priced under the Bates model with parameters: Strike $K = 100$, time to expiry $T = 0.5$

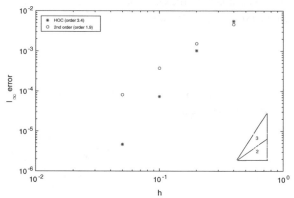

We conduct a numerical study to evaluate the rate of convergence of gamma. We refer to both the $l_2$-error $\epsilon_2$ and the $l_\infty$-error $\epsilon_\infty$ with respect to a numerical reference solution on a fine grid with $h_{\text{ref}} = 0.025$. For comparison we perform the same numerical study using a standard second-order central difference scheme. The results of these experiments are seen in Figs. 6 and 7.

The HOC scheme achieves convergence rates between three and four for the $l_2$- and $l_\infty$-errors, respectively. This is an improvement on the second-order scheme and suggests that the high-order scheme is beneficial when developing trading strategies which involve a gamma hedge.

## 3.4 Hedging Gamma

Hedges of gamma risk are often accompanied by a delta hedge, with delta being the first derivative of the option price with respect to the underlying asset. A delta hedged

**Table 2**  Percentage error in gamma hedge ratio

| Scheme | Mesh-size | Percentage error | Scheme | Mesh-size | Percentage error |
|---|---|---|---|---|---|
| HOC | 0.4 | 14.8885 | Second-order | 0.4 | 25.1112 |
| HOC | 0.2 | 2.3323 | Second-order | 0.2 | 6.3482 |
| HOC | 0.1 | 0.1281 | Second-order | 0.1 | 1.3304 |
| HOC | 0.05 | 0.0081 | Second-order | 0.05 | 0.2674 |

portfolio is not subject to risk owing to a change in the price of the underlying asset, the gamma hedge is a re-adjustment of this delta hedge.

Delta-gamma hedging strategies often require frequent adjustments and hence are subject to high trading costs. However, if executed correctly they can enable the holder to exploit positions with positive theta, meaning the position is profitable over short time durations.

### 3.4.1  Hedging Example 2

An analyst at an investment fund looks to create a strategy with positive theta against the funds currently held assets. They choose a ratio write spread, which involves writing options at a higher strike price than they are purchased. The analyst is wary of the positions risk related to move in the underlying asset and hence adjusts the ratio of short to long options to eliminate the net gamma.

The resulting position will have a delta value which must be hedged before the analyst can assess any profitability from the positive theta of the spread. The delta of the two option positions long and short is totalled and if positive or negative underlying assets are sold or bought, respectively.

The resulting theta is calculated and if positive the analyst can recommend the strategy as a short term trade for the investment fund.

We propose that using the HOC scheme the investment fund can utilise the high-order convergence in gamma to achieve a more accurate gamma hedge ratio. To measure this we compare the ratio used for each mesh size, $h$, with the fine reference grid and examine the resulting percentage error.

The results for the high-order scheme and those for a comparative second-order scheme are shown in Table 2. The high-order scheme offers better results at all mesh-sizes, this improvement is particularly important in hedged positions which require repeat computation and regular adjustments.

**Acknowledgements**  BD acknowledges partial support by the Leverhulme Trust research project grant 'Novel discretisations for higher-order nonlinear PDE' (RPG-2015-69). AP has been supported by a studentship under the EPSRC Doctoral Training Partnership (DTP) scheme (grant number EP/M506667/1).

# References

1. Bates, D.S.: Jumps and stochastic volatility: exchange rate processes implicit Deutsche mark options. Rev. Financ. Stud. **9**, 637–654 (1996)
2. Cont, R., Tankov, P.: Financial Modelling with Jump Processes. Chapman & Hall/CRC, Boca Raton, FL (2004)
3. Düring, B., Fournié, M.: High-order compact finite difference scheme for option pricing in stochastic volatility models. J. Comp. Appl. Math. **236**, 4462–4473 (2012)
4. Düring, B., Pitkin, A.: High-order compact finite difference scheme for option pricing in stochastic volatility jump models. Submitted for publication. arXiv:1704.05308 (2017)
5. Salmi, S., Toivanen, J., von Sydow, L.: An IMEX-scheme for pricing options under stochastic volatility models with jumps. SIAM J. Sci. Comp. **36**(5), B817–B834 (2014)

# An Explicit Optimal Strategy for Flow Trades at NASDAQ Around Its Close

Christoph Frei and Chad Yan

**Abstract** For many investors, such as mutual fund managers, the closing price of a stock is an important benchmark. Closing prices for stocks traded at NASDAQ and many other stock exchanges are determined through auctions. Each day and for each stock traded at NASDAQ, the projected order imbalance of the auction is announced beginning ten minutes before the close. We introduce a tractable model for stock price dynamics that takes the order imbalance announcements into account. In a mean-variance framework with the closing price as benchmark, we derive an explicit formula for the optimal trading strategy. We find that it is not beneficial for the investor to trade after the imbalance announcement. However, in addition to participating in the auction, the investor trades before the imbalance announcement to benefit from prices which do not reflect the later impact of the investor's own auction order.

**Keywords** Optimal trade execution · NASDAQ · Closing price · Benchmark

## 1 Introduction

Closing prices of stocks are important and often serve as reference points for investors to determine their performance. Closing prices are particularly relevant to managers of mutual funds. For mutual funds, flow trades correspond to inflows or outflows of cash when clients decide to buy or sell shares of the fund. Regardless of the specific time the transactions are taking place on a trading day, the mutual fund will receive from or pay to the client the closing price on that day. Hence, managers of such funds

C. Frei (✉)
University of Alberta, Mathematical and Statistical Sciences,
Edmonton, AB T6G 2G1, Canada
e-mail: cfrei@ualberta.ca

C. Yan
Alberta Investment Management Corporation, 1100-10830 Jasper Avenue,
Edmonton, AB T5J 2B3, Canada
e-mail: Chad.Yan@aimco.alberta.ca

© Springer Nature Switzerland AG 2018
D. M. Kilgour et al. (eds.), *Recent Advances in Mathematical
and Statistical Methods*, Springer Proceedings in Mathematics & Statistics 259,
https://doi.org/10.1007/978-3-319-99719-3_45

use the closing price as their benchmark: they aim to achieve a price that is as close as possible to the closing price and, if possible, more favourable than the closing price.

At stock exchanges in many emerging markets and almost all developed markets (see FTSE Russell [7] for an overview), the closing price is determined through an auction. The auction mechanisms and rules are similar for different markets. For this note, we focus on NASDAQ, where all traders are granted access to the same information. Each day until 3:50 p.m. Eastern Time, traders can submit orders to the closing auction at NASDAQ without any restriction. At 3:50 p.m., NASDAQ publishes an initial imbalance announcement, with information on the projected imbalance of the auction. Afterwards, NASDAQ publishes imbalance information every five seconds until 4:00 p.m. Between 3:50 p.m. and 4:00 p.m., restrictions on the possibility to submit orders to the closing auction apply, so to reduce the projected imbalance. At 4:00 p.m., the closing price is determined such that the most orders submitted to the auction are matched. Figure 1 gives an overview of the closing auction at NASDAQ. The goal of this note is to introduce a tractable stock price model around the close and to study what an optimal execution strategy is for a trader targeting the closing price. This work is in the area of algorithmic trading, the analysis and implementation of mathematical and computational algorithms to conduct trading decisions and asset management. Mathematical studies for algorithmic trading started with seminal papers by Bertsimas and Lo [3], who set up a discrete-time model to minimize expected slippage, and by Almgren and Chriss [1], who focused on the trading strategy targeting the arrival price benchmark including risk considerations. An overview of trading algorithms targeting different benchmarks can be found in the recent books by Cartea et al. [4], and Lehalle and Laruelle [9]. While trading strategies for many benchmarks, such as arrival price, VWAP (volume weighted average price), TWAP (time weighted average price) and POV (percentage of volume), have been well studied, there is only sparse literature on execution problems with a closing price benchmark. Frei and Westray [6] consider the particular situation in Hong Kong, where the closing price of stocks is computed as the median of five prices over the last minute of trade. Kan and Park [8] derive an opti-

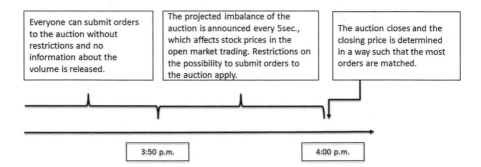

**Fig. 1** Timeline of the closing auction at NASDAQ

mal trading strategy in a continuous-time model with a mean-variance optimization criterion. Also using a mean-variance optimization criterion, but in a discrete-time setting, Labadie and Lehalle [10] find recursive formulae when considering arrival and closing price benchmarks.

In contrast to all these works, we include in our model the imbalance announcement, which provides crucial information when targeting the closing auction price. We find an explicit formula for the optimal execution strategy, which trades a part of the order before the imbalance announcement. This is because the trader benefits from favourable prices before the imbalance announcement by front running the impact of the trader's own participation in the closing auction. After the imbalance announcement, prices reflect the imbalance information so that, for our trader, it is not favourable to execute further orders. This result of not trading after the imbalance announcement is in line with observations in Bacidore et al. [2], who discuss issues surrounding trading in and around the closing auction.

## 2 Problem Formulation

Our market model consists of $T - 1$ periods in the open market, with $T$ the closing time of the auction. Let $\tau < T$ be the time of the initial imbalance announcement. At NASDAQ, $\tau$ and $T$ correspond to 3:50 p.m. and 4:00 p.m., respectively. We consider a trader with a buy order of $W$ units of some stock. The trader can split the order into $v_1, v_2, \ldots, v_T$ with $\sum_{t=1}^{T} v_t = W$, where $v_1, v_2, \ldots, v_{T-1}$ are the volumes of orders submitted to the open market and $v_T$ is submitted to the closing auction.

We suppose that the order imbalance is cleared immediately and there are no orders in the closing auction after 3:50 p.m., which are stylized features close to what we observe at NASDAQ. For a given initial price $\tilde{P}_0$, the prices excluding our market impact are modelled by

$$\tilde{P}_t = \tilde{P}_{t-1} + Z_t \quad \text{for } t \in \{1, \ldots, \tau - 1, \tau + 1 \ldots, T - 1\},$$
$$\tilde{P}_\tau = \tilde{P}_{\tau-1} + Z_\tau + \alpha N,$$
$$\tilde{P}_T = \tilde{P}_{T-1} + Y,$$

where

- $Z_t$, modelling the stock price fluctuations in the open market, are independent and identically distributed with mean zero and finite variance $\sigma_Z^2$.
- $Y$, modelling the fluctuations from the last price in the open market to the auction price, is independent from $Z_t$ with mean zero and finite variance $\sigma_Y^2$.
- $N = \tilde{N} + v_T$ is the auction imbalance (a positive value means more buy than sell orders at the current stock price), consisting of our auction order submission, $v_T$,

and that of all other market participants, $\tilde{N}$. We assume that $\tilde{N}$ is independent from $Z_t$ and $Y$, and it has mean zero and finite variance $\sigma_{\tilde{N}}^2$.

- $\alpha > 0$ reflects the impact of the auction imbalance on stock prices.

Assumptions similar to the above independence between auction volume and price increments have been made in the literature and are empirically justified; see for example Fig. 1 in Frei and Westray [5].

We assume that the trader's orders have a temporary market impact so that they affect stock prices at the execution time, but have no influence on subsequent stock prices. This means that the trader effectively pays a price

$$P_t = \tilde{P}_t + \beta v_t \text{ for } t \in \{1, 2, \ldots, T - 1\},$$

where $\beta > 0$ is the coefficient of temporary market impact. We set $P_T = \tilde{P}_T$ because our order placed in the closing auction, $v_T$, is already reflected in the earlier price $\tilde{P}_\tau$ through $N = \tilde{N} + v_T$.

The trader targets the closing price $P_T$. As is standard in the literature on algorithmic trading and in line with [1, 6, 8–10], we consider a mean-variance formulation. Thus, the objective is to minimize, over $v_t \geq 0$ with $\sum_{t=1}^{T} v_t = W$,

$$E\left[\sum_{t=1}^{T} v_t P_t - W P_T\right] + \lambda VAR\left[\sum_{t=1}^{T} v_t P_t - W P_T\right]$$

for a given mean-variance tradeoff parameter $\lambda > 0$, modelling the trader's risk aversion. This means that we minimize a combination of average costs and deviations to the closing price benchmark.

## 3   Main Result

Our main result gives an explicit formula for the optimal strategy.

**Theorem 1** *The optimal strategy is given by*

$$v_1 = \frac{\alpha W}{2(\beta + m_1 + \sum_{i=2}^{\tau-1} m_i p_i)},$$

$$v_t = p_t v_1 \quad for \ t = 2, 3, \ldots, \tau - 1,$$

$$v_k = 0 \quad for \ k = \tau, \tau + 1, \ldots, T - 1,$$

$$v_T = W - \left(1 + \sum_{i=2}^{\tau-1} p_i\right) v_1,$$

*where*

$$m_t := (T-t)\lambda\sigma_Z^2 + \lambda\sigma_Y^2 + \lambda\alpha^2\sigma_{\tilde{N}}^2 + \alpha,$$

$$p_t := \left(\frac{\lambda\sigma_Z^2}{\beta} + 1 - x_-\right)\frac{x_+^t}{x_+^2 - 1} + \left(\frac{\lambda\sigma_Z^2}{\beta} + 1 - x_+\right)\frac{x_-^t}{x_-^2 - 1},$$

$$x_\pm := 1 + \frac{\lambda\sigma_Z^2}{2\beta} \pm \sqrt{\frac{\lambda\sigma_Z^2}{\beta}\left(1 + \frac{\lambda\sigma_Z^2}{4\beta}\right)}.$$

The theorem shows that the portion $\frac{2(\beta+m_1+\sum_{i=2}^{\tau-1} m_i p_i)-\alpha-\alpha\sum_{i=2}^{\tau-1} p_i}{2(\beta+m_1+\sum_{i=2}^{\tau-1} m_i p_i)} W$ of the total order $W$ is placed into the closing auction. The remaining part is submitted to the open market before the initial imbalance announcement, with small orders $v_1, v_2, \ldots, v_{\tau-1}$ that are exponentially increasing over time with basis $x_\pm$. It is not optimal to trade after the initial imbalance announcement.

*Remark 1* (1) If the trader's orders have no influence on the stock prices in the closing auction ($\alpha = 0$), then it is optimal to trade only in the closing auction, that is, $v_T = W$.

(2) If the trader's orders have no influence on the stock prices in the open market ($\beta = 0$), then the optimal trading in the open market occurs only at the moment before the initial imbalance announcement. In particular, we have $v_t = 0$ for all $t \neq \tau - 1, T$ and

$$v_{\tau-1} = \frac{\alpha W}{2\big((T - \tau + 1)\lambda\sigma_Z^2 + \lambda\sigma_Y^2 + \lambda\alpha^2\sigma_{\tilde{N}}^2 + \alpha\big)}, \quad v_T = W - v_{\tau-1}.$$

(3) The value of the mean-variance tradeoff parameter $\lambda$ determines how much focus the trader puts on minimizing deviations to the benchmark compared to minimizing average costs. If $\lambda$ is big, the trader will submit most of the order to the closing auction so to minimize deviations to the closing price. Indeed, in the limit as $\lambda \to \infty$, the theorem implies that $v_t \to 0$ for $t = 1, 2, \ldots, T - 1$ and $v_T \to W$, using that $m_t \to \infty$ for any $t$ as $\lambda \to \infty$. By contrast, for $\lambda \to 0$, we have $v_t \to \frac{\alpha W}{2\beta+2\alpha(\tau-1)}$ for $t = 1, 2, \ldots, \tau - 1$ and $v_T \to \frac{(2\beta+\alpha(\tau-1))W}{2\beta+2\alpha(\tau-1)}$, as we can show that $m_t \to \alpha$ and $p_t \to 1$ as $\lambda \to 0$. In this case of $\lambda \to 0$, the trader minimizes average costs.

(4) In a generalized setting when the assumptions that $\tilde{N}$, $Z_t$ and $Y$ have zero means are relaxed, we can find a recursive algorithm for the optimal strategy, generalizing the explicit formula from Theorem 1; see Yan [11] for details.

## 4 Sketch of the Proof of Theorem 1

Using the assumptions that $\tilde{N}$, $Z_t$ and $Y$ have zero means, we can rewrite the objective function as

$$\min \; \beta \sum_{t=1}^{T-1} v_t^2 + \alpha \sum_{t=1}^{\tau-1} v_t \sum_{t=1}^{T-1} v_t - \alpha W \sum_{t=1}^{\tau-1} v_t + \lambda \sigma_Z^2 \sum_{t=2}^{T-1} \left( \sum_{i=1}^{t-1} v_i \right)^2$$

$$+ \lambda \sigma_Y^2 \left( \sum_{t=1}^{T-1} v_t \right)^2 + \lambda \alpha^2 \sigma_{\tilde{N}}^2 \left( \sum_{t=1}^{\tau-1} v_t \right)^2$$

$$\text{subject to } \; W - \sum_{t=1}^{T-1} v_t \geq 0 \text{ and } v_t \geq 0 \text{ for all } t \in \{1, \dots, T-1\}.$$

We analyze the corresponding Lagrange function given by

$$L(v_1, v_2, \dots, v_{T-1}; \delta) = \beta \sum_{t=1}^{T-1} v_t^2 + \alpha \sum_{t=1}^{\tau-1} v_t \sum_{t=1}^{T-1} v_t - \alpha W \sum_{t=1}^{\tau-1} v_t + \lambda \sigma_Z^2 \sum_{t=2}^{T-1} \left( \sum_{i=1}^{t-1} v_i \right)^2$$

$$+ \lambda \sigma_Y^2 \left( \sum_{t=1}^{T-1} v_t \right)^2 + \lambda \alpha^2 \sigma_{\tilde{N}}^2 \left( \sum_{t=1}^{\tau-1} v_t \right)^2 + \delta \left( \sum_{t=1}^{T-1} v_t - W \right)$$

and examine its first-order condition with respect to the execution order $v_t$ at each point in time. To minimize the objective function, the following Karush-Kuhn-Tucker (KKT) conditions must hold:

$$v_t \frac{\partial L}{\partial v_t} = 0, \; v_t \geq 0, \; \frac{\partial L}{\partial v_t} \geq 0 \quad \text{for } t \in \{1, 2, \dots, T-1\},$$

$$\delta \frac{\partial L}{\partial \delta} = 0, \; \delta \geq 0, \; \frac{\partial L}{\partial \delta} \leq 0.$$

By using the KKT conditions, we can show that it is not optimal to trade after the initial imbalance announcement based on a proof by contradiction.

Using $v_t = 0$ for $t = \tau, \tau + 1, \dots, T - 1$, we can reduce the level of complexity in the system of equations from the KKT conditions. We solve the system of KKT equations recursively, that is, we rewrite it such that each of its equations gives a linear relation between $v_t$, $v_{t-1}$ and $v_{t-2}$. By applying the concept of characteristic equation to this recursive system of equations, we can derive the explicit optimal trading strategy for every period before the initial imbalance announcement, given in Theorem 1.

## 5   Implementation Example

In this section, we use data on intraday stock prices and imbalance volumes during the closing auction to estimate input parameters, and then illustrate the optimal trading strategies for an investment in Amazon.com Inc. (AMZN). We choose the time increment in trading periods to be one second. The overall trading horizon consists of the last half hour before market close, which means the considered trading begins at 3:30 p.m. To estimate model parameters, we use a date set from Nov. 1, 2016 to Jan. 27, 2017, with intraday stock price, volume and imbalance data from NASDAQ. In this estimation, we find $\alpha = 5.72 \times 10^{-6}$, $\sigma_{\tilde{N}}^2 = 6.6 \times 10^9$, $\sigma_Z^2 = 1.96 \times 10^{-8}$ and $\sigma_Y^2 = 3.21 \times 10^{-8}$ while we set $\lambda = 5 \times 10^{-4}$ and $\beta = 10^{-6}$ in line with Sect. 3.4 of Almgren and Chriss [1]. We assume that the goal is to purchase $W = 100,000$ shares of the AMZN stock on January 30, 2017.

Figure 2 shows the cumulative trading volume based on the strategy of Theorem 1. After the initial imbalance announcement, the cumulative trading volume remains constant, until a spike occurs at 4:00 p.m., which reflects the order placed in the closing auction.

Figure 3 shows the different paths for AMZN's stock prices. The blue path corresponds to the actual historical stock prices on Jan. 30, 2017. We added two different price paths that incorporate our trading decisions. The red path models the stock prices if we purchased the entire 100,000 shares in the closing action while the green path displays the prices under our optimal strategy from Theorem 1. The price impact induced by the proposed strategy is considerably lower than that of the benchmark strategy. In this example, implementation costs of the strategy using only the closing auction are $83,095,241 while the optimal strategy entails implementation costs of $82,846,209, which reflects a cost reduction of $249,032, or 30 basis points. A more extensive analysis of the performance across 15 stocks listed at NASDAQ is contained in Yan [11]. In that study, the proposed strategy yields a positive and sta-

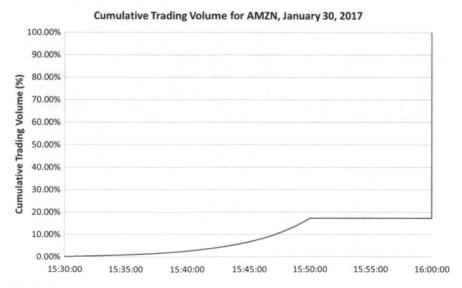

**Fig. 2** Cumulative trading volume for AMZN based on the strategy of Theorem 1

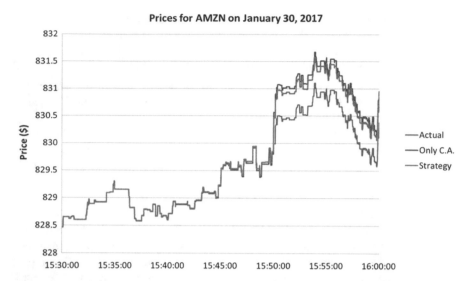

**Fig. 3** AMZN price dynamics for the different scenarios: observed prices (blue: 'Actual'), prices with an additional order entirely submitted to the closing auction (red: 'Only C.A.'), and prices with an additional order submitted based on the strategy of Theorem 1 (green: 'Strategy')

ble performance across different stocks. While the strategy may lead to temporary losses on some trading days, it showed an outperformance compared to trading in only the closing auction for all tested stocks over a one-month test period. Because the trading strategy is available in explicit form, its computation time for one stock and one trading day is only a couple of seconds on a standard personal computer.

The optimal strategy depends also on the chosen values for the mean-variance tradeoff parameter $\lambda$ and the coefficient $\beta$ of temporary market impact. A higher value of $\lambda$ means that the trader is more risk averse, and thus, trades a bigger portion in the closing auction. This is indeed the case, as we observe in Fig. 4 for a comparison with different values of $\lambda$: $10^{-4}$ (low), $5 \times 10^{-4}$ (default), and $10^{-3}$ (high), using the same other parameters as described at the beginning of this section. A higher value of the coefficient $\beta$ means that the trader has a bigger impact on prices in the open market. When $\beta$ is high, the trader will spread the orders more evenly during the period of the open market to reduce price impact while taking more risk from price fluctuations. This is confirmed in Fig. 5, which shows a comparison for different values of $\beta$: $10^{-7}$ (low), $10^{-6}$ (default), and $10^{-5}$ (high), with the other parameters the same as described at the beginning of this section.

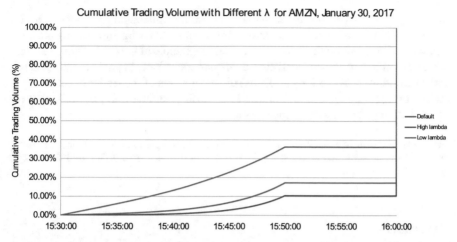

**Fig. 4** Cumulative trading volume for AMZN compared for different values of $\lambda$: $10^{-4}$ (low; green), $5 \times 10^{-4}$ (default; blue), and $10^{-3}$ (high; red)

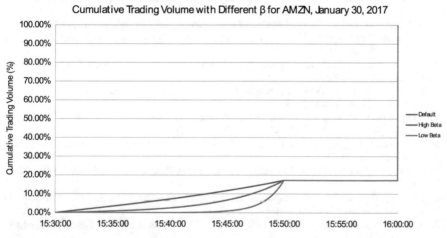

**Fig. 5** Cumulative trading volume for AMZN compared for different values of $\beta$: $10^{-7}$ (low; green), $10^{-6}$ (default; blue), and $10^{-5}$ (high; red)

## 6  Conclusion

In this note, we derived an explicit optimal strategy for a trader who targets the closing prices of stocks listed at NASDAQ. The trader attempts to minimize a combination of average costs and deviations to the closing price benchmark. We introduced a tractable model, which takes the key microstructural features into account, namely, fluctuations in stock prices and the impact of the order imbalance announcement. The optimal strategy puts a major part into the closing auction and smaller, exponentially increasing fractions in the open market before the imbalance announcement. No execution is done after the imbalance announcement. Using historical imbalance volume and intraday stock prices, we showed an example of how our optimal strategy can be implemented. Further statistical analysis done in Yan [11] indicate, persistently across different stocks of NASDAQ and different levels of the trader's risk aversion, an improvement compared to trading in the closing auction only; in particular, our optimal strategy has lower average costs.

**Acknowledgements** We thank an anonymous referee for helpful comments. Financial support by the Natural Sciences and Engineering Council of Canada under grant RGPIN/402585-2011 is gratefully acknowledged.

# References

1. Almgren, R., Chriss, N.: Optimal execution of portfolio transactions. J. Risk **3**, 5–40 (2001)
2. Bacidore, J., Polidore, B., Xu, W., Yang, C.: Trading around the close. J. Trading **8**, 48–57 (2012)
3. Bertsimas, D., Lo, A.: Optimal control of execution costs. J. Fin. Markets **1**, 1–50 (1998)
4. Cartea, Á., Jaimungal, S., Penalva, J.: Algorithmic and High-Frequency Trading. Cambridge University Press (2015)
5. Frei, C., Westray, N.: Optimal execution of a VWAP order: a stochastic control approach. Math. Fin. **25**, 612–639 (2015)
6. Frei, C., Westray, N.: Optimal execution in Hong Kong given a market-on-close benchmark. Quant. Fin. **18**, 655–671 (2018)
7. FTSE Russell: Closing prices used for index calculation, Version 1.8. Available at http://www.ftse.com/products/indices/Index-Support-Guides (2016)
8. Kan, Y.H., Park, S.: Optimal closing-price strategy: peculiarities and practicalities. J. Investment Strat. **6** (2016)
9. Lehalle, C.-A., Laruelle, S.: Market Microstructure in Practice. World Scientific Publishing (2013)
10. Labadie, M., Lehalle, C.-A.: Optimal starting times, stopping times and risk measures for algorithmic trading. J. Investment Strat. **3** (2014)
11. Yan, C.: Algorithms for flow trades at NASDAQ around its close. M.Sc. Thesis, University of Alberta (2017)

# Optimal Selection of Assets and Portfolios

**Bowen Hu and Roman N. Makarov**

**Abstract** In this paper, we propose a new method that allows an investor to rank available financial securities such as equities and exchange-traded funds (ETFs) in accordance with his or her risk preferences. We have demonstrated that using a linear combination of several risk measures and performance metrics as a ranking function can help us to select the most suitable efficient portfolio that is meeting risk preferences of an investor. We use three different methods to evaluate long-term values of metrics for each asset. After applying the ranking system to select most suitable assets from a large pool of securities, an optimal portfolio is formed by maximizing the ranking function. Past 5–10 years data with U.S. ETFs and S&P500 stocks have been extracted using a Bloomberg terminal.

**Keywords** Asset ranking · Portfolio optimization · Occupation time
Risk measures · Performance metrics · Value at risk · Expected shortfall
Sharpe ratio

## 1 Introduction

Different investors may have different preferences regarding the risk and performance of their portfolios that cannot be captured by a single metric such as the volatility or the Sharpe ratio. To find an optimal portfolio, the investor needs to first select assets from an extensive collection of securities that are meeting his or her criteria. Second, the investor needs to find optimal allocation weights for the assets selected. In this paper, we develop a ranking system to solve the selection problem by forming a linear combination of several risk and performance metrics. The ranking function attempts

B. Hu
University of Waterloo, Waterloo, ON, Canada
e-mail: b9hu@uwaterloo.ca

R. N. Makarov (✉)
Wilfrid Laurier University, Waterloo, ON, Canada
e-mail: rmakarov@wlu.ca

© Springer Nature Switzerland AG 2018
D. M. Kilgour et al. (eds.), *Recent Advances in Mathematical and Statistical Methods*, Springer Proceedings in Mathematics & Statistics 259,
https://doi.org/10.1007/978-3-319-99719-3_46

to quantify the fitness of assets such as exchange trading funds (ETF) and equities to a specific investor. The list of performance metrics includes the expected daily log-return rate and the Sharpe ratio. The list of risk metrics consists of the standard deviation, the Value-at-Risk (VaR) and the Expected Shortfall (ES) also known as the conditional Value-at-Risk (CVaR). Since the ranking function is a continuous-valued function, ties (equal scores) are not an issue. Later, the same ranking function can be used in the portfolio optimization problem.

In this paper, the analysis was mostly done on U.S. Equity ETFs and the stocks included in the S&P500 index. Our first step was to extract prices of all securities from Bloomberg for the period from June 2010 to June 2015. We imported data for all ETFs and deleted those of them that had less than five years worth of data and were not traded too frequently. In the end there were 537 ETFs left including the following: 67 U.S. Fixed income ETFs, 145 Global Equity ETFs, 117 Commodity ETFs and 208 U.S. Equity ETFs.

Here, we use daily logarithmic returns, which are calculated by

$$r_j = \ln \left( \frac{V_j}{V_{j-1}} \right), \tag{1}$$

where $r_j$ and $V_j$ are, respectively, the daily log-return and the asset value on day $j$. Here, we assume that for each asset the daily log-returns are independent and identically distributed (iid).

We will use $\mu(r) = E[r]$ to denote the expected daily log-return rate. It measures the growth rate of a fund or an equity one can expect. The average rate can be approximated by the sample mean $\hat{\mu}$ as follows:

$$\mu(r) \approx \hat{\mu} = \frac{1}{T} \sum_{j=1}^{T} r_j, \tag{2}$$

where $T$ is the size of the sample data set.

In the financial field, the standard deviation of asset's returns, denoted by $\sigma(r) = \sqrt{Var(r)}$, is a popular indicator to represent the risk of a financial asset. A riskier asset is having a larger standard deviation of its return. We use the following formula to calculate the sample standard deviation $\hat{\sigma}$:

$$\sigma(r) \approx \hat{\sigma} = \sqrt{\frac{1}{T-1} \sum_{j=1}^{T} (r_j - \hat{\mu})^2}. \tag{3}$$

The Sharpe Ratio is probably the most popular performance metric used by investors. It takes not only the expected return of a fund into account but also the risk associated with it. The formula of the Sharpe ratio, which was revised by Sharpe in [7], is

$$SR(r) = \frac{E[r - r_0]}{\sqrt{Var[r - r_0]}}, \tag{4}$$

where $r$ is the return on the asset we are measuring, $r_0$ is the return on another fund which is used as a benchmark. It allows for comparing funds with different strategies. The benchmark used here is a risk-free asset. Since we deal with daily returns and the impact of interest rate in a short time period is insignificant, we assume here that $r_0$ is 0. Thus, the Sharpe ration can be estimated as follows:

$$SR(r) \approx \widehat{SR} = \frac{\frac{1}{T}\sum_{j=1}^{T} r_j}{\sqrt{\frac{\sum_{j=1}^{T}(r_j - \hat{\mu})^2}{T-1}}} = \frac{\hat{\mu}}{\hat{\sigma}}. \tag{5}$$

The Value at Risk (VaR) is another important method to measure the risk of asset [1]. A $100\alpha\%$ VaR is the value of minimal loss in the worst $100(1-\alpha)\%$ scenarios. The formal definition of VaR is

$$VaR_\alpha(r) = \inf\{x \in \mathbb{R} : P(\ell > x) \leqslant 1 - \alpha\}, \tag{6}$$

where $\alpha$ is the probability that the portfolio will fall in value by more than $VaR_\alpha(r)$ and $\ell = -r$ is the loss.

The Expected Shortfall (ES) is another well-known risk measure. It captures the average loss given that one of the worst $100(1-\alpha)\%$ scenarios happens. The formula for ES is

$$ES_\alpha(r) = \frac{1}{\alpha} \int_0^\alpha VaR_t(r)dt. \tag{7}$$

We can approximate VaR and ES by the following nonparametric estimates [6]:

$$VaR_\alpha(r) \approx \widehat{VaR}_\alpha = r_{T:j}, \quad \text{for } 1 - \alpha \in \left(\frac{j-1}{T}, \frac{j}{T}\right], \quad 1 \leq j \leq T, \tag{8}$$

$$ES_\alpha(r) \approx \widehat{ES}_\alpha = \widehat{VaR}_\alpha + \frac{1}{\alpha}\frac{1}{T} \sum_{j=1}^{T} \left(r_i - \widehat{VaR}_\alpha\right)^+, \tag{9}$$

where $(x)^+ = \max\{x, 0\}$, and $r_{T:1} < \ldots < r_{T:T}$ are the order statistics of the sample.

## 2 Ranking System

In this section, we discuss techniques used to rank the funds and equities based on investor's risk preference. Three ranking schemes are introduced in the following subsections.

## 2.1 Standardization

The ranking function is to be defined as a linear combination of risk and performance metrics. However, the metrics have different ranges, and thus we need to set up an appropriate transformation to scale them up or down to the same range. For example, the expected daily return is usually between $-0.7\%$ and $0.7\%$ and the Sharpe ratio is typically changing from $-0.5$ to $0.7$. In this case, if we just simply added unadjusted values, the contribution of the expected daily return would be too small in comparison with the Sharpe ratio. In order to solve this problem, we apply the following method. Assume there are $N$ funds available for the investor. Let $\mu_n$ denote the expected daily return of fund $n$. To standardize $\mu$ for each fund, we need to find out the maximum and the minimum expected returns of all funds:

$$\mu_{\max} = \max\{\mu_n : 1 \leqslant n \leqslant N\}, \tag{10}$$

$$\mu_{\min} = \min\{\mu_n : 1 \leqslant n \leqslant N\}. \tag{11}$$

After that, the standardized expected return $\mu^s(r)$ of fund $n$ with return $r \equiv r^{(n)}$ is calculated as follows:

$$\mu^s(r) = \frac{\mu_n - \mu_{\min}}{\mu_{\max} - \mu_{\min}}. \tag{12}$$

The benefit of this formula is that it maps the expected return of any asset to a value between 0 and 1. The standardized expected return of the fund with the largest $\mu$ is 1 and 0 will be assigned to the lowest one. We use the same approach to standardize other risk and performance metrics:

$$\sigma^s(r) = \frac{\sigma - \sigma_{\min}}{\sigma_{\max} - \sigma_{\min}}, \tag{13}$$

$$SR^s(r) = \frac{SR(r) - SR_{\min}}{SR_{\max} - SR_{\min}}, \tag{14}$$

$$VaR_\alpha^s(r) = \frac{VaR_\alpha(r) - VaR_{\alpha,min}}{VaR_{\alpha,max} - VaR_{\alpha,min}}, \tag{15}$$

$$ES_\alpha^s(r) = \frac{ES_\alpha(r) - ES_{\alpha,min}}{ES_{\alpha,max} - ES_{\alpha,min}}, \tag{16}$$

where $\sigma_{\max}$ and $\sigma_{\min}$ are, respectively, the maximum and minimum standard deviations of the funds; similar notations are used for other metrics.

## 2.2 Coefficients for Metrics

We use a linear combination of several risk and performance metrics as a ranking function. Thus, we multiply each metric by some coefficient to adjust the contribution of each metric and then sum them up. The ranking function of return $r$ is defined as

$$F(r) = C_1 \cdot \mu^s(r) - C_2 \cdot \sigma^s(r) + C_3 \cdot SR^s(r) - C_4 \cdot VaR_\alpha^s(r) - C_5 \cdot ES_\alpha^s(r).$$
(17)

When selecting an optimal portfolio, a rational investor always prefers the one with high values of the expected return and the Sharp Ratio as well as with lower values of the volatility, the value at risk and the expect shortfall. Since we will assume that all the coefficients $C_i$ are non-negative, we have to put a negative sign in front of the risk measures we wish to be low. Same setting is also applied in (19), (24), and (26). This function can be used to compare different assets or investment portfolios. The higher objective value an asset has, the more suitable this asset is for the investor.

The multiplicative coefficients for metrics are adjusted for each individual investor according to his or her preferences. For example, if an investor is more concerned about risk, the coefficients for the volatility, VaR and ES, can be assigned higher values. To control the contribution of each metric easily, we set up the following constraints on the coefficients:

$$C_i \geqslant 0 \text{ for all } i \text{ and } \sum C_i = 1.$$
(18)

## 2.3 Static Value Method

The first approach used to calculate metrics is the static value method where all estimates are computed over the whole time period. In this method, the expected return rate $\mu$, the standard deviation $\sigma$, the Sharpe ratio, VaR and ES are calculated as sample estimates provided in (2), (3), (5), (8), (9), respectively.

Then, we need to standardize those values as described above. After we find the standardized values for all risk and performance metrics, we can put those values into the objective function and set up the coefficient for each metric:

$$F^s(r) = C_1 \cdot \hat{\mu}^s(r) - C_2 \cdot \hat{\sigma}^s(r) + C_3 \cdot \widehat{SR}^s(r) - C_4 \cdot \widehat{VaR}_\alpha^s(r) - C_5 \cdot \widehat{ES}_\alpha^s(r).$$
(19)

## 2.4 Occupation Time Method

The idea of the occupation time method is to compare the risk measures and performance metrics calculated for some asset with respective values computed for a benchmark over a 150-trading-day period. The selection of a benchmark depends on the asset class. For example, SPY, which is an ETF tracking the S&P500 market index, is used as the benchmark for the U.S. Equity class. We move the time window to update the metric values for both the asset and the benchmark and then calculate how many times the asset outperforms the benchmark. For example, we calculate a time series of expected return rates, $\{\hat{\mu}_t\}_{t \geqslant 1}$, by the following formula:

$$\hat{\mu}_t = \frac{1}{150} \sum_{j=0}^{149} r_{t+j} \, . \tag{20}$$

After applying the same formula to the benchmark, we can calculate the occupation-time metric as follows:

$$OT_\mu = \frac{1}{T_0} \sum_{t=1}^{T_0} \mathbb{1}_{\{\hat{\mu}_t \geqslant \hat{\mu}_t^b\}} \, , \tag{21}$$

where $\{\hat{\mu}_t\}$ is the time series for a fund of interest, $\{\hat{\mu}_t^b\}$ is the time series for the benchmark and $T_0 = T - 150$ is the length of those time series. Here, $\mathbb{1}_{\{\hat{\mu}_t \geqslant \hat{\mu}_t^b\}}$ is the indicator of event $\{\hat{\mu}_t \geqslant \hat{\mu}_t^b\}$ which is used to count the number of times $\mu_t$ is greater than $\mu_t^b$. Note that the summation in Eq. (21) is a discrete-time approximation of the occupation-time integral $\frac{1}{T_0} \int_0^{T_0} \mathbb{1}_{\{\mu_t \geqslant \mu_t^b\}} dt \approx \frac{1}{T_0} \sum_{t=1}^{T_0} \mathbb{1}_{\{\mu_t \geqslant \mu_t^b\}} \Delta_t$. Since we divide the whole time period into $T_0$ subintervals and the time is measured in days, we have $\Delta_t = 1$.

Similar formulas are used to calculate the occupation-time metrics for the standard deviation, the Sharpe ratio, VaR and ES:

$$OT_\sigma = \frac{1}{T_0} \sum_{t=1}^{T_0} \mathbb{1}_{\{\hat{\sigma}_t \geqslant \hat{\sigma}_t^b\}} \text{ where } \hat{\sigma}_t = \sqrt{\frac{\sum_{j=0}^{149} (r_{t+j} - \hat{\mu}_t)^2}{149}} \, , \tag{22}$$

$$OT_{SR} = \frac{1}{T_0} \sum_{t=1}^{T_0} \mathbb{1}_{\widehat{SR}_t \geqslant \widehat{SR}_t^b} \text{ where } \widehat{SR}_t = \frac{\hat{\mu}_t}{\hat{\sigma}_t} \, . \tag{23}$$

In order to normalize the contribution of each metric, we use the same approach as that in the previous subsection. Then, the objective function becomes:

$$F_{OT}^s(r) = C_1 \cdot OT_\mu^s(r) - C_2 \cdot OT_\sigma^s(r) + C_3 \cdot OT_{SR}^s(r) ,$$
$$- C_4 \cdot OT_{VaR_\alpha}^s(r) - C_5 \cdot OT_{ES_\alpha}^s(r) \, . \tag{24}$$

## 2.5 Occupation Area Method

The occupation area method is similar to the previous one. The key difference is that we calculate the occupation area between returns of a fund and the benchmark instead of the occupation time. The formula for the occupation area is

$$OA_\mu = \sum_{t=1}^{N} (\mu_t - \mu_{t,b}) . \tag{25}$$

The summation above is a discrete-time approximation of the integral $\int_0^{T_0} (\mu_t - \mu_{t,b}) dt$. The occupation-area formulae for other metrics are defined similarly. After we calculate the occupation-area metrics, the standardization is applied to all of them, and our objective function becomes

$$F_{OA}^s(r) = C_1 \cdot OA_\mu^s(r) - C_2 \cdot OA_\sigma^s(r) + C_3 \cdot OA_{SR}(r) ,$$
$$- C_4 \cdot OA_{VaR_\alpha}^s(r) - C_5 \cdot OA_{ES_\alpha}^s(r) . \tag{26}$$

## 3 Portfolio Optimization

Using one of the ranking functions (19), (24) and (26), we can select the top assets with highest rankings. It is obvious that the performance of portfolio will be better if it involves more stocks or funds in it. But handling too many stocks or funds is always unrealistic, we will restrict the number of funds in the portfolio within a reasonable number. In this paper, we assume that the top five ETFs (or stocks) have been selected. The next step is find an optimal portfolio in those five assets [4, 5].

Let $\{\omega_k\}_{k=1,2,3,4,5}$ denote the portfolio weights for the top five funds. As usual, we have $\sum \omega_k = 1$. If no short selling is allowed, then all weights are nonnegative. The weights $\{\omega_k\}_{k=1,2,3,4,5}$ of an optimal portfolio are to be found by maximizing the same ranking function that was used to select the top five assets. The ranking function is calculated for the portfolio return. For example, for the static value ranking function, the optimizing problem is

$$C_1 \cdot \mu^s(\omega) - C_2 \cdot \sigma^s(\omega) + C_3 \cdot SR^s(\omega) - C_4 \cdot VaR_\alpha^s(\omega) - C_5 \cdot ES_\alpha^s(\omega) \to \max_{\omega_k}$$
$$\text{s.t. } \omega_k \geqslant 0 \ \forall \ k = 1, 2, 3, 4, 5; \qquad \sum_{k=1}^{5} \omega_k = 1 ,$$

where $\mu^s(\omega)$ is the standardized expected rate of return on the portfolio with weights $\{\omega_k\}$ and similar notations are used for the other metrics. In order to standardize the portfolio performance and risk metrics, we use following formula:

$$M_i^s = \frac{M_i - M_{\min}}{M_{\max} - M_{\min}} , \tag{27}$$

where $M_i$ is a metric of asset $i$ and $M_{\max}$ and $M_{\min}$ denotes the maximal and minimal values of this metric calculated for the whole collection of assets. Although in the optimization stage, we only use the top 5 assets to form a portfolio, it is possible that the calculated value of a portfolio metric may be out of the range $[M_{\min}, M_{\max}]$. As a result the standardized value of a metric may not be between 0 and 1. To solve this issue, we find the maximal and minimal values of each portfolio metric by simulation and use those values in place of $M_{max}$ and $M_{min}$. As a result, the range of each performance or risk metric is still within the interval $[0, 1]$.

## 3.1  Bootstrapping Method

Essentially, the bootstrapping method is random sampling with replacement from a sample. Here, we deal with 5-year data available for each asset. We divided each data set into two parts. The first two years are used to rank assets and calibrate the optimization model for the top five funds or stocks. In all our numerical tests, we assumed a multivariate normal model. The last three years are used for sampling with replacement to simulate the portfolio behaviour. After simulating 1000 paths, we calculate the average values of metrics for the aggregate rate of return.

Here, $\{a, b, c\}$ denotes the following selection of parameters: $C_1 = a$, $C_2 = 0$, $C_3 = b$, $C_4 = 0$ and $C_5 = c$. Since we wish to verify if the performance of the portfolio will be affected by changing the coefficients, we select seven combinations as given in Tables 1 and 2. The first three are the cases when we only emphasize one single risk measure and put less weights on the other two measures. The next three combinations represent the situation when the investor is equally concerned about two measures and less concerned about the third one. The last combination is the case when the investor wishes to have a balanced portfolio. We have used two different datasets to test our algorithms. The first data set consists of the U.S. equity ETFs (June 2010–June 2015) and the second one is formed of the stocks contained in the S&P500 index (June 2010–June 2015). Although the length of each data set is 5 years, we only use the first two years data to rank assets and then use the last three years data in the bootstrapping method to test the future performance of our portfolio. All computations were done in R [2, 3].

### 3.1.1  Bootstrap Method Results for ETFs

As is seen from Table 1, we can construct optimal portfolios whose performances correlate with the parameters $\{a, b, c\}$ used. When we assign a larger weight to some metric, the optimal portfolio demonstrates a larger value of this metric in comparison with portfolios that have lower weights for the same metrics. For example, if the weights of SR and ES are larger than that of the expected return, the respective optimal portfolio is less risky. Unfortunately, our results do not allow us to make a general conclusion about which of the three methods is superior to the other two.

**Table 1** Application of the bootstrapping method to optimal ETFs portfolios with different coefficient settings. All values have been calculated for the three-year testing period

| Methods | $E[\mu]$ | $Var(\mu)$ | $E[SR]$ | $Var(SR)$ | $E[ES]$ | $Var(ES)$ |
|---|---|---|---|---|---|---|
| {.10, .10, .80} | | | | | | |
| Static | 0.4091437 | 0.03005339 | 0.0848539 | 0.001317085 | 0.01666016 | 1.50E−06 |
| Area | 0.4064643 | 0.03049992 | 0.08409062 | 0.00132626 | 0.01645895 | 1.65E−06 |
| Time | 0.4825162 | 0.03219531 | 0.09618697 | 0.001315382 | 0.01743876 | 1.23E−06 |
| {.10, .80, .10} | | | | | | |
| Static | 0.9511721 | 0.08165433 | 0.1250022 | 0.001452523 | 0.02608739 | 3.39E−06 |
| Area | 0.951139 | 0.08165433 | 0.1249978 | 0.001452521 | 0.02608743 | 3.39E−06 |
| Time | 0.9512173 | 0.08165433 | 0.1250081 | 0.001452526 | 0.02608733 | 3.39E−06 |
| {.80, .10, .10} | | | | | | |
| Static | 1.860952 | 0.49827 | 0.0958098 | 0.001372627 | 0.06777416 | 1.41E−05 |
| Area | 1.860955 | 0.49827 | 0.09580995 | 0.001372627 | 0.06777415 | 1.41E−05 |
| Time | 0.9587738 | 0.07924474 | 0.1260501 | 0.00142009 | 0.02601282 | 3.22E−06 |
| {.10, .45, .45} | | | | | | |
| Static | 0.8453735 | 0.0534542 | 0.1274899 | 0.001261965 | 0.02249692 | 2.06E−06 |
| Area | 0.6377875 | 0.0348291 | 0.1195583 | 0.001259684 | 0.01797712 | 1.11E−06 |
| Time | 0.6236637 | 0.03689596 | 0.1132767 | 0.001257914 | 0.01880658 | 9.56E−07 |
| {.45, .10, .45} | | | | | | |
| Static | 0.9581441 | 0.07184301 | 0.1257108 | 0.001282808 | 0.02603708 | 3.16E−06 |
| Area | 0.7003136 | 0.04045489 | 0.123548 | 0.001304535 | 0.01895667 | 1.22E−06 |
| Time | 0.8451697 | 0.05558618 | 0.1262633 | 0.001288165 | 0.02280545 | 2.05E−06 |
| {.45, .45, .10} | | | | | | |
| Static | 0.9640664 | 0.08146813 | 0.1265162 | 0.001456916 | 0.02604171 | 3.16E−06 |
| Area | 0.9640664 | 0.08146813 | 0.1265162 | 0.001456916 | 0.02604171 | 3.16E−06 |
| Time | 0.9640664 | 0.08146813 | 0.1265162 | 0.001456916 | 0.02604171 | 3.16E−06 |
| $\{\frac{1}{3}, \frac{1}{3}, \frac{1}{3}\}$ | | | | | | |
| Static | 0.9637661 | 0.07707189 | 0.1265918 | 0.001364749 | 0.02601397 | 3.17E−06 |
| Area | 0.800439 | 0.05360915 | 0.1273716 | 0.001391171 | 0.02108558 | 1.59E−06 |
| Time | 0.9265383 | 0.07062004 | 0.1271646 | 0.001366118 | 0.02488673 | 2.72E−06 |

**Table 2** Application of the bootstrapping method to optimal S&P500 stocks portfolios with different coefficient settings. All values have been calculated for the three-year testing period

| Methods | $E[\mu]$ | $Var(\mu)$ | $E[SR]$ | $Var(SR)$ | $E[ES]$ | $Var(ES)$ |
|---|---|---|---|---|---|---|
| {.10, .10, .80} | | | | | | |
| Static | 0.2626813 | 0.03404591 | 0.0509578 | 0.001289538 | 0.01795316 | 2.28E−06 |
| Area | 0.240569 | 0.03793836 | 0.04460797 | 0.00130799 | 0.01839741 | 2.41E−06 |
| Time | 0.1699602 | 0.04280512 | 0.03024206 | 0.001354304 | 0.01944491 | 2.70E−06 |
| {.10, .80, .10} | | | | | | |
| Static | 0.6566828 | 0.08835436 | 0.07997939 | 0.001303884 | 0.02606091 | 4.17E−06 |
| Area | 0.6566865 | 0.08835974 | 0.07997722 | 0.001303877 | 0.02606187 | 4.17E−06 |
| Time | 0.5609439 | 0.08806012 | 0.06906744 | 0.001317608 | 0.0249141 | 1.22E−06 |
| {.80, .10, .10} | | | | | | |
| Static | 0.7442291 | 0.1813149 | 0.06483054 | 0.001357688 | 0.03874738 | 1.07E−05 |
| Area | 0.7501041 | 0.1900891 | 0.06362852 | 0.001346189 | 0.03942093 | 9.86E−06 |
| Time | 0.661071 | 0.3984292 | 0.03772193 | 0.001289366 | 0.05419707 | 2.65E−05 |
| {.10, .45, .45} | | | | | | |
| Static | 0.4954457 | 0.06210857 | 0.07258444 | 0.001326988 | 0.02107827 | 1.35E−06 |
| Area | 0.4953065 | 0.0620733 | 0.07258416 | 0.001326992 | 0.0210743 | 1.35E−06 |
| Time | 0.503649 | 0.04042229 | 0.09019538 | 0.001304144 | 0.01907546 | 2.27E−06 |
| {.45, .10, .45} | | | | | | |
| Static | 0.6435807 | 0.09188279 | 0.07708096 | 0.001305725 | 0.02663781 | 4.24E−06 |
| Area | 0.5200333 | 0.07083103 | 0.07150622 | 0.001327822 | 0.02122669 | 1.12E−06 |
| Time | 0.405451 | 0.04739122 | 0.07057698 | 0.001446054 | 0.01905418 | 1.22E−06 |
| {.45, .45, .10} | | | | | | |
| Static | 0.6747057 | 0.1533039 | 0.0613858 | 0.001246811 | 0.03666783 | 1.01E−05 |
| Area | 0.6897843 | 0.1876729 | 0.05713474 | 0.001263258 | 0.04062 | 1.19E−05 |
| Time | 0.6533471 | 0.1284967 | 0.06742812 | 0.001348751 | 0.02921698 | 2.94E−06 |
| $\{\frac{1}{3}, \frac{1}{3}, \frac{1}{3}\}$ | | | | | | |
| Static | 0.6711223 | 0.0872366 | 0.08114371 | 0.00125501 | 0.02618213 | 3.97E−06 |
| Area | 0.6711296 | 0.08724839 | 0.08113867 | 0.00125499 | 0.02618424 | 3.97E−06 |
| Time | 0.4472853 | 0.04934969 | 0.07406981 | 0.001353427 | 0.01985187 | 1.61E−06 |

### 3.1.2  Bootstrap Method Results for S&P500 Stocks

As is seen from Table 2, the results are quite close to what was calculated for ETF-s portfolios, although the estimates are a bit less consistent relative to coefficient settings than those from the previous example.

# 4 Conclusion

In this project, we mainly focused on setting up a new ranking and optimization method that can take more than one risk or performance measure into account. We also compared three different schemes for ranking funds and stocks such as ETFs and S&P500 stocks. Each scheme has its own advantage, although, based on the results obtained using those three schemes, we can not identify the best one. Some funds always stay in the top five no matter what scheme we use. We applied the backtesting technique to verify the performance of portfolios generated by our method, and it turned out that our optimizer allowed for achieving the predefined objective. The main advantage of our optimizer is that it can provide investors with more choices than a traditional optimizer which often focused on the minimization of the variance of the maximization of the Sharpe ratio. The question of how to determine the coefficients for risk and performance measures to match investor's risk preferences is left for the future research.

**Acknowledgements** R. Makarov and B. Hu wish to acknowledge the generous support of the NSERC Discovery Grant, the NSERC Engage Grant and the NSERC Industrial Postgraduate Scholarships Program.

# References

1. Alexander, C.: Market Risk Analysis, Value at Risk Models, vol. 4. Wiley & Sons, London (2009)
2. Carmona, R.: Statistical Analysis of Financial Data in R, vol. 2. Springer, Berlin (2014)
3. Daróczi, G., Puhle, M., Berlinger, E., Csóka, P., Havran, D., Michaletzky, M., Tulassay, Z., Váradi, K., Vidovics-Dancs, A.: Introduction to R for Quantitative Finance. Packt Publishing Ltd, Birmingham (2013)
4. Markowitz, Harry: Portfolio selection. J. Fin. **7**(1), 77–91 (1952)
5. Prigent, J.L.: Portfolio Optimization and Performance Analysis. CRC Press, Boca Raton (2007)
6. Remillard, B.: Statistical Methods for Financial Engineering. CRC Press, Boca Raton (2013)
7. Sharpe, W.F.: The sharpe ratio. J. Portfolio Manage. **21**(1), 49–58 (1994)

# Kinetic Models of Need-Based Transfers

K. Kayser, D. Armbruster and C. Ringhofer

**Abstract** Kinetic exchange models of markets utilize microscopic binary descriptions of wealth transfers to derive a Boltzmann-like equation describing the evolution of the corresponding wealth distribution. We develop such a model to describe a binary form of welfare called need-based transfer (NBT), inspired by the gift-giving of cattle practiced among the Maasai of East Africa. Variants of such welfare schemes can be attributed to other human and animal communities. Specifically, we consider NBTs relative to a given welfare threshold such that individuals with surplus give to individuals with need in order to preserve the recipient's continued viable participation in the economy. Our NBT kinetic model considers redistribution rules parameterized to vary between regressive and progressive redistribution.

**Keywords** Kinetic exchange models · Welfare · Need-based transfers

## 1 Introduction

Need-based transfers are purpose-driven binary donations, given in order to preserve recipients' viable participation in an economy. They establish a sort of risk pool. Natural wealth evolution may cause past recipients to establish surplus and past donors to have deficit, and so gifts may end up being naturally reciprocated directly or indirectly [1, 11, 12]. This NBT wealth redistribution mechanism-featuring gift-giving based on need as determined by some threshold - has been used to describe

K. Kayser (✉) · D. Armbruster · C. Ringhofer
School of Mathematical and Statistical Sciences, Arizona State University,
Tempe, AZ 85287-1804, USA
e-mail: kirk.kayser@asu.edu

D. Armbruster
e-mail: armbruster@asu.edu

C. Ringhofer
e-mail: ringhofer@asu.edu

© Springer Nature Switzerland AG 2018
D. M. Kilgour et al. (eds.), *Recent Advances in Mathematical
and Statistical Methods*, Springer Proceedings in Mathematics & Statistics 259,
https://doi.org/10.1007/978-3-319-99719-3_47

the cattle-gifting practice of the Maasai pastoralists of East Africa [1, 2, 11], and could be used to describe other community practices such as food sharing among vampire bats [19, 20].

To explain the evolution of reciprocal altruism and cooperation among rational and strategic agents in a community, game theoretic perspectives are often taken and models like the repeated prisoner's dilemma are utilized [4, 5, 7, 17]; however, such models do not describe the distribution of wealth in an economy, but focus on the evolving prevalence of interactive strategies in a population. Agent-based models allow for consideration of complex socioeconomic interactions like account-keeping [1], various sharing network topologies [11, 12], and various transfer policies [12]. However, mean statistics from experiments repeated many times are relied on to describe the aspects of the economy rather than rigorously proved results.

The kinetic exchange model framework features relatively more simple binary socioeconomic interactions. The resulting Boltzmann-like equation is an integro-differential equation which allows for proving results about the macroscopic distribution of wealth, e.g. whether the tail of the wealth distribution is fat and obeys a Pareto power law or is slim. Sometimes in the hydrodynamic limit the Boltzmann equation is equivalent to a solvable Fokker-Plank equation [10, 15]. With discrete wealths or amounts of coins, a stochastic processes approach has also been used to describe the macroscopic wealth distribution corresponding to simple microscopic interactions [14].

As the NBT transfers we consider are naturally binary gifts, using tools from Econophysics - namely kinetic theory and Boltzmann-like equations - is not only a natural approach that has not yet been considered, it is an appropriate approach to take to focus on how many microscopic binary donations of the NBT type evolve the shape of the community distribution of wealth. In this paper, we begin to develop such kinetic models and examine aspects of numerical solutions. Future work will feature more analytical results like how moment evolution equations describe the shape of the shape of the wealth distribution [13].

## 1.1   Kinetic Exchange Models of Markets

Kinetic exchange models of markets utilize Boltzmann-like equations where individuals exchanging money in a trade are considered analogous to gas particles changing velocities after a collision [6, 10, 15, 16]. Commonly, rules are determined to describe random fractional amounts of individuals' wealths to be exchanged in a trade in order to recover realistic wealth distributions, namely with a log-normal distribution of a majority of wealth and a Pareto power law tail for the very rich [8]. The microscopic rules for such models can be described as follows: Where $v$ and $w$ are two individuals' respective wealths before a trade, the individuals' post-trade wealths are given by

$$v^* = p_1 v + q_1 w, \qquad w^* = q_2 v + p_2 w. \tag{1}$$

The coefficients $p_i$, $q_i$ are the non-negative random variables whose laws determine the shape of the steady state distribution [10].

The relative density of individuals with wealth $w \geq 0$ at time $t$ is given by $f(t; w)$, which evolves according to the following Boltzmann-like equation

$$\partial_t f = Q_+(f, f) + Q_-(f, f), \tag{2}$$

where $Q_+(f, f)$ is the collisional gain operator that gives the gains at wealth $w$ resulting from collisions, $Q_-$ gives the losses at wealth $w$ resulting from collisions, and $f(0, w) = f_0(w)$ is the initial wealth distribution. For models fitting the description of (1), a characteristic function has been defined which can classify the tail of the steady state distribution according to the given coefficients $p_i$, $q_i$ [10]. Also, wealth redistribution has been considered where the natural wealth redistribution process described above is still used, but in addition, portions of individuals' wealths are extracted via a tax on transfers and redistributed via a redistribution operator [6].

## 1.2  Need-Based Transfers

We develop a kinetic exchange model that examines wealth redistribution in a different way. Namely, we consider a fixed welfare threshold which determines the relative surplus or deficit of each individual; then we consider deterministic binary transfers in which individuals with surplus give to individuals with deficit in order to bring those who are below the welfare threshold up to it. Such a version of binary community welfare is inspired by the risk-pooling mechanism called *osotua* utilized among the Maasai in East Africa and has previously been examined via agent-based modeling under the name of need-based transfers (NBTs) [1, 2, 11, 12]. A microscopic description of NBTs with the welfare threshold $\theta \in \mathbb{R}$ and pre-trade wealths $v, w \in \mathbb{R}$ is the following:

$$v^* = v + H(v + w - 2\theta)\big[(\theta - v)H(\theta - v) - (\theta - w)H(\theta - w)\big]$$
$$w^* = w + H(v + w - 2\theta)\big[(\theta - w)H(\theta - w) - (\theta - v)H(\theta - v)\big]. \tag{3}$$

In (3), $H$ is the standard Heaviside step function, and as the rule is invariant under the permutation $w \leftrightarrow v, w^* \leftrightarrow v^*$, it allows for the assumption of statistical independence for many identical individuals. Essentially, the rule determines that wealths will change only if there is enough total wealth for both of them to be at or above threshold after the transfer, i.e. transfers where donors are caused to go below threshold are not allowed. Then, if there is enough total wealth for a transfer to occur, the individual with surplus gives from his/her surplus whatever the deficit of the needy individual is.

Multiple agent-based studies have examined variants of the NBT donations described in (3). Among the claims of these papers is that NBTs describe a reasonable welfare mechanism that is found in practice among the Maasai of East Africa [1, 2, 11] and that asking the wealthiest individuals with preference is generally socially optimal [12]. When NBTs are considered in an environment where needs are the result of random processes and thus people have needs due to no fault of their own, those with surplus at one time may have deficit at another time. In that way, gifts may be reciprocated directly or indirectly even without an account-keeping mechanism [1, 2]. Other forms of reciprocal gift-giving such as vampire bats sharing food [19, 20] can also be thought of as consisting of NBTs. Understanding the evolution of the wealth or fitness distribution of such communities is of interest, and a preliminary step is to model the welfare mechanism.

The binary transfers of NBTs have natural interpretation in the kinetic context, and we bring this form of welfare into the kinetic exchange model environment in order to (i) compare numerical results from the kinetic model to observations made in the agent-based studies and contribute new observations, (ii) control for desirable wealth distributions, and (iii) potentially prove some results in the integro-differential equation framework. In this paper we focus on item (i).

## 2   Kinetic Model of NBT Policies

Given a welfare threshold $\theta \in \mathbb{R}$, and assuming collisions occur at rate 1, the Boltzmann-like wealth distribution evolution equation corresponding to the microscopic transfers described in (3) is

$$\partial_t f(t; w) = \int_{-\infty}^{\theta} \int_{2\theta - u}^{\infty} \left[ -\delta(w - u) - \delta(w - v) + \delta(w - \theta) + \delta(w - u - v + \theta) \right]$$
$$\times f(t; v) f(t; u) \, dv \, du,$$
(4)

where $f(t; w)$ is the relative density of individuals with wealth $w \in \mathbb{R}$ at time $t \geq 0$. Note that here wealth is allowed to be negative, which can be understood as distance from threshold if $\theta = 0$, or as some form of debt if $\theta \neq 0$.

Equation (4) can be understood as $u$ denoting the wealth of a below-threshold individual and $v$ denoting the wealth of a donor (individual with enough surplus to cover the deficit $\theta - u$ and still be above threshold, i.e. $v > 2\theta - u$). Thus, when these individuals interact, there are density losses at their pre-trade wealths and density gains at their post-trade wealths, $u^* = \theta$ and $v^* = v - (\theta - u)$.

Integrating (4) with a test function $\phi(w)$ gives

$$\int_{-\infty}^{\infty} \phi(w) \partial_t f(t; w)\, dw = \lambda \int_{-\infty}^{\theta} \int_{2\theta - u}^{\infty} \Big[ -\phi(u) - \phi(v) + \phi(\theta) + \phi(u + v - \theta) \Big]$$
$$\times f(t; v) f(t; u)\, dv\, du.$$
(5)

Hence, for the particular cases of $\phi(w) = 1$, and $\phi(w) = w$, $\partial_t \int_{-\infty}^{\infty} f(t; w)\, dw = \partial_t \int_{-\infty}^{\infty} w f(t; w)\, dw = 0$ confirms that the mean wealth and total wealth are conserved for this model.

However, with (4) there is no preferential donor selection. For example, if an individual has a deficit of 1, and there are just as many individuals with a surplus of 2 as there are individuals with a surplus of 4, no preference is given between the individuals with less surplus or those with more. To introduce preferential donor selection based on donor wealths, which defines regressive to progressive transfer policies as in [12], first *exact-match* transfers are described.

## 2.1 Exact-Match Transfers

Let $\theta \in \mathbb{R}$, and $\varepsilon_0 \geq 0$, where $\varepsilon_0$ is not necessarily small. A corresponding exact-match transfer will only take place if the transfer will cause the recipient to go to the welfare threshold $\theta$ and the donor to go to the donor threshold $\theta + \varepsilon_0$. Hence, the microscopic description of exact transfers, given $\theta$, $\varepsilon_0$, is

$$v^* = v + \delta(v + w - 2\theta - \varepsilon_0)\big[(\theta - v)H(\theta - v) - (\theta - w)H(\theta - w)\big]$$
$$w^* = w + \delta(v + w - 2\theta - \varepsilon_0)\big[(\theta - w)H(\theta - w) - (\theta - v)H(\theta - v)\big], \quad (6)$$

and the macroscopic Boltzmann-like equation is

$$\partial_t f(t; w) = [\delta(w - \theta - \varepsilon_0) + \delta(w - \theta)] \int_{\theta + \varepsilon_0}^{\infty} f(v) f(2\theta + \varepsilon_0 - v)\, dv$$
$$- [H(w - \theta - \varepsilon_0) + H(\theta - w)]\, f(w) f(2\theta + \varepsilon_0 - w). \quad (7)$$

Choosing a donor threshold $\theta + \varepsilon_0$ automatically guarantees that no individuals with wealth below that threshold will be able to give. Thus, a higher donor threshold corresponds to only wealthier individuals being able to give. In this sense, an exact-match transfers with large donor thresholds could be consider as describing a more progressive wealth redistribution than a policy with a smaller donor threshold. We extend this by describing policies which incorporate what we call donor preference.

## 2.2    NBT Policies: Donor Preference

Donor preference is established by assuming the existence of a probability density function $p$ such that $p(\varepsilon_0)d\varepsilon$ is the probability a donor threshold will be selected between $\theta + \varepsilon_0$ and $\theta + \varepsilon_0 + d\varepsilon$. Thus, the donor preference, or transfer policy is defined by $p$ and the corresponding wealth evolution equation is

$$\partial_t f(t; w) = \lambda \int_0^\infty p(\varepsilon) \Bigg( [\delta(w - \theta - \varepsilon) + \delta(w - \theta)] \int_{\theta+\varepsilon}^\infty f(v)f(2\theta + \varepsilon - v)\,dv$$

$$-[H(w - \theta - \varepsilon) + H(\theta - w)]f(w)f(2\theta + \varepsilon - w) \Bigg) d\varepsilon.$$

$$(8)$$

For numerical results, we assume some maximal surplus $L > 0$ and define a parameterized probability density function $p_\alpha : [0, L) \to (0, \infty)$ as

$$p_\alpha(\varepsilon) = \left( \frac{\alpha}{e^{\alpha L} - 1} \right) e^{\alpha \varepsilon}.$$

$$(9)$$

If $\alpha$ is positive, increasing $p$ implies larger donor thresholds are more likely chosen and thus the policy would be progressive. For the rest of the paper, we will refer to $\alpha = -0.05$ as defining the *regressive* policy, $\alpha = 0.05$ as the *progressive* policy, and $\alpha \approx 0$ as the *flat* policy. $p_\alpha$ for these policies is illustrated in Fig. 1, where $L = 100$.

The flat policy ($\alpha \approx 0$) indicates no distinct preference for donor threshold and thus should correspond to the microscopic description of (3). Figure 2 shows a comparison of the numerical steady state solution of the flat policy and the wealth distribution resulting from agent-based simulation using the microscopic description of Eq. (3); the initial wealth distribution was chosen to be gamma, considered qualitatively realistic for natural wealth distributions [3, 8].

**Fig. 1** Policy illustration. The equation for these parameterized donor threshold probability distributions is given in (9)

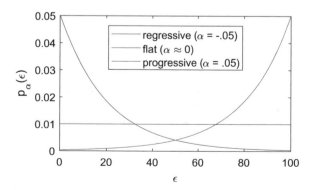

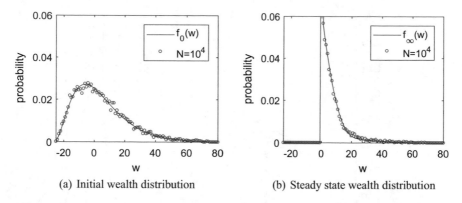

(a) Initial wealth distribution  (b) Steady state wealth distribution

**Fig. 2** Flat policy comparison with agent-based simulation. A gamma initial condition is used for $f_0(w)$ and $10^4$ agents are sampled from this distribution as well. Equation (8) is used with $\alpha \approx 0$ to find the steady state solution of the Boltzmann-like equation; for the agents, interactions are randomly generated and transfers are conducted according to the microscopic description of Eq. (3) until all $10^4$ agents are at or above threshold

## 3  Numerical Experiments

It is important to clarify that (8) does not incorporate any *natural* wealth process, but merely models the NBT welfare/risk pooling redistribution operator; future work will attempt to include *natural* wealth evolution processes such as economic growth and disasters in order to examine how NBTs function in those contexts. This being the case, steady state solutions to (8) are very dependent on initial condition.

For numerical experiments, $\theta = 0$ is considered and two different initial conditions are used: (i) gamma distribution and (ii) uniform distribution. Again, the gamma distribution is chosen as qualitatively representative of naturally observed wealth distributions [3, 8]. The uniform distribution is chosen because it allows for comparability of effectiveness of each policy in meeting the needs of below-threshold individuals.

For all results in Figs. 3 and 4, 'steady state' is considered to have been reached at time $T$ such that $\|f(T; w) - f(T - \Delta t; w)\|_2 < 10^{-5}$; in the tables, $T$ is rescaled by the minimum $T$ value for comparability. $\Delta t = 1$ is used for simulations. Gini index is calculated in the standard way [9], but only for the above-threshold wealth distribution. Smaller Gini indexes correspond to less inequality. Population below threshold is found as $\int_{-\infty}^{0} f(T; w)\, dw$ for Fig. 4 and is considered essentially 0 for Fig. 3.

In Figs. 3 and 4, the steady state distributions of each policy are qualitatively, and in terms of inequality, predictable or reinforce the regressive/progressive natures of the policies. Also, the rate of convergence for the regressive policy is greater than for the progressive policy. This is a new observation with respect to the work of [1, 2, 11, 12] but intuitively makes sense as the higher donor thresholds preferred in the progressive model reduce the number of potential donors.

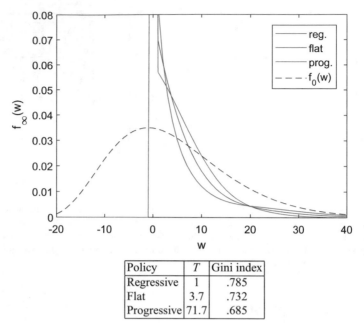

**Fig. 3** Steady state distributions and data for parameterized kinetic NBT policies with initial condition $f_0(w) \sim$ Gamma

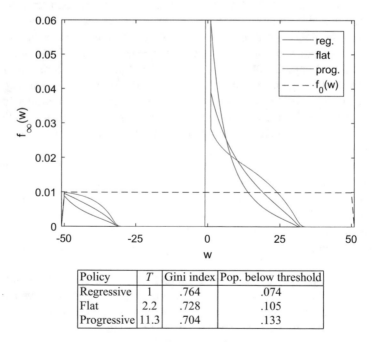

**Fig. 4** Steady state distributions and data for parameterized kinetic NBT policies with initial condition $f_0(w) \sim$ Uniform

Figure 4 echoes an observation made in [12], where regressive transfers were found to be a sort of cutting-stock optimization heuristic [18] for best matching all of the deficits to surpluses. We see that here also the regressive policy results in more individuals above threshold in steady state than the other policies. Essentially, by matching the deficits with the closest fitting surpluses in the regressive policy, larger surpluses are reserved for individuals with larger deficits. In contrast, the progressive policy cuts into large surpluses quickly leaving no large matching surplus available for a binary transfer to an individual with a large deficit.

## 4  Discussion

This paper considers economies that are assumed to practice altruistic welfare donations called need-based transfers. A parameterized kinetic model of regressive to progressive NBTs is developed in order to examine the influence of the details of NBT implementation on the wealth distribution of a society. Focusing on the transfer mechanism (absent natural wealth evolution processes), steady state solutions are very dependent on initial condition and conform to expectation with regard to inequality as well as with policy efficiency when compared to the cutting-stock observation made in [12]. Also, the rate at which successful transfers occur varies between transfer policies; this may be understood as reflecting the varying difficulty in finding aid given the restrictions of donor preference.

This model introduces kinetic theory to existing need-based transfer literature, and in this realm it provides an initial structure for examining how reciprocal gift-giving societies' wealth distributions evolve. Too, when various natural wealth evolution mechanisms are added to the model, questions about how NBTs affect disaster recovery, inequality, and economic growth may begin to be examined. Such questions will be considered in future work [13]; analytical properties and control perspectives will also be studied.

**Acknowledgements**  We thank Athena Aktipis and Lee Cronk for introducing us to the Osotua NBT concept, and we thank Michael Herty for valuable discussion. K.K. and D.A. gratefully acknowledge support through NSF grant DMS-1515592 and travel support through the KI-Net grant, NSF RNMS grant No. 1107291.

## References

1. Aktipis, A., De Aguiar, R., Flaherty, A., Iyer, P., Sonkoi, D., Cronk, L.: Cooperation in an uncertain world: for the Maasai of East Africa, need-based transfers outperform account-keeping in volatile environments. Hum. Ecol. **44**(3), 353–364 (2016)
2. Aktipis, C.A., Cronk, L., de Aguiar, R.: Risk-pooling and herd survival: an agent-based model of a Maasai gift-giving system. Hum. Ecol. **39**(2), 131–140 (2011)
3. Angle, J.: The surplus theory of social stratification and the size distribution of personal wealth. Soc. Forces **65**(2), 293–326 (1986)

4. Axelrod, R., Dion, D., et al.: The further evolution of cooperation. Science **242**(4884), 1385–1390 (1988)
5. Axelrod, R., Hamilton, W.D.: The evolution of cooperation. Science **211**(4489), 1390–1396 (1981)
6. Bisi, M., Spiga, G., Toscani, G.: Kinetic models of conservative economies with wealth redistribution. Commun. Math. Sci. **7**(4), 901–916 (2009)
7. Boyd, R.: Is the repeated prisoner's dilemma a good model of reciprocal altruism? Ethol. Sociobiol. **9**(2–4), 211–222 (1988)
8. Chakrabarti, B.K., Chakraborti, A., Chakravarty, S.R., Chatterjee, A.: Econophysics of Income and Wealth Distributions. Cambridge University Press, Cambridge (2013)
9. Dorfman, R.: A formula for the gini coefficient. Rev. Econ. Stat. **61**(1), 146–149 (1979)
10. Düring, B., Matthes, D., Toscani, G.: Kinetic equations modelling wealth redistribution: a comparison of approaches. Phys. Rev. E **78**(5), 056103 (2008)
11. Hao, Y., Armbruster, D., Cronk, L., Aktipis, C.A.: Need-based transfers on a network: a model of risk-pooling in ecologically volatile environments. Evol. Hum. Behav. **36**(4), 265–273 (2015)
12. Kayser, K., Armbruster, D.: Social Optima of Need-based Transfers. Submitted (2017)
13. Kayser, K., Armbruster, D.: Kinetic Models of Conservative Economies with Need-based Transfers as Welfare. In preparation, ASU (2018)
14. Lanchier, N., Reed, S.: Rigorous Results for the Distribution of Money on Connected Graphs. arXiv preprint arXiv:1801.00485 (2018)
15. Pareschi, L., Toscani, G.: Interacting Multiagent Systems: Kinetic Equations and Monte Carlo Methods. OUP, Oxford (2013)
16. Slanina, F.: Inelastically scattering particles and wealth distribution in an open economy. Phys. Rev. E **69**(4), 046102 (2004)
17. Trivers, R.L.: The evolution of reciprocal altruism. Q. Rev. Biol. **46**(1), 35–57 (1971)
18. Wäscher, G., Gau, T.: Heuristics for the integer one-dimensional cutting stock problem: a computational study. Oper. Res. Spektrum **18**(3), 131–144 (1996)
19. Wilkinson, G.S.: Reciprocal food sharing in the vampire bat. Nature **308**(5955), 181–184 (1984)
20. Wilkinson, G.S.: Reciprocal altruism in bats and other mammals. Ethol. Sociobiol. **9**(2–4), 85–100 (1988)

# Optimal Static Hedging of Non-tradable Risks with Discrete Distributions

Adam W. Kolkiewicz

**Abstract** We consider the problem of optimal static hedging of a non-tradable risk. Under general model assumptions, we find a representation of an optimal hedging option on a traded security that can be used to mitigate such a risk. Since we use the expectation of the shortfall as the criterion, the resulting hedging methods guard better against large losses when compared with a more traditional approach based on the quadratic criterion. We illustrate our method by applying it to the problem of hedging a multiple-barrier option.

**Keywords** Financial derivatives · Hedging · Shortfall risk
Path-dependent options

## 1 Introduction

In the paper we consider the problem of optimal static hedging of a non-tradable risk. For a fixed time interval $[0, T]$, the hedger's objective is to create a static portfolio, which includes European style options[1] on a traded security and possibly a bank account, so that its value at time $T$ replicates as closely as possible a liability $L$. The portfolio is constructed under the constraint that its initial cost does not exceed a given budget $V_I$.

Let $S(T)$ denote the price of the underlying traded security at time $T$. Since the terminal value of any static hedging portfolio can be represented as $h(S(T))$ for a certain function $h$, the hedger's objective is to find an admissible function $h$ so that the hedging error $L - h(S(T))$ meets his or her risk management objectives. In this paper we focus on strategies that minimize the shortfall risk, which we define as the expectation of the shortfall

$$E^P[(L - h(S(T)))^+].$$

---

[1]To simplify our presentation, we shall refer to path-independent options as European options.

A. W. Kolkiewicz (✉)
Department of Statistics and Actuarial Science,
University of Waterloo, Waterloo, Canada
e-mail: wakolkie@uwaterloo.ca

© Springer Nature Switzerland AG 2018
D. M. Kilgour et al. (eds.), *Recent Advances in Mathematical and Statistical Methods*, Springer Proceedings in Mathematics & Statistics 259,
https://doi.org/10.1007/978-3-319-99719-3_48

531

Thus, the payoff function $h_{opt}$ of the optimal hedging option must solve

$$h_{opt} := \arg \inf_{h \in \mathscr{H}_\mathscr{A}} E^P[(L - h(S(T)))^+], \tag{1}$$

where $\mathscr{H}_\mathscr{A}$ represents the set of admissible payoff functions.

The distribution of the hedging error is completely characterized by the join distribution of $L$ and $S(T)$, but for the purpose of solving (1) it will be convenient to use an alternative description. Let $\mathscr{S}$ denote the set of possible values of $S(T)$. Conditionally on $S(T) = s$, $s \in \mathscr{S}$, the size of a possible shortfall, when hedging $L$ with $h(S(T))$, depends only on the conditional distribution $L \mid S(T) = s$. Thus, if we introduce variables $L(s)$ in the following way

$$L(s) \overset{\mathscr{D}}{=} L \mid S(T) = s, \tag{2}$$

where "$\overset{\mathscr{D}}{=}$" denotes equality in law, then the hedging error can be completely described by the set

$$\mathscr{L}(T) := \{L(s) : s \in \mathscr{S}\} \tag{3}$$

and the distribution of the terminal price $S(T)$.

Under the assumptions that the distributions of $L(s)$, $s \in \mathscr{S}$, are continuous, the problem (1) has been solved in [4]. In Sect. 2 of this paper, we present a theorem that extends this result to the case when $L(s)$, $s \in \mathscr{S}$, follow discrete distributions.

To give an example of a situation where such distributions arise, consider the problem of discrete-time hedging of a path-dependent option using European options only. Suppose that under the empirical measure $P$ the value of the underlying security $S$ follows the process

$$dS(t) = S(t)(\mu dt + \sigma dW(t)), \quad S(0) = S_0, \tag{4}$$

where $\{W(t)\}$ is a standard Brownian motion. Let us denote the price of the option at any time $t$ between its inception at zero and maturity $T_M$ by

$$C(S(\cdot), t) \equiv C(S(u)_{u \in [0,t]}, t), \quad t \in [0, T_M]. \tag{5}$$

Under the model (4), any path-dependent option can be replicated by trading continuously the underlying security and a risk-less bond. In practice, however, only discrete-time hedging is possible, and hence the option writer is faced with the problem of searching for strategies that reduce the hedging error. If the hedging period ends at $T \leq T_M$, then this problem can be cast in the general framework described above by taking

$$L = C(S(\cdot), T).$$

In Sect. 3, we illustrate our approach by applying it to a roll-down call, which is a path-dependent option whose payoff depends on breaching some barriers during the life of the contract. Due to the presence of these barriers, the residuals risks $L(s), s \in \mathscr{S}$, follow discrete distributions.

Briefly we want to mention other applications of the main result presented in this paper. In the case when the distributions $L(s), s \in \mathscr{S}$, are continuous, the optimal hedge must be typically obtained through numerical methods. To avoid this, we can discretize these distributions and then use the optimal solution presented in this paper, which is quite straightforward to implement. Another potential application of the presented result is the determination of the optimal static hedge when CVaR is used as the criterion for selection. For a related approach, we refer to [7].

In Sect. 3 we compare our approach with hedging based on minimization of the mean-square value of the hedging error. If we restrict hedging strategies to linear functions of $S(T)$, then this criterion has been used by, among others, [2, 3] to determine local risk minimizing hedging methods. When this criterion is applied to the problem of hedging of a more general liability $L$, then the payoff function $h_{MSE}$ of the optimal hedging option solves

$$h_{MSE} := \arg \inf_{h \in \mathscr{L}^2(S(T))} E^P[(L - h(S(T)))^2],$$

where $\mathscr{L}^2(S(T))$ denotes the set of square integrable functions of $S(T)$. The solution to this problem admits the well-known representation given by $h_{MSE}(s) := E^P[L|S(T_h) = s], s \in \mathscr{S}$. More details about this approach, and examples of its applications to some insurance products, can be found in [5].

## 2  Optimal Hedging Strategy

We assume that for each $s \in \mathscr{S} \subset \mathscr{R}^+$ the distribution of the residual risk $L(s)$ is discrete and of the following form

$$P(L(s) = l_i(s)) = \pi_i(s), \ i = 0, 1, \ldots, N, \tag{6}$$

where $l_0 \equiv 0$, the functions $l_1, \ldots, l_N$ and $\pi_1, \ldots, \pi_N$ are continuous on $\mathscr{S}$, and for each $s \in \mathscr{S}$ they satisfy $0 < l_i(s) < l_{i+1}(s)$ and $\pi_i(s) > 0$. In (6) we allow $N = \infty$, which would correspond to a distribution with an infinite but countable number of possible outcomes.

For a given initial capital $V_I$, let $V_0 := \exp(rT)V_I$, where $r$ is an instantaneous short interest rate. In order to define admissible payoff functions, we first define the set

$$\mathscr{H}^0 := \{ \text{functions } h \text{ on } \mathscr{S} \text{ such that } h(s) \in [0, h_U(s)] \text{ for } s \in \mathscr{S} \},$$

where $h_U$ is a function that satisfies

($\mathscr{C}$1)   $V_0 \leq E^Q[h_U(S(T))] < \infty$
($\mathscr{C}$2)   $E^P[h_U(S(T))] < \infty$.

The superscripts $Q$ refers to the risk-neutral measure obtained, for example, from market prices of traded vanilla options on $S(T)$. Under this measure, the discounted price process $\{S(t)\}$ is a martingale.

In practice, $h_U$ can be chosen along selected quantiles of the conditional distributions of the residual risk $L(s), s \in \mathscr{S}$. To simplify the exposition, we are going to assume that this is indeed possible, and for this we shall adopt the following condition:

($\mathscr{C}$3) There exists $K$ such that for $h_U := l_K$ the conditions ($\mathscr{C}$1) − ($\mathscr{C}$2) are satisfied.

If $N$ is finite, then we can take $K = N$, assuming that $E^P[l_K(S(T))] < \infty$ and $E^Q[l_K(S(T))] < \infty$.

Now we can define the set of admissible payoff functions $h$ as

$$\mathscr{H} := \{h \in \mathscr{H}^0 : E^Q[h(S(T))] \leq V_0\}.$$

Then the optimal hedging option is the function $h_{opt}$ that solves the problem

$$h_{opt} := \arg\inf_{h \in \mathscr{H}} E^P[(L - h(S(T)))^+]. \tag{7}$$

Let $P^*$ and $Q^*$ denote the distribution of $S(T)$ under the measures $P$ and $Q$, respectively. In order to ensure uniqueness of the optimal hedging option, we will need the following condition.

($\mathscr{C}$4)   For each strictly positive $c$, the Lebesgue measure of the sets

$$B_c(i) := \{s \in \mathscr{S} : c = \sum_{j=i}^K \pi_j(s)\frac{dP^*}{dQ^*}(s)\}, \quad i = 1, \ldots, K, \tag{8}$$

is zero.

This assumption is satisfied, for example, when the functions

$$g_i(s) := \sum_{j=i}^K \pi_j(s)\frac{dP^*}{dQ^*}(s), \quad i = 1, \ldots, K,$$

are continuously differentiable and their derivatives are zero only at a finite number of points from $\mathscr{S}$.

**Theorem 1** *Under the assumptions (𝒞3)–(𝒞4), the payoff function of the optimal hedging option is given by*

$$
h_{opt} = \begin{cases} l_K(s) & \text{for } s: \quad \pi_K(s)\frac{dP^*}{dQ^*}(s) > c \\ l_i(s) & \text{for } s: \quad \sum_{j=i+1}^{K} \pi_j(s)\frac{dP^*}{dQ^*}(s) < c \leq \sum_{j=i}^{K} \pi_j(s)\frac{dP^*}{dQ^*}(s) \\ 0 & \text{for } s: \quad (1-\pi_0)\frac{dP^*}{dQ^*}(s) < c, \end{cases}
$$

*where c is the smallest number such that $E^Q[h_{opt}(S(T))] \leq V_0$.*

*Proof* To simplify the notation, we denote the random variable $S(T)$ by $S$. First we show that the solution to the optimization problem (7) can be represented in terms of the following auxiliary function

$$
g(s, z) := \frac{g_0(s, zh_U(s) - h_U(s))}{h_U(s)}, \quad (s, z) \in \mathscr{S} \times [0, 1], \tag{9}
$$

where

$$
g_0(s, z) := E^P[(L(s) + z)^+], \quad (s, z) \in \mathscr{S} \times [-h_U(s), 0]. \tag{10}
$$

Observe that each admissible function $h$ from $\mathscr{H}$ can be represented as $h = \gamma h_U$, where $\gamma$ is a function on $\mathscr{S}$ with values in $[0, 1]$. Using this representation, and conditioning on $S$, we can rewrite the optimization problem (7) in the following way

$$
\arg\min_{\gamma \in \mathscr{I}} E^P[E^P[((L(R, S) - \gamma(S)h_U(S))^+|S]]
$$
$$
= \arg\min_{\gamma \in \mathscr{I}} E^{P^*}[h_U(S)E^P[(\frac{L(R, S) - h_U(S)}{h_U(S)} + 1 - \gamma(S))^+|S]],
$$
$$
= \arg\min_{\gamma \in \mathscr{I}} E^{P^*}[h_U(S)g(S, 1 - \gamma(S))], \tag{11}
$$

where $\mathscr{I}$ represents Borel measurable functions on $\mathscr{S}$ with values in $[0, 1]$.

By (𝒞3), we can introduce a new probability measure $\tilde{Q}$ on $\mathscr{S}$ in the following way

$$
d\tilde{Q} = \text{const} \cdot h_U dQ^*.
$$

Then the constraint $E^{Q^*}[h(S)] \leq V_0$ implies that the optimal function $\gamma_{opt}$ in (11) must satisfy

$$
E^{\tilde{Q}}[\gamma_{opt}(S)] \leq \tilde{H}_0 := \frac{V_0}{E^{Q^*}[h_U(S)]}. \tag{12}
$$

Due to our assumptions about the distributions of $\{L(s), s \in \mathscr{S}\}$, it is possible to find explicit representations of the functions $g_0$ and $g$. In particular, we have

$$
g_0(s, z) = \sum_{j:l_j(s)+z\geq 0} (l_j(s) + z)\pi_j(s), \quad (s, z) \in \mathscr{S}_L \times [-h_U(s), 0],
$$

which for each $s$ is a piecewise linear, strictly increasing and continuous function of $z$. It can be rewritten in the following way

$$g_0(s, z) =$$
$$\sum_{i=1}^{K} \left[ \sum_{j=i}^{K} l_j(s)\pi_j(s) + z \sum_{j=i}^{K} \pi_j(s) \right] \mathbf{1}_{[-l_i(s), -l_{i-1}(s))}(z) + E^P[(L(s))^+]\mathbf{1}_{\{0\}}(z),$$

where $\mathbf{1}_A$ denotes the indicator function of a set $A$. From this, we can find the following representation of $g(s, z)$ for $(s, z) \in \mathscr{S} \times [0, 1]$:

$$g(s, z) =$$
$$\sum_{i=1}^{K} \left[ \sum_{j=i}^{K} (\frac{l_j(s)}{h_U(s)} - 1)\pi_j(s) + z \sum_{j=i}^{K} \pi_j(s) \right] \mathbf{1}_{[1-\frac{l_i(s)}{h_U(s)}, 1-\frac{l_{i-1}(s)}{h_U(s)})}(z) + E^P[(L(s))^+]\mathbf{1}_{\{1\}}(z).$$

For each $s$ the above function is piecewise linear, strictly increasing and continuous. Based on this representation we can find that the partial derivative of $g$ with respect to $z$ is given by

$$g_z(s, z) = \sum_{i=1}^{K} [\sum_{j=i}^{K} \pi_j(s)]\mathbf{1}_{(1-\frac{l_i(s)}{h_U(s)}, 1-\frac{l_{i-1}(s)}{h_U(s)})}(z), \quad \text{for} \quad (s, z) \in \mathscr{S} \times (0, 1),$$

which is a piecewise constant and nondecreasing function. For each $s$, partial derivatives are not determined at the points $1 - \frac{l_i(s)}{h_U(s)}$, $i = 0, \dots, K$.

We solve the problem (11)–(12) by reducing it to the form for which the Neyman-Pearson lemma can be applied. For this we use the method presented by [6], which is based on a characterization of the minimum in terms of directional derivatives. For two given functions $\tilde{\gamma}$ and $\gamma$ from $\mathscr{I}$, let

$$\gamma_\varepsilon = (1 - \varepsilon)\tilde{\gamma} + \varepsilon\gamma, \quad \text{for} \quad \varepsilon \in [0, 1].$$

It can be verified that the function

$$F(\varepsilon; \tilde{\gamma}, \gamma) = E^{P^*}[h_U(S)g(S, 1 - \gamma_\varepsilon(S))], \quad \varepsilon \in [0, 1],$$

is convex. Therefore any local solution will be also a global one, although uniqueness is not guaranteed. We will show that $\tilde{\gamma}$ is optimal for the problem (11) by demonstrating that for any $\gamma$ the corresponding function $\varepsilon \to F(\varepsilon; \tilde{\gamma}, \gamma)$ attains its minimum at $\varepsilon = 0$. This condition can be expressed by using a one-sided derivative of $F$. The latter can be found by taking the derivative inside the expectation, which can be justified by using our assumptions ($\mathscr{C}3$)–($\mathscr{C}4$). This leads to

$$F'(0+; \tilde{\gamma}, \gamma) = E^{P^*}[h_U(S)g_z(S, 1 - \tilde{\gamma}(S); p)(\tilde{\gamma}(S) - \gamma(S))].$$

Using this derivative, the condition for $\tilde{\gamma}$ to be optimal becomes

$$F'(0+; \tilde{\gamma}, \gamma) \geq 0, \quad \text{for any } \gamma \in \mathscr{I},$$

or equivalently,

$$E^{P^*}[h_U(S)g_z(S, 1 - \tilde{\gamma}(S))\tilde{\gamma}(S)] \geq E^{P^*}[h_U(S)g_z(S, 1 - \tilde{\gamma}(S))\gamma(S)] \qquad (13)$$

for any $\gamma \in \mathscr{I}$. Let us observe that this condition will hold regardless of how we define the derivatives $g_z(s, z)$ at the points $1 - \frac{l_i(s)}{h_U(s)}$, $i = 1, \ldots, K$.

Let us introduce a new measure $\tilde{P}$ in the following way

$$d\tilde{P} = \text{const} \cdot h_U(s) \cdot g_z(s, 1 - \tilde{\gamma}(s))dP^*.$$

Then the problem of finding $\tilde{\gamma}$ that satisfies (13) and the constraint (12) can be recognized as looking for the most powerful test for the hypothesis $\tilde{Q}$ against the alternative $\tilde{P}$ at the level $\alpha := \tilde{H}_0$. The structure of the optimal test $\tilde{\gamma}$ is given by the Neyman-Pearson lemma in terms of the likelihood ratio

$$\frac{d\tilde{P}}{d\tilde{Q}} = \text{const} \cdot g_z(s, 1 - \tilde{\gamma})\frac{dP^*}{dQ^*}.$$

For a given constant $c$, the optimal test should be equal to one on the set

$$\{d\tilde{P}/d\tilde{Q} > c\} = \{s : \cdot\pi_K(s)\frac{dP^*}{dQ^*}(s) > c\} \qquad (14)$$

and zero on the set

$$\{d\tilde{P}/d\tilde{Q} < c\} = \{s : (1 - \pi_0)\frac{dP^*}{dQ^*}(s) < c\}. \qquad (15)$$

On the set

$$\{d\tilde{P}/d\tilde{Q} = c\} = \{s : \cdot g_z(s, 1 - \tilde{\gamma}(s))\frac{dP^*}{dQ^*}(s) = c\} \qquad (16)$$

the optimal test $\tilde{\gamma}$ should be defined so that the level condition is satisfied.

Below we show that under ($\mathscr{C}4$) the optimal test is unique and given by $h_{opt}$. For a given $c$, suppose that the set

$$C_c := \{s : \pi_K(s)\frac{dP^*}{dQ^*}(s) \leq c \leq (1 - \pi_0)\frac{dP^*}{dQ^*}(s)\}$$

is non-empty. Since by (14) and (15) the optimal test is determined uniquely on $\mathscr{S} - C_c$, we focus on the definition of the test on $C_c$ only. Let

$$A_c(i) := \{s : \sum_{j=i+1}^{K} \pi_j(s)\frac{dP^*}{dQ^*}(s) < c < \sum_{j=i}^{K} \pi_j(s)\frac{dP^*}{dQ^*}(s)\}, \; i = 1, \ldots, K-1.$$

On each non-empty set $A_c(i)$, $i = 1, \ldots, K-1$, the condition

$$g_z(s, 1 - \tilde{\gamma}(s))\frac{dP^*}{dQ^*}(s) = c$$

will hold if we take $\tilde{\gamma}(s) = \frac{l_i(s)}{h_U(s)}$. This is possible since we have the freedom to choose values of the derivative at the points $1 - \frac{l_i(s)}{h_U(s)}, i = 1, \ldots, K-1$. Thus, the optimal test is uniquely determined on $\cup_{i=1}^{K-1}A_c(i)$. In addition, it is of the same form as $h_{opt}$.

Now let us consider the sets $B_c(i)$, $i = 1, \ldots, K$, defined in (8). For each $i$ for which the set $B_c(i)$ is non-empty, the test is not uniquely determined, as it can take any value from the interval $[-\frac{l_i(s)}{h_U(s)}, -\frac{l_{i-1}(s)}{h_U(s)}]$. However, under the assumption ($\mathscr{C}3$), the Lebesgue measure of the set of $s$ for which this occurs is zero.

Since it can be easily verified that $E^Q[h_{opt}(S(T))]$ is a decreasing function of $c$, the optimal $c$ should be selected as the smallest number for which $E^Q[h_{opt}(S(T))] \le V_0$. $\qquad\square$

## 3   Example: Roll-Down Call

To illustrate our approach, in this section we find the payoff function of the optimal static hedge for a roll-down call with two barriers. Such a contract involves barriers $b_1 > b_2$ that are below the spot price and strike, that is, $S_0 > b_1$ and $K_0 > b_1$. If the higher barrier is not reached before maturity $T$, then a roll-down call has the same terminal payoff as a standard call with strike price $K_0$. However, if the barrier $b_1$ is reached prior to maturity, then the strike price is rolled down to a new level $K_1 \in (b_1, K_0)$, and a new out-barrier becomes active at the level $b_2$. For more details about such contracts, we refer to [1].

If we define the following two stopping times

$$\tau_1 = \inf\{z : S(z) = b_1\} \quad \text{and} \quad \tau_2 = \inf\{z : S(z) = b_2\},$$

then the payoff function of a roll-down call can be written compactly as

$$(S(T) - K_0)^+\mathbf{1}_{\{\tau_1 > T\}} + (S(T) - K_1)^+\mathbf{1}_{\{\tau_1 < T \text{ and } \tau_2 > T\}}.$$

In order to determine the distributions of the residual risk, we assume that the underlying asset follows the Black-Scholes model (4). Then the distribution of $S(T)$ is lognormal, while the distributions of the residual risks depend on Brownian bridges. For a precise description, let us introduce $W^d(t) := (\mu - \frac{1}{2}\sigma^2)t + \sigma W(t)$, $t \geq 0$. Since $S(t) = S(0)e^{W^d(t)}$, conditioning on $S(T)$ is equivalent to conditioning on the terminal value of the Brownian motion $\{W^d(t), t \in [0, T]\}$. It is known that the law a Brownian motion conditioned on its terminal value does not depend on its drift and is described by a Brownian bridge. Therefore the law of the process $\{W^d(t), t \in [0, T]\}$ conditioned on $W^d(T) = u$ is the same as the law of $\{\frac{u}{T}t + \sigma W_{[0,T]}(t), t \in [0, T]\}$, where $\{W_{[0,T]}(t), t \in [0, T]\}$ is a standard Brownian bridge on $[0, T]$, that is a standard Brownian motion conditioned on $W(T) = 0$. Thus, under the Black-Scholes model, the distribution of each conditional residual risk can be represented as

$$L(s, T) \overset{\mathscr{D}}{=} C(S_0 \exp(\frac{u}{T}t + \sigma W_{[0,T]}(t))_{t \in [0,T]}, T), \tag{17}$$

where $u = \ln(s/S_0)$, $s \in \mathscr{R}^+$, and $C$ is a proper functional.

If we denote by $S_s$ the process $S$ conditioned on $S(T) = s$, then, using the notation from Sect. 2, the set of $s$ for which the residual risk is non-zero is given by $\mathscr{S} = [K_1, \infty)$. In addition, for $s \geq K_0$ we have

$$l_1(s) = s - K_0,$$
$$\pi_1(s) = P(\min_{z \in (0,T]} S_s(z) > b_1),$$

while for $s \geq K_1$, we have $l_2(s) = s - K_1$, with

$$\pi_2(s) = P(S_s(u) \leq b_1 \text{ for some} u \in [0, T) \text{ and } \min_{z \in (0,T]} S_s(z) > b_2).$$

In our implementation we have used the following values: $S_0 = K_0 = 100$, $b_1 = K_1 = 95$, $b_2 = 90$, $\sigma = 0.2$, $T = 0.25$, and $r = 0.04$. To approximate the probabilities $\pi_1(s)$, $s \geq K_0$, and $\pi_2(s)$, $s \geq K_1$, we have used Monte Carlo simulation with 50,000 repetitions.

The resulting payoff functions of the MSE-optimal and the ES-optimal hedging options, together with quantile functions of the conditional residual risks, are presented in Fig. 1. As the graphs suggest, the payoff functions of the MSE-optimal and the ES-optimal hedging options have very different characters, since the former is a continuous and strictly increasing function, while the latter is a piecewise linear function with a jump at a single point (equal to 101.85). Using the Monte Carlo method we have also found that the hedging method based on $h_{opt}$ reduces the expected shortfall by about 18.5% when compared with the MSE-optimal hedging option.

From these graphs it also follows that the ES-optimal option hedges perfectly the residual risk for any terminal value $S(T)$ that is below 101.85. Above this threshold value, the residual risk is hedged only partially. On the other hand, the MSE-optimal hedging option never hedges completely loss corresponding to the level $l_2$, but it pro-

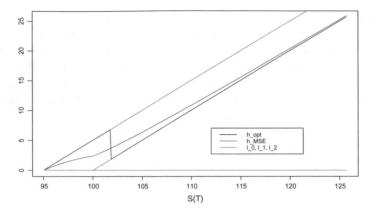

**Fig. 1** Payoff functions of the MS-optimal hedging option ($h_{MSE}$) and the ES-optimal option ($h_{opt}$), together with quantile functions of the conditional residual risks for a roll-down call option

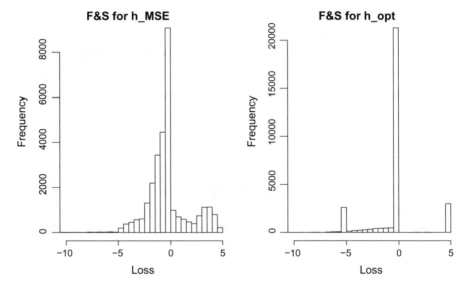

**Fig. 2** Frequencies of losses for MS-optimal and ES-optimal hedging options

vides more protection than $h_{opt}$ for terminal values $S(T)$ that are above the threshold $S(T) = 101.85$. These differences in hedging are well captured by the graphs of frequencies of losses for the two strategies, which we present in Fig. 2.

**Acknowledgements** This research was partially supported by the Natural Sciences and Engineering Research Council of Canada.

# References

1. Carr, P., Ellis, K., Gupta, V.: Static hedging of exotic options. J. Fin. **53**, 1165–1190 (1998)
2. Föllmer, H., Schweizer, M.: Hedging by sequential regression: an introduction to the mathematics of option trading. ASTIN Bull. **18**, 147–60 (1988)
3. Föllmer, H., Sondermann, D.: Hedging of non-redundant contingent claims. In: Hildenbrand, W., Mas-Colell, A. (eds.) Contributions to Mathematical Economics, pp. 205–223. North-Holland, Dordrecht (1986)
4. Kolkiewicz, A.W.: Efficient hedging of path-dependent options. Int. J. Theor. Appl. Fin. **19**, 1650032 (2016)
5. Kolkiewicz, A.W., Liu, Y.: Semi-static hedging for GMWB in variable annuities. N. Am. Actuarial J. **16**(1), 112–140 (2012)
6. Karlin, S.: Mathematical Methods and Theory in Games, Programming and Economics, vol. 2. Addison-Wesley, Massachusetts (1959)
7. Melnikov, A., Smirnov, I.: Dynamic hedging of conditional value-at-risk. Insurance Math. Econ. **51**, 182–190 (2012)

# Population and Pollution Interactions in a Spatial Economic Model

Davide La Torre, Danilo Liuzzi and Simone Marsiglio

**Abstract** We analyze the spatio-temporal dynamics of a simple model of economic geography in which population and pollution dynamics are mutually interdependent. Pollution by reducing the carrying capacity of the natural environment, which determines the maximum amount of people a given location can effectively bear, affects labor force dynamics which in turn alter pollution emissions. Such mutual links determine the development path followed by different locations, and spatial interactions further complicate the picture. We show that neglecting the existence of spatial externalities can lead to misleading predictions about the development path followed by different locations in the spatial economy.

**Keywords** Population dynamics · Pollution · Spatial model · Sustainability

## 1 Introduction

Sustainable development has become a very popular research topic lately, and the main research question in this context consists of understanding how to address the economy along a sustainable development path [1, 2]. Sustainability ultimately requires to satisfy *"the needs of the present without compromising the ability of*

D. La Torre (✉) · D. Liuzzi
Department of Economics, Management, and Quantitative Methods,
University of Milan, 20122 Milan, Italy
e-mail: davide.latorre@unimi.it

D. Liuzzi
e-mail: danilo.liuzzi@unimi.it

D. La Torre
Dubai Business School, University of Dubai, 14143 Dubai, UAE
e-mail: dlatorre@ud.ac.ae

S. Marsiglio
School of Accounting, Economics and Finance,
University of Wollongong, Wollongong, NSW 2522, Australia
e-mail: simonem@uow.edu.au

© Springer Nature Switzerland AG 2018
D. M. Kilgour et al. (eds.), *Recent Advances in Mathematical
and Statistical Methods*, Springer Proceedings in Mathematics & Statistics 259,
https://doi.org/10.1007/978-3-319-99719-3_49

*future generations to meet their own needs*" [3], demanding thus to take into account the population and environment relation. The channels through which the human population affects the natural environment in which it lives and how in turn the environment may alter the evolution of human population have been long discussed in literature since [4] seminal work (see among others [5–7]). However, none of the existing works is able to relate the issue to geographical and spatial characteristics, since they all assume that the economy is simply a unique point in space and thus eventual heterogeneities are completely ruled out. This is clearly a strong simplification of reality. While understanding the implications of geographical heterogeneity on the development path followed by a spatial-extended notion of economy is a very active and recent research topic, following [8] seminal work (see [9–13]). The goal of this paper consists of analyzing the population and environment relation from a spatial point of view, taking into account thus that the dynamics of population and the environment mutually affect each other not only over time but also across space.

Our work thus combine together two different streams of literature: the sustainability and the economic geography ones. From the latter we borrow the analytical framework by considering a spatial economic growth model with environmental and demographic interactions; the setup most similar to ours is [14], but differently from them we allow for population growth and labor migration. From the former, instead, we borrow the interest in understanding whether sustainable development can effectively occur; [5, 7] are closely related to our work, but differently from them our focus is not on natural resources but on pollution and we do not restrict our analysis to the temporal dynamics only since we allow also for spatial interactions. Our main results show that by neglecting the existence of spatial spillovers the possible predictions about the development path followed by different locations in the spatial economy may be misleading, suggesting thus that geographic externalities may be an important determinant of economic development.

The paper proceeds as follows. Section 2 introduces our spatio-temporal dynamic model, summarized by two partial differential equations. In Sect. 3 we derive some analytical results in absence of spatial diffusion, while in Sect. 4 we focus on the fully-fledged model in which spatial diffusion plays an active role. Section 5 concludes and presents directions for future research.

## 2   The Model

We consider a simple model of economic geography in which agents consume all their income and inelastically supply labor. Since there is no unemployment, the population size and the labor force perfectly coincide. Economic production generates pollution which by affecting the carrying capacity of the natural environment in which human population lives determines the evolution of the labor force, which is an essential input in the production of final output. We assume a continuous space structure to represent that the spatial economy develops along a linear city (see [15]), where the population is mobile across different locations and pollution, even if

generated in a specific location, diffuses across the whole economy [14]. We denote
with $L(x, t)$ and $P(x, t)$ respectively the population size and pollution stock in the
position $x$ at date $t$, in a compact interval $[x_a, x_b] \subset \mathbb{R}$, and $t \geq 0$. We also assume
that the initial population and pollution distribution, $L(x, 0)$ and $P(x, 0)$, are known
and there is no migration or pollution flow through the boundary of $[x_a, x_b]$ namely
the directional derivative is null, $\frac{\partial L(x,t)}{\partial x} = \frac{\partial P(x,t)}{\partial x} = 0$, at $x = x_a$ and $x = x_b$ ([11, 16].

The economic and environmental setup to a large extent resembles [14], but d-
ifferently from theirs, our model focuses on the dynamic evolution of population
and its interaction with pollution. Output is produced according to a Cobb-Douglas
production function employing capital and labor as $Y(x, t) = AK(x, t)^\alpha L(x, t)^{1-\alpha}$,
where $A > 0$ denotes the total factor productivity and $0 < \alpha < 1$ the capital share
of income. We abstract from capital accumulation and without loss of generality the
capital stock is normalized to unity, $K(x, t) = 1, \forall x, t$. Production activities generate
emissions which increase linearly the stock of pollution and $\theta > 0$ measures the degree of such environmental inefficiency. These emissions are dampened by (spatially
heterogeneous) public abatement activities, which reduce a share $u(x) \in [0, 1]$ of total emissions, thus $1 - u(x)$ represents unabated emissions. Apart from abatement
activities, the pollution stock tends to decrease at the constant rate $\delta_P > 0$ representing
the natural decay rate of pollution. Agents are subject to (location-specific) proportional income taxation, $\tau(x) > 0$, which is used to finance the abatement activities
needed to reduce the environmental effects associated with pollution; agents are assumed to consume completely their disposable income, implying that $C(x, t) = [1 -
\tau(x)]Y(x, t)$. We assume that the (local) government wishes to maintain a balanced
budget at any point in time, such that the tax revenue is totally devoted to reduce pollution. At location $x$ the tax revenue is $T(x, t) = \tau(x)Y(x, t)$, while abatement activities,
$M(x, t)$, decrease a certain share of pollution, $u(x) \in [0, 1]$, by employing a certain
amount of not consumed output with the following cost $M(x, t) = \mathscr{C}[u(x)]Y(x, t)$,
where $\mathscr{C}(\cdot)$ is the cost function of abatement activities, taking the following form
$\mathscr{C}[u(x)] = 1 - [1 - u(x)]^\varepsilon$ with $\varepsilon < 1$ [17]. By equating the tax revenue and abatement we obtain a one-to-one relationship between the tax rate and the share of abat-
ed emissions, $\tau(x) = \mathscr{C}[u(x)]$, implying that consumption is given by the following
expression: $C(x, t) = [1 - u(x)]^\varepsilon Y(x, t)$. Population evolves according to a logistic
equation, where $L^c(x) > 0$ represents the (spatially heterogeneous) carrying capacity
of the natural environment, which is affected by pollution flows, through the following damage function $D(x, t) = \frac{1}{1+BP(x,t)^\beta}$ with $B > 0$ being a scale parameter and
$\beta > 0$ measuring the magnitude of the pollution externality on population dynamic-
s. Note that the share of abatement activities rules the economic-environmental trade
off: a larger abatement improves the environmental outcome (by reducing pollution)
at the cost of deteriorating the economic one (by reducing consumption).

The spatio-temporal dynamic model can thus be summarized by the following
system of two partial differential equations:

$$\frac{\partial P(x, t)}{\partial t} = d_P \frac{\partial^2 P(x, t)}{\partial x^2} + \theta[1 - u(x)]AL(x, t)^{1-\alpha} - \delta_P P(x, t) \tag{1}$$

$$\frac{\partial L(x, t)}{\partial t} = d_L \frac{\partial^2 L(x, t)}{\partial x^2} + \left[\frac{L^c(x)}{1 + BP(x, t)^\beta} - L(x, t)\right]L(x, t) \tag{2}$$

Equation (1) describes the evolution of pollution over time and across space. The engine of pollution accumulation is represented by economic production activities; a fraction of the emissions is abated from the outset, through cleaning activities represented by term $1 - u$, while a constant part of the pollution stock is eliminated by the self-cleaning capacity of the natural environment, represented by $\delta_P P$. The spatial externality, representing the extent to which the outcome in specific locations affects the outcomes in other locations as well, is captured by the diffusion term: the intensity of the diffusion process is measured by the diffusion coefficient $d_P \geq 0$, quantifying the extent to which pollution no matter where it is originally generated spreads across the whole spatial economy [14].

Equation (2) describes the evolution of the human population over time and across space. In absence of pollution, the population size would grow according to a logistic law with constant carrying capacity $L^c$ [18]. By taking into account the negative pollution externality, the demographic law of motion is still logistic, but the maximum value of the population size that the natural environment can bear is represented by the term $\frac{L^c}{1+BP^\beta}$. As for the case of pollution, the spatial externality is represented by the diffusion term, where $d_L \geq 0$, represents the diffusion coefficient, measuring the extent to which population tends to migrate across different locations in the spatial economy.

## 3   The Model with No Diffusion

We first analyze the behavior of the above system without diffusion, but preserving the spatial structure. This allows us to compare the outcome with what arises in the diffusion case which we will analyze in the next section. In the case with no diffusion, that is $d_P = d_L = 0$, the partial differential equations (1) and (2) boil down to the following parametric system of ordinary differential equations:

$$\frac{dP(t)}{dt} = \theta[1 - u]AL(t)^{1-\alpha} - \delta_P P(t) \tag{3}$$

$$\frac{dL(t)}{dt} = \left[\frac{L_x^c}{1 + BP(t)^\beta} - L(t)\right]L(t) \tag{4}$$

The system (1)–(2) is characterized by several parameters, each of which could be space dependant, but we restrict our analysis to the effects of spatial heterogeneity on $L^c$. It is thus quite natural to suppose that the carrying capacity of the natural environment can vary across different locations, and thus it is reasonable to expect some spatial heterogeneity due to such inherent characteristic of specific locations. Since we are especially interested in discussing the implications of the population and environment relation, understanding the specific spatial characteristics of such a parameter, $L_x^c = L^c(x)$, is essential to comment on the interplay between human population and the natural environment. Specifically, this parameter captures the pollution feedback on population, and we wish to analyze how the location-specific carrying capacity $L_x^c$ along with the diffusion terms $d_i \frac{\partial^2}{\partial x^2}$ where $i = L, P$, shape the time evolution of population and pollution. Note first that the system (3)–(4) is actually a continuous set of systems of ordinary differential equations, because of the presence of the space dependant parameter $L_x^c$: each point in the spatial domain has its own time dynamics, but there is no interaction between adjacent locations. Next proposition offers a concise description of the properties of this continuous set of systems, stating that $\forall x \in [x_a, x_b]$ the system (3)–(4) has a unique and stable non-trivial equilibrium.

**Proposition 1** *The system (3)–(4) admits a unique nontrivial equilibrium, $(\overline{P}, \overline{L}) \in \mathbb{R}_{++}^2$, $\forall x \in [x_a, x_b]$:*

$$\overline{P} = \left[ \frac{\theta A(1 - u)}{\delta_P} \right] \overline{L}^{1-\alpha}$$

$$\overline{L} = RootOf \left\{ B \left[ \frac{\theta A(1 - u)}{\delta_P} \right]^\beta L^{(1-\alpha)\beta+1} + L - L_x^c = 0 \right\}.$$

*Moreover $(\overline{P}, \overline{L})$ is asymptotically stable.*

Proposition 1 can be proved by using a classical linearization approach. The Jacobian matrix associated with the non-trivial equilibrium, $J(\overline{P}, \overline{L})$, is given by:

$$J(\overline{P}, \overline{L}) = \begin{bmatrix} -\delta_P & A(1-\alpha)(1-u)\overline{L}^{-\alpha} \\ -\beta BL_x^c \overline{L}\overline{P}^{\beta-1}(1 + B\overline{P}^\beta)^{-2} & -\overline{L} \end{bmatrix} \tag{5}$$

It is not difficult to determine the signs of each element. $a_{11}$ is obviously negative. Since $\overline{L}$ and $\overline{P}$ are both positive, $a_{12}$ is positive while $a_{21}$ and $a_{22}$ are both negative. It follows that both the eigenvalues of the Jacobian matrix are negative. Figure 1 represents the phase portrait for the following parametrization: $u = 0.5$, $\theta = 0.2$, $\delta_P = 0.05$, $A = 1$, $B = 1$, $\alpha = 0.33$, $\beta = 1.5$ (see [14]), showing that whatever is the pair of initial conditions, $(P_0, L_0)$, the system converges to its unique nontrivial equilibrium. The existence of a steady state in which both human population and pollution attain a strictly positive value suggests that despite the pollution feedback on population dynamics each location in the spatial economy develops along a trajectory which could be deemed as sustainable in some minimal sense. In absence of spatial interactions, the spatial economy is overall able to proceed its process of economic development along a smooth path, independently on the spatial parameter $L_x^c$. Even if an analytical expression for the steady state values cannot be obtained, it is possible

**Fig. 1** Phase portrait in the
no diffusion case
$(d_P = d_L = 0)$

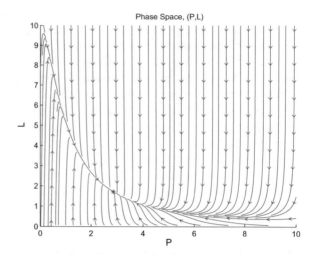

to infer from the steady state expressions above how they do depend on such a spatial
parameter and thus how the heterogeneity in the carrying capacity is likely to affect
the long run equilibrium of both population and pollution.

## 4   The Model with Diffusion

We now turn to the analysis of the full model in which diffusion and thus spatial
externalities are explicitly taken into account. In particular, we wish to understand
whether the presence of such spatial interactions can alter our previous predictions
about the development path followed by different locations in the spatial economy.
Given the spatial structure of the economy, the analysis of transitional dynamics
can be performed only numerically, thus we now focus on numerical simulations in
order to illustrate the spatial implications of pollution accumulation and population
growth. Even if the numerical simulations that follow are based upon a specific set
of parameters and initial conditions, reported in (6), it is possible to show that, since
the nontrivial equilibrium is unique (see [14], for a discussion of how the presence
of spatial externalities differently affect the system dynamics in the case of unique or
multiple equilibria), even under different parametrizations the following qualitative
results will hold true.

$$\begin{cases} u = 0.5, \ \theta = 0.2, \ x_a = -1, \ x_b = 1, \ \delta_P = 0.05, \\ A = 1, \ B = 1, \ \alpha = \frac{1}{3}, \ \beta = 1.5, \ d_P = 0.1, \ d_L = 0.1, \\ P(x, 0) = 1 + x, \ L(x, 0) = 1 + x, \\ \sigma_{L^c}^2 = 0.1, \ L^c = 10, \ L^c(x) = L^c e^{-\frac{x^2}{\sigma_{L^c}^2}}. \end{cases} \quad (6)$$

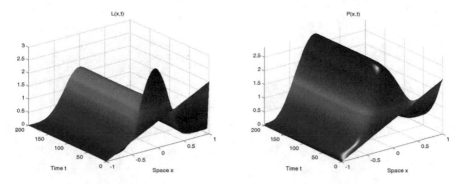

**Fig. 2** Evolution of pollution and population: no diffusion case ($d_P = d_L = 0$)

Most parameters take the same values as in [14] consistently with empirical evidence (see references therein), apart from those which are set to unity without loss of generality, and those which are specifically set in order to make our graphical illustrations as clear as possible. The share of abated emissions $u$ is a candidate to be a control variable, that is a policy variable optimally chosen by the social planner in order to keep under control the level of pollution stock and thus to limit its impacts on population. We do not analyze the associated optimal control problem, thus for the sake of simplicity we assume that it takes the central value in the control space, namely $u = 0.5$. We assume the initial distribution of pollution, $P(x, 0) = P_x = 1 + x$, to mimic to the initial distribution of population, $L(x, 0) = L_x = 1 + x$. We set the carrying capacity as follows $L^c(x) = L^c e^{-\frac{x^2}{\sigma_{Lc}^2}}$, meaning that in the central locations it is larger than in the lateral ones. The results of our simulations are shown in Figs. 2 and 3.

Figure 2 describes the evolution over time and across space of population (left panel) and pollution (right panel) in the case in which diffusion is absent, that is $d_P = d_L = 0$, consistently with what discussed in Sect. 3. Given the shape of $L^c(x)$, it is clear that the central locations, where a higher carrying capacity is assumed, establish their primacy over time. There is no interaction among locations (no spatial externality), and for each location $x$ the system (3)–(4) reaches its non-trivial and stable steady state. Figure 3 presents the same simulations in the case in which there is diffusion, that is $d_P = d_L > 0$. The overall dynamics of the system (1)–(2) is analogous to what seen before but there are notable differences that underline the role of diffusion as a spatial externality, justifying thus the introduction of a spatial model to the study of the dynamic relation between pollution and population. Indeed, even if the shape of the initial condition for both population and pollution increases linearly from the leftmost to the rightmost locations, the spatial profiles of both population and pollution over time change to end up mimicking the spatial pattern of the carrying capacity, which by being the only spatially-dependent parameter completely determines the spatial pattern at the equilibrium.

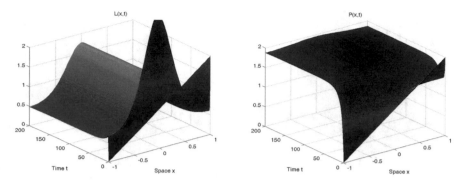

**Fig. 3** Evolution of pollution and population: diffusion case ($d_P = d_L = 0.1$)

By comparing Figs. 2 and 3, it is possible to notice that diffusion has a twofold effect on the dynamics and steady states of pollution: the central and the lateral locations witness less and more pollution accumulation, respectively, with respect to the case without diffusion. This is because of the inherent tendency of diffusion to smooth differences out [9, 14]. Pollution diffusion does have a beneficial effect for the initially most polluted locations and a detrimental effect for the less polluted ones: ignoring spatial externalities can thus result in macroscopic modeling errors, since not only the dynamics, but even the steady states are affected by this type of spatial interaction. It is also clear that when diffusion is present the overall population becomes larger: on the one hand, the central locations reach a higher demographic concentration, on the other hand, the lateral locations are an order of magnitude bigger, with respect to the no-diffusion scenario. This is apparently in contrast with what happens to pollution: pollution has a negative impact on the growth of population via its carrying capacity dampening factor. At the steady state, in the central locations there is less pollution such that the population concentration tends to increase: the reaction term, ($\frac{1}{1+BP^\beta}$), prevails on the smoothing tendency of diffusion, $d_L \frac{\partial^2}{\partial x^2}$. In the lateral locations we would expect a symmetrical behavior, that is pollution to increase while population to decrease; what instead happens is that diffusion prevails on reaction and the population in the lateral locations can benefit from migration from the central ones. Clearly, the introduction of diffusion enriches the dynamics and affects the steady states: the overall effects are the results of the dynamical tension between the reaction and the diffusion components of the system (1)–(2).

In Fig. 4 we show the long run per capita pollution in the case with no (left panel) and with (right panel) diffusion. At the beginning of the time horizon per capita pollution is identically equal to 1 across the spatial domain in both the cases by assumption. In both the cases, over time per capita pollution increases everywhere, but the locations who suffer the most are lateral ones, due to the extremely low value of the environmental carrying capacity that tends to keep population down. A few words on the long run spatial distribution of per capita pollution in the two different frameworks are needed. Per capita pollution is bounded, such that in the long run the spatial

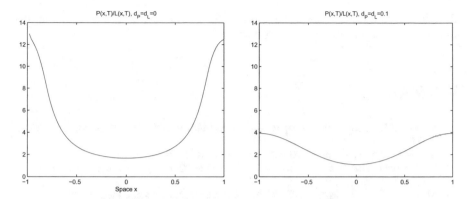

**Fig. 4** Steady state per capita pollution: no diffusion and positive diffusion cases

economy can be considered sustainable. Comparing the left and the right panels, it is clear that the central locations performs better in terms of per capita pollution, in both scenarios: the combined effect of reaction and diffusion previously mentioned turns out to be favorable to the central locations, as long as per capita pollution is deemed to be a proxy of the health status of the environment. The major difference between the two cases results in the higher level of pollution per capita taken in the no-diffusion scenario. As seen before, both pollution and population increase in the lateral locations when spatial externality are taken into account; however, now we can compare such relative increases: population increases more than pollution, resulting in lower per capita pollution than in the no-diffusion case.

## 5 Conclusion

This paper analyzes the mutual interactions between population and pollution in a spatio-temporal dynamic economic geography model. We develop a dynamic macroeconomic model to analyze the extent to which population and pollution may affect each other not only over time but also across space. We show that the population and pollution feedback may be important in order to assess the development path that different locations in the spatial economy will follow. This means that neglecting any spatial implication may give rise to misleading predictions about the environment and population relation. Thus, from a policy point of view, spatial externalities represent an important aspect which deserves further attention. Indeed, the analysis performed in this paper cannot be considered exhaustive, since important issues have not be taken into account. Specifically, the pure dynamic setup of the model does not allow us to assess how optimally defined policies may alter our conclusions about the development path followed by single locations in the spatial economy. Extending the analysis in order to consider the associated optimal control problem along the lines of [14] is a priority for future research.

# References

1. Solow, R.M.: Intergenerational equity and exhaustible resources. Rev. Econ. Stud. **41**, 29–45 (1974)
2. Stokey, N.: Are there limits to growth? Int. Econ. Rev. **39**, 1–31 (1998)
3. World Commission on Environment and Development: Our Common Future. Oxford University Press, Oxford (1987)
4. Malthus, T.R.: An Essay on the Principle of Population. J. Johnson, London (1798)
5. Marsiglio, S.: On the relationship between population change and sustainable development. Res. Econ. **65**, 353–364 (2011)
6. Marsiglio, S.: A simple endogenous growth model with endogenous fertility and environmental concern. Scottish J. Polit. Econ. **64**, 263–282 (2017)
7. Nerlove, M.: Population and the environment: a parable of firewood and other tales. Am. J. Agric. Econ. Agric. Appl. Econ. Assoc. **73**(5), 1334–1347 (1991)
8. Krugman, P.: Increasing returns and economic geography. J. Polit. Econ. **99**, 483–499 (1991)
9. Boucekkine, R., Camacho, C., Zou, B.: Bridging the gap between growth theory and economic geography: the spatial Ramsey model. Macroecon. Dyn. **13**, 20–45 (2009)
10. Camacho, C., Zou, B.: The spatial Solow model. Econ. Bull. **18**, 111 (2004)
11. Capasso, V., Engbers, R., La Torre, D.: On a spatial Solow model with technological diffusion and non-concave production function. Nonlinear Anal.: Real World Appl. **11**(5), 3858–3876 (2010)
12. Fujita, M., Thisse, J.F.: Economics of Agglomeration. Cambridge University Press, Cambridge (2002)
13. Xepapadeas, A.: Modeling complex systems. Agric. Econ. **41**, 181–191 (2010)
14. La Torre, D., Liuzzi, D., Marsiglio, S.: Pollution diffusion and abatement activities across space and over time. Math. Soc. Sci. **78**, 48–63 (2015)
15. Hotelling, H.: Stability in competition. Econ. J. **39**, 41–57 (1929)
16. Anita, S., Capasso, V., Kunze, H., La Torre, D.: Optimal control and long-run dynamics for a spatial economic growth model with physical capital accumulation and pollution diffusion. Appl. Math. Lett. **26**, 908–912 (2013)
17. Bartz, S., Kelly, D.L.: Economic growth and the environment: theory and facts. Resour. Energy Econ. **30**, 115–149 (2008)
18. Verhulst, P.F.: Notice sur la loi que la population suit dans son accroissement. Correspondance Mathmatique et Physique **10**, 113–121 (1838)

# Price Bounds in Jump-Diffusion Markets Revisited via Market Completions

## Anne MacKay and Alexander Melnikov

**Abstract** It is well known that incomplete markets generally admit infinitely many equivalent (local) martingale measures (EMMs), and that the resulting no-arbitrage price of a contingent claim is not unique. The bounds on no-arbitrage prices for a given contingent claim can be obtained by considering the set of EMMs on the market. In some cases, incomplete markets can be completed by adding specific sets of assets. Market completion techniques have been mentioned in various publications and can be used to simplify optimal investment and hedging problems. In this paper, we consider a multidimensional jump-diffusion market with predictable jump sizes and we revisit the no-arbitrage price bounds via market completions. We review the conditions under which a given set of assets can complete the original market, and we present a set of market completions that can be used to obtain the range of no-arbitrage prices.

**Keywords** Incomplete markets · Jump-diffusion markets · Market completions No-arbitrage price

## 1 Introduction

The absence of arbitrage in a market allows for the existence of at least one equivalent (local) martingale measure (EMM) that can be used to price contingent claims. In a complete market, such a measure is unique and claims can be perfectly replicated by trading in the available assets; the value of the replicating portfolio is the unique no-arbitrage price of the claim. In an incomplete market, there exists more than one such pricing measure, and some contingent claims cannot be perfectly replicated

A. MacKay (✉)
Université du Québec à Montréal, Montréal H3C 3P8, Canada
e-mail: mackay.anne@uqam.ca

A. Melnikov
University of Alberta, Edmonton T6G 2R3, Canada
e-mail: melnikov@ualberta.ca

© Springer Nature Switzerland AG 2018
D. M. Kilgour et al. (eds.), *Recent Advances in Mathematical and Statistical Methods*, Springer Proceedings in Mathematics & Statistics 259,
https://doi.org/10.1007/978-3-319-99719-3_50

by investing in the market. These claims do not have a unique no-arbitrage price. Instead, there exists a range of no-arbitrage prices that are acceptable for both the buyer and the seller of the claim.

The theory of no-arbitrage pricing in incomplete markets is well developed. An important result is that the range of no-arbitrage prices admitted by an incomplete market can be obtained by taking the infimum and the supremum of the no-arbitrage price over the set of EMMs.

In this paper, we discuss market completions as a way to describe the set of EMMs. The idea of market completions is to associate each equivalent local martingale measure with a set of fictitious assets which forms a complete market when combined with the original incomplete one. The idea of adding fictitious assets to investigate pricing and hedging problems in the Black-Scholes model first appeared in [9], and was used in various works since then. For example, [14] showed how these arguments can be also adapted to American options in a multidimensional diffusion market. Market completion techniques were also independently developed in the framework of multinomial markets in Appendix 3 of [11].

Market completion techniques have also been used to solve precise problems. [6] make external risk tradable via market completion, and use the method to price weather derivatives. In a diffusion model, [10] study pricing and hedging problems by completing a market where incompleteness is due to different borrowing and lending rates (see also [3]). Kane and Melnikov [8] extend the results to a jump-diffusion model. Finally, [4] consider market completion techniques in the setting of a general Lévy model.

In this paper, we consider a multidimensional jump-diffusion model with predictable jump sizes, in which incompleteness stems from a larger number of risk sources than traded assets. We review results on the set of EMMs in this particular model, and describe the assets that can be used to complete the market. We show the equivalence between the set of all EMMs admitted by the market, and a subset of possible market completions. Note that this is only possible because we assume that the jump sizes are predictable (see [12] for details).

The paper is organized as follows. In Sect. 2, we present the market model and recall specific results on market arbitrage and completeness. We discuss the link between the set of EMMs and market completions in Sect. 3. Section 4 concludes.


## 2    Review of Basic Definitions and Concepts

In this section, we introduce the market model and review some key results on no-arbitrage and market completeness conditions in the context of our model.

## 2.1  Market Model

We work on a probability space $(\Omega, \mathscr{F}, P)$ with a finite time horizon $T \in \mathbb{R}$. On the probability space, we assume the existence of a $d$-dimensional Brownian motion $W = (W_1, \ldots, W_d)^\top$ and a multivariate Poisson process $N = (N_1, \ldots, N_{n-d})^\top$ with intensity $\lambda = (\lambda_1, \ldots, \lambda_{n-d})^\top$, independent of $W$. We denote by $\mathbb{F} = \{\mathscr{F}_t\}_{t \leq T}$ the filtration generated by $W$ and $N$, and augmented by the $P$-null sets. The intensity $\lambda$ can be stochastic, but is assumed to be predictable in $t$.

We define a market $(B, S) = (B, S_1, \ldots, S_k)$, in which $B$ denotes the bank account process (considered to be risk-free) and $S = (S_1, \ldots, S_k)$ represents the value of $k$ risky assets. Throughout the paper, we assume that $k \leq n$. The $k + 1$ assets have the following dynamics

$$
\begin{aligned}
dB(t) &= B(t)\, r(t)\, dt, \\
dS_i(t) &= S_i(t_-) \left( \mu_i(t)\, dt + \sigma_i^V(t)\, dW(t) + \sigma_i^J(t)\, dM(t) \right)
\end{aligned}
\tag{1}
$$

with $B(0) = 1$ and $S^i(0) = s_0^i \in \mathbb{R}_+$ for $i \in \{1, \ldots, k\}$, and where $M(t) = N(t) - \int_0^t \lambda(s)\, ds$. The risk-free interest rate $r(t) \geq 0$, as well as the appreciation rate $\mu = (\mu_1, \ldots, \mu_k)^\top$ and the matrix-valued processes $\sigma^V$ and $\sigma^J$, with $i$th row given by the vectors $\sigma_i^V = (\sigma_{i1}^V, \ldots, \sigma_{id}^V)$, and $\sigma_i^J = (\sigma_{i1}^J, \ldots, \sigma_{i(n-d)}^J)$, respectively, for $i = 1, \ldots, k$, are predictable with respect to the filtration $\mathbb{F}$. Going forward, we assume that $r(t) \equiv 0$ for all $t \in [0, T]$, so that $B(t) = 1$ for all $t \in [0, T]$. In other words, we consider that the price processes are discounted by the bank account numéraire.

We also assume that $\mu$, $\sigma^V$ and $\sigma^J$ are uniformly bounded in $(t, \omega) \in [0, T] \times \Omega$, and that $\sup_{t \leq T} \lambda_l(t) \leq K$, for some $K < \infty$, for all $0 \leq l \leq m$. Under these assumptions, (1) has a unique solution. In order for the risky asset prices to remain positive, we further assume that $\sigma_{il}^J(t) \in [0, 1]$ and $\lambda_l(t) > 0$ and bounded uniformly in $t$, for $1 \leq i \leq k$ and $1 \leq l \leq n - d$.

Finally, we denote by $\sigma = [\sigma^V\ \sigma^J]$ the $k \times n$ matrix containing the volatility coefficients. We assume that $\sigma$ has full rank, so that $\det(\sigma(t)\sigma^\top(t)) \neq 0$ $P$-a.s. for all $t \in [0, T]$. This allows us to define the process $\theta = [\theta_V\ \theta_J]^\top$ by

$$
\theta(t) = \sigma^\top(t)(\sigma(t)\sigma^\top(t))^{-1}\mu(t),
\tag{2}
$$

for $t \in [0, T]$.

We let the $\mathbb{R}^{(k+1)}$-valued process $\pi = (\pi_0(t), \pi_1(t), \ldots, \pi_k(t))_{0 \leq t \leq T}$ represent a *(portfolio) strategy*, and we assume that $\int_0^T \|\pi(t)\|^2\, dt < \infty$, $P$-a.s. We denote the value process of the resulting portfolio by $X^\pi$, with

$$
X^\pi(t) = \pi_0(t)\, B(t) + \sum_{i=1}^k \pi_i(t)S_i(t), \quad \text{for all } 0 \leq t \leq T.
$$

A portfolio strategy is called *admissible* if its value process satisfies $X^\pi(t) \geq -K$ for some $K = K(\pi) \geq 0$. We denote the class of admissible portfolio strategies with initial capital $x$ by

$$\mathscr{A}(x) = \{\pi \in \mathbb{R}^{k+1} : X^\pi(0) = x,\ X^\pi(t) \geq -K \text{ for all } t \leq T\}.$$

An admissible portfolio strategy $\pi$ is called *self-financing* if the following holds:

$$X^\pi(t) = X^\pi(0) + \int_0^t \pi_0(t)dB(t) + \sum_{i=1}^k \int_0^t \pi_i(t)dS_i(t), \qquad \text{for all } 0 \leq t \leq T. \quad (3)$$

Note that under our assumption that $r(t) \equiv 0$, the second term on the right-hand side of (3) is always 0, and will therefore be omitted going forward.

As is usually the case, we only consider arbitrage-free markets. That is, we assume that for any self-financing strategy $\pi$ in $\mathscr{A}(0)$, for all $0 \leq t \leq T$,

$$P(X^\pi(t) = 0) = 1, \qquad P(X^\pi(t) \geq 0) = 1 \qquad \Rightarrow \qquad P(X^\pi(t) = 0) = 1.$$

The existence of an equivalent martingale measure (EMM), i.e. a measure equivalent to $P$ under which the value of any self-financing strategy is a local martingale, is a sufficient condition for our market to be arbitrage-free. Such a measure exists if the market allows for at least one predictable process $\gamma = (\gamma^V, \gamma^J)^\top$ with $\gamma^J = (\gamma_1^J, \ldots, \gamma_{n-d}^J)$ strictly positive that satisfies

$$\sigma^V(t)\gamma^V(t) + \sigma^J(t)\lambda(t) \cdot (\mathbf{1} - \gamma^J(t)) = \mu(t) = \sigma(t)\theta(t), \qquad (4)$$

where $\mathbf{1}$ denotes a vector of ones, and where the second equality follows from (2). Heuristically, this condition ensures that the drift of the discounted asset prices "disappears" under an EMM. It is analogous to the no-arbitrage condition in a multidimensional diffusion market, and comes from similar arguments. Going forward, we will assume the existence of at least one process $\gamma$ as described above.

It is possible to show that any solution $\gamma$ to (4), with $\gamma_l^J > 0$ for $l \in \{1, \ldots, n - d\}$, defines a probability measure. Indeed, for such a solution $\gamma$, we can define the process $L_\gamma = L_\gamma^V L_\gamma^J$, with

$$L_\gamma^V(t) = \exp\left\{-\int_0^t \gamma^V(s)^\top dW(s) - \frac{1}{2}\int_0^t \|\gamma^V(s)\|^2 ds\right\},$$

$$L_\gamma^J(t) = \exp\left\{-\int_0^t \lambda(s) \cdot (1 - \gamma^J(s))ds\right\}\prod_{l=1}^{n-d}\prod_{s \leq t} \gamma_l^J(s)\Delta N_l(s), \qquad \text{for } t \leq T.$$

Then $L_\gamma$ is a non-negative local martingale with $E[L_\gamma(t)] = 1$ for all $t \in [0, T]$. We are only interested in the solutions $\gamma$ such that $L_\gamma$ is a true martingale, and we define this set by

$\Gamma = \{\gamma : \gamma \text{ solves (4)}, \gamma_l^J > 0 \text{ for } l \in \{1, \ldots, n - d\}, L_\gamma \text{ is a martingale}\}.$

It is well known by now that the set $\Gamma$ characterizes the set of all possible EMMs on the $(B, S)$ market (see for example [2]). This result is summarized in the following proposition.

**Proposition 2.1** (Theorem 4.2 of [2]) *Let $\mathcal{Q}$ denote the set of all EMMs on the $(B, S)$ market and let $\frac{dQ_\gamma}{dP}\Big|_{\mathscr{F}_t} = L_\gamma(t)$. Then, $Q_\gamma \in \mathcal{Q}$ if and only if $\gamma \in \Gamma$.*

The reader is referred to [2] for the proof of this proposition.

## 2.2 Market (In)Completeness and Hedging Contingent Claims

Jumps in the stock price process are often a source of incompleteness. In our particular case, the size of the jumps is predictable, and the market is incomplete only when there are less assets than sources of risk. Next, we review the concept of market (in)completeness and discuss it in the context of the $(B, S)$ market.

Market completeness is closely linked to the perfect replication of contingent claims. We define a *contingent claim* as an $\mathscr{F}_T$-measurable random variable $f_T = f_T(\omega)$ that satisfies $\mathbb{E}_Q[f_T] < \infty$ for all $Q \in \mathcal{Q}$.

A contingent claim is called *replicable* if there exists an initial capital $x$ and an admissible, self-financing strategy $\pi$ that satisfies

$$X^\pi(T) = x + \sum_{i=1}^k \int_0^T \pi_i(t) dS_i(t) = f_T, \qquad P - \text{a.s.}$$

A market is called *complete* if any contingent claim is replicable. In a complete market, the *perfect hedging price* (or *fair price*) $\mathbf{C}(f_T)$ of a replicable contingent claim $f_T$ is defined as the lowest initial capital needed to perfectly replicate the claim at $T$:

$$\mathbf{C}(f_T, P) = \inf\{x \geq 0 : \exists \pi \in \mathscr{A}(x) \text{ s.t. } X_T^\pi = f_T, P - \text{a.s.}\}.$$

The perfect hedging price is also obtained as the expectation of the (discounted) claim under the unique EMM, that is

$$\mathbf{C}(f_T) = \mathbb{E}_Q[f_T]. \tag{5}$$

A well-known necessary and sufficient condition for market completeness is the uniqueness of the EMM. In our setting, this is equivalent to the set $\Gamma$ being a singleton. In other words, if (4) has only one solution such that $\gamma_l^J > 0$ for $l \in \{1, \ldots, n - d\}$ and $L_\gamma$ is a martingale, then the market is complete.

Note that (4) can be written as a system of $k$ equations, and $\gamma$ is a vector of length $n$. Thus, when $k < n$, the solution cannot be unique. It is only possible for our market to be complete when $k = n$, that is, when there are as many assets as sources of risk.

In the case where $k = n$, the unique element of $\Gamma$ is given by $\gamma^V(t) = \theta^V(t)$ and $\gamma^J(t) = \lambda^{-1}(t) \cdot (\lambda(t) - \theta^J(t))$, if $\theta^J(t) < \lambda(t)$ for all $t \in [0, T]$. When the bound on $\theta^J(t)$ is not satisfied, the market does not admit any martingale measure. This result is discussed, for example, in [1, 7].

In this paper, our goal is to study no-arbitrage price bounds in incomplete markets. Henceforth, we assume $k < n$, which results in market incompleteness.

As recalled previously, in an incomplete market, some contingent claims are not perfectly replicable. That is, it is impossible to find a self-financing admissible trading strategy whose value at $T$ is equal to $f_T$ $P$-almost surely. Therefore, we extend the set of admissible strategies to consider investment strategies with consumption. Such strategies will be represented by a $(k + 2)$-dimensional $\mathbb{F}$-adapted process $(\pi, c) = (\pi_0(t), \pi_1(t), \ldots, \pi_k(t), c(t))_{t \leq T}$, where $c(t) \geq 0$ for $t \leq T$. The value process of the strategy $(\pi, c)$ is given by

$$X^{\pi,c}(t) = X^{\pi,c}(0) + \sum_{i=1}^{k} \int_0^t \pi_i(s)dS_i(s) - \int_0^t c(s)ds.$$

The strategy $(\pi, c)$ with initial capital $x$ is a (super-)hedge for the contingent claim $f_T$ if its value process satisfies $X^{\pi,c}(T) \geq f_T, P - $ a.s..

An investor selling the contingent claim $f_T$ will require its price to be at least sufficient to build a (super-)hedging portfolio for the claim. Thus, in the $(B, S)$ market, we call the *upper hedging price* (or *seller price*) $\mathbf{C}^*(f_T)$ the smallest initial capital needed by the investor to set up such a portfolio for $f_T$:

$$\mathbf{C}^*(f_T) = \inf\{x \geq 0 : \exists(\pi, c) \in \mathscr{A}(x) : X^{\pi,c}(T) \geq f_T, P - \text{a.s.}\} \qquad (6)$$

An investor buying the contingent claim $f_T$ will not want to pay more than the amount that she will be able to recover by time $T$, by investing in a strategy with consumption. Therefore, the largest amount allowing for such result is called *lower hedging price* (or *buyer price*) $\mathbf{C}_*(f_T)$ is given by:

$$\mathbf{C}_*(f_T) = \inf\{x \geq 0 : \exists(\pi, c) \in \mathscr{A}(-x) : X^{\pi,c}(T) \geq -f_T, P - \text{a.s.}\} \qquad (7)$$

Claims that cannot be perfectly replicated in an incomplete market do not have a unique, perfect hedging price as defined by (5). Indeed, each measure $Q \in \mathscr{Q}$ yields a different arbitrage price $\mathbb{E}_Q[f_T]$. It is well known that the lower and upper hedging prices correspond to the lower and upper bounds of the set of arbitrage prices (for more details on this result, the reader is referred to [5]).

The upper and lower hedging prices for a contingent claim $f_T$ can thus be obtained by taking the infimum and the supremum over the set of EMMs admitted by an incomplete market:

$$\mathbf{C}^*(f_T) = \sup_{Q \in \mathcal{Q}} \mathbb{E}_Q[f_T], \qquad \mathbf{C}_*(f_T) = \inf_{Q \in \mathcal{Q}} \mathbb{E}_Q[f_T].$$

# 3 Pricing Via Market Completions

In this section, we show how the upper and lower hedging prices can be represented in terms of market completions, or additional assets added to complete the original $(B, S)$ market. In particular, in the market defined in Sect. 2.1, we characterize the set of completions that should be considered to obtain the no-arbitrage price bounds.

## 3.1 Market Completions

Let $S^c$ be an $(n - k)$-dimensional process representing the value of $(n - k)$ assets that will be added to the original market. We assume that the new assets have dynamics similar to the first $k$ ones, that is, for $i \in \{k + 1, \ldots, n\}$,

$$dS_i(t) = S_i(t_-) \left( v_i(t)\, dt + \rho_i^V(t)\, dW(t) + \rho_i^J(t)\, dM(t) \right),$$

with $S_i(0) = s_0^i \in \mathbb{R}_+$, and where $W$ and $M$ are defined as in Sect. 2.1. The $(n - k)$-dimensional appreciation rate process $v$ and the matrix-valued processes $\rho^V$ and $\rho^J$, with $i$th row given by $\rho_i^V = (\rho_{i1}^V, \ldots, \rho_{id}^V)$, and $\rho_i^J = (\rho_{i1}^J, \ldots, \rho_{i(n-d)}^J)$, respectively, for $i = 1, \ldots, n - k$, are predictable with respect to the filtration $\mathbb{F}$. As in the original market, we assume that $v$ and $\rho = [\rho^V\ \rho^J]$ are uniformly bounded in $(t, \omega) \in [0, T] \times \Omega$, and that $\rho_{il}^J \in [0, 1]$, for $k + 1 \leq i \leq n$ and $1 \leq l \leq n - d$.

We denote $\tilde{S} = (S, S^c)$, $\tilde{\mu} = (\mu, v)^\top$ and $\tilde{\sigma} = (\binom{\sigma}{\rho})$, and only consider completions $S^c$ such that the augmented market $(B, \tilde{S})$ is complete. That is, for a given market augmented with the completion $S^c$, we assume that $\det \tilde{\sigma} \neq 0$, and we define $\tilde{\theta} = (\tilde{\theta}^V, \tilde{\theta}^J)$ by

$$\tilde{\theta} = \tilde{\sigma}^\top \left( \tilde{\sigma}\tilde{\sigma}^\top \right)^{-1} \tilde{\mu}, \tag{8}$$

and $\tilde{\gamma} = (\tilde{\gamma}^V, \tilde{\gamma}^J)$ by

$$\tilde{\gamma}^V = \tilde{\theta}^V \qquad \tilde{\gamma}^J = \lambda^{-1} \cdot \left( \lambda - \tilde{\theta}^J \right). \tag{9}$$

If $\tilde{\theta}^J(t) < \lambda(t)$ for all $t \in [0, T]$, then $L_{\tilde{\gamma}}$ is a true martingale and the $(B, \tilde{S})$ market is complete.

Then, $Q_{\widetilde{\gamma}}$, defined by $\frac{dQ_{\widetilde{\gamma}}}{dP} = L_{\widetilde{\gamma}}$, is the unique EMM on the completed market $(B, \widetilde{S})$. It immediately follows that a contingent claim $f_T$ has the unique no-arbitrage price $E[L_{\widetilde{\gamma}} f_T]$ in the completed market.

## 3.2  A Special Set of Market Completions

In this section, we want to express the upper and lower hedging prices defined in (6) and (7) in terms of market completions. To do so, we follow ideas similar to those used by [14] in a multivariate diffusion setting.

We let $\mathscr{R}_\rho$ be defined as the set of $(n - k) \times n$ matrix-valued $\mathbb{F}$-adapted process uniformly bounded in $(t, \omega) \in [0, T] \times \Omega$, with $\rho_{il}^j \in [0, 1]$, for $k + 1 \le i \le n$ and $1 \le l \le n - d$, such that $\det\begin{pmatrix} \sigma \\ \rho \end{pmatrix} \neq 0$ $P$-a.s.

For each $\rho \in \mathscr{R}_\rho$, we denote by $\mathscr{D}_\rho$ the set of appreciation rate processes $\nu$ for which the associated market is complete. Therefore, we have

$$\mathscr{D}_\rho := \{\nu : \nu \text{ is } \mathbb{F}\text{-predictable, uniformly bounded, s.t. } \widetilde{\theta}^J(t) < \lambda(t) \; \forall \, t \in [0, T]\}.$$

For a given $\rho \in \mathscr{R}_\rho$, we define the *upper* and *lower completion prices* $\widetilde{\mathbf{C}}^*(f_T; \rho)$ and $\widetilde{\mathbf{C}}_*(f_T; \rho)$ by

$$\widetilde{\mathbf{C}}^*(f_T; \rho) = \sup_{\nu \in \mathscr{D}_\rho} E[L_{\widetilde{\gamma}}(\nu, \rho) f_T], \qquad \widetilde{\mathbf{C}}_*(f_T; \rho) = \inf_{\nu \in \mathscr{D}_\rho} E[L_{\widetilde{\gamma}}(\nu, \rho) f_T].$$

In the above, the density process $L_{\widetilde{\gamma}}(\nu, \rho) = L_{\widetilde{\gamma}}^V(\nu, \rho) L_{\widetilde{\gamma}}^J(\nu, \rho)$ defines the unique EMM on the market completed using assets with appreciation rate vector $\nu$ and diffusion coefficient matrix $\rho$.

As it is the case in the multidimensional diffusion market (see [14]), the upper and lower completion prices do not depend on the choice of $\rho$.

**Proposition 3.1** *Fix* $\rho$ *and* $\rho' \in \mathscr{R}_\rho$. *Then,*

$$\widetilde{\mathbf{C}}^*(f_T; \rho) = \widetilde{\mathbf{C}}^*(f_T; \rho'), \qquad \widetilde{\mathbf{C}}_*(f_T; \rho) = \widetilde{\mathbf{C}}_*(f_T; \rho').$$

*Proof* The proof is very similar to the proof of Proposition 2.1 of [14]. Take the $(n - k) \times k$ and $(n - k) \times (n - k)$ predictable matrix valued processes $C$ and $D$ with $\det(D) \neq 0$ satisfying

$$\begin{pmatrix} \sigma \\ \rho' \end{pmatrix} = \begin{pmatrix} I & 0 \\ C & D \end{pmatrix} \begin{pmatrix} \sigma \\ \rho \end{pmatrix},$$

where $I$ denotes the identity matrix. Then it is possible to show that

$$
\widetilde{\theta}_{v,\rho'} = \begin{pmatrix} \sigma \\ \rho' \end{pmatrix}^{\mathsf{T}} \left( \begin{pmatrix} \sigma \\ \rho' \end{pmatrix} \begin{pmatrix} \sigma \\ \rho' \end{pmatrix}^{\mathsf{T}} \right)^{-1} \begin{pmatrix} \mu \\ v \end{pmatrix} = \widetilde{\theta}_{v',\rho},
$$

with $v' = D^{-1}(v - C\mu) \in \mathscr{D}_\rho$. The result follows. $\qquad\square$

Since the upper and lower completion prices are independent of $\rho$, it is natural to only consider the market completions associated with a particular matrix-valued process $\rho$. Henceforth, we fix $\bar{\rho} \in \mathscr{R}_\rho$ satisfying

$$
\sigma\bar{\rho}^{\mathsf{T}} = 0 \quad \text{and} \quad \bar{\rho}\bar{\rho}^{\mathsf{T}} = I. \tag{10}
$$

It follows that $\widetilde{\theta}_{v,\bar{\rho}} = \theta + \vartheta_v$ with $\vartheta_v = \bar{\rho}^{\mathsf{T}}(\bar{\rho}\bar{\rho}^{\mathsf{T}})^{-1}v$ for any $v \in \mathscr{D}_{\bar{\rho}}$.

The density process $L_{\widetilde{\gamma}}(v, \bar{\rho})$ of the EMM associated with each market completion with parameters $\bar{\rho}$ and $v \in \mathscr{D}_{\bar{\rho}}$ can then be written as

$$
L_{\widetilde{\gamma}}(t; v, \bar{\rho}) = e^{-\int_0^t \gamma^V(s)^{\mathsf{T}} dW(s) - \int_0^t \vartheta_v^V(s)^{\mathsf{T}} dW(s) - \frac{1}{2}\int_0^t \|\theta^V(s) + \vartheta_v^V(s)\|^2 ds}
$$

$$
\times e^{-\int_0^t \theta^J(s)\, ds - \int_0^t \vartheta_v^J(s)\, ds} \prod_{l=1}^{n-d} \prod_{s\leq t} \lambda^{-1}(s) \cdot \left( \lambda(s) - \theta^J(s) - \vartheta_v^J(s) \right) \Delta N_l(s).
$$

In the above, $\theta = (\theta^V, \theta^J)$ is as defined in (2), and is therefore independent of the market completion.

## 3.3 Completion Price Bounds

Finally, we highlight the equivalence between the set of EMMs $\mathscr{Q}$ of the original market and the set of market completions associated with the fixed matrix process $\rho$ satisfying (10).

**Lemma 1** Fix $\rho \in \mathscr{R}_\rho$. Then for any $\gamma \in \Gamma$, it is possible to find $v \in \mathscr{D}_\rho$ such that

$$
\gamma^V = \widetilde{\theta}_{v,\rho}^V, \qquad \gamma^J = \lambda^{-1} \cdot (\lambda - \widetilde{\theta}_{v,\rho}^J).
$$

*Proof* To find such a $v \in \mathscr{D}_\rho$, it suffices to let $\widetilde{\theta}^V = \gamma^V$ and $\widetilde{\theta}^J = \lambda - \lambda \cdot \gamma^J$.

Then, since $\widetilde{\sigma}^{\mathsf{T}}(\widetilde{\sigma}\widetilde{\sigma}^{\mathsf{T}})^{-1}$ is an $n \times n$ matrix, there is only one solution $\widetilde{\mu} = (\mu, v)$ that satisfies

$$
\widetilde{\theta} = \widetilde{\sigma}^{\mathsf{T}}(\widetilde{\sigma}\widetilde{\sigma}^{\mathsf{T}})^{-1}\widetilde{\mu}. \tag{11}
$$

Indeed, this solution is given by $\widetilde{\mu} = \widetilde{\sigma}\widetilde{\theta}$, and $v \in \mathscr{D}_\rho$ by definition.

It follows from Lemma 1 that any measure $Q \in \mathcal{Q}$ can be recovered by completing the market using a market completion $S^c$ with parameters $\bar{\rho}$ and $v$, for some $v \in \mathcal{D}_{\bar{\rho}}$. We can also show that any $v \in \mathcal{D}_{\bar{\rho}}$ defines an element $\gamma \in \Gamma$.

**Lemma 2** *Fix $\rho \in \mathcal{R}_\rho$, with $\rho$ satisfying (10). Then for any $v \in \mathcal{D}_\rho$, the resulting $\tilde{\gamma}$, as defined by (8) and (9) is an element of $\Gamma$.*

*Proof* From (10), we have $\tilde{\theta} = \theta + \vartheta$, and the resulting $\tilde{\gamma}$ solves (4), since $\sigma\theta^\top = \mu$ and $\sigma\vartheta^\top = 0$.

Therefore, the unique EMM resulting from any market completion $S^c$ with parameters $\bar{\rho}$ and $v$, with $v \in \mathcal{D}_{\bar{\rho}}$ is an element of $\mathcal{Q}$.

Lemmas 1 and 2 confirm that the set of market completions with diffusion coefficient matrix $\rho$ fixed spans the set of EMMs $\mathcal{Q}$ on the complete market. It is therefore possible to express the range of no-arbitrage prices for a contingent claim $f_T$ in terms of the set of market completions.

**Proposition 3.2** *The upper and lower hedging prices $\mathbf{C}^*(f_T)$ and $\mathbf{C}_*(f_T)$ coincide with the upper and lower completion prices $\tilde{\mathbf{C}}^*(f_T)$ and $\tilde{\mathbf{C}}_*(f_T)$, and we have*

$$\mathbf{C}^*(f_T) = \sup_{v \in \mathcal{D}_\rho} E[L_{\tilde{\gamma}}(T; v, \rho) f_T], \qquad \mathbf{C}_*(f_T) = \inf_{v \in \mathcal{D}_\rho} E[L_{\tilde{\gamma}}(T; v, \rho) f_T].$$

## 4   Concluding Remarks

In a pure diffusion market, the process $L_{\tilde{\gamma}}(v, \rho)$ can be expressed as the product of two (local) martingales; one pertaining to the original market, and the other one associated with the market completion. This makes market completion techniques very useful in the context of hedging and portfolio optimization problems. The addition of jumps in the market generally removes the possibility of such an expression, as is remarked at the end of Sect. 1 of [13].

**Acknowledgements** Both authors aknowledge funding from IFSID grant number R2091 and from the Natural Sciences and Engineering Research Council of Canada.

## References

1. Bardhan, I., Chao, X.: Martingale analysis for assets with discontinuous returns. Math. Oper. Res. **20**(1), 243–256 (1995)
2. Bardhan, I., Chao, X.: On martingale measures when asset returns have unpredictable jumps. Stochast. Process. Appl. **63**(1), 35–54 (1996)
3. Bergman, Y.Z.: Option pricing with differential interest rates. Rev. Fin. Stud. **8**(2), 475–500 (1995)
4. Corcuera, J.M., Nualart, D., Schoutens, W.: Completion of a Lévy market by power-jump assets. Finance Stochast. **9**(1), 109–127 (2005)

5. El Karoui, N., Quenez, M.C.: Dynamic programming and pricing of contingent claims in an incomplete market. SIAM J. Control Optim. **33**(1), 29–66 (1995)
6. Hu, Y., Imkeller, P., Müller, M.: Partial equilibrium and market completion. Int. J. Theor. Appl. Finance **8**(04), 483–508 (2005)
7. Jeanblanc-Picque, M., Pontier, M.: Optimal portfolio for a small investor in a market model with discontinuous prices. Appl. Math. Optim. **22**(1), 287–310 (1990)
8. Kane, S., Melnikov, A.: On pricing contingent claims in a two interest rates jump-diffusion model via market completions. Theory Probab. Math. Stat. **77**, 57–69 (2008)
9. Karatzas, I., Lehoczky, J.P., Shreve, S.E., Xu, G.L.: Martingale and duality methods for utility maximization in an incomplete market. SIAM J. Control Optim. **29**(3), 702–730 (1991)
10. Korn, R.: Contingent claim valuation in a market with different interest rates. Zeitschrift für Oper. Res. **42**(3), 255–274 (1995)
11. Melnikov, A.: Financial Markets: Stochastic Analysis and the Pricing of Derivative Securities. Translations of Mathematical Monographs. American Mathematical Society, Boston (1999)
12. Runggaldier, W.J.: Jump-diffusion models. Handbook of Heavy Tailed Distributions in Finance **1**, 169–209 (2003)
13. Schweizer, M.: A minimality property of the minimal martingale measure. Stat. Probab. Lett. **42**(1), 27–31 (1999)
14. Wang, G.: Pricing and hedging of American contingent claims in incomplete markets. Acta Mathematicae Applicatae Sinica **15**(2), 144–152 (1999)

# Part VIII
# Theory and Applications
# of Dynamical Systems

# Error Expansion for a Symplectic Scheme for Stochastic Hamiltonian Systems

Cristina Anton

**Abstract** We consider a stochastic autonomous Hamiltonian system for which the flow preserves the symplectic structure. Numerical simulations show that for stochastic Hamiltonian systems symplectic schemes produce more accurate results for long term simulations than non-sysmplectic numerical schemes. We study the approximation error corresponding to a symplectic weak scheme of order one. A backward error analysis is done at the level of the Kolmogorov equation associated with the initial stochastic Hamiltonian system. We obtain an expansion of the error in terms of powers of the discretization step size and the solutions of the modified Kolmogorov equation.

**Keywords** Backward error analysis · Stochastic Hamiltonian systems Kolmogorov equation · Weak symplectic scheme

## 1 Introduction

Numerical simulations [5, 9, 11] show that for stochastic Hamiltonian systems (SHS) symplectic schemes give more accurate results for long term simulation that non-symplectic schemes, but, to the best of our knowledge, no theoretical proof was done in the stochastic case. For a SHS and a first weak order symplectic scheme, in [2] we present an expansion of the global approximation error in powers of the discretization step size. Comparing this expansion with the global error expansion obtained in [13] for the Euler scheme (which has also weak order one), we justify the superior performance of the symplectic scheme for the simple linear SHS corresponding to the Kobo oscillator [2]. However, this justification can not be easily extended for general non-linear SHSs. Here we use backward error analysis to find an expansion of error for the symplectic scheme in terms of the powers of the discretization step size and the solutions of the modified Kolmogorov equation [3].

C. Anton (✉)
MacEwan University, 5-103C, 10700 - 104 Avenue Edmonton,
Edmonton, AB T5J 4S2, Canada
e-mail: popescuc@macewan.ca

© Springer Nature Switzerland AG 2018
D. M. Kilgour et al. (eds.), *Recent Advances in Mathematical and Statistical Methods*, Springer Proceedings in Mathematics & Statistics 259,
https://doi.org/10.1007/978-3-319-99719-3_51

Backward error analysis was successfully applied to study long term behavior of deterministic Hamiltonian systems [4]. Recently, backward error analysis was extended to stochastic differential equations (SDE). Modified SDEs associated with various numerical schemes are presented in [1, 10, 14]. A SDE defined on the $n$-dimensional torus and its approximation by the explicit Euler scheme are studied using backward error analysis in [3].

We follow the same approach as in [3], and we construct the modified equation not at the level of the SDE, but at the level of the associated Kolmogorov equation. Compared with [3] we consider a fully implicit scheme instead of an explicit one, and we consider a SHS with additive or multiplicative noise defined on $R^{2n}$ instead of the compact $n$ dimensional torus. Implicit numerical schemes are also considered in [6, 7], but for Langevin SDEs on $R^n$ with additive noise. Studying the multiplicative noise case is more difficult, especially for a fully implicit numerical scheme.

In the next section we present some preliminary results regarding the solution of the SHS and the approximate solution given by the numerical scheme. The steps followed for the backward error analysis are included in Sect. 3. The last section contains the conclusions.

## 2   Assumptions and Preliminary Results

We introduce a few definitions and notations. We denote $N = \{1, 2, \ldots\}$, $N^* = \{1, 2, \ldots\}$ and for any $x = (x_1, \ldots, x_n)^T \in R^n$, $|x|$ represents the Euclidean norm.

For any multi-index $\alpha = (\alpha_1, \ldots, \alpha_r) \in N^r$ with length $|\alpha| = \alpha_1 + \cdots + \alpha_r$, let $\partial_\alpha = \frac{\partial^{|\alpha|}}{\partial_1^{\alpha_1} \cdots \partial_r^{\alpha_r}}$ denote the partial derivative of order $|\alpha|$.

We define the following space of functions with polynomial growth:

$$C_{pol}^\infty(R^{2n}) = \left\{ f \in C^\infty(R^{2n}) \text{ such that } f \text{ and all its derivatives have polynomial growth} \right\}$$

For any $k, l \in N$, we denote

$$C_k^l(R^{2n}) = \left\{ f \in C^l(R^{2n}) : \text{ there exists } C_{l,k} > 0 \text{ such that for all } x \in R^{2n} \text{ and any index} \right.$$

$$\left. \alpha \in N^{2n}, |\alpha| \le l, |\partial_\alpha f(x)| \le C_{l,k}(1 + |x|^{2k}) \right\}.$$

On $C_k^l(R^{2n})$ we define [7] the norm $\| \cdot \|_{l,k}$ and the semi norm $| \cdot |_{l,k}$:

$$\|f\|_{l,k} = \sup_{\alpha, |\alpha| \le l} \frac{|\partial_\alpha f(x)|}{1 + |x|^{2k}}, \quad |f|_{l,k} = \sup_{\alpha, 1 \le |\alpha| \le l} \frac{|\partial_\alpha f(x)|}{1 + |x|^{2k}}. \tag{1}$$

Notice that if $\phi \in C_{pol}^\infty(R^{2n})$, then for all $d \in N$, there exists $r_d \in N$ such that $\phi \in C_{r_d}^d(R^{2n})$.

We consider the following stochastic Hamiltonian system

$$dP = -\partial_Q H_0(P, Q)dt - \sum_{r=1}^{m} \partial_Q H_r(P, Q) \circ dw_t^r, \quad P(0) = p$$

$$dQ = \partial_P H_0(P, Q)dt + \sum_{r=1}^{m} \partial_P H_r(P, Q) \circ dw_t^r, \quad Q(0) = q, \tag{2}$$

where $P, Q, p, q$ are $n$-dimensional column vectors, $w_t^r, r = 1, \ldots, m$ are independent standard Wiener processes, and for any function $f$ defined on $R^n \times R^n$, $\partial_P f$ and $\partial_Q f$ denote the column vectors with components $(\partial f/\partial P_i), 1 \le i \le n$ and $(\partial f/\partial Q_i), 1 \le i \le n$, respectively. The stochastic flow $(p, q) \longrightarrow (P, Q)$ of the SHS (2) preserves the symplectic structure [9]: $dP \wedge dQ = dp \wedge dq$, where the differential 2-form $dp \wedge dq = dp_1 \wedge dq_1 + \cdots + dp_n \wedge dq_n$.

The system (2) can be re-written in the Ito formulation:

$$dP = a(P, Q)dt + \sum_{r=1}^{m} \sigma^r(P, Q)dw_t^r, \quad P(0) = p \tag{3}$$

$$dQ = b(P, Q)dt + \sum_{r=1}^{m} \gamma^r(P, Q)dw_t^r, \quad Q(0) = q, \tag{4}$$

where

$$a = -\partial_Q H_0 + \frac{1}{2} \sum_{r=1}^{m} \sum_{j=1}^{n} \left( \frac{\partial H_r}{\partial Q_j} \partial_Q \left( \frac{\partial H_r}{\partial P_j} \right) - \frac{\partial H_r}{\partial P_j} \partial_Q \left( \frac{\partial H_r}{\partial Q_j} \right) \right)$$

$$b = \partial_P H_0 + \frac{1}{2} \sum_{r=1}^{m} \sum_{j=1}^{n} \left( -\frac{\partial H_r}{\partial Q_j} \partial_P \left( \frac{\partial H_r}{\partial P_j} \right) + \frac{\partial H_r}{\partial P_j} \partial_P \left( \frac{\partial H_r}{\partial Q_j} \right) \right)$$

$$\sigma^r = -\partial_Q H_r, \quad \gamma^r = \partial_P H_r.$$

Here everywhere the arguments are $(P, Q)$, and $a, b, \sigma^r, \gamma^r, r = 1, \ldots, m$ are $n$-dimensional column vectors.

The Kolmogorov generator $L(p, q, \partial_p, \partial_q)$ associated with the SHS (3)–(4) has the following form [12]

$$L(p, q, \partial_p, \partial_q)\phi(p, q) = \sum_{j=1}^{n} \left( a_j \frac{\partial}{\partial p_j} \phi(p, q) + b_j \frac{\partial}{\partial q_j} \phi(p, q) \right) + \frac{1}{2} \sum_{r=1}^{m} \sum_{i,j=1}^{n} \left( \sigma_i^r \sigma_j^r \right.$$

$$\frac{\partial^2}{\partial p_i p_j} \phi(p, q) + \gamma_i^r \gamma_j^r \frac{\partial^2}{\partial q_i q_j} \phi(p, q) + 2\sigma_i^r \gamma_j^r \frac{\partial^2}{\partial p_i q_j} \phi(p, q) \right), \phi \in C^\infty(R^{2n})$$

Throughout the paper we make the same assumptions as in [12, 13]:

A1. The derivatives of any order of $H_i \in C^\infty$, $i = 1, \ldots, m$ are bounded, and the derivative of any order $k \geq 2$ of $H_0 \in C^\infty$ are bounded.

A2. The operator $L$ is uniformly elliptic: there exists a constant $\alpha > 0$ such that for all $x = (p, q)^T \in R^{2n}$ we have

$$
\alpha |x|^2 \leq \sum_{r=1}^{m} \sum_{i,j=1}^{n} \left( \sigma_i^r \sigma_j^r p_i p_j + \gamma_i^r \gamma_j^r q_i q_j + 2\sigma_i^r \gamma_j^r p_i q_j \right) \tag{5}
$$

A3. There exists a constant $\beta > 0$ and a compact set $K$ such that for all $x = (p, q)^T \in R^{2n} - K$ we have $p \cdot a(x) + q \cdot b(x) \leq -\beta |x|^2$.

Notice that assumption A1 implies that we have a Lipschitz condition, i.e. there exists $L_1 > 0$ such that for all $X = (P, Q)^T$, $x = (p, q)^T \in R^{2n}$ we have

$$
\sum_{j=0}^{m} \left| \left( \partial_P H_j, \partial_Q H_j \right)^T (X) - \left( \partial_p H_j, \partial_q H_j \right)^T (x) \right| \leq L_1 |X - x|. \tag{6}
$$

## 2.1 Results Regarding the Solution of the Stochastic Hamiltonian System

Proceeding as in Proposition 3.1 in [12], under the assumptions A1-A3 we can prove the following result regarding the solution $\left( X^{0,x_0}(t) \right) = \left( (P(t, p_0, q_0), Q(t, p_0, q_0))^T \right)$ of the SHS (2) with the initial condition $x_0 = (p_0, q_0)^T \in R^{2n}$.

**Lemma 1** *The Markov process $\left( X^{0,x_0}(t) \right)$ is ergodic. The unique invariant probability measure $\mu$ has finite moments of any order and a density $\rho \geq 0$. Moreover, for any $k \in N$ there exist $C_k, \gamma_k > 0$ such that for any $x_0 = (p_0, q_0)^T \in R^{2n}$, and any $t \geq 0$ we have:*

$$
E(|X^{0,x_0}(t)|^k) \leq C_k \left( 1 + |x_0|^k \exp(-\gamma_k t) \right). \tag{7}
$$

We consider any function $\phi \in C_{pol}^\infty(R^{2n})$, and for all $x = (p, q)^T \in R^{2n}$ and all $t > 0$ we define $u(t, p, q) := E[\phi(X^{0,x}(t))]$. Notice that Lemma 1 implies that $u$ is well defined. It is well known [12] that $u(t, p, q)$ is a classical solution of the Kolmogorov equation

$$
\frac{du}{dt}(t, p, q) = Lu(t, p, q), \quad u(0, p, q) = \phi(p, q), (p, q)^T \in R^{2n}, t > 0. \tag{8}
$$

For any function $f \in C_{pol}^\infty(R^{2n})$ we denote the average

$$
< f > := \int f(x) d\mu(x)
$$

The results included in the following lemma show the exponential convergence of $u$ and its derivatives and are essential for the backward error analysis presented in this paper. The proof is an extension of the proof of Theorem 3.4 in [12], based on Theorem 2.5 in [8].

**Lemma 2** *Let $k \in \mathbf{N}$, $k \geq 1$, and $\phi \in C_{pol}^{\infty}(\mathbf{R}^{2n}) \cap C_{r_{k+n+1}}^{k+n+1}(\mathbf{R}^{2n})$, $r_{k+n+1} \in \mathbf{N}$. Then there exist $\gamma_k > 0$, $C_k > 0$ and $l_k \in \mathbf{N}$ such that $l_k > r_{k+n+1}$ and for any $0 < \gamma < \gamma_k$ and all $t \geq 0$ we have*

$$|u(t,x)|_{k,l_k} \leq C_k \|\phi - <\phi>\|_{k+n+1,r_{k+n+1}} \exp(-\gamma t). \tag{9}$$

$$\|u(t,x) - <\phi>\|_{0,l_0} \leq C_0 \|\phi - <\phi>\|_{n+1,r_{n+1}} \exp(-\gamma t). \tag{10}$$

## 2.2  Results Regarding the Symplectic Scheme

We consider the following one-step approximation [9] for the system (2):

$$P_{k+1} = P_k - h\left(\partial_Q H_0 + \frac{1}{2}\sum_{r=1}^{m}\partial_Q G_{(r,r)}\right) - \sqrt{h}\sum_{r=1}^{m}\varsigma_{rk}\partial_Q H_r, \quad P_0 = p_0 \tag{11}$$

$$Q_{k+1} = Q_k + h\left(\partial_P H_0 + \frac{1}{2}\sum_{r=1}^{m}\partial_P G_{(r,r)}\right) + \sqrt{h}\sum_{r=1}^{m}\varsigma_{rk}\partial_P H_r \quad Q_0 = q_0 \tag{12}$$

where $G_{(r,r)} = \sum_{i=1}^{n}\frac{\partial H_r}{\partial Q_i}\frac{\partial H_r}{\partial P_i}$, the random variables $\varsigma_{rk}$ are mutually independent identically distributed according to the law, $P(\varsigma_{rk} = \pm 1) = 1/2$, and everywhere the arguments are $(P_{k+1}, Q_k)$.

Notice that the first equation (11) is implicit. Let denote $\delta := \sqrt{h}$ and $F(p,q) = \left(H_0(p,q) + \frac{1}{2}\sum_{r=1}^{m}G_{(r,r)}(p,q)\right)$. Then we can reformulate the scheme (11)–(12) as follows:

$$P_{k+1} = P_k - \delta^2\partial_Q F(P_{k+1}, Q_k) - \delta\sum_{r=1}^{m}\varsigma_{rk}\partial_Q H_r(P_{k+1}, Q_k) \tag{13}$$

$$Q_{k+1} = Q_k + \delta^2\partial_P F(P_{k+1}, Q_k) + \delta\sum_{r=1}^{m}\varsigma_{rk}\partial_P H_r(P_{k+1}, Q_k) \tag{14}$$

Using the Lipschitz condition (6) and proceeding as in the proof of Theorem 4.6.1 in [9] we can show that the scheme (13)–(14) is well defined:

**Lemma 3** *There exist $h_{01} > 0$, $C > 0$ such that for any $0 < h \leq h_{01}$ and any $(p,q)^t \in \mathbf{R}^{2n}$ there exists a unique $z \in \mathbf{R}^n$ such that $z = p - h\partial_q F(z,q) - \sqrt{h}\sum_{r=1}^{m}\varsigma_{rk}\partial_q H_r(z,q)$ which satisfies $|z - p| \leq C(1 + |p|)\sqrt{h}$.*

Moreover, Theorem 4.6.1 in [9] shows that implicit method (13)–(14) is symplectic and of first weak order: for any $T > 0$, and any $\phi \in C_{pol}^{\infty}(\mathbf{R}^{2n})$ we have

$$|E(\phi(P_k, Q_k)) - E(\phi(X^{0,x_0}(kh)))| \le c(\phi, T)h, k = 0, \ldots, \lfloor T/h \rfloor, c(\phi, T) > 0.$$
(15)

We define the function $\phi_\delta$ which associate to $(q, p) \in \mathbb{R}^{2n}$ the solution $z = (z_1, z_2)^T \in \mathbb{R}^{2n}$ of $f(\delta, q, p, z_1, z_2) = 0$, where

$$f(\delta, q, p, z) = \begin{bmatrix} z_1 - p + \delta^2 \partial_q F(z_1, q) + \delta \sum_{r=1}^m \varsigma_r \partial_q H_r(z_1, q) \\ z_2 - q - \delta^2 \partial_p F(z_1, q) - \delta \sum_{r=1}^m \varsigma_r \partial_p H_r(z_1, q) \end{bmatrix}$$
(16)

where the random variables $\varsigma_r$ are mutually independent identically distributed according to the law, $P(\varsigma_r = \pm 1) = 1/2$, Since the scheme (13)–(14) is well defined, the function $\phi_\delta$ is also well defined for any $\delta \in (0, \sqrt{h_{01}})$. Using A1 it is easy to show that there exists $h_{03} \le h_{01}$ such that $\partial_z f(\delta, q, p, z) = I - B(\delta, p, q, z)$ where $\|B(\delta, p, q, z)\| < 1$ for any $(\delta, p, q, z) \in (0, \sqrt{h_{03}}) \times \mathbb{R}^{2n} \times \mathbb{R}^{2n}$. Thus, $\partial_z f(\delta, q, p, z)$ is invertible, and from the Implicit Functions Theorem we obtain that the function defined by $(\delta, p, q) \to \phi_\delta(p, q)$ is $C^\infty$ on a neighborhood of each point of $(0, \sqrt{h_{03}}) \times \mathbb{R}^{2n}$.

Following the same approach as in the proof of Proposition 7.1 in [12] we can show that the moments of the approximating process $(P_k, Q_k)$ satisfy a similar property with (7):

**Lemma 4** *There exist* $0 < h_{02} \le h_{01}$ *such that the symplectic scheme* (11)–(12) *with any initial condition* $(p, q)^t \in \mathbb{R}^{2n}$ *and any* $0 < h \le h_{02}$ *satisfies for any* $l \in \mathbb{N}^*$

$$E_{p,q}(|P_k|^{2l} + |Q_k|^{2l}) \le C_l \left(1 + (|p|^{2l} + |q|^{2l}) \exp(-\alpha_l kh)\right), \quad C_l > 0, \alpha_l > 0.$$
(17)

## 3 Asymptotic Expansion of the Weak Error

Using a Taylor expansion and the fact that $u$ is a solution of the Kolmogorov equation (8) we obtain the following expansion.

**Proposition 1** *Let consider any* $N \in \mathbb{N}$ *and any* $\phi \in C^\infty_{pol}(\mathbb{R}^{2n}) \cap C^{2N+n+3}_{r_{2N+n+3}}(\mathbb{R}^{2n})$, $r_{2N+n+3} \in \mathbb{N}$. *There exist* $c(N) > 0$ *and* $l_N \in \mathbb{N}$, $l_N > r_{2N+n+3}$ *such that for all* $h > 0$ *and* $(p, q)^T \in \mathbb{R}^{2n}$ *we have*

$$|u(h, p, q) - \sum_{k=0}^N \frac{h^k}{k!} L^k \phi(p, q)| \le c(N) h^{N+1} \|\phi- <\phi> \|_{2N+3+n, r_{2N+3+n}}$$
$$(1 + |p|^{2l_N} + |q|^{2l_N})$$
(18)

Let $h_0 = \min\{h_{02}, h_{03}\}$. We study the first step of the approximating process $(P_k, Q_k)$, and later we will use the Markov property to extend the results at all steps. The following result gives an expansion for the symplectic scheme, similar with the expansion (18).

**Proposition 2** *For any $k \in \mathbb{N}$ there exists an operator $A_k$ of order $2k$ with coefficients in $C^\infty_{pol}(\mathbb{R}^{2n})$ such that for any $N \in \mathbb{N}$ and any $\phi \in C^\infty_{pol}(\mathbb{R}^{2n}) \cap C^{2N+2}_{r_{2N+2}}(\mathbb{R}^{2n})$, $r_{2N+2} \in$
$\mathbb{N}$, there exist $C_N > 0$ and $l_N \in \mathbb{N}$ such that for all $0 < h \le h_0$ and $(p, q)^T \in \mathbb{R}^{2n}$ we
have $A_0 = I$, $A_1 = L$, and*

$$|E(\phi(Q_1, P_1)) - \sum_{k=0}^{N} h^k A_k(p, q)\phi(p, q)| \le C_N h^{N+1}(1 + |p|^{2l_N} + |q|^{2l_N})|\phi|_{2N+2, r_{2N+2}}$$

*Proof* Firstly we use Taylor expansions to obtain expansions for $P_1$ and $Q_1$ (see also
the proof of Lemma 3.4 in [6]). Then the proof can be done using the same approach
as in the proof of Proposition 3.2 in [6]. □

## 3.1 The Modified Generator

Following the same approach as in [3], we want to construct a formal series $\mathscr{L} =$
$L + hL_1 + \cdots + h^k L_k + \cdots$ such that formally the solution $v(h, p, q)$ of the equation

$$\partial_t v(t, p, q) = \mathscr{L}v(t, p, q), t > 0, \quad v(0, p, q) = \phi(p, q), (p, q)^T \in \mathbb{R}^{2n},$$

coincides in the sense of asymptotic expansion with the transition semigroup $E(\phi(P_1, Q_1))$ studied in Proposition 2. In order to have

$$\exp(h\mathscr{L})\phi = \phi + \sum_{k \ge 1} h^k A_k \phi$$

we define the $L_k$ operator as

$$L_k = A_{k+1} + \sum_{l=1}^{k} \frac{B_l}{l!} \sum_{k_1 + \cdots + k_{l+1} = k-l} L_{k_1} \ldots L_{k_l} A_{k_{l+1}+1} \tag{19}$$

$B_l$ are the Bernoulli numbers and $L_k$ is an operator of order $2k + 2$ with coefficients
in $C^\infty_{pol}(\mathbb{R}^{2n})$ and $L_k 1 = 0$. We also have

$$A_k = \sum_{l=1}^{k} \frac{1}{l!} \sum_{k_1 + \cdots + k_l = k-l} L_{k_1} \ldots L_{k_l}. \tag{20}$$

We define the modified generator

$$L^{(N)} = L + \sum_{k=1}^{N} h^k L_k, \quad N \in \mathbb{N}^*. \tag{21}$$

Since we do not know if the modified equation

$$\partial_t v^{(N)}(t, p, q) = L^{(N)} v^{(N)}(t, p, q), t > 0, \quad v^{(N)}(0, p, q) = \phi(p, q), (p, q)^T \in \mathbb{R}^{2n},$$

has a solution, we construct an approximate solution associated to (21).

**Proposition 3** *Let $\phi \in C_{pol}^{\infty}(\mathbb{R}^{2n})$. For all $k \in \mathbb{N}$ there exist functions $v_k(t, \cdot) \in C_{pol}^{\infty}(\mathbb{R}^{2n})$ defined for all $t \geq 0$ such that $v_0(0, \cdot) = \phi(\cdot)$, $v_k(0, \cdot) = 0$, $k \geq 1$, and*

$$\partial_t v_k(t, p, q) - L v_k(t, p, q) = \sum_{l=1}^{k} L_l v_{k-l}(t, p, q), \quad t \geq 0. \tag{22}$$

*Moreover, for all $k \in \mathbb{N}$, $j \in \mathbb{N}^*$ there exist $\gamma_{k,j} > 0$ and positive integers $\alpha_{k,j}$ and $l_{k,0}$ such that for all $t \geq 0$ we have*

$$|v_k(t)|_{j,\alpha_{k,j}} \leq Q_{k,j}(t) e^{-\gamma_{k,j} t} \|\phi - <\phi>\|_{j+(n+1)(k+1)+4k, r_{j+(n+1)(k+1)+4k}}, \tag{23}$$

$$\|v_k(t)\|_{0, l_{k,0}} \leq C_{0,k} \|\phi - <\phi>\|_{(n+1)(k+1)+4k, r_{(n+1)(k+1)+4k}}, \tag{24}$$

*Here $Q_{k,j} : [0, \infty) \to [0, \infty)$ are polynomial functions with positive coefficients and the constants $C_{0,k}$ do not depend on t.*

*Proof* The proof is similar with the proof of Theorem 4.1 in [6]. Inequalities (23)–(24) are a consequence of the results presented in Lemma 2.

For any $N \geq 0$, we define the approximate solution of the modified flow as:

$$v^{(N)}(t, p, q) = \sum_{k=0}^{N} h^k v_k(t, p, q). \tag{25}$$

We can easily show that for all $t \geq 0$ we have

$$\partial_t v^{(N)}(t, p, q) = L^{(N)} v^{(N)}(t, p, q) - R^{(N)}(t, p, q), \quad v^{(N)}(0, p, q) = \phi(p, q), \tag{26}$$

where

$$R^{(N)}(t, p, q) = \sum_{i=N+1}^{2N} h^i \sum_{k=i-N}^{N} L_k v_{i-k} \tag{27}$$

is of order $O(h^{N+1})$. The following result can be proved similarly with Theorem 4.1 in [3].

**Proposition 4** *Let* $\phi \in C_{pol}^{\infty}(\mathbf{R}^{2n})$. *For any* $N \in \mathbf{N}^*$ *there exist* $C_N > 0$ *and* $l_N$, $k_{2N+2} \in \mathbf{N}$ *such that for all* $t \geq 0$, $0 < h \leq h_0$, $(p, q) \in \mathbf{R}^{2n}$ *we have*

$$\left| E(v^{(N)}(t, P_1, Q_1) - v^{(N)}(t + h, p, q)) \right|$$

$$\leq h^{N+1} C_N (1 + |p|^{2l_N} + |q|^{2l_N}) \sup_{\substack{s \in [0,h] \\ k=0,\dots,N}} |v_k(t + s, \cdot)|_{2N+2, k_{2N+2}}. \tag{28}$$

## 3.2 Main Result

We now study the long time behavior of the numerical solution. We obtain an expansion similar with the one for the exact solution, given in Proposition 1.

**Theorem 1** *Let* $N \in \mathbf{N}$ *be fixed, and let* $(P_k, Q_k)$ *be the discrete process defined by the symplectic scheme. Let* $0 < h \leq h_0$, $\alpha_N = 6N + 8 + (n + 1)(N + 2)$ *and* $\phi \in C_{pol}^{\infty}(\mathbf{R}^{2n}) \cap C_{r_{\alpha_N}}^{\alpha_N}$. *Then there exist* $C_N > 0$ *and* $l_N \in \mathbf{N}$ *such that for all* $k \in \mathbf{N}$

$$|E(\phi(P_k, Q_k)) - v^{(N)}(kh, p, q)| \leq h^{N+1} C_N (1 + |p|^{2l_N} + |q|^{2l_N}) \| \phi - <\phi> \|_{\alpha_N, r_{\alpha_N}}.$$

*Proof* Let $t_k = kh$. By the Markov property of $(P_k, Q_k)$ we have

$$|E(\phi(P_k, Q_k)) - v^{(N+1)}(t_k, p, q)| = |E(v^{(N+1)}(0, P_k, Q_k)) - v^{(N+1)}(t_k, p, q)| =$$

$$\left| E \left( \sum_{j=0}^{k-1} E \left( v^{(N+1)}(t_j, P_{k-j}, Q_{k-j}) - v^{(N+1)}(t_{j+1}, P_{k-j-1}, Q_{k-j-1}) \Big| P_{k-j-1}, Q_{k-j-1} \right) \right) \right|$$

$$\leq \sum_{j=0}^{k-1} \left| E \left( E \left( v^{(N+1)}(t_j, P_1(P_{k-j-1}, Q_{k-j-1}), Q_1(P_{k-j-1}, Q_{k-j-1})) - v^{(N+1)}(t_{j+1}, \right. \right. \right.$$

$$\left. \left. \left. P_{k-j-1}, Q_{k-j-1}) \Big| P_{k-j-1}, Q_{k-j-1} \right) \right) \right|,$$

where $(P_1(p, q), Q_1(p, q))$ is the first step of the scheme (11)–(12) when the initial condition is $(p, q)$. Using inequalities (17), (23), and (28), with $t = t_j$, $j = 0, \dots, k - 1$, we deduce that there exist positive integers $l_N$, $k_N$ such that

$$\|E(v^{(N+1)}(0, P_k, Q_k)) - v^{(N+1)}(t_k, p, q)\|_{0, l_N} \leq h^{N+2} c \sum_{j=0}^{k-1} \sup_{\substack{s \in [0,h] \\ i=0,\dots,N+1}} |v_i(t_j + s, \cdot)|_{2N+4, k_N}$$

$$\leq h^{N+2} c \|\phi - <\phi> \|_{\alpha_N, r_{\alpha_N}} \sum_{j=0}^{k-1} Q_{2N+4}(t_j) e^{-\lambda_{2N+4} t_j}$$

$$\leq h^{N+2} c \|\phi - <\phi> \|_{\alpha_N, r_{\alpha_N}} \sum_{j=0}^{k-1} e^{-\tilde{\lambda}_{2N+4} t_j},$$

where $c > 0$, $0 < \tilde{\lambda}_{2N+4} < \lambda_{2N+4}$ and $Q_{2N+4}$ is a polynomial function with positive coefficients. Notice that for a fixed constant $\lambda > 0$ we have

$$\sum_{j=0}^{k-1} e^{-\lambda t_j} \leq \frac{1}{1 - e^{-\lambda h}} \leq \frac{c_1}{h},$$

where the constant $c_1$ depends on $\lambda$ and $h_0$. Hence, using the previous inequality and (24) we get

$$\|E(\phi(P_k, Q_k) - v^{(N)}(t_k, p, q)\|_{0,l_N} = \|E(v^{(N+1)}(0, P_k, Q_k) - v^{(N+1)}(t_k, p, q)$$
$$+ h^{N+1} v_{N+1}(t_k, p, q)\|_{0,l_N} \leq h^{N+1} c_2 \|\phi - < \phi >\|_{\alpha_N, r_{\alpha_N}} + h^{N+1} \|v_{N+1}(t_k, p, q)\|_{0,l_N}$$
$$\leq h^{N+1} c_2 \|\phi - < \phi >\|_{\alpha_N, r_{\alpha_N}} + h^{N+1} C_{0,N+1} \|\phi - < \phi >\|_{(n+1)(N+2)+4(N+1), r_{\alpha_N}}$$
$$\leq h^{N+1} C_N \|\phi - < \phi >\|_{\alpha_N, r_{\alpha_N}}$$

## 4 Conclusions and Future Work

We have presented a weak backward error analysis for a SHS system and a symplectic scheme of first weak order. The main tools are the exponential convergence to equilibrium of the solution of the Kolmogorov equation, and the uniform ellipticity of the associated operator. We plan to do a backward error analysis under less restrictive assumptions. The main difficulty is that the symplectic schemes are fully implicit, and for SDEs with multiplicative noise and unbounded coefficients, methods from Malliavin calculus are needed.

**Acknowledgements** This work is supported by the NSERC grant DDG-2015-00041.

## References

1. Abdulle, A., Cohen, D., Vilmart, G., Zygalakis, K.: High weak order methods for stochastic differential equations based on modified equations. SIAM J. Sci. Comput. **34**(3), 1800–1823 (2012)
2. Anton, C., Wong, Y., Deng, J.: On global error of symplectic schemes for stochastic Hamiltonian systems. Int. J. Numer. Anal. Model. Ser. B **4**(1), 80–93 (2013)
3. Debussche, A., Faou, E.: Weak backward error analysis for SDEs. SIAM J. Numer. Anal. **50**(3), 1735–1752 (2012)
4. Hairer, E., Lubich, C., Wanner, G.: Geometric Numerical Integration: Structure-Preserving Algorithms for Ordinary Differential Equations. Springer, Berlin (2006)
5. Hong, J., Sun, L., Wang, X.: High order conformal symplectic and ergodic schemes for the stochastic Langevin equation via generating functions. SIAM J. Numer. Anal. **55**(6), 3006–3029 (2017)
6. Kopec, M.: Weak backward error analysis for Langevin process. BIT Numer. Math. **55**(4), 1057–1103 (2015)

7.  Kopec, M.: Weak backward error analysis for overdamped Langevin processes. IMA J Numer. Anal. **35**(2), 583–614 (2015)
8.  Mattingly, J., Stuart, A., Higham, D.J.: Ergodicity for SDEs and approximations: locally Lipschitz vector fields and degenerate noise. Stochast. Process. Appl. **2**(101), 185–232 (2002)
9.  Milstein, G.N., Tretyakov, M.V.: Stochastic Numerics for Mathematical Physics. Springer, Berlin (2004)
10. Shardlow, T.: Modified equations for stochastic differential equations. BIT Numer. Math. **46**(1), 111–125 (2006)
11. Sun, L., Wang, L.: Stochastic symplectic methods based on the Pade approximations for linear stochastic Hamiltonian systems. J. Comp. Appl. Math. **311**, 439–456 (2017)
12. Talay, D.: Second order discretization schemes of stochastic differential systems for the computation of the invariant law. Stochast. Stochast. Rep. **29**(1), 13–36 (1990)
13. Talay, D., Tubaro, L.: Expansion of the global error for numerical schemes solving stochastic differential equations. Stochast. Anal. Appl. **8**(4), 483–509 (1990)
14. Wang, L., Hong, J., Sun, L.: Modified equations for weakly convergent stochastic symplectic schemes via their generating functions. BIT Numer. Math. **56**, 1131–1162 (2016)

# Rogue Waves in the Generalized Davey-Stewartson System

Mervenur Belin and Irma Hacinliyan

**Abstract** In this study, we consider rogue waves, which appear and disappear suddenly with large amplitudes, in the generalized Davey-Stewartson (GDS) system found in acoustics and discuss their dynamic structure. For the rogue wave solutions, we first obtain the Hirota bilinear form of the GDS system through rational and bilogarithmic transformations. Then, forming the solutions of the GDS system through determinants of matrices, we obtain three types of rogue wave solutions depending on the size of the matrices ($N \times N$) and the order of the $N$-rational solutions: fundamental (line), multi- and higher-order rogue waves. We report the behavior and differences of these three types of rogue waves and explain the change in the waves with respect to time.

**Keywords** Solution · Rogue waves · Davey-Stewartson system

## 1 Introduction

Rogue waves, often called freak waves or giant waves, are those that appear from nowhere and then suddenly disappear without any trace [1]. Researchers considered modulational instability to be the reason for the formation of rogue waves [2, 3]. Peregrine first obtained a fundamental rogue wave for the nonlinear Schrödinger (NLS) equation involving water waves in 1983 [4]. For this reason, the solution is also called the Peregrine soliton. Subsequently, rogue waves have been observed in many other nonlinear wave phenomena, such as water, optical and acoustic waves [3, 5–7]. Ohta and Yang have recently established rogue waves in the Davey-Stewartson (DS) equations [8–10]:

M. Belin · I. Hacinliyan (✉)
Istanbul Technical University, Istanbul, Turkey
e-mail: hacinliy@itu.edu.tr

M. Belin
e-mail: mervenurbelin@gmail.com

© Springer Nature Switzerland AG 2018
D. M. Kilgour et al. (eds.), *Recent Advances in Mathematical and Statistical Methods*, Springer Proceedings in Mathematics & Statistics 259,
https://doi.org/10.1007/978-3-319-99719-3_52

$$iu_\zeta = u_{\xi\xi} + \gamma u_{\eta\eta} + \chi |u|^2 u + \beta u v_\xi,$$
$$v_{\xi\xi} + \alpha v_{\eta\eta} = (|u|^2)_\xi, \tag{1}$$

where $u$ is the complex wave amplitude and $v$ is a real field. Also, $\zeta$ is the time coordinate and $(\xi, \eta)$ denotes spatial coordinates. The coefficients in (1) depend on the frequency, wave number, group velocity and gravity. If $(\gamma, \alpha) = (1, -1)$, the DS system is known as DSI; for $(\gamma, \alpha) = (-1, +1)$ it is DSII. Ohta and Yang eventually classified rogue wave solutions for DSI in three forms: Fundamental (line) rogue waves, Multi-rogue waves and Higher-order rogue waves. Fundamental rogue waves, the simplest rogue waves, have line profiles in the $(\xi, \eta)$-plane and therefore, they are also called line rogue waves. Their initially constant amplitude suddenly increases, reaches a maximum value, and then returns to the initial value. Multi-rogue waves occur when multiple fundamental rogue waves interact with each other. In this case, it is observed that fundamental rogue waves interfere and vanish back into the constant background. In contrast, higher-order rogue waves cannot approach the constant background uniformly as $\zeta \to \infty$. Only some parts of the waves approach uniformly the constant background [9].

In the current study, we focus on the generalized Davey-Stewartson (GDS) system in acoustics given as

$$iu_\zeta = u_{\xi\xi} + \gamma_1 u_{\eta\eta} + \gamma_2 u_{\xi\eta} + \chi |u|^2 u + u(\beta_1 \partial_\xi + \beta_2 \partial_\eta)v,$$
$$\alpha_{11} v_{\xi\xi} + \alpha_{22} v_{\eta\eta} = -2(\beta_1 \partial_\xi + \beta_2 \partial_\eta)|u|^2, \tag{2}$$

where

$$\gamma_2 = \frac{4\beta_1 \beta_2 \gamma_1}{\beta_2^2 + \beta_1^2 \gamma_1}, \quad \alpha_{11} = \frac{\beta_2^2 - \beta_1^2 \gamma_1}{\beta_2^2 + \beta_1^2 \gamma_1},$$
$$\alpha_{22} = -\gamma_1 \left( \frac{\beta_2^2 - \beta_1^2 \gamma_1}{\beta_2^2 + \beta_1^2 \gamma_1} \right), \quad \chi = -\frac{\beta_2^2 + \beta_1^2 \gamma_1}{\gamma_1}.$$

This system for $(\gamma_2, \beta_2) = (0, 0)$ reduces to the DS system (1). The GDS system is obtained for the weakly nonlinear modulation of a wave originated by the interaction between a long wave-length acoustic mode and a high frequency mode given in [11]. Therefore, the real mode $v$ represents a mean motion induced by the oscillatory wave packet, which has the complex amplitude $u$. This system can be classified in two categories depending on the relationship between the coefficients: the GDSI (elliptic-hyperbolic) system if $\gamma_2^2 - 4\gamma_1 < 0$ and $\alpha_{11}\alpha_{22} < 0$, and the GDSII (hyperbolic-elliptic) system if $\gamma_2^2 - 4\gamma_1 > 0$ and $\alpha_{11}\alpha_{22} > 0$. With the constraints $\gamma_1 > 0$ and $\beta_2 - \beta_1 \sqrt{\gamma_1} < 0$, the GDSI system is obtained. In this study, we find fundamental, multi- and higher-order rogue waves in the GDSI system (2) by following a similar approach to the DS system in [9, 10]. In the next section, the main theorem which presents the rational solutions of the GDSI system is stated and proved. Rogue wave solutions are also mentioned in Sect. 2. Simulations of these solutions are presented in Sect. 3.

## 2 The Non-singular Rational Solutions of GDSI

**Theorem 1** *The non-singular rational solutions of the GDSI Eq. (2) are given by*

$$u = \frac{\sqrt{2\gamma_1}}{\sqrt{\beta_2^2 + \beta_1^2\gamma_1}} \frac{\tau_1}{\tau_0}, \quad v = \frac{2-\beta_2}{\beta_1}\xi + \eta + \frac{4\gamma_1}{\beta_2^2 + \beta_1^2\gamma_1}(\beta_1\partial_\xi + \beta_2\partial_\eta)log\tau_0, \quad (3)$$

*where $\tau_n$ is a determinant of the $N \times N$ matrix $\left(m_{ij}^{(n)}\right)$ whose entries are*

$$m_{ij}^{(n)} = \sum_{k=0}^{n_i} c_{ik}\left(n + \mu_i' + p_i\partial_{p_i}\right)^{n_i-k}$$

$$\times \sum_{l=0}^{n_j} c_{jl}^*\left(-n + (\mu_j')^* + p_j^*\partial_{p_j^*}\right)^{n_j-l}\frac{1}{p_i+p_j^*}, \quad (4)$$

*with*

$$\mu_i' = \frac{\sqrt{\beta_2^2 + \beta_1^2\gamma_1}}{2}\left(\frac{1}{p_i(\beta_2 + \beta_1\sqrt{\gamma_1})} - \frac{p_i}{\beta_2 - \beta_1\sqrt{\gamma_1}}\right)\xi$$

$$+ \frac{\sqrt{\beta_2^2 + \beta_1^2\gamma_1}}{2\sqrt{\gamma_1}}\left(\frac{1}{p_i(\beta_2 + \beta_1\sqrt{\gamma_1})} + \frac{p_i}{\beta_2 - \beta_1\sqrt{\gamma_1}}\right)\eta + \frac{p_i^2 + p_i^{-2}}{\sqrt{-1}}\zeta. \quad (5)$$

*Proof* Substituting the transformation

$$u = \frac{\sqrt{2\gamma_1}}{\sqrt{\beta_2^2 + \beta_1^2\gamma_1}} \frac{G}{F}, \quad v = \frac{2-\beta_2}{\beta_1}\xi + \eta + \frac{4\gamma_1}{\beta_2^2 + \beta_1^2\gamma_1}(\beta_1\partial_\xi + \beta_2\partial_\eta)logF,$$

where $G$ is complex and $F$ is real valued function, into (2) implies the following bilinear form of GDSI:

$$(-iD_\zeta + D_\xi^2 + \gamma_1 D_\eta^2 + \gamma_2 D_\xi D_\eta)GF = 0,$$

$$(\alpha_{11}D_\xi^2 + \alpha_{22}D_\eta^2)(FF) = \frac{2\chi\gamma_1}{\beta_2^2 + \beta_1^2\gamma_1}|G|^2 + 2FF. \quad (6)$$

On other hand, there is an auxiliary bilinear form,

$$(D_{x_1}D_{x_{-1}} - 2)\tau_n\tau_n = -2\tau_{n+1}\tau_{n-1},$$

$$(D_{x_1}^2 - D_{x_2})\tau_{n+1}\tau_n = 0,$$

$$(D_{x_{-1}}^2 + D_{x_{-2}})\tau_{n+1}\tau_n = 0, \quad (7)$$

which is reduced to (6) by the independent variables transformation

$$x_1 = \frac{\sqrt{\beta_2^2 + \beta_1^2 \gamma_1}}{2(\beta_2 - \beta_1 \sqrt{\gamma_1})}\left(-\xi + \frac{1}{\sqrt{\gamma_1}}\eta\right), \qquad x_2 = -\frac{i\zeta}{2}$$

$$x_{-1} = \frac{-\sqrt{\beta_2^2 + \beta_1^2 \gamma_1}}{2(\beta_2 + \beta_1 \sqrt{\gamma_1})}\left(\xi + \frac{1}{\sqrt{\gamma_1}}\eta\right), \qquad x_{-2} = \frac{i\zeta}{2}, \tag{8}$$

with $\tau_0 = F$, $\tau_1 = G$ and $\tau_{-1} = G^*$ (* denotes the complex conjugate of the indicated term). The form of solutions for the system (7) is given by the following lemma.

**Lemma 1** *[9] If the functions $m_{ij}^{(n)}$, $\varphi_i^{(n)}$, and $\psi_j^{(n)}$ of $x_1$, $x_2$, $x_{-1}$ and $x_{-2}$ satisfy the differential equations*

$$\partial_{x_1} m_{ij}^{(n)} = \varphi_i^{(n)} \psi_j^{(n)},$$

$$\partial_{x_2} m_{ij}^{(n)} = \varphi_i^{(n+1)} \psi_j^{(n)} + \varphi_i^{(n)} \psi_j^{(n-1)},$$

$$\partial_{x_{-1}} m_{ij}^{(n)} = -\varphi_i^{(n-1)} \psi_j^{(n+1)},$$

$$\partial_{x_{-2}} m_{ij}^{(n)} = -\varphi_i^{(n-2)} \psi_j^{(n+1)} - \varphi_i^{(n-1)} \psi_j^{(n+2)},$$

$$\partial_{x_k} \varphi_i^{(n)} = \varphi_i^{(n+k)},$$

$$\partial_{x_k} \psi_j^{(n)} = -\psi_j^{(n-k)} \qquad (k = -2, -1, 1, 2) \tag{9}$$

*and the difference relation*

$$m_{ij}^{(n+1)} = m_{ij}^{(n)} + \varphi_i^{(n)} \psi_j^{(n+1)}, \tag{10}$$

*then the bilinear Eq. (7) are satisfied by the determinant $\tau_n = \det_{1 \le i, j \le N}\left(m_{i,j}^{(n)}\right)$.*

It is easy to observe that the transformation (8) and Lemma 1 lead to the complex conjugate conditions

$$\tau_n^* = \tau_{-n}, \qquad m_{ij}^{(n)*} = m_{ji}^{(-n)}. \tag{11}$$

We now define the appropriate functions $\varphi_i^{(n)}$, $\psi_j^{(n)}$ and $m_{i,j}^{(n)}$ to obtain rational solutions:

$$\varphi_i^{(n)} = A_i p_i^n e^{\mu_i}, \qquad \psi_j^{(n)} = B_j(-q_j)^{-n} e^{\lambda_j},$$

$$m_{ij}^{(n)} = A_i B_j \frac{1}{p_i + q_j}\left(-\frac{p_i}{q_j}\right)^n e^{\mu_i + \lambda_j}, \tag{12}$$

where $A_i$ and $B_j$ denote differential operators of order $n_i$ and $n_j$ with respect to $p_i$ and $q_j$ as

$$A_i = \sum_{k=0}^{n_i} c_{ik}(p_i \partial_{p_i})^{n_i - k} \quad \text{and} \quad B_j = \sum_{l=0}^{n_j} d_{lj}(q_j \partial_{q_j})^{n_j - l} \tag{13}$$

for which $c_{ik}, d_{lj}$ are complex numbers and $n_i$ and $n_j$ are positive integers. The functions in (12) satisfy Eqs. (9) and (10). Thus $\tau_n$ is a solution of the auxiliary form (7).

To find the matrix $m_{ij}^{(n)}$, the reduction formulas

$$\left(q_j \partial_{q_j}\right)\left(-q_j\right)^{-n} e^{\lambda_j} = \left(-q_j\right)^{-n} e^{\lambda_j}\left(-n + \frac{2x_{-2}}{q_j^2} - \frac{x_{-1}}{q_j} + q_j x_1 - 2q_j^2 x_2 + q_j \partial_{q_j}\right),$$

$$\left(p_i \partial_{p_i}\right) p_i^n e^{\mu_i} = p_i^n e^{\mu_i}\left(n - \frac{2x_{-2}}{p_i^2} - \frac{x_{-1}}{p_i} + p_i x_1 + 2p_i^2 x_2 + p_i \partial_{p_i}\right) \qquad (14)$$

are applied to (12); restrictions $d_{jl} = c_{ik}^*$ and $q_j = p_j^*$ are assumed because of the conditions (11). After straightforward but long computations, we obtain the expression of $m_{ij}^{(n)}$ as:

$$m_{ij}^{(n)} = \left(-\frac{p_i}{p_j^*}\right)^n e^{\mu_i + \mu_j^*} \sum_{k=0}^{n_i} c_{ik}\left(n + \mu_i' + p_i \partial_{p_i}\right)^{n_i - k}$$

$$\times \sum_{l=0}^{n_j} c_{jl}^*\left(-n + (\mu_j')^* p_j^* \partial_{p_j^*}\right)^{n_j - l} \frac{1}{p_i + p_j^*}, \qquad (15)$$

where $\mu_i = x_{-2}/p_i^2 + x_{-1}/p_i + p_i x_1 + p_i^2 x_2$ and $\mu_i' = -2x_{-2}/p_i^2 - x_{-1}/p_i + p_i x_1 + 2p_i^2 x_2$. Then, we use the gauge freedom of $\tau_n$ to get Eq. (4).

Finally, we discuss nonsingularity of rational solutions (3). The aim of this part is to prove $\tau_0 = \det(m_{ij}^{(0)}) > 0$. To do this, integrating the first differential equation in (9) and using the fact that $B_j^* = A_j$ gives us

$$m_{ij}^{(0)} = \int_{-\infty}^{x_1} A_i A_j^* e^{\mu_i + \mu_j^*} \, dx_1. \qquad (16)$$

The antiderivative of $\exp(\mu_i + \mu_j^*)$ with respect to $x_1$ disappears as $x_1 \to -\infty$, if the real part of $p_i$ is positive. Then, we find that the matrix $m_{ij}^{(0)}$ is positive definite since we have

$$v\left(m_{ij}^{(0)}\right)_{i,j=1}^{N} (v^*)^T = \int_{-\infty}^{x_1} \left|\sum_{i=1}^{N} v_i A_i e^{\mu_i}\right|^2 dx_1 > 0, \qquad (17)$$

for every non-zero vector $v = (v_1, v_2, v_3, \ldots, v_N)$ and its conjugate transpose $(v^*)^T$. This means that $\det(m_{ij}^{(0)}) > 0$. In the same manner, it is possible to prove that the solution is nonsingular for the case $\mathrm{Re}(p_i) < 0$. (For details, see [10].) $\qquad \square$

The dynamical behavior of the rational solutions for the DSI equations was investigated in [9]. As a result, it was found that these solutions become rouge waves if $p_i$'s are real. Since the GDSI system for the case $\beta_1 = -1$, $\beta_2 = 0$ and $\gamma_1 = 1$ is reduced to DSI in [9], we continue the work with assumption $p_i^* = p_i$.

In order to observe that the 1- dimensional rational solution of the first order ($N = 1$ and $n_1 = 1$) forms a fundamental rogue wave, we substitute $N = 1, n_1 = 1$, $c_{10} = 1$ and $p_1^* = p_1$ to the rational solution (3). Then, we have

$$u = \frac{\sqrt{2\gamma_1}}{\sqrt{\beta_2^2 + \beta_1^2 \gamma_1}} \left( 1 - \frac{1 + 2i\text{Im}(\mu)}{|\mu|^2 + \frac{1}{4}} \right),$$

$$v = \frac{2 - \beta_2}{\beta_1} \xi + \eta + \frac{4\gamma_1}{\beta_2^2 + \beta_1^2 \gamma_1} (\beta_1 \partial_\xi + \beta_2 \partial_\eta) \log \left( \frac{4|\mu|^2 + 1}{8p_1} \right), \qquad (18)$$

where

$$\mu = c_{11} - \frac{1}{2} + \frac{\sqrt{\beta_2^2 + \beta_1^2 \gamma_1}}{2} \left( \frac{1}{p_1(\beta_2 + \beta_1 \sqrt{\gamma_1})} - \frac{p_1}{\beta_2 - \beta_1 \sqrt{\gamma_1}} \right) \xi$$

$$+ \frac{\sqrt{\beta_2^2 + \beta_1^2 \gamma_1}}{2\sqrt{\gamma_1}} \left( \frac{1}{p_1(\beta_2 + \beta_1 \sqrt{\gamma_1})} + \frac{p_1}{\beta_2 - \beta_1 \sqrt{\gamma_1}} \right) \eta - i \left( p_1^2 + p_1^{-2} \right) \zeta.$$

The coefficients of $\xi$ and $\eta$ in $\mu$ are real and the coefficient of $\zeta$ in $\mu$ is purely imaginary, so the solution $u$ is in the form of a line. The line wave is oriented in the direction $((p_1^2 - 1)\beta_1 + (p_1^2 + 1)\beta_2/\sqrt{\gamma_1}, (p_1^2 + 1)\beta_1\sqrt{\gamma_1} + (p_1^2 - 1)\beta_2)$ of the $(\xi, \eta)$-plane. However, the line profile does not show up at all times in the $(\xi, \eta)$-plane, since $u$ approaches to uniformly constant background $\sqrt{2\gamma_1}/\sqrt{\beta_2^2 + \beta_1^2 \gamma_1}$ as $\zeta \to \pm\infty$. Moreover, the form of $|u|$ is two-dimensional counterparts of the Peregrine solution [4].

We now proceed with a consideration of multi- and higher-order rogue waves. Due to the involved nature of these waves and for brevity, we will limit our discussion to the selected special cases.

Considering the $N = 2$ rogue wave, $p_1$ and $p_2$ are arbitrary real parameters. We take $n_i = c_{i0} = 1$, for $i = 1, 2$ and $c_{11}$ and $c_{21}$ as arbitrary complex parameters. Then, the solution is:

$$u = \frac{\sqrt{2\gamma_1}}{\sqrt{\beta_2^2 + \beta_1^2 \gamma_1}} \frac{\begin{vmatrix} m_{11}^{(1)} & m_{12}^{(1)} \\ m_{21}^{(1)} & m_{22}^{(1)} \end{vmatrix}}{\begin{vmatrix} m_{11}^{(0)} & m_{12}^{(0)} \\ m_{21}^{(0)} & m_{22}^{(0)} \end{vmatrix}}, \qquad (19)$$

where

$$m_{ij}^{(0)} = \frac{1}{p_i + p_j} \left( \left( \mu_i' + c_{i1} - \frac{p_i}{p_i + p_j} \right) \left( \mu_j' \right)^* + c_{j1}^* - \frac{p_j}{p_i + p_j} \right) + \frac{p_i p_j}{\left( p_i + p_j \right)^2} \right)$$

$$m_{ij}^{(1)} = \frac{1}{p_i + p_j} \left( \left( \mu_i' + 1 + c_{i1} - \frac{p_i}{p_i + p_j} \right) \right.$$
$$\times \left. \left( \left( \mu_j' \right)^* - 1 + c_{j1}^* - \frac{p_j}{p_i + p_j} \right) + \frac{p_i p_j}{(p_i + p_j)^2} \right).$$

As defined by Ohta and Yang [9, 10] multi-rogue waves result from the interaction of multiple fundamental rogue waves.

For an example of higher-order rogue waves, we impose the condition $N = 1$ and $n_1 = 2 > 1$. Taking $c_{10} = 1$, $c_{11} = 0$, $c_{12} = 0$ and $c_{21} = 0$, we get the second-order rogue wave $u = \sqrt{2\gamma_1}\tau_1 / \left( \sqrt{\beta_2^2 + \beta_1^2 \gamma_1} \, \tau_0 \right)$, where

$$\tau_0 = \left( \mu_1' + p_1 \partial_{p_1} \right)^2 \left( \left( \mu_1' \right)^* + p_1^* \partial_{p_1^*} \right)^2 \frac{1}{p_1 + p_1^*} ,$$

$$\tau_1 = \left( 1 + \mu_1' + p_1 \partial_{p_1} \right)^2 \left( -1 + \left( \mu_1' \right)^* + p_1^* \partial_{p_1^*} \right)^2 \frac{1}{p_1 + p_1^*} . \tag{20}$$

Substituting $N = 1$ and any $n_1 > 1$ in (3), other examples of higher-order rogue waves are obtained. Thus, solutions are generated from a higher-order differential operator.

## 3  Simulations of Rogue Waves

In this section, all types of rogue waves for $(\gamma_1, \beta_1, \beta_2) = (1, 1, 0.5)$ are simulated and their behavior are shown.

### 3.1  Fundamental (Line) Rogue Waves

In Fig. 1. the line rogue wave solutions (18) are simulated. In the intermediate time $\zeta = 0$, $|u|$ reaches the maximum amplitude $6\sqrt{2/5} \approx 3.79473$. However, as $\zeta \to \pm\infty$, the solution $|u|$ approaches to the constant background which is approximately $2\sqrt{2/5} \approx 1.26491$ in the $(\xi, \eta)$-plane. We see that the fundamental rogue wave appears and disappears suddenly.

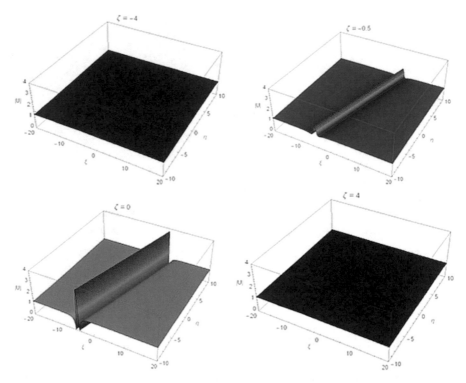

**Fig. 1** The fundamental rogue wave solution for the case $(\gamma_1, \beta_1, \beta_2) = (1, 1, 0.5)$ with $p_1 = 1$

## 3.2 Multi-rogue Waves

In Fig. 2, two fundamental rogue waves (19) are given by taking $p_1 = 1$, $p_2 = 1.5$ and $c_{11} = c_{21} = 0$. Starting from the usual constant background of 1.26491, the local maximum amplitude 3.94784 is reached at $\zeta = -1$. After this amplitude fades, the two fundamental rogue waves in the far field appear to be with their maximum amplitude of 3.95446 at $\zeta = 0$. The wave fronts at this stage are well separated. Due to the interaction of two fundamental rogue waves, curvy wave fronts are formed. When $\zeta$ becomes larger, the waves go back to the constant background as seen at $\zeta = -10$ and $\zeta = 10$. In all cases, the amplitude does not reach four times the constant value. Thus, this means that the interaction does not guarantee very high peaks.

In order to see the situation in more than two rouge waves, setting $p_1 = 1$, $p_2 = 1.5$, $p_3 = 2$ and $c_{i1} = 0$ for $i = 1, 2, 3$, three interacting rogue waves are obtained in Fig. 3. However, we get a more complicated outcome from the case of two-rogue waves. In the graphics, we see that three rogue waves at $\zeta = 0$ individually reach a maximum amplitude. After a while the rogue wave disappears without any trace.

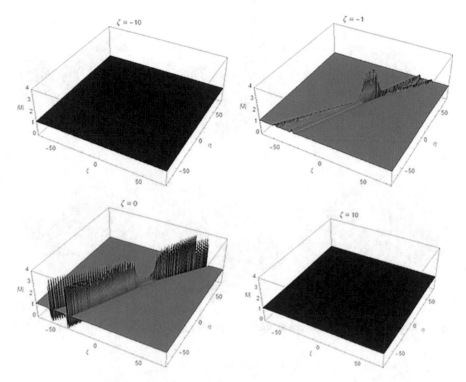

**Fig. 2** The two-rogue wave solution for the case $(\gamma_1, \beta_1, \beta_2) = (1, 1, 0.5)$ with $p_1 = 1$ and $p_2 = 1.5$

## 3.3 Higher-Order Rogue Waves

The higher-order rogue wave (20) is formed as in Fig. 4. Unlike fundamental rogue wave and multi-rogue wave, in this case the rogue wave does not disappear without any trace. For instance, at $\zeta = -5, \zeta = 5$ and $\zeta = 10$ parts of waves still exist. When the graphs are examined, it can be said that in the case that $\zeta$ approaches $-2.5$, the solution tends to lump. As $\zeta$ increases further, the lump begins to split into two branch rogue waves. When $\zeta$ goes to 0, the branches become dominant. Then the lump dissipates.

In conclusion, rogue waves in GDSI system (2) which is derived in acoustics are obtained. The results show that the properties of the waves in the solution are compatible with Ohta and Yang's classification of rogue waves as fundamental rogue wave, multi-rogue wave and higher-order rogue wave for the DS system. With the additional term in the GDSI system, the results from the DS system are qualitively similar.

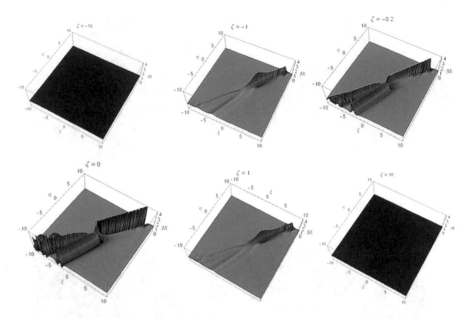

**Fig. 3** The three-rogue wave solution for the case $(\gamma_1, \beta_1, \beta_2) = (1, 1, 0.5)$ with $p_1 = 1, p_2 = 1.5$ and $p_3 = 2$

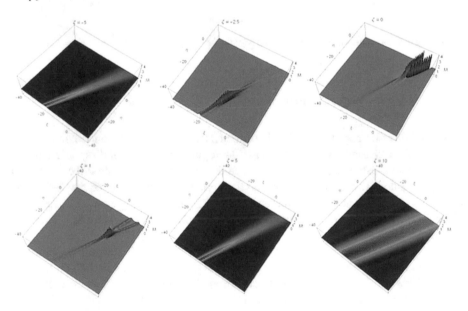

**Fig. 4** The higher-order rogue wave solution for the case $(\gamma_1, \beta_1, \beta_2) = (1, 1, 0.5)$ with $p_1 = 1$

# References

1. Akhmediev, N., Ankiewicz, A., Taki, M.: Waves that appear from nowhere and disappear without a trace. Phy. Lett. A **373**(6), 675–678 (2009)
2. Akhmediev, N., Soto-Crespo, J.M., Ankiewicz, A.: Extreme waves that appear from nowhere: on the nature of rogue waves. Phys. Lett. A **373**(25), 2137–2145 (2009)
3. Yurova, A.: A hidden life of Peregrine's soliton: rouge waves in the oceanic depths. Int. J. Geom. Methods Mod. Phys. **11**(6), 1450057 (2014)
4. Peregrine, D.H.: Water waves, nonlinear Schrödinger equations and their solutions. J. Austral. Math. Soc. B. **25**, 1643 (1983)
5. Bailung, H., Sharma, S.K., Nakamura, Y.: Observation of peregrine solitons in a multicomponent plasma with negative ions. Phys. Rev. Lett. **107**, 255005 (2011)
6. Liu, Y.K., Li, B.: Rogue waves in the (2+ 1)-dimensional nonlinear schrödinger equation with a parity-time-symmetric potential. Chin. Phys. Lett. **34**(1), 010202 (2017)
7. Solli, D.R., Ropers, C., Koonath, P., Jalali, B., Peregrine, D.H.: Optical rogue waves. Nature **450**, 10541057 (2007)
8. Davey, A., Stewartson, K.: On three-dimensional packets of surface waves. Proc. R. Soc. Lond. A. **338**, 101–110 (1974)
9. Ohta, Y., Yang, J.: Rogue waves in the Davey-Stewartson I equation. Phys. Rev. E **86**(3), 036604 (2012)
10. Ohta, Y., Yang, J.: Dynamics of rogue waves in the Davey-Stewartson II equation. J. Phys. A: Math. Theor. **46**(10), 105202 (2013)
11. Huang, G., Konotop, V.V., Tam, H.W., Hu, B.: Nonlinear modulation of multidimensional lattice waves. Phys. Rev. E. **64**(5), 056619 (2001)

# Linearization and Local Topological Conjugacies for Impulsive Systems

Kevin E. M. Church and Xinzhi Liu

**Abstract** The celebrated Hartman-Grobman theorem for ordinary differential equations states that the phase portrait nearby a hyperbolic equilibrium point of a nonlinear system is equivalent to that of its linearization by a conjugation. Hartman and Grobmans theorem has been extended in numerous ways to accommodate more general classes of dynamical systems. For instance, generalizations have been proven for finite-dimensional nonautonomous systems, impulsive systems, and impulsive differential equations in Banach spaces. All of the aforementioned generalized results, however, require global Lipschitz assumptions on the vector field and jump map, as well as intimate knowledge of the dichotomy properties of the linearized system. Since many systems encountered in applied fields are nonlinear and not globally Lipschitz, there is a need to weaken the assumptions. We show that one can localize such linearization theorems near a hyperbolic equilibrium point, provided sufficient smoothness conditions are satisfied and time-varying terms are suitably bounded. Global assumptions on the nonlinearity are no longer necessary and one does not require as detailed an analysis of the linearized system to apply the result.

**Keywords** Impulsive differential equation · Topological conjugacy
Hartman-Grobman theorem

## 1 Introduction and Background

Impulsive differential equations see applications in numerous fields where the systems of study exhibit rapid jumps in state. Such jumps may be intrinsic to the system, such as in the firing of a neuron in a biological neural network, or synthetic, such as the application of an insecticide or antibiotic treatment in a biological model.

K. E. M. Church (✉) · X. Liu
University of Waterloo, 200 University Ave W, Waterloo, ON N2L 3G1, Canada
e-mail: k5church@uwaterloo.ca

X. Liu
e-mail: xzliu@uwaterloo.ca

© Springer Nature Switzerland AG 2018
D. M. Kilgour et al. (eds.), *Recent Advances in Mathematical
and Statistical Methods*, Springer Proceedings in Mathematics & Statistics 259,
https://doi.org/10.1007/978-3-319-99719-3_53

Arguably, one of the most common applications of the theory of impulsive differential equations arises in the latter case, where a continuous autonomous system is perturbed by impulses in an impulsive control setting. Specifically, there are many applications involving systems of the form

$$\dot{x} = Ax + f(x), \quad t \neq \tau_k \tag{1}$$

$$\Delta x = Bx + g(x), \quad t = \tau_k, \tag{2}$$

where (1) describes the continuous evolution of the system, and (2) the discontinuous impulsive control. We will call such a system an *impulsive system with autonomous right-hand side*. To be precise, such a system consists of a continuous evolution defined by the differential equation (1) coupled with jumps at times $\tau_k$ indexed by $k \in \mathbb{Z}$, according to Eq. (2). The notation $\Delta x$ stands for $\Delta x = x(\tau_k^+) - x(\tau_k)$, where $x(\tau_k^+)$ denotes the limit from the right at time $\tau_k$. In particular, the Eq. (2) should be understood as

$$x(\tau_k^+) - x(\tau_k) = Bx(\tau_k) + g(x(\tau_k)).$$

Frequently in applications, the sequence $\tau_k$ is periodic, and in this case, there are a wealth of techniques available to study the complete impulsive system. Specifically, the following elementary tools are available.

1. A linearized stability theorem.
2. A local bifurcation theory of fixed points and periodic orbits.
3. A local topological equivalence (Hartman-Grobman) theorem.

Linearized stability principles for finite-dimensional impulsive systems have been known for quite some time; see the monographs [1, 2] and the literature cited therein for relevant background information on finite-dimensional impulsive systems and stability, and [3] for background on stability of impulsive delay differential equations. In applications, Poincaré maps and numerical continuation methods have been used to study bifurcations of fixed points and periodic orbits: see [4–7] for recent applications of these methods and [8] for an outline of analytical techniques based on Poincaré maps.

The Hartman-Grobman Theorem [9] was originally proven for finite-dimensional ordinary differential equations and difference equations. The theorem yields topological information about the phase portrait near a hyperbolic equilibrium point. Since then, the theorem has been extended to different classes of systems. Recent advances include variants of the theorem for hyperbolic evolution equations [10] and dynamic equations on time scales [11]. There are several generalizations of the Hartman-Grobman theorem to impulsive systems [12–14]. However, the latter results and seemingly all published Hartman-Grobman-type linearization theorems for impulsive systems assume global boundedness and Lipschitz conditions on the vector field and jump map, as well as a detailed analysis of the linearization. In these proceedings, we show how these assumptions can be weakened in favour of local smoothness assumptions, resulting in a direct analogue of the local, classical Hartman-Grobman theorem.

## 1.1   The Linearization Theorem of Fenner and Pinto

The starting point for our result will be the linearization theorem of Fenner and Pinto [13]. We will later show how this theorem can be localized near an equilibrium point. To begin, we remind the reader of the definition of exponential dichotomy [1].

**Definition 1**   Consider the linear impulsive system

$$\dot{x} = A(t)x, \quad t \neq \tau_k$$
$$\Delta x = B_k x, \qquad t = \tau_k, \tag{3}$$

with Cauchy (fundamental) matrix solution $X(t, s)$. We say the system (3) has *exponential dichotomy* if there exist $K \geq 1$, $\alpha > 0$ and a family $P(t)$ of projection matrices such that for all $t \geq s$ one has $X(t, s)P(s) = P(t)X(t, s)$ and the following inequalities:

$$\|X(t, s)P(s)\| \leq Ke^{-\alpha(t-s)},$$
$$\|X(t, s)^{-1}[I - P(t)]\| \leq Ke^{-\alpha(t-s)}.$$

The $K$ and $\alpha$ are admissible *constants* and *exponents* of the dichotomy. In this case, we will also say that $X(t, s)$ has exponential dichotomy.

A brief reminder: system (3) is *periodic with period $T$ and $c$ impulses per period* if $A(t + T) = A(t)$, $B_{k+c} = B_k$ and $\tau_{k+c} = \tau_k + T$ for all $t \in \mathbb{R}$ and $k \in \mathbb{Z}$. When (3) is periodic, the existence of an exponential dichotomy is equivalent to an eigenvalue condition. Namely, if one computes the monodromy matrix $M = X(\tau_0 + T, \tau_0)$ for period $T > 0$, the linear system has exponential dichotomy if and only if $M$ has no eigenvalues with unit modulus [1]. Exponential dichotomy is also guaranteed if (3) is exponentially stable, regardless of periodicity assumptions.

We will also need a notion of accumulation of the sequence of impulses. We will say that $\{\tau_k\}$ has *upper density bound $N$* if $\#\{\tau_k \in [n, n + 1) : n \in \mathbb{Z}\} \leq N$. That is, in each unit interval starting at an integer, there are at most $N$ impulse times.

Fenner and Pinto's linearization theorem [13] is stated in terms of $(h, k)$-dichotomies, which are more general than exponential dichotomies. To keep the presentation elementary, we will refrain from using this notion here. Then, a special case of the aforementioned theorem is as follows: it is stated with respect to the quasilinear system

$$\dot{x} = A(t)x + f(t, x), \quad t \neq \tau_k \tag{4}$$
$$\Delta x = B_k x + g_k(x), \qquad t = \tau_k, \tag{5}$$

and its *formal linearization*

$$\dot{x} = A(t)x, \quad t \neq \tau_k \tag{6}$$

$$\Delta x = B_k x, \quad t = \tau_k. \tag{7}$$

**Proposition 1** (Fenner and Pinto, [13]) *Consider the periodic impulsive system (4)–(5) and the linear equation (6)–(7). Suppose the linear system has exponential dichotomy with constant $K$ and exponent $\alpha$. Assume for all $x, y \in \mathbb{R}^n$, the following inequalities are satisfied:*

$$\|f(t, x)\|\| \leq \mu, \quad \|f(t, x) - f(t, y)\| \leq \gamma \|x - y\|,$$

$$\|g_k(x)\| \leq \mu, \quad \|g_k(x) - g_k(y)\| \leq \gamma \|x - y\|.$$

*If the sequence $\{\tau_k\}$ of impulse times has upper density bound $N$ and the inequality*

$$2K\gamma \left( \frac{1}{\alpha} + N \frac{2 - e^{-\alpha}}{1 - e^{-\alpha}} \right) < 1 \tag{8}$$

*holds, then there exists a function $H : \mathbb{R} \times \mathbb{R}^n \to \mathbb{R}^n$ with the following properties:*

1. *For all $t \in \mathbb{R}$, $x \mapsto H_t(x) = H(t, x)$ is a homeomorphism,*
2. *$H_t(x(t))$ is a solution of the linear equation whenever $x(t)$ is a solution of the quasilinear equation,*
3. *$H_t^{-1}(y(t))$ is a solution of the quasilinear equation whenever $y(t)$ is a solution of the linear equation,*
4. *For all $(t, x) \in \mathbb{R} \times \mathbb{R}^n$, $H_t(x) - x$ is uniformly bounded with*

$$|H_t(x) - x| \leq 4K\mu \left( \frac{1}{\alpha} + N \frac{2 - e^{-\alpha}}{1 - e^{-\alpha}} \right). \tag{9}$$

Clearly, if the conditions of the proposition are satisfied, then the quasilinear system (4)–(5) admits at most one solution that is bounded for all time. This is to be expected, since the time-varying topological conjugacy $H_t$ induces a *global* equivalence of the quasilinear system with its formal linearization, and the latter is exponentially dichotomous and therefore admits only one bounded solution: the trivial solution.

## 2   Localized Impulsive Linearization

In this section, we demonstrate how Proposition 1 can be localized near a given fixed point. The result is that one needs no longer verify the inequality (8), and so the constant and exponent of the exponential dichotomy need not be known explicitly. Next, we obtain a parameter-dependent analogue.

## 2.1  Main Result and Proof

Given the quasilinear system (4)–(5), we will say that the formal linearization (6)–(7) is *hyperbolic* [15] if it has exponential dichotomy. Before stating our main result, we will need one more definition.

**Definition 2** Let $x(\cdot; s, x_s) : I \to \mathbb{R}^n$ denote the solution of the quasilinear impulsive system (4)–(5) satisfying $x(s; s, x_s) = x_s$, where $I$ denotes the maximal interval of existence. The partial function $\varphi : \mathbb{R} \times \mathbb{R} \times \mathbb{R}^n \to \mathbb{R}^n$ defined by $\varphi(t, s, y) = x(t; s, y)$ is the *process* associated to (4)–(5), and we will write $\varphi(t, s)y := \varphi(t, s, y)$.

**Theorem 1** *Let $f : \mathbb{R} \times \mathbb{R}^n \to \mathbb{R}^n$ be differentiable in its second variable and let $g_k : \mathbb{R}^n \to \mathbb{R}^n$ be differentiable. Assume $t \mapsto Df(t, r(t))$ is locally integrable for all continuous functions $r(t)$ sufficiently small, and for each $\alpha \in \mathbb{R}$ there exists a continuously differentiable $H_\alpha : U \to \mathbb{R}^+$ for some open set $U$ containing the origin, satisfying $H_\alpha(0) = 0$ and $DH_\alpha(0) = 0$, and a continuous $N_\alpha : U \to \mathbb{R}^+$ with $N_\alpha(0) = 0$ such that*

$$\sup_{t \in [\alpha, \infty)} |f(t, x)| + \sup_{\tau_k \geq \alpha} |g_k(x)| \leq H_\alpha(x), \tag{10}$$

$$\sup_{t \in [\alpha, \infty)} ||Df(t, x)|| + \sup_{\tau_k \geq \alpha} ||Dg_k(x)|| \leq N_\alpha(x), \tag{11}$$

*on $U$. Consider the impulsive system (4)–(5) with process $\varphi$ and the linearized equation (6)–(7) with process $L$. Suppose the linearization is hyperbolic and the sequence of impulses has an upper density bound. Let $\xi > 0$ be given. There exists a family of homeomorphisms $H_t : \mathbb{R}^n \to \mathbb{R}^n, t \in \mathbb{R}$, satisfying the bound $|H_t x - x| \leq \xi$ and the following additional properties:*

- *For all $u \leq v \in \mathbb{R}$, there exists $\delta > 0$ such that for all $||x|| < \delta$, one has $H_t \circ \varphi(t, s)x = L(t, s)H_s x$ for all $[s, t] \subseteq [u, v]$.*
- *If $x^* = 0$ is either linearly or nonlinearly stable, then for all $s \in \mathbb{R}$, there exists $\delta > 0$ such that $H_t \circ \varphi(t, s)x = L(t, s)H_s x$ for $||x|| < \delta$ and $s \leq t < \infty$.*

*Proof* Let $\epsilon > 0$ be a constant that has yet to be chosen. By the mean-value theorem and the assumptions on $f$ and $g_k$, one can show that

$$||\varphi(t, u, x)|| \leq ||x|| + \int_u^t M_{u,v}||\varphi(r, u, x)||dr + \sum_{u \leq \tau_k < t} M_{u,v}||\varphi(\tau_k, u, x)||,$$

$$M_{u,v} = \sup_{[u,v]} ||A(t)|| + \max_{\tau_k \in [u,v]} ||B_k|| + \max_{||x|| \leq \epsilon} F_u(x),$$

provided $||x|| \leq \epsilon_2 < \epsilon$ for some $\epsilon_2$ and $t > u$ is small enough. By Gronwall's inequality for impulsive systems [1], it follows that

$$||\varphi(t, s, x)|| \leq ||x||(1 + M_{u,v})^{N(\lceil t \rceil - \lfloor s \rfloor)} e^{M_{u,v}(t-s)} := ||x||C_{s,t}$$

for $t - s > 0$ small enough. One obtains $||\varphi(t, s, x)|| \leq \epsilon$ for $[s, t] \subseteq [u, v]$ provided $||x|| \leq \epsilon_2 = \epsilon C_{u,v}^{-1}$.

Let $r^\epsilon : U \to [0, 1]$ be a smooth cutoff function satisfying $r^\epsilon|_{||x|| \leq \epsilon} = \text{Id}$, $r^\epsilon|_{||x|| \geq 2\epsilon} = 0$ and $||\nabla r^\epsilon|| \leq 2/\epsilon$ on the annulus $\epsilon \leq ||x|| \leq 2\epsilon$, where we assume without loss of generality that $U$ contains the closed ball of radius $2\epsilon$ centered at the origin. Define the time-varying cutoff vector fields and jump maps as follows:

$$f^\epsilon(t, x) = \begin{cases} f(t, x)r^\epsilon(x), & t \geq s \\ 0, & t < s, \end{cases} \qquad g_k^\epsilon(x) = \begin{cases} g_k(x)r^\epsilon(x), & s \leq \tau_k \\ 0, & s > \tau_k. \end{cases}$$

By the mean-value theorem and the chain rule, we obtain the estimates

$$\max\{||Df^\epsilon||, ||Dg_k^\epsilon||\} \leq \sup_{||x|| \leq 2\epsilon} ||N_u(x)|| + 4 \sup_{||x|| \leq 2\epsilon} ||DH_u|| := A(\epsilon),$$

uniformly, for all $t \in \mathbb{R}, k \in \mathbb{Z}$ and $x \in \mathbb{R}^n$. Choose $\epsilon$ small enough so that inequality (8) is satisfied with $\gamma = A(\epsilon)$ and apply Proposition 1 to the quasilinear system

$$\dot{x} = A(t)x + f^\epsilon(t, x), \qquad t \neq \tau_k$$
$$\Delta x = B_k x + g_k^\epsilon(x), \qquad t = \tau_k,$$

to obtain the family of conjugacies $H_t$. Then, $H_t \circ \varphi^\epsilon(t, s)x = L(t, s) \circ H_s x$ for all $x \in \mathbb{R}$ and $t \geq s$. In particular, it holds for $||x|| < \delta = \epsilon C_{u,v}^{-1}$ and $[s, t] \subseteq [u, v]$. Since it is known that $||\varphi(t, s)x|| \leq \epsilon$ whenever these same constraints hold, we obtain the equality $H_t \circ \varphi(t, s)x = L(t, s) \circ H_s x$ for $||x||\delta$ and $[s, t] \subseteq [u, v]$, as claimed in the theorem.

Now we prove the assertions concerning stability. We prove only that linear stability implies nonlinear stability, since the other direction is similar. Suppose $x^* = 0$ is linearly stable. To begin, let some $s \in \mathbb{R}$ be given and let $\epsilon > 0$, where we may assume without loss of generality that $\epsilon$ is small enough for inequality (8) holds with $\gamma = A(\epsilon)$. By linear stability, let $\delta_1 > 0$ be small enough so that $\rho = \sup_{||y|| \leq \delta_1} ||L(t, s)y||_{t \geq s}$ satisfies inequality

$$4K\rho \left( \frac{1}{\alpha} + N \frac{2 - e^{-\alpha}}{1 - e^{-\alpha}} \right) < \frac{\epsilon}{2}.$$

By triangle inequality and the conjugation property, we have

$$||\varphi_\epsilon(t, s)x|| \leq ||(H_t^{-1} - id)L(t, s)H_s x|| + ||L(t, s)H_s x||. \tag{12}$$

From inequality (9), it follows that for $||y|| \leq \delta_1$ one has $||H_t y - y|| \leq \epsilon/2$, and by homeomorphism, one obtains $||H_t^{-1}y - y|| \leq \epsilon/2$ as well. By continuity of $H_s$, the same holds true with $y = H_s x$ provided $||x||$ is small enough. Stability of $L(t, s)$ and continuity of $H_s$ once again yield $||L(t, s)H_s x|| < \epsilon/2$ for $||x||$ s-mall enough. It then follows that there exists some $\delta > 0$ such that, in light of inequality (12), $||\varphi_\epsilon(t, s)x|| < \epsilon$ whenever $||x|| < \delta$ and $t \geq s$. But this implies that $\varphi_\epsilon(t, s)x = \varphi(t, s)x$ for all such $||x|| < \delta$.

In the periodic case, the inequality conditions of Theorem 1 are satisfied under reasonable smoothness assumptions on the vector field and jump map. The following corollary makes this concrete, and the proof is obvious.

**Corollary 1** *Inequalities* (10)–(11) *can be replaced with one of the following stronger assumptions.*

- *The quasilinear system* (4)–(5) *is periodic, each $g_k$ is $C^1$, and $f$ and $Df$ are continuous at $(t, x)$ unless $t = \tau_k$, where they are continuous from the left and have right limits in $t$.*
- *The "nonlinearities" $f$ and $g_k$ of the quasilinear system are autonomous and $C^1$.*

## 2.2 An Application to Bifurcation Theory

Consider the system

$$\dot{x} = f(t, x, p), \quad t \neq \tau_k \tag{13}$$
$$\Delta x = g_k(x, p), \quad t = \tau_k, \tag{14}$$

together with its linearization at the origin

$$\dot{y} = Df(0, t, p)y, \quad t \neq \tau_k \tag{15}$$
$$\Delta y = Dg_k(0, p)y, \quad t = \tau_k, \tag{16}$$

dependent on a parameter $p \in \Pi \subseteq \mathbb{R}^m$, and suppose that 0 is an equilibrium point for all $p \in B_r(\pi)$ for some $r > 0$ and some given $\pi \in \Pi$. Generally, if one possesses a parameter-dependent family of periodic orbits or equilibrium points (or, more generally, complete bounded solutions) $x_p^*(t)$, the time- and parameter-dependent change of variables $x = y + x_p^*$ transforms the system to one in which 0 is an equilibrium point, independent of $p$. One then has the following theorem.

**Theorem 2** *Suppose $f : \mathbb{R} \times \mathbb{R}^n \times \Pi \to \mathbb{R}^n$ and $g_k : \mathbb{R}^n \times \Pi \to \mathbb{R}^n$ are $C^1$ and $f(t, 0, p) = g_k(0, p) = 0$ for all $t \in \mathbb{R}$ and $k \in \mathbb{Z}$; that is, 0 is an equilibrium point of* (13)–(14). *Let $\pi \in \Pi$ be given, and assure for each $\alpha \in \mathbb{R}$, there exists $P \subseteq \Pi$ with $\pi \in P$, a continuously differentiable $H_\alpha : U \times P \to \mathbb{R}^+$ satisfying $H_\alpha(0, p) = 0$ and $DH_\alpha(0, p) = 0$, and a continuous $N_\alpha : U \times P \to \mathbb{R}^+$ satisfying $N_\alpha(0, p) = 0$, such that*

$$\sup_{t \in [\alpha, \infty)} |F(t, x, p)| + \sup_{\tau_k \geq \alpha} |G_k(x, p)| \leq H_\alpha(x, p), \tag{17}$$

$$\sup_{t \in [\alpha, \infty)} ||DF(t, x, p)|| + \sup_{\tau_k \geq \alpha} ||DG_k(x, p)|| \leq N_\alpha(x, p), \tag{18}$$

on $\mathbb{R}^n \times P$, where $F(t, x, p) = f(t, x, p) - Df(t, 0, \pi)x$ and $G_k(x, p) = g_k(x, p) - Dg_k(0, \pi)x$. For a given parameter $p \in \Pi$, let $\varphi^p$ denote the process associated to the impulsive system (13)–(14), and $L^p$ the process of its associated linearized equation (15)–(16). Suppose $L^\pi$ is hyperbolic and the sequence $\tau_k$ has a upper density bound. Then, there exists $\eta > 0$ such that for all $p_1, p_2 \in (\pi - \eta, \pi + \eta)$, there exists a family of homeomorphisms $H_t : \mathbb{R}^n \to \mathbb{R}^n$, $t \in \mathbb{R}$, with the following properties:

- For all $[u, v] \subset \mathbb{R}$ bounded, there exists $\delta > 0$ such that for all $||x|| < \delta$, one has $H_t \circ \varphi^{p_1}(t, s)x = \varphi^{p_2}(t, s)H_s x$ for all $[s, t] \subseteq [u, v]$.
- If $x^* = 0$ is linearly stable at parameter $\pi$, the previous conclusion holds, but the interval $[u, v]$ can be unbounded on the right.

*Proof* Write system (13)–(14) equivalently, for each parameter $p$, let $E(p)$ denote the system,

$$\dot{x} = Df(t, 0, \pi)x + F(t, x, p), \quad t \neq \tau_k$$
$$\Delta x = Dg_k(0, \pi)x + G_k(x, p), \quad t = \tau_k,$$

where $F(t, x, p) = f(t, x, p) - Df(t, 0, \pi)x$ and $G_k(x, p) = g_k(x, p) - Dg_k(0, \pi)x$. Also, denote by $L(\pi)$ its formal linearization

$$\dot{x} = Df(t, 0, \pi)x, \quad t \neq \tau_k$$
$$\Delta x = Dg_k(0, \pi)x, \quad t = \tau_k.$$

Broadly, the idea of the proof is as follows. We locally conjugate the process associated to $E(p_1)$ to $L(\pi)$ by a family of homeomorphism $H_t$, and also conjugate the process associated to $E(p_2)$ to $L(\pi)$ by a family of homeomorphism $G_t$. The family of compositions $G_t^{-1} \circ H_t$ will then be a local conjugacy of $E(p_1)$ with $E(p_2)$. Therefore, it is enough to emulate the proof of Theorem 1 with a parameter, establishing the existence of the conjugacy of $E(p_1)$ with $L(\pi)$ provided $|p_1 - \pi|$ is small enough, since the other conjugacy is obtained by the same method.

Let $\varphi$ denote the process associated with $E(p_1)$. Let $\epsilon > 0$ be a constant that has yet to be chosen. One has

$$||\varphi(t, u, x)|| \leq ||x|| + \int_u^t M(p)||\varphi(r, u, x)||dr + \sum_{u \leq \tau_k < t} M(p)||\varphi(\tau_k, u, x)||,$$

$$M(p) = \sup_{t \in [u,v]} ||Df(t, 0, \pi)|| + \max_{\tau_k \in [u,v]} ||Dg_k(0, \pi)||$$

$$+ \sup_{||x|| \leq \epsilon} H_u(x, p) + \sup_{||x|| \leq \epsilon} N_u(x, p),$$

provided $||x|| \leq \epsilon_2 < \epsilon$ for some $\epsilon_2$ and $t > u$ is small enough. By Gronwall's inequality for impulsive systems [1], it follows that

$$||\varphi(t, s, x)|| \leq ||x||(1 + M(p))^{N(\lceil t \rceil - \lfloor s \rfloor)} e^{M(p)(t-s)} := ||x||C_{s,t}(p)$$

for $t > s$ small enough. One obtains $||\varphi(t, s, x)|| \leq \epsilon$ for $[s, t] \subseteq [u, v]$ provided $||x|| \leq \epsilon_2 = \epsilon C_{u,v}(p)^{-1}$. As in the previous proof, set

$$A(\epsilon, \eta) = \sup_{(x,p)\in D} ||N_u(x, p)|| + 4 \sup_{(x,p)\in D} ||DH_u(x, p)||$$

with $D = \{(x, p) : ||x|| \leq 2\epsilon, |p - \pi| \leq \eta\}$, and choose $\eta > 0$ and $\epsilon > 0$ small enough so that inequality (8) is satisfied with $\gamma = A(\epsilon, \eta)$ for all $||x|| \leq 2\epsilon$ and $|p - \pi| < \eta$. Defining the cutoff process $\varphi_\epsilon$ at this $\epsilon > 0$ and choosing $p_1 \in (\pi - \eta, \pi + \eta)$, the proof proceeds in essentially the same way as that of Theorem 1, with the only difference being that $\eta$ and $\epsilon$ may need to be chosen smaller to accomodate for the restrictions $|F(t, x, p_1)| \leq \mu$ and $|G_k(x, p_1)| \leq \mu$ for the second point concerning stability. Again, the argument is analogous to the one for Theorem 1, and is omitted.

An obvious variant of Corollary 1 holds for Theorem 2.

**Corollary 2** *Inequalities* (17)–(18) *can be replaced with one of the following stronger assumptions.*

- *The nonlinear system* (13)–(14) *is periodic, each $g_k(x, p)$ is $C^1$, $f$ and $Df$ are continuous at $(t, x, p)$ unless $t = \tau_k$, where they are continuous from the left and have right limits in $t$.*
- *The vector field and jump map $f$ and $g_k$ of the nonlinear system are autonomous and $C^1$*

We should make a remark concerning the change of variables $x = y + x_p^*(t)$ preceding the statement of Theorem 2 that serves to translate the family of bounded parameter-dependent solutions $x_p^*(t)$ to the origin. After performing the change of variables, the vector field, for instance, becomes

$$\dot{y} = \tilde{f}(t, y, p) := f(t, y, p) - f(t, x_p^*(t), p).$$

One hypothesis of Theorem 2 is that $\tilde{f}$ is $C^1$, and since the bounded solution $x_p^*(t)$ depends on the parameter, it becomes necessary to study the smoothness of $p \mapsto x_p^*(t)$. If the functions $f$ and $g_k$ are $C^1$, the differentiability of $p \mapsto x_p^*(t)$ at a given parameter $\pi$ is equivalent [15] to the *variational equation*

$$\dot{z} = Df(t, x_\pi^*(t), \pi)z, \qquad\qquad t \neq \tau_k$$
$$\Delta z = Dg_k(x_\pi^*(\tau_k), \pi)z, \qquad\qquad t = \tau_k,$$

having exponential dichotomy, which in the new coordinate system is one one of the assumptions of Theorem 2: namely, that $L^\pi$ is hyperbolic, where $L^\pi$ is the process associated to the linearization. Conveniently, the linearization in this case is precisely the variational equation.

# 3   Conclusions

Theorem 1 provides a local topological conjugacy theorem for hyperbolic fixed points of finite-dimensional impulsive differential equations. The result is also applicable to hyperbolic periodic orbits and bounded solutions by first applying the changes of coordinates to map these orbits to the origin. Like the classical Hartman-Grobman theorem, our theorem requires only local smoothness properties of the vector field (and jump map). Other topological conjugacy theorems for impulsive systems assume strong global Lipschitz conditions, boundedness, and inequality conditions concerning the linearization, making our result more flexible.

Theorem 2 is a robustness result. It states that the dynamics near a hyperbolic equilibrium point or periodic orbit are robust with respect to parameter variation. Namely, the phase portraits are topologically conjugate. This strengthens a result of Church and Liu [15] concerning the absence of bifurcations at equilibrium points.

**Acknowledgements**  Kevin E. M. Church acknowledges the support of Natural Sciences and Engineering Research Council of Canada through the Alexander Graham Bell Canada Graduate Scholarships-Doctoral Program.

# References

 1. Bainov, D.D., Simeonov, P.S.: Impulsive Differential Equations: Periodic Solutions and Applications. Longman Scientific & Technical, Burnt Mill (1993)
 2. Samoilenko, A.M., Perestyuk, N.A.: Impulsive Differential Equations. World Scientific Publishing, Singapore (1995)
 3. Stamova, I.: Stability Analysis of Impulsive Functional Differential Equations. Walter de Grutyer GmBH & Co., Berlin (2009)
 4. Banerjee, C., Das, P.: Impulsive effect on tri-trophic food chain model with mixed functional responses under seasonal perturbations. Differ. Equ. Dyn. Syst. **26**(1–3), 157–176 (2018)
 5. Chávez, J.P., Jungmann, D., Siegmund, S.: Modeling and analysis of integrated pest control strategies via impulsive differential equations. Int. J. Differ. Equ. **2017**, 1820607 (2017)
 6. Huang, W., et al.: Dynamics of a saturation incidence SIRS epidemic model with pulses at different moments. In: 13th International Conference on Computational Intelligence and Security (CIS) (2017). https://doi.org/10.1109/CIS.2017.00086
 7. Wei, C., Liu, J., Chen, L.: Homoclinic bifurcation of a ratio-dependent predator-prey system with impulsive harvesting. Nonlinear Dyn. **89**(3), 2001–2012 (2017)
 8. Church, K.E.M., Liu, X.: Bifurcation analysis and application for impulsive systems with delayed impulses. Int. J. Bifurcat. Chaos **27**(12), 1750186 (2017)
 9. Chicone, C.: Ordinary Differential Equations with Applications. Springer, New York (1999)
10. Hein, M., Prüss, J.: The Hartman-Grobman theorem for semilinear hyperbolic evolution equations. J. Differ. Equ. **261**(8), 4709–4727 (2016)
11. Reinfelds, A., Šteinberga, D.: Dynamical equivalence of quasilinear dynamic equations on time scales. J. Math. Anal. **7**(1), 115–120 (2016)
12. Palmer, K.J.: A generalization of Hartman's linearization theorem. J. Math. Anal. Appl. **41**(3), 753–758 (1973)
13. Fenner, J.L., Pinto, M.: On a Hartman linearization theorem for a class of ODE with impulse effect. Nonlinear Anal. **38**(3), 307–325 (1999)

14. Reinfelds, A., Šteinberga, D.: Dynamical equivalence of impulsive quasilinear equations. Tatra Mt. Math. Publ. **63**(1), 237–346 (2015)
15. Church, K.E.M., Liu, X.: Bifurcation of bounded solutions of impulsive differential equations. Int. J. Bifurcat. Chaos **26**(14), 1650242 (2016)

# Oscillations in Low-Dimensional Cyclic Differential Delay Systems

### Anatoli F. Ivanov and Zari A. Dzalilov

**Abstract** Nonlinear autonomous $N$-dimensional systems of cyclic differential e-quations with delays and overall negative feedback are considered. Such systems serve as mathematical models of numerous real world phenomena in physics and laser optics, physiology and mathematical biology, economics and life sciences a-mong others. In the case of lower dimensions $N = 2$ and $N = 3$ sufficient conditions are derived for the oscillation of all solutions about the unique equilibrium. Open problems and conjectures are discussed for the higher dimensional case $N \geq 4$ and for more convoluted sign feedbacks.

**Keywords** Differential delays equations · Cyclic systems
Overall negative feedback · Unique equilibrium · Oscillatory solutions

## 1 Introduction

We consider a system of delay differential equations of the form

$$x_i'(t) = -\alpha_i x_i(t) + f_i(x_{i+1}(t - \tau_{i+1})), \ 1 \leq i \leq N, \tag{1}$$

where the functions $f_i(u)$ are real-valued and continuous on $\mathbf{R}$, $f_i \in C(\mathbf{R}, \mathbf{R})$, the decay rates $\alpha_i > 0$ are positive, and the delays $\tau_i$ are non-negative with the total delay $\tau = \sum_{i=1}^{N} \tau_i > 0$ being positive. The system is a cyclic one, with the variables $x_{N+1}$ and $\tau_{N+1}$ defined as $x_1$ and $\tau_1$, respectively, for the index value $i = N$.

Systems of form (1) are used in various applications, including physics and laser optics, physiology and mathematical biology, economics and life sciences among

A. F. Ivanov (✉)
Pennsylvania State University, Lehman, USA
e-mail: aivanov@psu.edu

Z. A. Dzalilov
Federation University, Ballarat, Australia
e-mail: z.dzalilov@federation.edu.au

© Springer Nature Switzerland AG 2018
D. M. Kilgour et al. (eds.), *Recent Advances in Mathematical
and Statistical Methods*, Springer Proceedings in Mathematics & Statistics 259,
https://doi.org/10.1007/978-3-319-99719-3_54

603

others. In particular, they naturally appear in physiology and mathematical biology [5, 7, 9, 10, 14], where they serve as models of enzyme production [6, 11] or of an intracellular circadian rhythm generator [12]. An extensive description of various applications can be found in e.g. [4, 5, 13, 14].

The problem of oscillatory behavior of all solutions in systems of type (1) is a very important one. From the applied point of view, when a system is a mathematical model of a real world phenomenon, it is essential to know whether solutions are monotone (and thus approaching an equilibrium) or they oscillate about the unique equilibrium. The oscillatory behavior is more typical in applied models; it also leads, under proper circumstances, to the existence of periodic motions in the model.

This work is devoted to derivation of sufficient conditions when all solutions of system (1) oscillate. Two partial cases of lower dimension $N = 2$ and $N = 3$ are studied.

## 2 Preliminaries

In this section we recall some basic notions and facts about system (1), introduce relevant definitions, and derive preliminary results necessary for the exposition and proof of our main results in Sect. 3.

The phase space of system (1) is the set $\mathbf{X} = C([-\tau_1, 0], \mathbf{R}) \times \cdots \times C ([-\tau_N, 0], \mathbf{R})$. For every initial function $\Phi = (\phi_1, \ldots, \phi_N) \in \mathbf{X}$, $\phi_i \in C([-\tau_i, 0], \mathbf{R})$, $1 \le i \le N$, there exists a unique solution $\mathbf{x} = \mathbf{x}(t) = \mathbf{x}(t, \Phi) = (x_1(t), \ldots, x_N(t))$ satisfying system (1) for all $t > 0$. The solution is built by the standard step-by-step integration procedure [1, 3, 8].

We also assume that each nonlinearity $f_i$ satisfies either the positive or negative feedback condition in the sense of the following definition.

**Definition 1** We say that function $f(u)$ satisfies the *positive* feedback condition on $\mathbf{R}$ if the following inequality holds

$$u \cdot f(u) > 0 \quad \text{for all} \quad u \in \mathbf{R}, \ u \ne 0. \tag{2}$$

Likewise, function $g(u)$ satisfies the *negative* feedback condition if the inequality holds

$$u \cdot g(u) < 0 \quad \text{for all} \quad u \in \mathbf{R}, \ u \ne 0. \tag{3}$$

When $i = N$ we set $i + 1 = 1$. If the number of nonlinearities in system (1) satisfying the negative feedback assumption (3) is odd we say that the system possesses the *overall negative feedback*. If it is even (including zero) the system is said to have the *overall positive feedback*.

It is easy to see that the sign assumptions (2) and (3) together with the continuity of $f_i$ imply that $f_i(0) = 0$, $1 \le i \le N$. Therefore, system (1) admits the only constant solution $\mathbf{0} = (0, \ldots, 0)$.

We shall make an additional assumption about the smoothness of functions $f_i$ in a neighborhood of zero: each $f_i$ is continuously differentiable for all $u$ such that $|u| \leq \delta$ for some $\delta > 0$. Their derivatives satisfy $f_i'(0) = a_i \neq 0, 1 \leq i \leq N$. The latter inequality describes a generic case for the nonlinearities $f_i$ around the zero equilibrium.

Note that system (1) can be reduced to a standard form where each of the nonlinearities $f_i, 1 \leq i \leq N - 1$, satisfies the positive feedback condition (2), while the last nonlinearity $f_N$ satisfies the negative feedback assumption (3) [2]. Indeed, assume that the $k$-th equation, $k < N$,

$$x_k'(t) = -\alpha_k x_k(t) + f_k(x_{k+1}(t - \tau_{k+1}))$$

is the first one in system (1) where the nonlinearity $f_k$ satisfies the negative feedback condition (3). Introduce then the new component $y_{k+1} =: -x_{k+1}$ and the new nonlinearity $\hat{f}_k(y_{k+1}) = f_k(-y_{k+1})$. One easily sees that $\hat{f}_k$ satisfies the positive feedback condition (2). The next $(k + 1)$-st equation of system (1) should also be rewritten in terms of the new $y_{k+1}$:

$$\begin{aligned} y_{k+1}'(t) &= -\alpha_{k+1} y_{k+1}(t) - f_{k+1}(x_{k+2}(t - \tau_{k+2})) \\ &= -\alpha_{k+1} y_{k+1}(t) + \hat{f}_{k+1}(x_{k+2}(t - \tau_{k+2})). \end{aligned}$$

If $\hat{f}_{k+1}, k + 1 < N$, satisfies the negative feedback condition, then one applies the same procedure of introducing the new variable $y_{k+2} = -x_{k+2}$ to this equation, and renaming the nonlinearity accordingly. If it satisfies the positive feedback condition then one moves to the next equation of the system, and so on until the last equation. The last $N$-th equation will satisfy the negative feedback assumption since the overall feedback in the system is negative.

**Definition 2** Let $\mathbf{x} = (x_1, \ldots, x_N)$ be a solution to system (1). We shall call its $k$-th component $x_k$ to be oscillatory (about zero) if there exists a sequence $t_n \to \infty, n \in \mathbf{N}$, such that $x_k(t_n) \cdot x_k(t_{n+1}) < 0$. The component $x_k$ will be called non-oscillatory if there exists $T \geq 0$ such that $|x_k(t)| > 0$ for all $t > T$. We exclude from consideration solutions which are identical zero for sufficiently large $t$: $\mathbf{x} = (0, \ldots, 0) \forall t \geq T$ for some $T \geq 0$.

**Lemma 1** *Let $\mathbf{x} = (x_1, \ldots, x_N)$ be an arbitrary solution to system (1).*

*(i) If its $k$-th component $x_k$ is oscillatory then any other component $x_i, i \neq k$, is oscillatory as well;*

*(ii) If its $k$-th component $x_k$ is non-oscillatory, so that $x_k(t) \geq 0$ or $x_k(t) \leq 0$ holds for all $t \geq T_1 \geq 0$, then there exists $T_2 \geq T_1$ such that $x_k(t) > 0$ or $x_k(t) < 0$ holds respectively for all $t \geq T_2$;*

*(iii) If its $k$-th component $x_k$ is of eventually definite sign, i.e. $x_k(t) > 0$ or $x_k(t) < 0$ for all $t > T$ and some $T \geq 0$, then any other component $x_i, i \neq k$, is also of eventually definite sign;*

*(iv) Every component $x_k$ of any non-oscillatory solution $\mathbf{x}$ satisfies*

$$\lim_{t \to \infty} x_k(t) = \lim_{t \to \infty} x'_k(t) = 0, \ 1 \le k \le N. \tag{4}$$

In order to prove Lemma 1 we need several simple facts about solutions of initial value problems for scalar first order ordinary differential equations.

**Proposition 1** *Consider the initial value problem*

$$u'(t) + \alpha u(t) = b(t), \quad u(t_0) = u_0, \quad t \ge t_0, \tag{5}$$

*where $\alpha > 0$ is a constant and $b(t)$ is a continuous real-valued function defined for $t \ge t_0$, $b \in C([t_0, \infty), \mathbf{R})$, with $b(t) \not\equiv 0$ for large values of $t$.*

*(i) If $u_0 \ge 0$ and $b(t) \ge 0$ for all $t \ge t_0$ then there exists $t_1 \ge t_0$ such that $u(t) > 0$ for all $t \ge t_1$. If $u_0 \le 0$ and $b(t) \le 0$ for all $t \ge t_0$ then there exists $t_2 \ge t_0$ such that $u(t) < 0$ for all $t \ge t_2$;*

*(ii) If $u_0 < 0$ and $b(t) \ge 0$ for all $t \ge t_0$ then either $u(t) < 0$ for all $t \ge t_0$, or there exists $t_1 \ge t_0$ such that $u(t_1) = 0$. Likewise, if $u_0 > 0$ and $b(t) \le 0$ for all $t \ge t_0$ then either $u(t) > 0$ for all $t \ge t_0$, or there exists $t_1 \ge t_0$ such that $u(t_1) = 0$. For either one of these two possibilities the solution $u(t)$ is of definite sign eventually (for all $t \ge T \ge t_0$ and some $T$).*

*Proof* The proof of this proposition easily follows from the integral representation of the solution of the initial value problem (5):

$$u(t) = u_0 \exp\{-\alpha(t - t_0)\} + \int_{t_0}^{t} \exp\{-\alpha(t - s)\} b(s) \, ds. \tag{6}$$

It is easily seen that when $u_0 > 0$ and $b(t) \ge 0$ then $u(t) > 0 \ \forall t \ge t_0$. When $u_0 = 0$ and $b(t) \ge 0$ (however, $b(t) \not\equiv 0$) then there exists point $t_1 \ge t_0$ such that $u(t) > 0 \ \forall t \ge t_1$ (since the integral value in (6) becomes positive for all large $t$). The remaining possibilities are treated analogously.

**Proposition 2** *Consider the initial value problem*

$$\beta v'(t) + v(t) = c(t), \quad v(t_0) = v_0, \quad t \ge t_0, \tag{7}$$

*where $\beta > 0$ is a constant and $c(t)$ is a continuous function, $c \in C([t_0, \infty), \mathbf{R})$, such that the limit $\lim_{t \to \infty} c(t) = c_0$ is finite. Then the solution $v(t)$ of the initial value problem (7) also has the same limit $\lim_{t \to \infty} v(t) = c_0$ (for any initial value $v_0 \in \mathbf{R}$ and any positive parameter value $\beta > 0$).*

*Proof* To prove the limit for any solution we shall show that for arbitrary $\varepsilon > 0$ there exists $t_\varepsilon \ge t_0$ such that the solution $v(t)$ satisfies the inclusion $v(t) \in [c_0 - \varepsilon, c_0 + \varepsilon]$ for all $t \ge t_\varepsilon$.

We shall show first that if a solution enters a sufficiently small neighborhood of value $c$ then it must stay there for all forward times. That is if the above claim about the solution $v(t)$ is not valid for a particular choice of $\beta > 0$, $v_0 \in \mathbf{R}$, and a sufficiently small $\varepsilon_0 > 0$ then the solution $v(t)$ must satisfy $v(t) \notin [c_0 - \varepsilon_0, c_0 + \varepsilon_0]$ for all $t \geq T_1 \geq t_0$ for some $T_1$. Indeed, given $\varepsilon_0 > 0$ one can choose $T_1$ large enough such that the inclusion $c(t) \in (c_0 - \varepsilon_0, c_0 + \varepsilon_0)$ holds for all $t \geq T_1$. If there exists a point $t_1 \geq T_1$ such that $v(t_1) \in [c_0 - \varepsilon_0, c_0 + \varepsilon_0]$ then $v(t) \in [c_0 - \varepsilon_0, c_0 + \varepsilon_0]$ must hold for all $t \geq t_1$. Indeed, assume that $t_2 \geq t_1$ is the first point of exit of the solution $v(t)$ from the interval $[c_0 - \varepsilon_0, c_0 + \varepsilon_0]$. To be definite, assume that $v(t_2) = c_0 + \varepsilon_0$, and $v(t) > c_0 + \varepsilon_0$ for all $t \in (t_2, t_2 + \delta)$ for some $\delta > 0$. Then the interval $(t_2, t_2 + \delta)$ also contains a point $t_3$ such that $v(t_3) > c_0 + \varepsilon_0$ and $v'(t_3) > 0$. On the other hand, according to the equation, $v'(t_3) = \frac{1}{\beta}[c(t_3) - v(t_3)] < 0$, a contradiction. The other possibility $v(t_2) = c_0 - \varepsilon_0$ leads to a contradiction in a similar way.

Therefore, we can assume next that there exists $T_2 \geq t_0$ such that $c(t) \in [c_0 - \varepsilon_0, c_0 + \varepsilon_0]$ and $v(t) \notin [c_0 - \varepsilon_0, c_0 + \varepsilon_0]$ for all $t \geq T_2$. To be definite, assume that $v(t) > c_0 + \varepsilon_0 \ \forall t \geq T_2$. Equation (7) then implies that $\beta v'(t) = c(t) - v(t) < 0$ for $t \geq T_2$, therefore the solution $v(t)$ is monotone decreasing. Set $v_0 = \lim_{t \to \infty} v(t) \geq c_0 + \varepsilon_0$. By using the limit values for functions $c(t)$ and $v(t)$ the last inequality yields

$$\beta v'(t) = c(t) - v(t) < c_0 + \sigma - (v_0 - \sigma) = c_0 - v_0 + 2\sigma < 0$$

for any sufficiently small $\sigma > 0$ and all $t \geq t_\sigma$ for some large $t_\sigma$. The latter implies that $\lim_{t \to \infty} v(t) = -\infty$, a contradiction with $v(t) \to v_0 \geq c_0 + \varepsilon_0$. The other possibility $v(t) < c_0 - \varepsilon_0 \ \forall t \geq T_2$ is treated analogously leading to a contradiction in a similar way. This completes the proof of the proposition.

Note that Proposition 2 can also be proved by using the variation of constant formula for the solution of the initial value problem (7).

Now we are in position to prove Lemma 1.

*Proof* We shall prove first that when a solution $\mathbf{x} = (x_1, \ldots, x_N)$ to system (1) is non-oscillatory, so either $x_k(t) \geq 0$ or $x_k(t) \leq 0$ holds for all $t \geq T_1$ and some $k \in \{1, 2, \ldots, N\}$, then there exists $T_2 \geq T_1$ such that in fact the strict inequalities hold: either $x_k(t) > 0$ or $x_k(t) < 0$ for all $t \geq T_2$. Besides, for every other component $x_i$, $i \neq k$, there exists time moment $s_i$ such that either $x_i(t) > 0$ or $x_i(t) < 0$ holds for all $t \geq s_i$.

To be definite, assume that $x_1(t) \geq 0 \ \forall t \geq T_1$ and $x_1(t) \not\equiv 0$ (other possibilities are considered similarly). Then the inequality $f_N(x_1(t - \tau_1)) \leq 0$ (and $\not\equiv 0$) holds for all large $t$. The last equation of system (1) can be represented in the integral form as follows

$$x_N(t) = x_N(t_0) \exp\{-\alpha_N(t - t_0)\} + \int_{t_0}^{t} \exp\{-\alpha_N(t - s)\} f_N(x_1(s - \tau_1)) \, ds. \quad (8)$$

One applies now Proposition 1 to conclude that either $x_N(t) > 0$ or $x_N(t) < 0$ holds eventually, since the kernel of the integral in the representation (8) is non-positive and is not identical zero eventually. Note that similarly to formula (8) any other equation of system (1) has its integral representation as follows

$$x_k(t) = x_k(t_0) \exp\{-\alpha_k(t - t_0)\} + \int_{t_0}^{t} \exp\{-\alpha_k(t - s)\} f_k(x_{k+1}(s - \tau_{k+1})) \, ds.$$

$$(9)$$

Using next the $(N - 1)$-st equation of the system, and its analogous representation in the form of integral Eq. (9) one finds that either $x_{N-1}(t) > 0$ or $x_{N-1}(t) < 0$ holds eventually. Going up along equations of system (1) one completes the proof of the claim for all the components $x_k$, $1 \le k \le N$.

We shall show next that all the components $x_i$, $1 \le i \le N$, of the non-oscillatory solution $\mathbf{x} = (x_1, \ldots, x_N)$ converge to zero together with their derivatives. To be definite assume that $x_1(t) > 0 \; \forall t \ge t_0$. Consider the last equation of system (1). Suppose first that $x_N(t) > 0$ holds for all $t \ge t_N$. Then $x'_N(t) = -\alpha_N x_N(t) + f_N(x_1(t - \tau_1)) < 0$ is satisfied for all large $t$. Therefore, the finite limit $\lim_{t\to\infty} x_N(t) = x_N^0 \ge 0$ exists. By using the second from the last equation of system (1), $x'_{N-1}(t) = -\alpha_{N-1} x_{N-1}(t) + f_{N-1}(x_N(t - \tau_N))$, its integral representation in the form of (9), and Proposition 2, one sees that the limit of the component $x_{N-1}(t)$ exists with $\lim_{t\to\infty} x_{N-1}(t) = (1/\alpha_{N-1}) f_{N-1}(x_N^0) =: x_{N-1}^0$. Likewise, $\lim_{t\to\infty} x_{N-2}(t) = (1/\alpha_{N-2}) f_{N-2}(x_{N-1}^0) =: x_{N-2}^0$, and finally the limit of the first component is $\lim_{t\to\infty} x_1(t) = (1/\alpha_2) f_2(x_2^0) =: x_1^0$. Using again the last equation of system (1) and Proposition 2 one finds that $\lim_{t\to\infty} x_N(t) = (1/\alpha_N) f_N(x_1^0) =: x_N^0$. Therefore, the constant $x_N^0$ satisfies the recursive equation

$$x_N^0 = \frac{1}{\alpha_N} f_N(x_1^0) = \frac{1}{\alpha_N} f_N \circ \frac{1}{\alpha_1} f_1(x_2^0) = \cdots = \frac{1}{\alpha_N} f_N \circ \frac{1}{\alpha_1} f_1 \circ \ldots \circ \frac{1}{\alpha_{N-1}} f_{N-1}(x_N^0).$$

Since function $F(u) = (1/\alpha_N) f_N \circ (1/\alpha_1) f_1 \circ \ldots \circ (1/\alpha_{N-1}) f_{N-1}(u)$ satisfies the negative feedback condition (3) the only solution of the equation $F(u) = u$ is $u = 0$. Therefore, $x_1^0 = x_2^0 = \cdots = x_N^0 = 0$. Also, one easily finds next that $\lim_{t\to\infty} x'_k(t) = \lim_{t\to\infty}[-\alpha_k x_k(t) + f_k(x_{k+1}(t - \tau_{k+1}))] = 0$. This completes the proof of the lemma.

## 3  Main Results

In this section we consider two particular cases of system (1) when $N = 2$ and $N = 3$. We establish sufficient conditions for the oscillatory behavior of all solutions in the system. The complete proof is provided for the case $N = 2$. The very same ideas for the proof are applicable for the three-dimensional system, however, an outline is only given for the more involved case $N = 3$, due to the length of considerations.

### 3.1  Two Dimensional Systems

Consider the two-dimensional case $N = 2$ of system (1)

$$x_1'(t) = -\alpha_1 x_1(t) + f_1(x_2(t - \tau_2))$$
$$x_2'(t) = -\alpha_2 x_2(t) + f_2(x_1(t - \tau_1)). \tag{10}$$

Since it is in the standard form $f_1$ satisfies the positive feedback assumption (2) while $f_2$ satisfies the negative feedback assumption (3). Introduce the following quantities: $a = -a_1 \cdot a_2 > 0$, $\tau_1 + \tau_2 = \tau > 0$, where $f_1'(0) = a_1 > 0$, $f_2'(0) = a_2 < 0$.

**Theorem 1** *Suppose that the inequality $a\tau > \max\{\alpha_1, \alpha_2\}$ is satisfied. Then all nontrivial solutions of system (10) oscillate.*

*Proof* Consider consecutively all the possibilities for non-oscillatory solutions of system (10).

(i) Assume first that inequalities $x_1(t) > 0$ and $x_2(t) > 0$ hold eventually. Then by Lemma 1 (iv) one has that

$$\lim_{t\to\infty} x_1(t) = \lim_{t\to\infty} x_2(t) = \lim_{t\to\infty} x_1'(t) = \lim_{t\to\infty} x_2'(t) = 0. \tag{11}$$

The second equation of system (10) shows that $x_2'(t) < 0$ eventually, so $x_2(t)$ is monotone decreasing to zero for large $t$. The first equation of (10) can be written in the form $(1/\alpha_1)x_1'(t) = -x_1(t) + (1/\alpha_1)f_1(x_2(t - \tau_2))$. Since $(1/\alpha_1)f_1(x_2(t - \tau_2)) > 0$ and is decreasing to zero as $x_2 \to 0^+$ one sees that the inequality $x_1(t) \leq (1/\alpha_1)f_1(x_2(t - \tau_2))$ holds for all sufficiently large $t$.

Assume now that for arbitrary $\varepsilon_1 > 0$ and $\varepsilon_2 > 0$ the values of $t$ are chosen to be large enough, $t \geq T$, so that the following inequalities hold:

$$f_2(x_1(t - \tau_1)) \leq [f_2'(0) + \varepsilon_1] x_1(t - \tau_1) \text{ and } f_1(x_2(t - \tau_2)) \geq [f_1'(0) - \varepsilon_2] x_2(t - \tau_2).$$

Integrate now the second equation of system (10) over the interval $[t - \tau, t]$:

$$x_2(t) - x_2(t - \tau) = -\alpha_2 \int_{t-\tau}^{t} x_2(s)\, ds + \int_{t-\tau}^{t} f_2(x_1(s - \tau_1))\, ds \leq$$

$$-\alpha_2 x_2(t)\tau + [f_2'(0) + \varepsilon_1] \int_{t-\tau}^{t} x_1(s - \tau_1)\, ds \leq$$

$$-\alpha_2 x_2(t)\tau + [f_2'(0) + \varepsilon_1] \frac{1}{\alpha_1} \int_{t-\tau}^{t} f_1(x_2(s - \tau))\, ds \leq$$

$$-\alpha_2 x_2(t)\tau + \frac{\tau}{\alpha_1} [f_2'(0) + \varepsilon_1][f_1'(0) - \varepsilon_2] x_2(t - \tau)).$$

Therefore, we obtain the inequality

$$x_2(t)[1 + \alpha_2\tau] \leq x_2(t - \tau)\left\{1 + \frac{\tau}{\alpha_1}[f_2'(0) + \varepsilon_1][f_1'(0) - \varepsilon_2]\right\}.$$

In the case when $1 + \frac{\tau}{\alpha_1}[f_2'(0) + \varepsilon_1][f_1'(0) - \varepsilon_2] < 0$ is satisfied we arrive at a contradiction with $x_2(t) > 0$. This will clearly be the case when the inequality $\tau a > \alpha_1$ is satisfied and $\varepsilon_1, \varepsilon_2$ are sufficiently small.

(ii) Assume next that inequalities $x_1(t) > 0$ and $x_2(t) < 0$ are satisfied eventually. As in part (i) one has the limits (11). The first equation of system (10) shows that $x_1'(t) < 0$ so $x_1(t)$ is decreasing to zero. The second equation of the system implies that $x_2'(t) > 0$ eventually, so $x_2(t)$ is increasing with $x_2(t) \le (1/\alpha_2)f_2(x_1(t - \tau_1))$ satisfied for all large $t$. Now integrate the first equation of the system over the interval $[t - \tau, t]$, assuming similar smallness of $\varepsilon_1, \varepsilon_2$ as in part (i) above:

$$x_1(t) - x_1(t - \tau) = -\alpha_1 \int_{t-\tau}^t x_1(s) \, ds + \int_{t-\tau}^t f_1(x_2(s - \tau_2) \, ds \le$$

$$-\alpha_1 \tau x_1(t) \, ds + \int_{t-\tau}^t [f_1'(0) - \varepsilon_1] x_2(s - \tau_2) \, ds \le$$

$$-\alpha_1 \tau x_1(t) \, ds + [f_1'(0) - \varepsilon_1] \int_{t-\tau}^t (1/\alpha_2) f_2(x_1(s - \tau)) \, ds \le$$

$$-\alpha_1 \tau x_1(t) \, ds + \frac{1}{\alpha_2}[f_1'(0) - \varepsilon_1][f_2'(0) + \varepsilon_2] \int_{t-\tau}^t x_1(s - \tau) \, ds \le$$

$$-\alpha_1 \tau x_1(t) \, ds + \frac{\tau}{\alpha_2}[f_1'(0) - \varepsilon_1][f_2'(0) + \varepsilon_2] x_1(t - \tau).$$

The last inequality implies that the following estimate holds

$$x_1(t) [1 + \alpha_1 \tau] \le x_1(t - \tau) \left\{ 1 + \frac{\tau}{\alpha_2}[f_1'(0) - \varepsilon_1][f_2'(0) + \varepsilon_2] \right\}.$$

Therefore when the condition $a\tau > \alpha_2$ is satisfied the latest inequality leads to a contradiction with $x_1(t) > 0$.

(iii) Two remaining subcases, $\{x_1(t) < 0, x_2(t) < 0\}$ and $\{x_1(t) < 0, x_2(t) > 0\}$ are symmetric to those treated above in cases (i) and (ii), respectively. The details of the proof are derived along the same lines, with a contradiction obtained to the assumption that $x_1(t) < 0$. They are left to the reader.

## 3.2   Three Dimensional Systems

Consider the three-dimensional case $N = 3$ of system (1)

$$x_1'(t) = -\alpha_1 x_1(t) + f_1(x_2(t - \tau_2))$$
$$x_2'(t) = -\alpha_2 x_2(t) + f_2(x_3(t - \tau_3)) \qquad (12)$$
$$x_3'(t) = -\alpha_3 x_3(t) + f_3(x_1(t - \tau_1)).$$

Since it is in the standard form $f_1$ and $f_2$ satisfy the positive feedback assumption (2) while $f_3$ satisfies the negative feedback assumption (3). Introduce the following quantities: $a = -a_1 a_2 a_3 > 0$, $\tau_1 + \tau_2 + \tau_3 = \tau > 0$ where $f_1'(0) = a_1 > 0$, $f_2'(0) = a_2 > 0$, $f_3'(0) = a_3 < 0$.

**Theorem 2** *Suppose that the inequality* $a\tau > \max\{\alpha_1\alpha_2, \alpha_1\alpha_3, \alpha_2\alpha_3\}$ *is satisfied. Then all nontrivial solutions of system (10) oscillate.*

*Proof* The proof of this theorem in very similar to that of Theorem 1. One has to consider the following three principal subcases for the eventual signs of the components $x_1, x_2, x_3$ of a non-oscillating solution **x**: $\{x_1 > 0, x_2 > 0, x_3 > 0\}$, $\{x_1 > 0, x_2 > 0, x_3 < 0\}$, and $\{x_1 > 0, x_2 < 0, x_3 < 0\}$. The remaining five subcases are symmetric opposite or similar to those three, and are considered along the same lines. For example, the case $\{x_1 > 0, x_2 > 0, x_3 > 0\}$ leads to the following integral equation for the component $x_3$, when the last equation of the system is integrated over the interval $[t - \tau, t]$,

$$x_3(t) - x_3(t - \tau) = -\alpha_3 \int_{t-\tau}^{t} x_3(s)\, ds + \int_{t-\tau}^{t} f_3(x_1(s - \tau_1))\, ds,$$

and to the following two inequalities for the components $x_1$ and $x_2$

$$x_1(t) \geq \frac{1}{\alpha_1} f_1(x_2(t - \tau_2)), \quad x_2(t) \geq \frac{1}{\alpha_2} f_2(x_3(t - \tau_3)).$$

Substituting the latter into the integral equation, one derives a contradiction with the assumption $x_3(t) > 0$, when the inequality $\tau a > \alpha_1\alpha_2$ is satisfied. The other two principal subcases lead to a similar contradiction when the other two assumptions are in place, $\tau a > \alpha_1\alpha_3$ and $\tau a > \alpha_2\alpha_3$. We leave details to the reader.

# 4 Discussion

Theorems 1 and 2 provide simple and verifiable sufficient conditions for the oscillation of all solutions of system (1) in cases $N = 2$ and $N = 3$. In the case when the feedback functions $f_1, f_2, f_3$ are fixed, and the rates of decay of all the components are bounded above, $\max_i \alpha_i \leq \alpha_0$ for some fixed constant $\alpha_0 > 0$, a sufficiently large overall delay $\tau = \sum_{i=0}^{N}$ in the system forces all its solutions to oscillate. We believe that an analogue of these two theorems is valid in the case of general dimension $N$. However, we are not in a position to provide a complete proof at this time. The ideas used in the proof of Theorems 1 and 2 cannot be extended to the case $N \geq 4$, due to the variety and complexity of all the subcases. Therefore, we are only in a position to state the following conjecture.

Set $a = -a_1 a_2 \ldots a_{N-1} a_N > 0$ and $\tau = \tau_1 + \cdots + \tau_N > 0$, where $f_i'(0) = a_i > 0$, $1 \leq i \leq N - 1$ and $f_N'(0) = a_N < 0$. Given positive $\alpha_1, \ldots, \alpha_N$ introduce the following quantities: $\Lambda_i = \prod_{k \neq i} \alpha_k$, $1 \leq i \leq N$.

**Conjecture 1** Suppose that the inequality $a\tau > \max\{ \Lambda_1, \ldots, \Lambda_N \}$ is satisfied. Then all nontrivial solutions of system (1) oscillate.

Another interesting and challenging problem is to derive sufficient conditions for the oscillation of all solutions in cyclic type systems when either a positive or a negative type feedback is in place between any two consecutive components $x_k$ and $x_{k+1}$, however, all other components are also involved on every step. In the simplest case of dimension $N = 2$ such system would have the form

$$x_1'(t) = -\alpha_1 x_1(t) + f_1(x_1(t - \tau_1), x_2(t - \tau_2))$$
$$x_2'(t) = -\alpha_2 x_2(t) + f_2(x_1(t - \tau_1), x_2(t - \tau_2)),$$

where the nonlinearities $f_1$ and $f_2$ satisfy the positive and negative feedback assumptions, respectively, in the following sense:

$$v \cdot f_1(u, v) > 0 \ \ \forall (u, v) \in \mathbf{R}^2, v \neq 0 \ \ \ \ u \cdot f_2(u, v) < 0 \ \ \forall (u, v) \in \mathbf{R}^2, u \neq 0.$$

This problem can be generalized to the case of arbitrary dimension $N$. This oscillation problem and the above stated Conjecture 1 represent a program for future research.

**Acknowledgements** This work was initiated in the fall 2016 during A. Ivanov's visit and research stay at the University of Giessen, Germany, under the support of the Alexander von Humboldt Stiftung. In its final stages and during the preparation for publication A. Ivanov and Z. Dzalilov were supported by internal grants from the Federation University Australia (Ballarat, Victoria).

# References

1. Bellman, R., Cooke, K.L.: Differential-Difference Equations. Academic Press, New York (1963)
2. Bravermen, E., Hasik, K., Ivanov, A.F., Trofimchuk, S.I.: A cyclic system with delay and its characteristic equation. Discrete and Continuous Dynamical Systems, Ser. S (to appear); Preprint, July 2017, 22 p. (arXiv:1707.06726 [math.CA])
3. Diekmann, O., van Gils, S., Verdyn Lunel, S.M., Walther, H.-O.: Delay Equations: Complex, Functional, and Nonlinear Analysis. Springer, New York (1995)
4. Erneux, T.: Applied Delay Differential Equations, vol. 3. Series: Surveys and Tutorials in the Applied Mathematical Sciences. Springer, Berlin (2009)
5. Glass, L., Mackey, M.C.: From Clocks to Chaos. The Rhythms of Life. Princeton University Press, Princeton (1988)
6. Goodwin, B.C.: Oscillatory behaviour in enzymatic control process. Adv. Enzime Regul. **3**, 425–438 (1965)
7. Hadeler, K.P.: Delay equations in biology. Springer Lect. Notes Math. **730**, 139–156 (1979)
8. Hale, J.K., Verduyn Lunel, S.M.: Introduction to Functional Differential Equations. Applied Mathematical Sciences. Springer, Berlin (1993)

9. Hopfield, J.: Neural networks and physical systems with emergent collective computational abilities. Proc. Nat. Acad. Sci. USA **79**, 2554–2558 (1982)
10. Kuang, Y.: Delay Differential Equations with Applications in Population Dynamics, vol. 191. Series: Mathematics in Science and Engineering. Academic Press Inc., New York (2003)
11. Mahaffy, J.: Periodic solutions of certain protein synthesis models. J. Math. Anal. Appl. **74**, 72–105 (1980)
12. Scheper, T., Klinkenberg, D., Pennartz, C., van Pelt, J.: A mathematical model for the intracellular circadian rhythm generator. J. Neurosci. **19**(1), 40–47 (1999)
13. Smith, H.: An Introduction to Delay Differential Equations with Applications to the Life Sciences, vol. 57. Series: Texts in Applied Mathematics. Springer, Berlin (2011)
14. Wu, J.: Introduction to Neural Dynamics and Signal Transmission Delay. Nonlinear Anal. Appl., vol. 6, Walter de Gruyter & Co., Berlin (2001)

# Asynchronous Control of Switched Nonlinear Systems

**Jiaojiao Ren, Xinzhi Liu, Hong Zhu and Shouming Zhong**

**Abstract** This paper studies the problem of asynchronous control of switched nonlinear systems. The asynchronous control means that the switchings between the candidate controllers and system models are asynchronous. By using the piecewise Lyapunov function and average dwell time approach, the asynchronously switched stabilizing control problem for nonlinear systems is solved under the proposed switching law, which allows us to have a stable or unstable subnonlinear system. Illustrative examples are provided to show the effectiveness of the results.

**Keywords** Asynchronous control · Switched nonlinear system
Exponential stability · Average dwell time

## 1 Introduction

Switched systems [1, 2], consisting of a family of subsystems and a switching rule that orchestrates the switching between them, have been used to model many physical

J. Ren (✉)
School of Information Science and Engineering,
Chengdu University, Chengdu 610106, People's Republic of China
e-mail: jiaojiaoren06@163.com

J. Ren · X. Liu
Department of Applied Mathematics, University of Waterloo,
Waterloo, ON N2L 3G1, Canada
e-mail: xzliu@uwaterloo.ca

H. Zhu
School of Automation Engineering, University of Electronic Science
and Technology of China, Sichuan 611731, People's Republic of China
e-mail: zhuhong@uestc.edu.cn

S. Zhong
School of Mathematical Sciences, University of Electronic Science
and Technology of China, Sichuan 611731, People's Republic of China
e-mail: zhongsm@uestc.edu.cn

© Springer Nature Switzerland AG 2018
D. M. Kilgour et al. (eds.), *Recent Advances in Mathematical
and Statistical Methods*, Springer Proceedings in Mathematics & Statistics 259,
https://doi.org/10.1007/978-3-319-99719-3_55

or man-made systems displaying switching features. The diverse switching signals differentiate switched systems from general time-varying systems, since the solutions of the switched systems are dependent on not only the system's initial conditions but also the switching signals. This class of systems have numerous applications in the control of mechanical systems, the automotive industry, air traffic control, switching power converters and many other fields [2].

In switched systems, each subsystem is called a mode, and control problems are said to design a set of mode-dependent controllers or mode-independent controllers for the unforced system and find admissible switching signals such that the resulting systems is stable or satisfies certain performance criteria [2–4]. As we know, mode-dependent controller design is less conservative. However, for the control problem, it inevitably takes some time to identify the system modes and apply the matched controller. So, a very common assumption in the mode-dependent context, the controllers are switched synchronously with the switching of system modes, is quite unpractical. Therefore, the asynchronous phenomena between the system modes and the controller modes always exists. Recently, some efforts have been made to study asynchronous control problems [5–9]. In [5–8], each subsystem is stable. In [5], desirable controller is designed such that the energy function is decreasing in each switching interval (both mismatched period and matched period). This requirement is weakened in [6–8]. The energy function is not required decreasing in mismatched period any more. Most recently, in [9], the authors deal with asynchronous stabilization problem of switched system, which contains stable and unstable subsystems. However, the condition $\inf_{t \geq t_0} \left[ \frac{T^-(t)}{T^+(t)} \right] \geq -\frac{\beta}{\alpha}$ can not guarantee the condition $-\gamma t = T^-(t)\alpha + T^+(t)\beta$ holds, which only can guarantee $T^-(t)\alpha + T^+(t)\beta < 0$ holds, where, $T^-(t)$ and $T^+(t)$ represent, respectively, the total active time of subsystems that are stable, not stable subsystems over $(0, t)$; $\alpha$, $\beta$ and $\gamma$ are constants. Therefore, a switching law is need.

In this paper, the problem of asynchronous control of switched nonlinear systems is studied. By using the piecewise Lyapunov function and average dwell time approach, the asynchronously switched stabilizing control problem for nonlinear systems is solved under the proposed switching law , which allows us to have stable and unstable subnonlinear system. Some examples are provided to show the effectiveness of the results.

## 2 Problem Descriptions and Preliminaries

Consider the following switched nonlinear system:

$$\dot{x}(t) = f_{\sigma(t)}(x(t), u(t)), \tag{1}$$

where $x(t) \in R^n$ is a state vector and $u(t) \in R^m$ is a control input vector. $f_{\sigma(t)}$ are a set of regularly nonlinear functions. $\sigma(t) : [0, \infty) \to \mathbb{S}$ is the switching signal, i.e., $\sigma(t) = i_k \in \mathbb{S}$ for $t \in [t_k, t_{k+1})$, where $t_k$ is the $k$th switching time instant, $\mathbb{S} = \{1, 2, \ldots, s\}$, $s, k \in \mathbb{N}$. $0 = t_0 < t_1 < \ldots < t_k < \ldots$, $\lim_{k \to \infty} t_k = \infty$, which can rule out Zeno behavior automatically.

In fact, for the control problem, it inevitably takes some time to identify the system modes and apply the matched controller. Therefore, the asynchronous phenomena between the system modes and the controller modes always exists. In this paper, we assume that the time lag of controllers modes to system modes is $t_d > 0$ ($t_d < t_{k+1} - t_k$, $k \in N$). The state feedback control input can be written as $u(t) = K_{\sigma(t-t_d)} x(t)$.

Before proceeding further, the following definitions are introduced.

**Definition 2.1** [10] For a switching signal $\sigma(t)$ and any $t'' > t' > t_0$, let $N_\sigma(t', t'')$ be the switching numbers of $\sigma(t)$ over the interval $[t', t'')$. If $N_\sigma(t', t'') \leq N_0 + \frac{t'' - t'}{\tau_a}$ holds for $N_0 \geq 1$, $\tau_a > 0$, then $N_0$ and $\tau_a$ are called the chatter bound and the average dwell time, respectively.

**Note that**: When the active subsystems are changed at some time instant, a switching happens. Therefore, switching numbers mean the total numbers of switching.

**Definition 2.2** [6] The equilibrium point of system (1) is globally uniformly exponentially stable under certain switching signals $\sigma(t)$ if, for $u(t)$, there exist constants $K > 0$ and $\delta > 0$ such that the solution of the system satisfies $\|x(t)\| \leq Ke^{-\delta(t-t_0)} \|x(t_0)\|$, $\forall t \geq t_0$.

## 3 Main Results

In this section, we first proposed a switching law for the system (1). Under this switching law, the sufficient condition is given to guarantee the system (1) without control input is exponentially stable by using average dwell time. Second, the obtained result is extended to the system with control input.

### 3.1 Exponential Stability for the System (1) Without Control Input

**Switching law 3.1** [11] Let $0 = t^0 < t^1 < t^2 < \ldots$ ($\lim_{j \to \infty} t^j = \infty$) be a specified sequence of time instants satisfying $\sup_j \{t^{j+1} - t^j\} = T < \infty$. Determine the switching signal $\sigma(t)$ such that the inequality $T^-(t^j, t^{j+1})/T^+(t^j, t^{j+1}) \geq -(\beta + \alpha^*)/(\alpha + \alpha^*)$ holds on every time interval $[t^j, t^{j+1})$ ($j = 0, 1, \ldots$), where $0 < \alpha^* < -\alpha$, $\alpha$ and $\beta$ are given constants, $T^-(t^j, t^{j+1})$ and $T^+(t^j, t^{j+1})$ denote the total active time of stable and unstable subsystems respectively over $(t^j, t^{j+1})$.

Based on the given switching law 3.1, the following theorem is presented to guarantee the system is exponentially stable.

**Theorem 3.1** *For the given scalars $\alpha_{\sigma(t)}$ and $\mu \geq 1$, the system (1) with $u(t) = 0$, under the switching law 3.1, is exponentially stable if there exist Lyapunov functions $V_{\sigma(t)}(t) : R^n \rightarrow R$, and two positive constants $K_1$ and $K_2$ such that $\forall \sigma(t) = i \in \mathbb{S}$ the following inequalities hold*

$$K_1 \|x(t)\|^2 \leq V_i(t) \leq K_2 \|x(t)\|^2, \tag{2}$$

$$\dot{V}_i(t) \leq \alpha_i V_i(t), t \in [t_k, t_{k+1}) \tag{3}$$

$$V_{\sigma(t_k)}(t_k) \leq \mu V_{\sigma(t_k^-)}(t_k^-), \tag{4}$$

$$\tau_a > \frac{\ln \mu}{\alpha^*}. \tag{5}$$

*Proof* When $\forall t \in [t_k, t_{k+1})$, for $\sigma(t) = i \in \mathbb{S}, k \in N$, it means the switched system is active within the $i$th subsystem. From (3) and (4), we have

$$\begin{aligned} V_{\sigma(t)}(t) &\leq e^{\alpha_i(t-t_k)} V_{\sigma(t_k)}(t_k) \\ &\leq \mu e^{\alpha_i(t-t_k)} V_{\sigma(t_k^-)}(t_k^-) \\ &\leq \mu e^{\alpha_i(t-t_k)+\alpha_{\sigma(t_{k-1})}(t_k-t_{k-1})} V_{\sigma(t_{k-1})}(t_{k-1}) \\ &\leq \mu^2 e^{\alpha_i(t-t_k)+\alpha_{\sigma(t_{k-1})}(t_k-t_{k-1})} V_{\sigma(t_{k-1}^-)}(t_{k-1}^-) \\ &\leq \dots \\ &\leq \mu^{N_\sigma(t_0,t)} V_{\sigma(t_0)}(t_0) e^{\alpha T^-(t_0,t)+\beta T^+(t_0,t)}, \end{aligned} \tag{6}$$

where $\alpha = \sup_{i \in \mathbb{S}}\{\alpha_i : \alpha_i < 0\}$, $\beta = \sup_{i \in \mathbb{S}}\{\alpha_i : \alpha_i \geq 0\}$, $T^-(t_0, t)$ and $T^+(t_0, t)$ denote the total active time of those subsystems that are stable, not stable subsystems over $(t_0, t)$, respectively.

Suppose $0 = t^0 < t^1 < t^2 < \dots$ ($\lim_{j \to \infty} t^j = \infty$) be a specified sequence of time instants satisfying Switching law 3.1. For any $t$, we have two cases:

(1) For $t_0$ and $t$ satisfying $t^{j-1} < t_0 \leq t^j < t^{j+1} < \dots < t^k \leq t$, one has

$$\frac{T^-(t^j, t^{j+1})}{T^+(t^j, t^{j+1})} \geq -\frac{\beta + \alpha^*}{\alpha + \alpha^*}$$

$$\Rightarrow T^-(t^j, t^{j+1})(-\alpha - \alpha^*) \geq T^+(t^j, t^{j+1})(\beta + \alpha^*)$$

$$\Rightarrow -\alpha^*(T^-(t^j, t^{j+1}) + T^+(t^j, t^{j+1})) \geq \alpha T^-(t^j, t^{j+1}) + \beta T^+(t^j, t^{j+1})$$

$$\Rightarrow -\alpha^*(t^{j+1} - t^j) \geq \alpha T^-(t^j, t^{j+1}) + \beta T^+(t^j, t^{j+1}), \tag{7}$$

$$\frac{T^-(t^j, t^{j+1})}{T^+(t^j, t^{j+1})} \geq -\frac{\beta + \alpha^*}{\alpha + \alpha^*}$$

$$\Rightarrow T^-(t^j, t^{j+1})(-\alpha - \alpha^*) \geq T^+(t^j, t^{j+1})(\beta + \alpha^*)$$

$$\Rightarrow T^-(t^j, t^{j+1})(-\alpha - \alpha^*) + T^+(t^j, t^{j+1})(-\alpha - \alpha^*)$$

$$\geq T^+(t^j, t^{j+1})(\beta + \alpha^*) + T^+(t^j, t^{j+1})(-\alpha - \alpha^*)$$

$$\Rightarrow T^+(t^j, t^{j+1}) \leq \frac{-\alpha - \alpha^*}{\beta - \alpha} T, \tag{8}$$

and whether or not the activated subsystems over the interval $[t_0, t^j]$ and $[t^k, t]$ are stable subsystems, we consider that the activated subsystems over the interval $[t_0, t^j]$ and $[t^k, t]$ are unstable subsystems. Then, one obtain

$$e^{\alpha T^-(t_0,t)+\beta T^+(t_0,t)} \leq e^{\beta(t^j - t_0)+\sum_{q=j}^{k-1}[\beta T^+(t^q,t^{q+1})+\alpha T^-(t^q,t^{q+1})]+\beta(t-t^k)}$$

According to (7) and (8), one obtains

$$e^{\alpha T^-(t_0,t)+\beta T^+(t_0,t)} \leq e^{\beta(t-t^k)-\alpha^* \sum_{q=j}^{k-1}(t^{q+1}-t^q)+\beta(t^j - t_0)}$$

$$= e^{\beta(t-t^k)-\alpha^*(t^k - t^j)+\beta(t^j - t_0)}$$

$$= e^{(\beta+\alpha^*)(t-t^k+t^j - t_0)-\alpha^*(t - t_0)}$$

$$\leq e^{(\beta+\alpha^*)(T^+(t^k,t^{k+1})+T^+(t^{j-1},t^j))-\alpha^*(t - t_0)}$$

$$\leq e^{\gamma-\alpha^*(t - t_0)}, \tag{9}$$

where $\gamma = \frac{-2(\beta+\alpha^*)(\alpha+\alpha^*)}{\beta-\alpha} T$.

(2) For $t_0$ and $t$ satisfying $t^q \leq t_0 < t \leq t^{q+1}$, one has

$$e^{\alpha T^-(t_0,t)+\beta T^+(t_0,t)} \leq e^{\beta(t-t_0)}$$

$$= e^{(\beta+\alpha^*)(t-t_0)-\alpha^*(t-t_0)}$$

$$\leq e^{\gamma-\alpha^*(t-t_0)}, \tag{10}$$

where $\gamma$ has the same value as the one above.

Based on (6), (9) and (10) and average dwell time, for any $t$, the following inequality holds

$$V_{\sigma(t)}(t) \leq \mu^{N_\sigma(t_0,t)} V_{\sigma(t_0)}(t_0) e^{\alpha T^-(t_0,t)+\beta T^+(t_0,t)}$$

$$\leq e^{N_0 \ln \mu + \gamma} e^{(\frac{\ln \mu}{\tau_a}-\alpha^*)(t-t_0)} V_{\sigma(t_0)}(t_0). \tag{11}$$

From (2) and (5), we have

$$\|x(t)\| \leq K e^{-\kappa(t-t_0)} \|x(t_0)\|, \tag{12}$$

where $K = (\frac{K_2}{K_1} e^{N_0 \ln \mu + \gamma})^{1/2}$ and $\kappa = \frac{1}{2}(\alpha^* - \frac{\ln \mu}{\tau_a})$.

Therefore, the system (1) without control input is exponentially stable.

## 3.2    Exponential Stability for the System (1)
##         With Control Input

**Switching law 3.2** *Let* $0 = t^0 < t^1 < t^2 < \ldots (\lim_{j \to \infty} t^j = \infty)$ *be a specified sequence of time instants satisfying* $\sup_j \{t^{j+1} - t^j\} = T < \infty$. *Determine the switching signal* $\sigma(t)$ *such that the inequality* $(T^-(t^j, t^{j+1}) - N_\sigma^-(t^j, t^{j+1})t_d)/(T^+(t^j, t^{j+1}) + N_\sigma^-(t^j, t^{j+1})t_d) \geq -(\beta + \alpha^*)/(\alpha + \alpha^*)$ *holds on every time interval* $[t^j, t^j + 1)(j = 0, 1, \ldots)$, *where* $0 < \alpha^* < -\alpha$, $\alpha$ *and* $\beta$ *are given constants.* $T^-(t^j, t^{j+1})$, $T^+(t^j, t^{j+1})$ *and* $N_\sigma^-(t^j, t^{j+1})$ *denote the total active time of those subsystems that are stable, not stable subsystems and the total switching numbers of stable subsystems over* $(t^j, t^{j+1})$, *respectively.*

Based on the given switching law 3.2, the following theorem is presented to guarantee the system is exponentially stable.

**Theorem 3.2** *For the given scalars* $\alpha_{\sigma(t), \sigma(t-t_d)}$ *and* $\mu \geq 1$, *the system (1) with* $u(t) = K_{\sigma(t-t_d)}x(t)$, *under the switching law 3.2, is exponentially stable if there exist Lyapunov functions* $V_{\sigma(t), \sigma(t-t_d)}(t) : R^n \to R$, *and two positive constants* $\hat{K}_1$ *and* $\hat{K}_2$ *such that* $\forall \sigma(t) = i$, $\sigma(t - t_d) = p$, $\forall i, p \in \mathbb{S}$ *the following inequalities hold*

$$\hat{K}_1 \|x(t)\|^2 \leq V_{i,p}(t) \leq \hat{K}_2 \|x(t)\|^2, \tag{13}$$

$$\dot{V}_{i,p}(t) \leq \begin{cases} \alpha_{i,p} V_{i,p}(t), & t \in [t_k, t_k + t_d), i \neq p, \\ \alpha_{i,i} V_{i,i}(t), & t \in [t_k + t_d, t_{k+1}), i = p, \end{cases} \tag{14}$$

$$V_{\sigma(t_k), \sigma(t_k - t_d)}(t_k) \leq \hat{\mu} V_{\sigma(t_k^-), \sigma(t_k^- - t_d)}(t_k^-), \tag{15}$$

$$V_{\sigma(t_k+t_d), \sigma(t_k)}(t_k + t_d) \leq \hat{\mu} V_{\sigma(t_k^- + t_d), \sigma(t_k^-)}(t_k^- + t_d), \tag{16}$$

$$\tau_a > \frac{2 \ln \hat{\mu}}{\alpha^*}. \tag{17}$$

*Proof* When $\forall t \in [t_k + t_d, t_{k+1})$, $\sigma(t) = i \in \mathbb{S}$; $\forall t \in [t_k, t_k + t_d)$, $\sigma(t - t_s) = p \in \mathbb{S}$, $k \in N$. From (14), (15) and (16), we have

$$\begin{aligned}
V_{\sigma(t), \sigma(t-t_d)}(t) &\leq e^{\alpha_{i,i}(t-t_k-t_d)} V_{\sigma(t_k+t_d), \sigma(t_k)}(t_k + t_d) \\
&\leq \hat{\mu} e^{\alpha_{i,i}(t-t_k-t_d)} V_{\sigma(t_k^- + t_d), \sigma(t_k^-)}(t_k^- + t_d) \\
&\leq \hat{\mu} e^{\alpha_{i,i}(t-t_k-t_d) + \alpha_{i,p}t_d} V_{\sigma(t_k), \sigma(t_k-t_d)}(t_k) \\
&\leq \hat{\mu}^2 e^{\alpha_{i,i}(t-t_k-t_d) + \alpha_{i,p}t_d} V_{\sigma(t_k^-), \sigma(t_k^- - t_d)}(t_k^-) \\
&\leq \ldots \\
&\leq \hat{\mu}^{2N_\sigma(t_0,t)} e^{\alpha(T^-(t_0,t) - N_\sigma^-(t_0,t)t_d) + \beta(T^+(t_0,t) + N_\sigma^-(t_0,t)t_d)} \times \\
&\quad\; V_{\sigma(t_0), \sigma(t_0-t_d)} V(t_0),
\end{aligned} \tag{18}$$

where $\alpha = \sup_{i \in \mathbb{S}} \{\alpha_{i,i}, \alpha_{i,i} < 0\}, \beta = \sup_{i, p \in \mathbb{S}, i \neq p} \{\alpha_{i,p}, \alpha_{i,i} > 0\}, T^-(t_0, t), T^+(t_0, t)$ and $N_\sigma^-(t_0, t)$ denote the total active time of those subsystems that are stable, not stable subsystems and the total switching numbers of stable subsystems over $(t_0, t)$, respectively.

Combining Switching law 3.2 and following the similar proof procedure, we can conclude that the system (1) with $u(t) = K_{\sigma(t-t_d)} x(t)$, under the switching law 3.2, is exponentially stable.

# 4   Numerical Examples

*Example 1*   Consider the following switched nonlinear system without control input
**Switching Region 1**: $\sigma(t) = 1$

$$\dot{x}_1(t) = 0.2x_1(t) + 0.1x_2(t) - 0.15|sin(10x_2(t))|e^{-sin(10x_2(t))}x_2(t)$$
$$\dot{x}_2(t) = 0.7x_1(t) + 0.02x_2(t) \tag{19}$$

**Switching Region 2**: $\sigma(t) = 2$

$$\dot{x}_1(t) = -x_1(t)$$
$$\dot{x}_2(t) = -0.2|cos(10x_1(t))|x_1(t) - x_2(t) \tag{20}$$

Here, let $\alpha_1 = 1.5, \alpha_2 = -0.6, \alpha^* = 0.3$ and $\mu = 1.2$. According to Switching law 3.1, for $t \in [0, 12]$, the switching signal $\sigma(t)$ is given as follows:

$$\sigma(t) = 1: \quad t \in [0, 0.3), \quad [2.9, 3.4), \quad [6.8, 7.1), \quad [8.9, 9.4),$$
$$\sigma(t) = 2: \quad t \in [0.3, 2.9), \quad [3.4, 6.8), \quad [7.1, 8.9), \quad [9.4, 12],$$

where the specified sequence of time instants $\{t_n\}_{n=0}^4$ is given as $\{0, 3, 6, 9, 12\}$. Note that the condition $1.5 = \tau_a \geq \frac{\ln \mu}{\alpha^*} = 0.6077$ also holds. The simulation results are shown in Figs. 1 and 2, which well illustrate Theorem 3.1.

*Example 2*   Consider the following switched nonlinear system
**Switching Region 1**: $\sigma(t) = 1$

$$\dot{x}_1(t) = x_1(t) + 0.1x_2(t) + 0.15|sin(6x_1(t))|e^{-sin(6x_1(t))}x_2(t)$$
$$+ (0.1 + \frac{0.4}{e}|sin(6x_1(t))|e^{-sin(6x_1(t))})u_1(t)$$
$$\dot{x}_2(t) = 0.7x_1(t) + 0.2x_2(t), \tag{21}$$

**Fig. 1** The switching signal
$\sigma(t)$

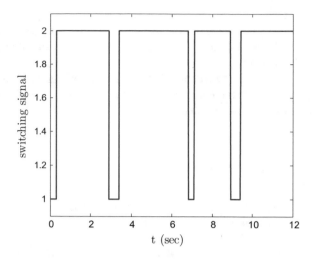

**Fig. 2** The state trajectories
of the system (3)

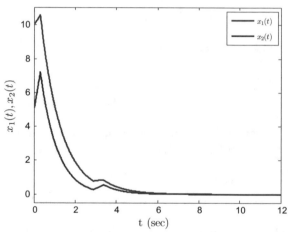

**Switching Region 2**: $\sigma(t) = 2$

$$\dot{x}_1(t) = 0.6x_1(t) + 0.3u_1(t) + 0.7|cos(6x_2(t))|u_1(t)$$
$$\dot{x}_2(t) = 0.2|cos(10x_2(t))|x_1(t) - 0.7x_2(t), \tag{22}$$

Here, let $\alpha_{11} = 0.2$, $\alpha_{12} = 0.5$, $\alpha_{21} = 0.1$, $\alpha_{22} = -0.3$, $\alpha^* = 0.2$, $\mu = 1.1$ and $t_d = 0.2$. According to Switching law 3.2, for $t \in [0, 12]$, the switching signal $\sigma(t)$ and $\sigma(t - t_d)$ are given as follows:

$$\sigma(t) = 1: \quad t \in [0, 0.3), \quad [2.9, 3.4), \quad [6.8, 7.1), \quad [9.0, 9.4),$$
$$\sigma(t) = 2: \quad t \in [0.3, 2.9), \quad [3.4, 6.8), \quad [7.1, 9.0), \quad [9.4, 12],$$

$$\sigma(t - t_d) = 1: \quad t \in [0, 0.5), \quad [3.1, 3.6), \quad [7.0, 7.3), \quad [9.2, 9.6),$$
$$\sigma(t - t_d) = 2: \quad t \in [0.5, 3.1), \quad [3.6, 7.0), \quad [7.3, 9.2), \quad [9.6, 12],$$

where the specified sequence of time instants $\{t_n\}_{n=0}^4$ is given as $\{0, 3, 6, 9, 12\}$. Note that the condition $1.5 = \tau_a \geq \frac{2 \ln \mu}{\alpha^*} = 0.9532$ also holds. The simulation results are shown in Figs. 3 and 4, which well illustrate Theorem 3.2.

**Fig. 3** The switching signal $\sigma(t)$

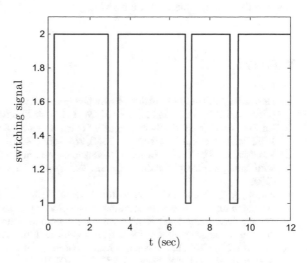

**Fig. 4** The state trajectories of the system (3)

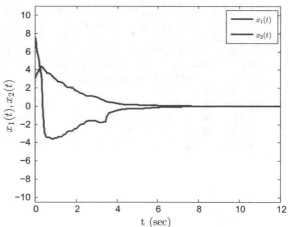

# 5    Conclusion

In this paper, the piecewise Lyapunov function and average dwell time approach have been used to investigate the problem of asynchronous control of switched nonlinear systems. By using the proposed switching law, the asynchronously switched stabilizing control problem for nonlinear systems has been solved, which allows us to have stable and unstable subnonlinear system. Illustrative examples have been provided to show the effectiveness of the results.

# References

1. Hespanha, J.P: Uniform stability of switched linear systems extensions of Lasalle's invariance principle. IEEE Trans. Autom. Control **49**(4), 470–482 (2004)
2. Lu, B., Wu, F., Kim, S.: Switching LPV control of an F-16 aircraft via controller state reset. IEEE Trans. Control Syst. Technol. **14**(2), 267–277 (2003)
3. Rinehart, M., Dahleh, M., Reed, D., Kolmanovsky, I.: Suboptimal control of switched systems with an application to the disc engine. IEEE Trans. Control Syst. Technol. **16**(2), 189–201 (2008)
4. Xu, X., Antsaklis, P.J.: Optimal control of switched systems based on parameterization of the switching instants. IEEE Trans. Autom. Control **49**(1), 2–16 (2004)
5. Zhang, Z.R., Wang, R.H.: Roust control for uncertain switched nonlinear systems with time delay under asynchronous swithching. IET Control Theor. Appl. **3**(8), 1041–1050 (2009)
6. Zhang, L.X., Gao, H.J.: Asynchronously switched control of switched linear systems with average dwell time. Automatic **46**, 953–958 (2010)
7. Xiang, M., Xiang, Z.R., Karimi, H.R.: Asynchronous $L_1$ control of delayed swithched positive systems with mode-dependent average dwell time. Inf. Sci. **278**, 703–714 (2014)
8. Ren, W., Xiong, J.L.: Stability and stabilization of switched stochastic systems under asynchronous switching. Syst. Control Lett. **97**, 184–192 (2016)
9. Mao, Y.B., Zhang, H.B., Xu, S.Y.: The exponential stability and asynchronous stabilization of a class of switched nonlinear system via the T-S fuzzy model. IEEE Trans. Fuzzy Syst. **22**(4), 817–828 (2014)
10. Hespanha, J.P., Morse, A.S.: Stability of switched systems with average dwell time. In: Proceedings of 38th Conference on Decision Control Phoenix, AZ 2655–2660 (1999)
11. Zhai, G.S., Hu, B., Yasuda, K., Michel, A.N.: Disturbance attenuation properties of time-controlled switched systems. J. Frankl. Inst. **338**, 765–779 (2001)

# FMPS of Master-Slave Dynamical Networks with Hybrid Feedback Control

Xin Wang, Xinzhi Liu, Kun She and Shouming Zhong

**Abstract** In this paper, the problem concerning function matrix projective synchronization (FMPS) for two different coupled complex dynamical networks with nonidentical nodes of different dimensions is investigated, in which the internal time delay is different from the coupling delay. With the aid of Lyapunov stability theory and mathematical induction, a hybrid feedback control protocol is proposed to achieve the FMPS. In contrast to most existing results, the symmetric or diffusive criteria for the coupling matrices are not needed. Numerical example is presented to illustrate the effectiveness and conservatism reduction of the proposed scheme.

**Keywords** Synchronization · Hybrid control · Complex networks

## 1 Introduction

Many large-scale systems in real world, such as biological neural networks, food webs, electrical power grid and social networks, can be described by complex networks. A complex dynamical network consists of coupling nodes, each node is a nonlinear dynamical system and interconnected by edges. In the past few decades,

X. Wang (✉) · K. She
School of Information and Software Engineering, University of Electronic Science
and Technology of China, Chengdu 610054, Sichuan, People's Republic of China
e-mail: xinwang201314@126.com

K. She
e-mail: kunshe@126.com

X. Liu
Department of Applied Mathematical, University of Waterloo,
Waterloo, ON N2L 3G1, Canada
e-mail: xzhi@uwaterloo.ca

S. Zhong
School of Mathematical Sciences, University of Electronic Science
and Technology of China, Chengdu 611731, Sichuan, People's Republic of China
e-mail: zhongsm@uestc.edu.cn

© Springer Nature Switzerland AG 2018
D. M. Kilgour et al. (eds.), *Recent Advances in Mathematical
and Statistical Methods*, Springer Proceedings in Mathematics & Statistics 259,
https://doi.org/10.1007/978-3-319-99719-3_56

the study of complex networks has attracted increasing attention from researchers in different fields [1–3]. In particular, synchronization as a typical collective dynamical behavior of coupled nonlinear systems has been widely investigated in [4–7].

In addition, a new type of synchronization phenomenon, called function projective synchronization (FPS), has been proposed and extensively investigated in [8–11]. FPS means that the master system and the slave system could be synchronization up to a scaling function matrix. FPS is a more general definition of chaotic synchronization. For example, if we let the scaling function matrix be unity or constant; one can get complete synchronization (CS) or projective synchronization (PS). Since the unpredictability of the scaling function matrix in FMPS can additionally enhance the security of communication [12, 13], recently, FPS has attracted the interest of many researchers in various fields. For example, on the basis of an adaptive control method, FPS for a class of chaotic systems with unknown parameters was studied in [14]. In [15], the authors addressed FPS in complex dynamical networks via hybrid feedback control. Furthermore, results on generalized matrix projective synchronization of general complex networks were considered in [16]. However, although synchronization of complex networks with identical or nonidentical dynamical systems have been studied extensively, the dimensions of node dynamics are always assumed to be identical. In reality, many systems are modeled by nonlinear dynamics which may be totally different, and the interactions among them can also be totally different. On the other hand, due to time and space characteristics of the complex networks, at the process of information transmission, the time delay that exists in a single network and the coupling delays between complex networks may be different at different times.

Motivated by the issues discussed above, based on the Lyapunov stability theory and mathematical induction scheme, we use a matrix as a bridge, for complex dynamical networks with nonidentical nodes of different dimensions, and achieve the synchronization via a hybrid feedback control protocol. Here, the symmetric or diffusive conditions for the coupling matrices are not needed. Finally, a numerical example is presented to illustrate the effectiveness and conservatism reduction of the proposed method.

**Notation**: The $diag\{\ldots\}$ denotes the block diagonal matrix. For a real symmetric matrix $P$, $\lambda_{min}(P)$ and $\lambda_{max}(P)$ denote the minimum and maximum eigenvalues of $P$, respectively. $\|\cdot\|$ denotes the Euclidean vector norm. $|\cdot|$ denotes the absolute value. The superscript $T$ denotes matrix or vector transposition. The symmetric terms in a symmetric matrix are denoted by $*$. Matrices, if not explicitly stated, are assumed to have compatible dimensions.

## 2 Preliminaries

Consider a general complex network with different internal time-varying delay and coupled time-varying delay:

$$\dot{x}_i(t) = f_i(x_i(t), x_i(t - \tau_1(t))) + \varepsilon \sum_{j=1}^{N} c_{ij} Q_{ij} x_j(t - \tau_2(t)), \tag{1}$$

where $i = 1, 2, \ldots, N$, $x_i(t) = (x_{i1}(t), x_{i2}(t), \ldots, x_{in_i}(t))^T \in \Re^{n_i}$ stands for the state vector of the $i$th node. $f_i(\cdot, \cdot) \in \Re^{n_i}$ is vector-valued function. $\varepsilon > 0$ is the coupling strength, $\tau_1(t)$ and $\tau_2(t)$ are the known internal time-varying delay and coupled time-varying delay. $Q_{ij} \in \Re^{n_i \times n_j}$ is the inner coupling matrix, $i, j \in \{1, 2, \ldots, N\}$, $C = (c_{ij})_{N \times N}$ is the outer coupling matrix satisfying: if there is a connection from node $j$ to node $i$ $(i \neq j)$, then $c_{ij} \neq 0$; otherwise $c_{ij} = 0$.

We refer to (1) as the drive network, the response network with suitable controllers will be described as follows:

$$\dot{y}_i(t) = g_i(y_i(t), y_i(t - \tau_1(t))) + \varepsilon \sum_{j=1}^{N} d_{ij} G_{ij} y_j(t - \tau_2(t)) + u_i(t), \tag{2}$$

where $i = 1, 2, \ldots, N$, $y_i(t) = (y_{i1}(t), y_{i2}(t), \ldots, y_{im_i}(t))^T \in \Re^{m_i}$ stands for the state vector of the $i$th node. $g_i(\cdot, \cdot) \in \Re^{m_i}$ is vector-valued function. $\varepsilon > 0$ is the coupling strength, $\tau_1(t)$ and $\tau_2(t)$ are the known internal time-varying delay and coupled time-varying delay. $u_i(t)$ is the control input. $G_{ij} \in \Re^{m_i \times m_j}$ is the inner coupling matrix, $i, j \in \{1, 2, \ldots, N\}$, $D = (d_{ij})_{N \times N}$ is the outer coupling matrix satisfying: if there is a connection from node $j$ to node $i$ $(i \neq j)$, then $d_{ij} \neq 0$; otherwise $d_{ij} = 0$.

**Definition 1** The FMPS between drive network (1) and response network (2) is achieved, if there exists a continuously differentiable scaling function matrix $M_i(t) \in \Re^{m_i \times n_i}$ such that

$$\lim_{t \to \infty} \|y_i(t) - M_i(t) x_i(t)\| = 0, \quad i = 1, 2, \ldots, N. \tag{3}$$

**Assumption 1** $0 \leq \tau_i(t) \leq \tau_i$ and $\dot{\tau}_i(t) \leq \mu_i < 1$ for $i = 1, 2$, where $\tau_i$ and $\mu_i$ are constants.

**Assumption 2** The function $\sigma(\cdot, \cdot) \in \Re^n$ is said to satisfy the QUAD condition, i.e., $\sigma \in QUAD(L, \Delta)$, if there exist positive diagonal matrices $L$ and $\Delta$ such that

$$(x - y)^T (\sigma(x, \tilde{x}) - \sigma(y, \tilde{y})) \leq (x - y)^T L(x - y) + (\tilde{x} - \tilde{y})^T \Delta(\tilde{x} - \tilde{y}). \tag{4}$$

for any $x, y, \tilde{x}, \tilde{y} \in \Re^n$.

**Lemma 1** For any $x, y \in \Re^n$ and positive definite matrix $R \in \Re^{n \times n}$, the following matrix inequality holds:

$$2x^T y \leq x^T R x + y^T R^{-1} y. \tag{5}$$

## 3  Main Results

In this section, we propose a hybrid feedback control method to achieve FMPS. Define the error vectors as follows:

$$e_i(t) = y_i(t) - M_i(t)x_i(t), \tag{6}$$

where $M_i(t) \in \Re^{m_i \times n_i}$ is the time-varying scaling matrix.

The hybrid controller is designed as

$$u_i(t) = u_i^1(t) + u_i^2(t), \tag{7}$$

where

$$u_i^1(t) = M_i(t)\dot{x}_i(t) + \dot{M}_i(t)x_i(t) - g_i(M_i(t)x_i(t), M_i(t - \tau_1(t))x_i(t - \tau_1(t)))$$

$$- \varepsilon \sum_{j=1}^{N} d_{ij} G_{ij} M_i(t - \tau_2(t))x_j(t - \tau_2(t)), \tag{8}$$

$$u_i^2(t) = -\beta_i(t)e_i(t), \tag{9}$$

and the adaptive law is

$$\dot{\beta}_i(t) = k_i e_i^T(t)e_i(t), \quad i = 1, 2, \ldots, N, \tag{10}$$

where $k_i$ is positive constant, $u_i^1(t)$ is the nonlinear controller, and $u_i^2(t)$ is the adaptive feedback controller.

Then, the error dynamical network can be obtained:

$$\dot{e}_i(t) = \dot{y}_i(t) - \dot{M}_i(t)x_i(t) - M_i(t)\dot{x}_i(t)$$

$$= \tilde{g}_i(e_i(t), e_i(t - \tau_1(t))) + \varepsilon \sum_{j=1}^{N} \tilde{G}_{ij} e_j(t - \tau_2(t)) - \beta_i(t)e_i(t), \tag{11}$$

where $\tilde{g}_i(e_i(t), e_i(t - \tau_1(t))) = g_i(y_i(t), y_i(t - \tau_1(t))) - g_i(M_i(t)x_i(t), M_i(t - \tau_1(t))x_i(t - \tau_1(t))), \tilde{G}_{ij} = d_{ij}G_{ij}$.

**Theorem 1** *Suppose that the Assumptions 1 and 2 hold, for given synchronization scaling function matrix $M_i(t) \in \Re^{m_i \times n_i}$, the drive network (1) and the response network (2) can achieve FMPS, if there exists sufficiently large positive constant $\beta^*$, such that the following inequality holds for $i = 1, 2, \ldots, N$,*

$$\lambda_{max}(\frac{\varepsilon}{2} \sum_{j=1}^{N} \tilde{G}_{ij} \tilde{G}_{ij}^T) + (1 - \mu_1)^{-1}\delta_{max} + \ell_{max} + \frac{N\varepsilon}{2(1 - \mu_2)} < \beta_i^*, \tag{12}$$

*Proof* Choose a Lyapunov functional as follows:

$$V(e_t) = V_1(e_t) + V_2(e_t) \tag{13}$$

$$V_1(e_t) = \frac{1}{2} \sum_{i=1}^{N} e_i^T(t)e_i(t) + \frac{1}{2} \sum_{i=1}^{N} \frac{(\beta_i(t) - \beta^*)^2}{k_i}$$

$$V_2(e_t) = \sum_{i=1}^{N} \int_{t-\tau_1(t)}^{t} e_i^T(s)P_i^{(1)}e_i(s)ds + \sum_{i=1}^{N} \int_{t-\tau_2(t)}^{t} e_i^T(s)P_i^{(2)}e_i(s)ds$$

where $\beta^*$ is a positive constant, $P_i^{(1)}$ and $P_i^{(2)} \in \Re^{m_i \times m_i}$ are the positive definite diagonal matrices to be determined.

Differentiating $V(e_t)$ along the trajectory of the system (11), we have

$$\dot{V}_1(e_t) = \sum_{i=1}^{N} e_i^T(t)\dot{e}_i(t) + \sum_{i=1}^{N}(\beta_i(t) - \beta^*)e_i^T(t)e_i(t)$$

$$= \sum_{i=1}^{N} e_i^T(t)\tilde{g}_i(e_i(t), e_i(t - \tau_1(t))) + \varepsilon \sum_{i=1}^{N}\sum_{j=1}^{N} e_i^T(t)\tilde{G}_{ij}e_j(t - \tau_2(t))$$

$$- \beta^* \sum_{i=1}^{N} e_i^T(t)e_i(t) \tag{14}$$

$$\dot{V}_2(e_t) = \sum_{i=1}^{N}[e_i^T(t)P_i^{(1)}e_i(t) - (1 - \dot{\tau}_1(t))e_i^T(t - \tau_1(t))P_i^{(1)}e_i(t - \tau_1(t))]$$

$$+ \sum_{i=1}^{N}[e_i^T(t)P_i^{(2)}e_i(t) - (1 - \dot{\tau}_2(t))e_i^T(t - \tau_2(t))P_i^{(2)}e_i(t - \tau_2(t))]$$

$$\tag{15}$$

$$\leq \sum_{i=1}^{N} e_i^T(t)(P_i^{(1)} + P_i^{(2)})e_i(t) - (1 - \mu_1) \sum_{i=1}^{N} e_i^T(t - \tau_1(t))P_i^{(1)}$$

$$e_i(t - \tau_1(t)) - (1 - \mu_2) \sum_{i=1}^{N} e_i^T(t - \tau_2(t))P_i^{(2)}e_i(t - \tau_2(t))$$

Notice that $\tilde{g}_i(\cdot, \cdot)$ satisfies the QUAD condition, thus there exist positive matrices $L_i$ and $\Delta_i$ such that

$$e_i^T(t)\tilde{g}_i(e_i(t), e_i(t - \tau_1(t)))$$
$$\leq e_i^T(t)L_ie_i(t) + e_i^T(t - \tau_1(t))\Delta_ie_i(t - \tau_1(t)) \tag{16}$$

where $L_i = diag(l_{i1}, l_{i2}, \ldots, l_{im_i})$, $\Delta_i = diag(\delta_{i1}, \delta_{i2}, \ldots, \delta_{im_i})$, $i = 1, 2, \ldots, N$. Moreover, by Lemma 1, we get

$$
2 \sum_{i=1}^{N} \sum_{j=1}^{N} e_i^T(t) \tilde{G}_{ij} e_j(t - \tau_2(t))
$$

$$
\leq \sum_{i=1}^{N} \sum_{j=1}^{N} e_i^T(t) \tilde{G}_{ij} \tilde{G}_{ij}^T e_i(t) + \sum_{i=1}^{N} \sum_{j=1}^{N} e_j^T(t - \tau_2(t)) e_j(t - \tau_2(t)) \qquad (17)
$$

$$
= \sum_{i=1}^{N} \sum_{j=1}^{N} e_i^T(t) \tilde{G}_{ij} \tilde{G}_{ij}^T e_i(t) + N \sum_{i=1}^{N} e_i^T(t - \tau_2(t)) e_i(t - \tau_2(t))
$$

Then, according to (14)–(17), it follows that

$$
\dot{V}(e_t) \leq \sum_{i=1}^{N} e_i^T(t) L_i e_i(t) + \sum_{i=1}^{N} e_i^T(t - \tau_1(t)) \Delta_i e_i(t - \tau_1(t))
$$

$$
+ \frac{\varepsilon}{2} \sum_{i=1}^{N} \sum_{j=1}^{N} e_i^T(t) \tilde{G}_{ij} \tilde{G}_{ij}^T e_i(t) + \frac{N\varepsilon}{2} \sum_{i=1}^{N} e_i^T(t - \tau_2(t)) e_i(t - \tau_2(t))
$$

$$
+ \sum_{i=1}^{N} e_i^T(t)(P_i^{(1)} + P_i^{(2)}) e_i(t) - (1 - \mu_1) \sum_{i=1}^{N} e_i^T(t - \tau_1(t)) P_i^{(1)} \qquad (18)
$$

$$
e_i(t - \tau_1(t)) - (1 - \mu_2) \sum_{i=1}^{N} e_i^T(t - \tau_2(t)) P_i^{(2)} e_i(t - \tau_2(t))
$$

$$
- \beta^* \sum_{i=1}^{N} e_i^T(t) e_i(t).
$$

Let $P_i^{(1)} = (1 - \mu_1)^{-1} \Delta_i$, $P_i^{(2)} = \frac{N\varepsilon}{2(1-\mu_2)} I_{m_i}$, then

$$
\dot{V}(e_t) \leq \sum_{i=1}^{N} e_i^T(t)[L_i + \frac{\varepsilon}{2} \sum_{j=1}^{N} \tilde{G}_{ij} \tilde{G}_{ij}^T + (1 - \mu_1)^{-1} \Delta_i + \frac{N\varepsilon}{2(1 - \mu_2)} I_{m_i}
$$

$$
- \beta^* I_{m_i}] e_i(t)
$$

$$
\leq [\lambda_{max}(\frac{\varepsilon}{2} \sum_{j=1}^{N} \tilde{G}_{ij} \tilde{G}_{ij}^T) + (1 - \mu_1)^{-1} \delta_{max} + \ell_{max} + \frac{N\varepsilon}{2(1 - \mu_2)} - \beta^*] \qquad (19)
$$

$$
\sum_{i=1}^{N} e_i^T(t) e_i(t)
$$

where $\delta_{max} = max\{\delta_{ij}\}$, $\ell_{max} = max\{l_{ij}\}$, $\mu_{min} = min\{\mu_i\}$, $i = 1, 2, \ldots, N$ and $j = 1, 2, \ldots, m_i$.

It follows from the condition (12), one can get $\dot{V}(e_t) \leq 0$, then the FMPS is achieved. The proof is completed. $\qquad\qquad\qquad\qquad\qquad\qquad\qquad\qquad\qquad\qquad\qquad$ $\square$

## 4 Numerical Example

In this section, a numerical example is given to illustrate the effectiveness and correctness of the proposed method.

Consider two different complex networks as follows: Firstly, the drive network is given by

$$\dot{x}_i(t) = f_i(x_i(t), x_i(t - \tau_1(t))) + \varepsilon \sum_{j=1}^{2} c_{ij} Q_{ij} x_j(t - \tau_2(t)), \qquad (20)$$

where $x_i(t) = (x_{in_1}, x_{in_2})^T$, $i = 1, 2$, $n_1 = 3$, $n_2 = 4$, $\tau_1(t) = \frac{e^t}{4(1+e^t)}$, $\tau_2(t) = \frac{e^t}{2(1+e^t)}$, $f_i(x_i(t), x_i(t - \tau_1(t))) = f_i(x_i(t)) + \frac{1}{2} sin(x_i(t - \tau_1(t)))$. Here, we consider the nonlinear functions $f_i(x_i(t))$ of these nonidentical nodes consist of the hyperchaotic Rossler system and hyperchaotic Lorenz system, that is

$$f_1(x_1(t)) = \begin{pmatrix} 36(x_{12}(t) - x_{11}(t)) \\ 20x_{12}(t) - x_{11}(t)x_{13}(t) \\ -3x_{13}(t) + x_{11}(t)x_{12}(t) \end{pmatrix}, \quad f_2(x_2(t)) = \begin{pmatrix} 10(x_{22}(t) - x_{21}(t)) + x_{24}(t) \\ 28x_{21}(t) - x_{22}(t) - x_{21}(t)x_{23}(t) \\ x_{21}(t)x_{22}(t) - \frac{8}{3}x_{23}(t) \\ 1.3x_{24}(t) - x_{21}(t)x_{23}(t) \end{pmatrix}.$$

The coupling matrices of system (14) are defined as

$$C = \begin{pmatrix} -0.3 & -0.2 \\ 0.1 & 0.4 \end{pmatrix}, Q_{11} = \begin{pmatrix} 0.4 & -0.2 & 0.3 \\ 0.2 & -0.3 & 0.4 \\ 0.3 & 0.2 & 0.1 \end{pmatrix}, Q_{12} = \begin{pmatrix} 0.2 & 0 & 0.3 & -0.5 \\ 0.1 & -0.3 & 0.4 & 0 \\ 0.3 & 0.2 & 0.1 & -0.2 \end{pmatrix},$$

$$Q_{21} = \begin{pmatrix} 0.2 & -0.1 & 0.3 \\ 0 & 0.3 & 0.2 \\ 0.4 & 0.2 & 0.1 \\ 0.1 & -0.2 & 0.5 \end{pmatrix}, Q_{22} = \begin{pmatrix} 0.1 & -0.2 & 0.3 & 0.1 \\ 0.4 & -0.3 & 0 & 0.2 \\ -0.3 & 0.2 & -0.1 & 0.1 \\ 0 & 0.2 & 0.1 & -0.2 \end{pmatrix}.$$

Moreover, the response network with suitable controllers is described as follows:

$$\dot{y}_i(t) = g_i(y_i(t), y_i(t - \tau_1(t))) + \varepsilon \sum_{j=1}^{2} d_{ij} G_{ij} y_j(t - \tau_2(t)) + u_i(t), \qquad (21)$$

$$u_i(t) = u_i^1(t) + u_i^2(t), \tag{22}$$

where

$$u_i^1(t) = M_i(t)\dot{x}_i(t) + \dot{M}_i(t)x_i(t) - g_i(M_i(t)x_i(t), M_i(t-\tau_1(t))x_i(t-\tau_1(t)))$$

$$- \varepsilon \sum_{j=1}^{N} d_{ij} G_{ij} M_i(t-\tau_2(t))x_j(t-\tau_2(t)),$$

$$u_i^2(t) = -\beta_i(t)e_i(t),$$

$$\dot{\beta}_i(t) = k_i e_i^T(t)e_i(t), \quad i = 1, 2,$$

$g_i(y_i(t), y_i(t-\tau_1(t))) = B_i y_i(t) + \frac{1}{2}(cos^2(y_i(t)) - y_i(t-\tau_1(t)))$, and the parameters of system (15) are given by

$$B_1 = \begin{pmatrix} 1 & -2 & 3 & 1 \\ 4 & 3 & -1 & 2 \\ -3 & 2 & -1 & 1 \\ 0 & 2 & 1 & -5 \end{pmatrix}, \quad B_2 = \begin{pmatrix} 1 & -2 \\ 3 & -4 \end{pmatrix}, \quad D = \begin{pmatrix} -0.5 & 0 \\ 0.3 & 0.4 \end{pmatrix},$$

$$G_{11} = \begin{pmatrix} 0.4 & 0 & 0 & -0.1 \\ 0.1 & 0.3 & 0 & -0.2 \\ 0 & 0 & 0.1 & 0 \\ -0.1 & 0.1 & -0.2 & 0.5 \end{pmatrix}, \quad G_{12} = \begin{pmatrix} -0.2 & 0.1 \\ 0.1 & 0 \\ -0.1 & 0.1 \\ 0 & -0.2 \end{pmatrix},$$

$$G_{21} = \begin{pmatrix} 0.1 & 0.1 & 0 & -0.1 \\ 0 & 0.1 & -0.1 & 0.2 \end{pmatrix}, \quad G_{22} = \begin{pmatrix} -0.1 & 0.1 \\ 0 & -0.3 \end{pmatrix},$$

Now, we take the time-varying scaling matrices as:

$$M_1(t) = \begin{pmatrix} 0 & 0 & 1 \\ 0 & 0.5sin2t & -1 \\ 2cost & 0 & 1 \\ 0 & 0 & 1-sint \end{pmatrix}, \quad M_2(t) = \begin{pmatrix} -2 & -1 & 1 & 0 \\ 0 & -0.5cos2t & -1 & 0 \end{pmatrix},$$

and $\varepsilon = 0.5, k_i = 5, \beta_i(0) = 0.5, i = 1, 2$. Choose the initial values state variables of drive-response networks randomly.

Figures 1 and 2 show the state trajectories of master system and slave system, respectively. It can be seen from Fig. 3 that the state trajectories of drive system and response system have been synchronization under the hybrid controller (16). Moreover, Fig. 4 shows the orbits of adaptive feedback gains $\beta_i(t)$.

**Fig. 1** The state trajectories of master system (14)

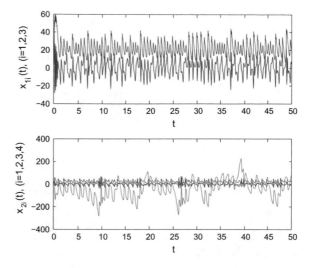

**Fig. 2** The state trajectories of slave system (15)

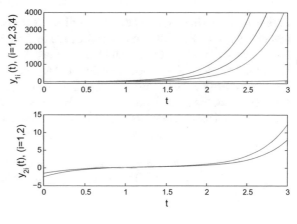

**Fig. 3** The orbits of synchronization errors $e_i(t)$

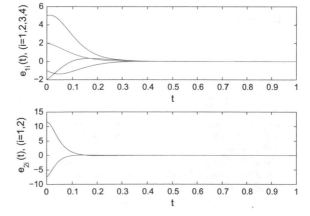

**Fig. 4** The orbits of adaptive feedback gains $\beta_i(t)$

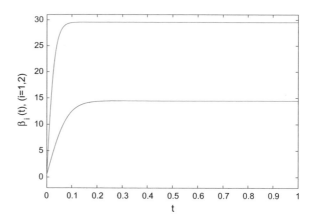

## 5 Conclusions

In this paper, we have studied the issue of FMPS for two different coupled complex dynamical networks with nonidentical nodes of different dimensions, in which the internal time delay is different from the coupling delay. Based on Lyapunov stability theory and mathematical induction, a hybrid feedback control protocol is proposed to achieve the FMPS. The symmetric or diffusive conditions for the coupling matrices are not needed. Finally, a numerical example is presented to illustrate the effectiveness and conservatism reduction of the proposed scheme. In the future, we will use the proposed approach to fractional-order complex networks.

**Acknowledgements** This research was financially supported by the National Natural Science Foundation of China (Nos. 61771004 and 61533006), the China Scholarship Council (CSC) and NSERC Canada.

## References

1. Albert, R., Barabsi, A.L.: Statistical mechanics of complex networks. Rev. Mod. Phys. **74**, 47–97 (2002)
2. Zhang, R., Liu, X., Zeng, D., Zhong, S., Shi, K.: A novel approach to stability and stabilization of fuzzy sampled-data markovian chaotic systems. Fuzzy Sets Syst. (2017). https://doi.org/10.1016/j.fss.2017.12.010
3. Zhang, R., Zeng, D., Zhong, S., Yu, Y.: Event-triggered sampling control for stability and stabilization of memristive neural networks with communication delays. Appl. Math. Comput. **310**, 57–74 (2017)
4. Yang, H., Wang, X., Zhong, S., Shu, L.: Synchronization of nonlinear complex dynamical systems via delayed impulsive distributed control. Appl. Math. Comput. **320**, 75–85 (2018)
5. Wang, X., Liu, X., She, K., Zhong, S.: Pinning impulsive synchronization of complex dynamical networks with various time-varying delay sizes. Nonlinear Anal.: Hybrid Syst. **26**, 307–318 (2017)

6. Wang, X., Liu, X., She, K., Zhong, S.: Finite-time lag synchronization of master-slave complex dynamical networks with unknown signal propagation delays. J. Frankl. Instit. **354**(12), 4913–4929 (2017)
7. Yang, H., Shu, L., Zhong, S.: Pinning lag synchronization of complex dynamical networks with known state time-delay and unknown channel time-delay. Nonlinear Dyn. **89**, 1793–1802 (2017)
8. Shi, Y., Zhu, P., Qin, K.: Projective synchronization of different chaotic neural networks with mixed time delays based on an integral sliding mode controller. Neurocomputing **123**, 443–449 (2014)
9. Shi, L., Zhu, H., Zhong, S., Shi, K., Cheng, J.: Function projective synchronization of complex networks with asymmetric coupling via adaptive and pinning feedback control. ISA Trans. **65**, 81–87 (2016)
10. Du, H., Zeng, Q., Wang, C., Ling, M.: Function projective synchronization in coupled chaotic systems. Nonlinear Anal.: Real World Appl. **11**, 705–712 (2010)
11. Al-mahbashi, G., Noorani, M., Bakar, S., Al-sawalha, M.: Robust projective lag synchronization in drive-response dynamical networks via adaptive control. Eur. Phys. J. Special Top. **225**, 51–64 (2016)
12. Wu, X., Wang, H., Lu, H.: Hyperchaotic secure communication via generalized function projective synchronization. Nonlinear Anal.: Real World Appl. **12**, 1288–1299 (2011)
13. Chee, C., Xu, D.: Secure digital communication using controlled projective synchronisation of chaos. Chaos, Solitons Fractals **23**, 1063–1070 (2005)
14. Du, H., Zeng, Q., Wang, C.: Function projective synchronization of different chaotic systems with uncertain parameters. Phys. Lett. A **372**, 5402–5410 (2008)
15. Du, H., Shi, P., Lü, N.: Function projective synchronization in complex dynamical networks with time delay via hybrid feedback control. Nonlinear Anal.: Real World Appl. **14**, 1182–1190 (2013)
16. Wu, Z., Xu, X., Chen, G., Fu, X.: Generalized matrix projective synchronization of general colored networks with different-dimensional node dynamics. J. Frankl. Inst. **351**, 4584–4595 (2014)

# Implicit State Dependent Delay in Range-Based Position Estimation and Navigation

**Erik I. Verriest**

**Abstract** The transmission delay present in sonar based navigation may present a problem. Typically one solves such navigation using a quasi-static assumption, by assuming that the position of the mobile unit (MU) does not change significantly over the time the signal travels between the MU and the beacon (and back, in case of two-way ranging). For fast moving units, this may pose a problem which is addressed in this paper. An extension of the Lagrange-Bürman inversion, dynamic inversion, and perturbation methods are proposed to solve the problem.

**Keywords** Transmission delay · State dependent delay · Lagrange inversion
Sonar based positioning

## 1 Problem Setting

We visit the problem of localization of underwater and/or surface vehicles by sonar. We limit our discussion to the position estimation and tracking given range measurements only, and solve two cases: The first considers one-way signaling: The mobile unit (MU) sends out signals, carrying transmission time information, which are received by the processing platforms (P). In the second scenario, two-way signaling is employed. The MU transmits to the platform, which reflects or repeats the signal back to the MU. In each scenario, multiple platforms may be employed (the long baseline (LBL) solution). The problem is that the signaling is *not* instantaneous, and as the speed of the MU may be a substantial fraction of the speed of sound, corrections need to be made for its motion. Although this problem has been dealt with in the recent literature (see [2, 3, 8] for an overview), we consider a new approach based on the Lagrange-Bürman inversion, which is exact in the absence of noise and in the assumption that the system is driven by an input modeled as an analytic function. In contrast, methods based on the Taylor expansion assuming piecewise constant delays are

E. I. Verriest (✉)
Georgia Institute of Technology, Atlanta, GA, USA
e-mail: erik.verriest@ece.gatech.edu

© Springer Nature Switzerland AG 2018
D. M. Kilgour et al. (eds.), *Recent Advances in Mathematical
and Statistical Methods*, Springer Proceedings in Mathematics & Statistics 259,
https://doi.org/10.1007/978-3-319-99719-3_57

known to give erroneous results [1]. In what follows it is assumed that the transmission delays can be measured, We also assume that signalling proceeds in straight line paths, thus neglecting bending of paths due to varying water temperature and salinity.

## 2   Observability

We shall focus on the problem consisting of a single MU. If the MU moves in a plane (ocean surface), it is well known from Euclidean geometry that the position of this MU can be determined uniquely from knowledge of the distances to three non-collinear observers provided the position of the observers is perfectly known. With only two observers, the location of the MU is at the intersection of two circles, but without side information, it cannot be known which of the two possible intersections (generically) is the right one.

If the MU can submerge, four non-planar observers are necessary to uniquely determine the position as the intersection of four spheres.

However distance measurements may be prone to observation noise, so that in general only a probability density for the position can be established, or in a deterministic setting, only a bounded region of space may be known to contain the MU.

In addition it may of interest to estimate the velocity and/or acceleration of the MU as well. This would involve differentiation of the range information which may be problematic in the presence of noise. We present an interpolation method to derive the velocity. We consider a sampled approach, and an induced continuous method.

### 2.1   Sampled Process

Assume that at times $-k\delta$, where $k \in \{0, 1, 2, \ldots, n\} \subseteq \mathbb{Z}_+$, the distances $|x(k\delta)|$ are known. From the Taylor approximation we obtain then for all $t$ and $k$ $x(-k\delta) = x(t) - (t + k\delta)\dot{x}(t) + \frac{(t+k\delta)^2}{2!}\ddot{x}(t) +$ h.o.t., where "h.o.t." refers to higher order terms. Neglecting the higher order terms, these relations can be collected in a matrix form, which evaluated at $t = 0$ is

$$
\underbrace{\begin{bmatrix} x(0) \\ x(-\delta) \\ \vdots \\ x(-n\delta) \end{bmatrix}}_{\mathbf{x}(\delta)} = \underbrace{\begin{bmatrix} 1 & 0 & \cdots & 0 \\ 1 & \frac{(-\delta)}{1!} & \cdots & \frac{(-\delta)^n}{n!} \\ \vdots & & \cdots & \vdots \\ 1 & \frac{(-n\delta)}{1!} & \cdots & \frac{(-n\delta)^n}{n!} \end{bmatrix}}_{T_n(\delta)} \underbrace{\begin{bmatrix} x \\ \mathbf{D}x \\ \vdots \\ \mathbf{D}^n x \end{bmatrix}_0}_{\mathscr{D}\,x(0)}. \tag{1}
$$

Hence, with the vectors and matrix identified above, $\mathscr{D}x(0) = T_n(\delta)^{-1}\mathbf{x}(\delta)$. The second component of $\mathscr{D}x(0)$ is the requested derivative. We note that the matrix $T_n(\delta)$ is invertible, so that $x$ and its derivatives at $t = 0$ are solvable. In fact $x(0)$ does not need to be estimated as it corresponds to the last sample value at $t = 0$.

## 2.2 Continuous Process

The continuous analog is obtained by setting up integral equations for the data. Thus let again for $-\delta < s < 0$ the Taylor expansion be $x(s) = x(t) + (s - t)\dot{x}(t) + \frac{(s-t)^2}{2!}\ddot{x}(t) + \text{h.o.t.}$ Integrating from $t - \delta$ to $t$. we get

$$\langle x \rangle \overset{\text{def}}{=} \int_{-\delta}^{0} x(s)\ \mathrm{d}s = \delta x(0) - \frac{\delta^2}{2!}\dot{x}(0) + \frac{\delta^3}{3!}\ddot{x}(0) + \text{h.o.t.}$$

Additional equations are created by considering the moments $\langle x \rangle_k = \int_{-\delta}^{0} s^k x(s)\ \mathrm{d}s$. A simple $2 \times 2$ system of equations is

$$\begin{bmatrix} \langle x \rangle_1 \\ \langle x \rangle_2 \end{bmatrix} = \begin{bmatrix} \delta & -\frac{\delta^2}{2} \\ -\frac{\delta^2}{2!} & \frac{\delta^3}{3!} \end{bmatrix} \begin{bmatrix} x(0) \\ \dot{x}(0) \end{bmatrix}.$$

By time shifting the equation, we obtain from this an estimate for the derivative

$$\widehat{\mathbf{D}x}(t) = -\frac{12}{\delta^3}\left[\frac{\delta}{2!}\langle x \rangle_1 + \langle x \rangle_2\right].$$

Thus, in principle the derivatives of $\|\mathbf{r}_i\|$ can be obtained by processing the observations $\|\mathbf{r}_i\|$. Using two observing stations, and letting $\mathbf{r}_2 = \mathbf{r}_1 - \mathbf{d}$, we get

$$\frac{\mathrm{d}}{\mathrm{d}t}\|\mathbf{r}_1\| = \mathbf{v} \cdot \mathbf{1}_{\mathbf{r}_1}, \quad \frac{\mathrm{d}}{\mathrm{d}t}\|\mathbf{r}_2\| = \mathbf{v} \cdot \mathbf{1}_{\mathbf{r}_1 - \mathbf{d}}.$$

This yields the components of the velocity of the MU in two different directions (generically), so that the vector $\mathbf{v}$ may be reconstructed from these projections. The 3-D case is similar. With two observing stations, A and B as in Fig. 1, one can nicely represent the observations in the following topological form. Represent the observed distances $r_i \geq 0$ in an orthogonal coordinate frame. See Fig. 2. Not all points of the quadrant correspond to a geometrically feasible case. The points $(r_1, r_2)$ are feasible distances for the MU problem only if they fall within a semi-infinite rectangular domain. If A and B are one unit apart, then their representations A′ and B′ respectively have coordinates $(1, 0)$ and $(0, 1)$. Points on the line of sight between A and B are represented by the line segment A′B′, while the external parts of the line is represented by the parallel lines orthogonal to A′B′. In fact each point in the rectangular domain of the representation corresponds to two points in the geometry, one lying above AB and one beneath. Hence the rectangle should be seen as two copies, connected at their boundaries, thus giving a "pita bread" like representation (with opening at the far end in the $(1, 1)$ direction.)

Lines of constant sum $r_1 + r_2$ are ellipses with A and B as foci in Fig. 1, while in Fig. 2 they are line segments parallel to A′B′. Lines of constant differences $r_1 - r_2$ are hyperbolae again with A and B as foci, while in the representation they are the

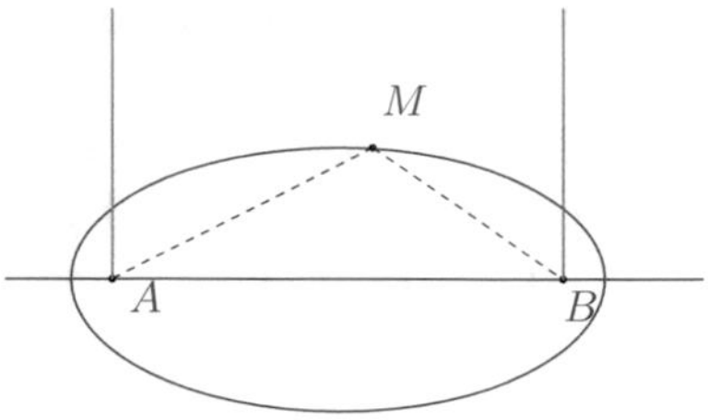

**Fig. 1** Geometry of the two observer problem (color online)

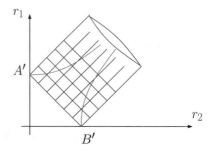

**Fig. 2** Topology of the two observer problem (color online)

straight lines at a 45 degree angle. The (green) lines orthogonal to AB in Fig. 1 map to the parts of (green) hyperbolae in Fig. 2 (color online). It should be emphasized that although the ellipses and hyperbolas are mutually orthogonal and map to orthogonal line bundles in the representation, the mapping is *not* conformal. It is easily shown that the Cauchy-Riemann conditions (when using a complex representation) are not satisfied.

Finally, if the signal propagation speed is not infinite, a delay will be incurred. This is of no consequence when the MU is stationary. However, when it is in motion, the signals to the observers will in general incur different path lengths, and the signals received by the stations at time $t$ will contain information about the position of the MU at *different past times*. It was shown in [5–7] that the history of position can be obtained from delay either graphically by construction, or analytically.

## 3  One-Way Signalling

The scenario is as follows. At a known time $t_0$, the MU is a known distance $r_0$ away from a platform P. For instance the MU is moored to another platform, or surfaced to get its precise coordinates via GPS. During its motion, the MU transmits time-stamped signals to the platform. This enables a processor at P to observe the delay between transmission and reception. This delay is the only available measurement to P at time $t$. Thus let the receiver (the platform) define the perceived delay at time $t$ as its output, $y(t) = \tau_r(t)$, and this delay reports information about the position of the MU at some *earlier* time $t - \tau_r(t)$. If this position is $r(t - \tau_r(t))$, then the delay was precisely $|r(t - \tau_r(t)) - R_P|/c$, where $R_P$ denotes the fixed position of the platform P. The observation constraint is therefore:

$$c\tau_r(t) = |r(t - \tau_r(t)) - R_P|. \tag{2}$$

This is an implicit equation for $\tau_r(t)$, given $r(t)$ or vice versa.

An alternate viewpoint is possible: with reference to the position, $r(t)$ of the MU at time $t$. A signal emitted from the MU at time $t$ will need a time $\tau_e(t) = |R_P - r(t)|/c$ to reach the platform. Since we're processing data from each platform separately, without loss of generality, we can set $R_P = 0$. Some reflection will elucidate that this second viewpoint then means that

$$c\tau_e(t) = |r(t)|, \tag{3}$$

and that the signal arrives at the platform at time $t' = t + \tau_e(t)$. It follows that $\tau_r(t + \tau_e(t)) = \tau_e(t)$, and inversely, $\tau_r(t') = \tau_e(t' - \tau_r(t'))$.

In practice, there always is the ubiquitous observation noise that further corrupts the measurements of $\tau_r(t)$ (Since $r(t)$ is the unknown position, $\tau_e(t)$ is actually a non-measured quantity). In addition the system equation (MU) may contain a driving noise term.

We propose two methods: The first (Sect. 3.1) focuses on the explicit form that can be obtained to express the observation in terms of the (delayed) state, so that a nonlinear observer (or methods akin to extended Kalman filtering in the stochastic case) can be used. The second method (Sect. 3.2) proceeds by expressing the state directly in terms of the measurement and its derivatives. Both methods fuse the delay information with *dead-reckoning*, the process of calculating one's position by advancing a prior known position based on an estimated velocity-vector over the elapsed time.

Preliminary ideas were presented in [5, 7] where a geometric construction was given. A similar equation is encountered in a pure physical problem involving the finite propagation speed of gravitation. In the weak field assumption, where space may still be considered flat, and the notion of simultaneity holds locally, a so-called post-Newtonian approach led to a useful approximation of effects due to general relativity. This was explored in [6]. The main idea was to extend the Lagrange-Bürman inversion to implicit equations.

## 3.1 Inversion for Implicit Equations

At each platform P the received signal relates to the range from P, say, $|r| = x \geq 0$, by a reduced one-dimensional implicit delay equation,

$$c\tau(t) = x(t - \tau(t)) \geq 0. \tag{4}$$

This allows the information at each platform to be preprocessed independently from the others, and therefore renders the problem one-dimensional. The "pinning" condition, $x(t_0) = x_0$, with $\tau(t_0) = \tau_0$, may be considered as a generalized initial condition: At time $t_0$ position and signal delay are known exactly, and $x(t) = x(t_0)$ for $t < t_0$, so that

$$c\tau(t_0) = x(t_0 - \tau(t_0)) = x_0. \tag{5}$$

If $\forall t < t_0, x(t) \neq x(t_0)$, then we assume that also all derivatives of $x$ are known at $t_0$.

### 3.1.1 Lagrange-Bürman Inversion for Implicit Equations

Given a more general relation between delay and output of the form

$$G(\tau) = F(y(t), y(t - \tau)), \tag{6}$$

where the functions $F$, $G$ and $y$ are all *analytic*, the following generalization of the Lagrange-Bürman inversion holds: (see [5] for a proof.).

**Theorem 1** *If $G'(\tau) + F_2(y(t), y(t))$ is nonzero at $t$, then $\tau(t)$ is expressed by the power series*

$$\tau(t) = \sum_{k \geq 1} \frac{(G(0) + F(y(t), y(t)))^k}{k!} \left\{ \left(\frac{\mathrm{d}}{ds}\right)^{k-1} \left(\frac{s}{f(s)}\right)^k \right\}_{s=0}, \tag{7}$$

*where*

$$f(\tau) = G(\tau) - G(0) - F(x(t), x(t - \tau)) + F(x(t), x(t)). \tag{8}$$

Unfortunately, methods based on the implicit function theorem and the Lagrange-Bürmann inversion are limited by the need of the explicit functional form of $x(t)$.

### 3.1.2 Application of the Lagrange-Bürman Inversion

Revisit the specific Eq. (4) where we may assume without loss of generality that $x(t) > 0$. Indeed, if $x = 0$, then $r = 0$ and the function $|r|$ fails to be analytic there. However, the case $r = 0$ obviously does not require position estimation. Hence one can restrict the problem to the two open half-lines where the inversion formula holds (locally). We get, letting $t = t_0 + \tilde{t}$, $\tau(t) = \tau(t_0 + \tilde{t}) = \tau_0 + \tilde{\tau}$ and with $s = \tilde{t} - \tilde{\tau}$

$$f(s) = x(t_0 - \tau_0 + s) - x(t_0 - \tau_0) + cs = c\tilde{t}. \tag{9}$$

This choice results in $f(0) = 0$ and $f'(0) = \dot{x}(t_0 - \tau_0) + c \neq 0$, where we also need to let $\tilde{t} \to 0$ if $s \to 0$. The inversion yields

$$s = c\tilde{t} \left[ \frac{\theta}{f(\theta)} \right]_{\theta=0} + \frac{c^2 \tilde{t}^2}{2} \left( \mathbf{D} \left[ \frac{\theta}{f(\theta)} \right]^2 \right)_{\theta=0} + \cdots \tag{10}$$

After some algebra, we obtain the expansion

$$\tau \left( t | \tau(t_0) = \frac{x_0}{c} \right) = \frac{x_0}{c} + (t - t_0) \frac{\dot{x}[x_0]}{c + \dot{x}[x_0]} + \frac{(t - t_0)^2}{2} \frac{c^2 \ddot{x}[x_0]}{(c + \dot{x}[x_0])^3} + \cdots$$

where $\dot{x}[x_0]$ stands for the derivative of $x$ when $x$ was at position $x_0$, thus in the past. A nonlinear observer is constructed from this output relation in continuous time with a discretized model of the dynamics.

## 3.2 Approximate Dynamic Inversion

The current range of the MU from the platform is approximated by a truncation of the Taylor series. This involves using derivatives of the observable delay $\tau(t)$. In principle the observability guarantees their existence. However, because of observation noise, the practicality of the method may be limited. Knowledge of when the mathematical problem has a solution still sheds light on the ultimate observability problem. In fact, not just position, but also velocity and acceleration may be recoverable. We start again from Eq. (2) and take successive derivatives. The exposition is streamlined by introducing the differentiation operator $\mathbf{D}$, and the evaluation functional $\sigma_t$, defined by $\sigma_t(x) = x(t)$ for almost all $t$, on piecewise continuous functions. Finally, introduce the concatenation operator $\circ$ concatenating two functions as follows $\sigma_t(x \circ \beta) = \sigma_{\beta(t)} x = x(\beta(t))$. Note the fundamental identity (chain rule)

$$\sigma_t \mathbf{D}(x \circ \beta) = \sigma_t[(\mathbf{D}x) \circ \beta] \cdot \mathbf{D}\beta, \quad \forall t,$$

implying that the identity can be lifted from the evaluations to the functions themselves $\mathbf{D}(x \circ \beta) = [(\mathbf{D}x) \circ \beta] \cdot \mathbf{D}\beta$.

This avoids a common ambiguity with the usual notation: Is $\dot{x}(2t)$ the derivative of $x$ evaluated at $2t$ or is it the derivative of the concatenation $x(2t)$ with respect to $t$? The interpretations differ by a factor of 2! Thus, Eq. (2) becomes, with $\beta(t) = t - \tau(t)$,

$$x \circ \beta = c\tau,$$

from which successive differentiation yields

$$c \begin{bmatrix} \tau \\ \mathbf{D}\tau \\ \mathbf{D}^2\tau \\ \vdots \end{bmatrix} = \begin{bmatrix} 1 \\ \mathbf{D}\beta \\ \mathbf{D}^2\beta & (\mathbf{D}\beta)^2 \\ \vdots & & \ddots \end{bmatrix} \begin{bmatrix} x \circ \beta \\ \mathbf{D}x \circ \beta \\ \mathbf{D}^2 x \circ \beta \\ \vdots \end{bmatrix} \tag{11}$$

Any analytic $x$ can be represented by its Taylor expansion. Consider here the expansion about $\beta(t)$, so that $x = x \circ \beta + \tau(\mathbf{D}x \circ \beta) + \frac{\tau^2}{2!}(\mathbf{D}^2x \circ \beta) + \cdots$ and by extension

$$
\begin{bmatrix} x \\ \mathbf{D}x \\ \mathbf{D}^2x \\ \vdots \end{bmatrix} = \begin{bmatrix} 1 & \tau & \tau^2/2! & \cdots \\ & 1 & \tau & \cdots \\ & & 1 & \cdots \\ & & & \ddots \end{bmatrix} \begin{bmatrix} x \circ \beta \\ \mathbf{D}x \circ \beta \\ \mathbf{D}^2x \circ \beta \\ \vdots \end{bmatrix}. \tag{12}
$$

The matrices in these systems (11) and (12) are triangular. The obvious observability condition, namely invertibility of the matrix in (11), boils down to $\mathbf{D}\beta \neq 0$. This is in fact the condition for *causality*, $\dot{\tau} < 1$, of the delay equation (see [4]). It follows then that (normalizing $c = 1$)

$$
\begin{bmatrix} x \\ \mathbf{D}x \\ \mathbf{D}^2x \\ \vdots \end{bmatrix} = \begin{bmatrix} 1 & \tau & \tau^2/2! & \cdots \\ & 1 & \tau & \cdots \\ & & 1 & \cdots \\ & & & \ddots \end{bmatrix} \begin{bmatrix} 1 & & & \\ \mathbf{D}\beta & & & \\ \mathbf{D}^2\beta & (\mathbf{D}\beta)^2 & & \\ \vdots & & \ddots & \end{bmatrix}^{-1} \begin{bmatrix} \tau \\ \mathbf{D}\tau \\ \mathbf{D}^2\tau \\ \vdots \end{bmatrix}. \tag{13}
$$

The present position, $x(t)$ is estimated by truncating the infinite series. For instance, the three-term series truncation yields the continuous time position estimate

$$
\hat{x}_{(3)}(t) = \frac{\tau}{1 - \dot{\tau}} + \frac{\tau^2 \ddot{\tau}}{2(1 - \dot{\tau})^3} + \frac{\tau^3(\ddot{\tau}^2 + \dddot{\tau}(1 - \dot{\tau}))}{6(1 - \dot{\tau})^5}.
$$

In practice, a discrete version would be sought, so that each time update allows for a new pinning condition, and the data fusion centers about this, thus avoiding problems with the smaller radius of convergence for the LB inversion.

## 4 Two-Way Problem

In the two-way problem, the MU emits the signal, which takes a time $\tau_1$ to propagate to the stationary platform where it is scattered (or repeated) and takes another $\tau_2$ seconds to reach the MU, which now is at another position. In this case only the total delay $\tau = \tau_1 + \tau_2$ is known and the geometry dictates

$$
c\tau(t) = \|r(t - \tau(t))\| + \|r(t)\|.
$$

Let again a pinning conditions be that at time $t_0$ the position $r_0$ (and velocity etc.) were exactly known, and that the MU emits a signal that is scattered and picked up by the MU $\tau_0$ seconds later. This means that $\|r(t_0 + \tau_0)\| + \|r_0\| = c\tau(t_0 + \tau_0) = c\tau_0$, with $\tau_0 = \tau(t_0 + \tau_0)$. The LB inversion starts now from the relation, setting $s = \tau - \tau_0$

$$cs - \|r(t - \tau_0 - s)\| + \|r(t - \tau_0)\| = \|r(t)\| + \|r(t - \tau_0)\| - c\tau_0.$$

Denoting the left hand side by $f(t, s)$, we note that $f(t, 0) = 0$ and $\frac{\partial}{\partial s} f(t, 0) = c + \dot{r}(t - \tau_0) \cdot \frac{r(t-\tau_0)}{\|r(t-\tau_0)\|}$. In the neighborhood of $r_0$, the LB inversion yields the relation between position and observed delay as

$$\tau = \tau_0 + \sum_{k \geq 1} \frac{(\|r(t)\| - \|r(t - \tau_0)\| - c\tau_0)^k}{k!} \Gamma_k \tag{14}$$

$$\Gamma_k = \lim_{s \to 0} \mathbf{D}^{k-1} \left( \frac{s}{f(t, s)} \right)^k. \tag{15}$$

Alternatively, the reverse relation may be derived to get the range and its derivatives as a nonlinear functional of the observed delay $\tau$.

We sketch two perturbation approaches as an alternative way to solve the problem. Let's focus on a decoupled spatial 1-D system, thus assuming that $x(\cdot) \geq 0$ so that the constraint equation is simply

$$c\tau(t) = x(t) + x(t - \tau(t)). \tag{16}$$

Approach 1

Rearrange (16) as follows using successive substitution

$$\begin{aligned}
x(t) &= c\tau(t) - x(t - \tau(t)) \\
&= c\tau(t) - c\tau(t - \tau(t)) + x(t - \tau(t) - \tau(t - \tau(t))) \\
&= c\tau(t) - c\tau(t - \tau(t)) + c\tau(t - \tau(t) - \tau(t - \tau(t))) - x(t - \tau(t) - \tau(t - \tau(t))) \\
&= \cdots
\end{aligned}$$

Reorganize this by defining first a sequence of times $\{t_k\}$ satisfying

$$t_{k+1}(t) = t_k(t) - \tau(t_k(t)), \quad t_0 = t. \tag{17}$$

so that the above series is $x(t) = c[\tau(t) - \tau(t_1) + \tau(t_2) - \cdots]$. We note that, since $\tau(t) < t$, the ratio $t_{k+1}(t)/t_k(t)$ equals to $1 - \tau(t_k)/t_k \in (0, 1)$. Hence the sequence $\{t_k\}$ is monotone and converges to zero, with $\tau(0) = 0$. Consequently the alternating series $\tau(t_0) - \tau(t_1) + \tau(t_2) - \cdots$ converges to a finite limit for all $t$.

Approach 2

Reorganize the constraint (16) as $c\tau(t) = 2x(t) - (x(t) - x(t - \tau(t)))$. The idea is that if $\tau$ is small, then $x(t) - x(t - \tau(t)) \approx -\dot{x}(t)\tau(t)$. This gives approximately $x(t) \approx \frac{c\tau(t)}{2} \left( 1 + \frac{\dot{x}(t)}{c} \right)$, suggesting a perturbation expansion for $x(t)$, initialized with $x_0(t) = \frac{c\tau(t)}{2}$. We established the following

**Theorem 2** *The constraint equation (16) is solved by the limit of*

$$x_{k+1}(t) = \frac{c\tau(t)}{2} - \frac{1}{2}\sum_{i=1}^{k}(-\tau(t))^i \frac{x_k^{(i)}(t)}{i!}. \tag{18}$$

*Proof* Suppose $x_k(t) \to x_\infty(t)$. The limit must solve $x_\infty(t) = -\frac{1}{2}\sum_{i=1}^{\infty}(-\tau(t))^i \frac{x_\infty^{(i)}(t)}{i!}$ $+ \frac{c\tau(t)}{2}$. But the rhs series is the expansion of $x_\infty(t-\tau) - x_\infty(t)$. Thus $x_\infty(t) = \frac{c\tau(t)}{2} - \frac{1}{2}(x_\infty(t-\tau) - x_\infty(t))$, and therefore satisfies the constraint. $\square$

## 5 Conclusions

We considered the one-way and the two-way sonar-based localization problems, where large vehicle speeds lead to implicit delay equations. Two methods were presented: One based on an extension of the Lagrange-Bürman inversion, and one based on dynamic inversion. Alternative perturbation-based approaches are also suggested for the two-way problem. We focused on the exact (noise-free) problem in order to gauge the ultimate feasibility. Simulations, reported in [8], hint at Approach 1 converging faster for high speeds compared to the signal speed $c$, but it seems to have problems when $\tau$ returns to zero. In contrast, the perturbation Approach 2 converged faster at slow speeds in the test case for $\tau(t) = t(1-t)/4$.

**Acknowledgements** This work was supported by NSF grant CPS-1544857.

## References

1. Insperger, T.: On the approximation of delayed systems by Taylor series expansion. J. Comput. Nonlinear Dyn. **10**(024503), 1–4 (2015)
2. Li, Z., Dosso, S.E., Sun, D.: Motion compensated acoustic localization for underwater vehicles. IEEE J. Oceanic Eng. **41**(4), 840–851 (2016)
3. Newman, P., Leonard, J.: Pure range-only sub-sea SLAM. In: Proceedings of the 2003 IEEE International Conference on Robotics & Automation, Taipei, Taiwan, 14–19 September, 2003, pp. 1921–1926
4. Verriest, E.I.: Inconsistencies in systems with time-varying delays and their resolution. IMA J. Math. Control Inf. **28**, 147–162 (2011)
5. Verriest, E.I.: Inversion of state-dependent delay. In: Malisoff, M., Pepe, P., Mazenc, F., Karafyllis, I. (eds.) Recent Results on Nonlinear Delay Control Systems, pp. 327–346. Springer, Berlin (2016)
6. Verriest, E.I.: Post-newtonian gravitation. In: Blair, J., Frigaard, I.A., Kunze, H., Makarov, R., Melnik, R., Spiteri, R.J. (eds.) Mathematical and Computational Approaches in Modern Science and Engineering, pp. 153–164. Springer, Berlin (2016)
7. Verriest, E.I., Ivanov, A.F.: Observation and observers for systems from delay convoluted observation. In: Proceedings of the 19th IFAC World Congress, Cape Town, South Africa, 24–29 August, 2014, pp. 3720–3725
8. Verriest, E.I., Lampe, B.: Range-only position estimation with delay correction via Lagrange-Bürman inversion. In: IFAC World Congress, Toulouse, France, 9–14 July, 2017, Paper-ID 3839

Printed in the United States
By Bookmasters